Health Care Advice

Patient Education for Children, Teens, and Parents

American Academy of Pediatrics
141 Northwest Point Blvd
Elk Grove Village, IL 60009-0927

BS

AAP Department of Marketing and Publications Staff

Maureen DeRosa, Director, Department of Marketing and Publications

Mark Grimes, Director, Division of Product Development
Diane Beausoleil, Senior Product Development Editor
Kate Simone, Electronic Publishing Manager

Sandi King, Director, Division of Publishing and Production Services
Jill Rubino, Manager, Editorial Services
Jason Crase, Editorial Specialist
Leesa Levin-Doroba, Manager, Print Production Services
Linda Diamond, Manager, Graphic Design
Peg Mulcahy, Graphic Designer

Jill Ferguson, Director, Division of Marketing and Sales
Susan Thompson, Manager, Consumer Product Marketing and Sales

Natalie Arndt, Department Coordinator

Library of Congress Control Number: 2002100193
ISBN: 1-58110-085-X
MA0197

The recommendations in this publication do not indicate an exclusive course of treatment or serve as a standard of medical care. Variations, taking into account individual circumstances, may be appropriate.

11/17/03

Introduction

Studies have shown that information handouts are effective educational tools and are an excellent means to reinforce verbal instructions. In the short term, handouts help to lessen parent anxiety, increase patient and parent compliance, and reduce the number of unnecessary telephone calls and office visits. Long-term benefits include increased knowledge of development, enhanced parent-child relationships, and increased parental self-confidence.

To support your efforts at effective patient and parent teaching, the American Academy of Pediatrics has compiled more than 150 patient education handouts into this handy reusable manual. This compendium includes the same information as our printed brochures, fact sheets, and *Patient Education on CD-ROM*. The manual is divided into 10 sections: Infants and Toddlers, Adolescents and School-age Children, Common Illnesses and Conditions, Feeding and Nutrition, Behavior and Psychosocial Issues, Developmental Issues, Safety and Prevention, TIPP® Bicycle Safety, Immunization Information, and Promoting Pediatric Care. Within each section, the handouts are arranged alphabetically. A list of brochures is included at the beginning of the manual and a helpful index can be found at the end of the manual. Also included is a handout checklist for use by parents and patients to indicate which handouts they would like to receive. A copy of the checklist can then be placed in a patient's chart as a patient education record. A Spanish-language version with identical features and content is also available (part number MA0201).

The pages of this manual are perforated and 3-hole punched. You may remove pages for duplication*, then store the originals in a binder for future use. A copyright line is included on each page. Permission to duplicate the pages for noncommercial purposes is granted and no additional or special permission is needed to copy and distribute the materials to your patients. There is space on most of the handouts for you to insert your practice information and personalized patient instructions.

After you have had a chance to use this manual, please take a moment to complete the product survey that was included. Your comments are valuable to us and will enable us to continue to develop products that best meet your needs.

Please note that you can set your copier at 103% to increase the print size of the pages.

Below is a listing of publications available from the American Academy of Pediatrics. Please check the publications that you would like to receive, and give this form to your health care professional.

Infants and Toddlers

- ☐ Baby Bottle Tooth Decay—How to Prevent It
- ☐ Baby Walkers
- ☐ Bed-wetting
- ☐ Car Safety Seats: A Guide for Families—2002
- ☐ Care of the Uncircumcised Penis
- ☐ Circumcision: Information for Parents
- ☐ Diaper Rash
- ☐ Early Arrival: Information for Parents of Premature Infants
- ☐ Fun in the Sun: Keep Your Baby Safe
- ☐ Infant Sleeping Position and SIDS
- ☐ Newborn Hearing Screening and Your Baby
- ☐ One-Minute Car Seat Safety Check-up
- ☐ Prevent Shaken Baby Syndrome
- ☐ Thumbs, Fingers, and Pacifiers: Guidelines for Parents
- ☐ Toilet Training

Adolescents and School-age Children

- ☐ Acne Treatment and Control
- ☐ ADHD and Your School-Aged Child
- ☐ Better Health and Fitness Through Physical Activity: Guidelines for Teens
- ☐ Breast Self-Exam
- ☐ The Correct Use of Condoms: A Message to Teens
- ☐ Deciding to Wait
- ☐ For Today's Teens: A Message From Your Pediatrician
- ☐ Gay, Lesbian, and Bisexual Teens: Facts for Teens and their Parents
- ☐ Health Care for College Students: What Your Pediatrician Wants You to Know
- ☐ Important Information for Teens Who Get Headaches: Guidelines for Teens
- ☐ Know the Facts About HIV and AIDS
- ☐ Making the Right Choice: Facts for Teens on Preventing Pregnancy—Guidelines for Teens
- ☐ The Pelvic Exam: Guidelines for Teens
- ☐ Puberty: Information for Girls
- ☐ Puberty: Information for Boys
- ☐ The Risks of Tobacco Use: A Message to Parents and Teens
- ☐ School Health Centers and Your Child
- ☐ Smokeless Tobacco: Guidelines for Teens
- ☐ Smoking: Straight Talk for Teens
- ☐ Steroids: Play Safe, Play Fair
- ☐ Substance Abuse Prevention: Part I What Every Parent Needs to Know
- ☐ Substance Abuse Prevention: Part II Additional Information
- ☐ Surviving: Coping With Adolescent Depression and Suicide—Guidelines for Parents
- ☐ Talking With Your Young Child about Sex
- ☐ Talking to Your Young Teen About Sex and Sexuality: Guidelines for Parents
- ☐ The Teen Driver: Guidelines for Parents
- ☐ Testicular Self-Exam
- ☐ Tips for Parents of Adolescents

Common Illnesses and Conditions

- ☐ Allergies in Children
- ☐ Anemia and Your Young Child: Guidelines for Parents
- ☐ Bronchiolitis and Your Young Child: Guidelines for Parents
- ☐ Common Childhood Infections: Part I Respiratory and Ear, Nose, and Throat Infections
- ☐ Common Childhood Infections: Part II Other Common Infections
- ☐ Croup and Your Young Child
- ☐ Diarrhea and Dehydration
- ☐ Ear Infections and Children: Part I Symptoms, Treatment, and Complications
- ☐ Ear Infections and Children: Part II Treatments for Repeated Ear Infections
- ☐ Febrile Seizures
- ☐ Fever and Your Child
- ☐ A Guide to Children's Medications: Part I Prescription Medications
- ☐ A Guide to Children's Medications: Part II Over-the-counter Medications
- ☐ How to Help Your Child With Asthma
- ☐ Influenza: Guidelines for Parents
- ☐ Lyme Disease
- ☐ Tonsils and the Adenoid
- ☐ Treating Jaundice in Healthy Newborns
- ☐ Urinary Tract Infections in Young Children
- ☐ Your Child and Antibiotics: Unnecessary Antibiotics CAN Be Harmful
- ☐ Your Child's Eyes: Part I Visual Development and Warning Signs
- ☐ Your Child's Eyes: Part II Specific Problems That Require Further Evaluation

Feeding and Nutrition

- ☐ Calcium and You: Facts for Teens
- ☐ Feeding Kids Right Isn't Always Easy: Tips for Preventing Food Hassles
- ☐ Growing Up Healthy: Fat, Cholesterol and More
- ☐ Right from the Start: ABC's of Good Nutrition for Young Children
- ☐ Starting Solid Foods
- ☐ What's to Eat?: Healthy Foods for Hungry Children

Behavior and Psychosocial Issues

- ☐ Adoption: Guidelines for Parents—Part I Adopting a Young Child
- ☐ Adoption: Guidelines for Parents—Part II Adopting an Older Child
- ☐ Adoption: Guidelines for Parents—Part III Additional Resources
- ☐ Alcohol: Your Child and Drugs
- ☐ Child Sexual Abuse: What It Is and How To Prevent it
- ☐ Choosing Child Care: What's Best for Your Family?
- ☐ Cocaine: Your Child and Drugs
- ☐ Discipline and Your Child
- ☐ Divorce and Children
- ☐ Eating Disorders: Part I Anorexia Nervosa
- ☐ Eating Disorders: Part II Bulimia Nervosa
- ☐ Gambling: Not a Safe Thrill
- ☐ Healthy Communication With Your Child
- ☐ Inhalant Abuse: Your Child and Drugs—Guidelines for Parents

☐ The Internet and Your Family

☐ Marijuana: Your Child and Drugs

☐ Media History

☐ The Ratings Game: Choosing Your Child's Entertainment

☐ Sex Education: A Bibliography of Educational Materials for Children, Adolescents, and Their Families

☐ Sibling Relationships: Part I Siblings, Step-siblings, Half-siblings, and Twins

☐ Sibling Relationships: Part II Preparing for a New Baby

☐ Single Parenting: Part I What You Need to Know

☐ Single Parenting: Part II Additional Resources

☐ Sleep Problems in Children: Part I Infants, Toddlers, and Preschoolers

☐ Sleep Problems in Children: Part II Common Sleep Problems

☐ Television and the Family

☐ Temper Tantrums: A Normal Part of Growing Up

☐ Understanding the Impact of Media on Children and Teens

Developmental Issues

☐ Helping Your Child Learn to Read

☐ Learning Disabilities and Children

☐ Learning Disabilities and Young Adults

☐ Your Child's Growth: Developmental Milestones

Safety and Prevention

☐ Air Bag Safety

☐ Anesthesia and Your Child

☐ Car Seat Shopping Guide for Children With Special Needs: Guidelines for Parents

☐ Choking Prevention and First Aid for Infants and Children

☐ Environmental Tobacco Smoke: A Danger to Children

☐ A Guide to Children's Dental Health

☐ Home Safety Checklist

☐ Keep Your Family Safe: Fire Safety and Burn Prevention at Home

☐ Keep Your Family Safe From Firearm Injury

☐ Lawn Mower Safety

☐ Lead Poisoning: Prevention and Screening

☐ Minor Head Injuries in Children

☐ A Parent's Guide to Water Safety: Part I Infants and Preschoolers

☐ A Parent's Guide to Water Safety: Part II School-age Children and Adolescents

☐ Playground Safety

☐ Protect Your Child From Poison: Part I Prevention and Treatment

☐ Protect Your Child From Poison: Part II Poison Proofing Your Home

☐ Raising Children to Resist Violence: What You Can Do

☐ Sports and Your Child

☐ Toy Safety: Part I Guidelines for Parents

☐ Toy Safety: Part II Age-Appropriate Toys and Toys to Avoid

☐ Trampolines

☐ When Your Child Needs Emergency Medical Services for Children

☐ Your Child and the Environment: Guidelines for Parents—Part I Where Children Live

☐ Your Child and the Environment: Guidelines for Parents—Part II What Children Eat and Drink

☐ Your Child and the Environment: Guidelines for Parents—Part III Where Children Learn and Play

TIPP® Bicycle Safety

☐ About Bicycle Helmets

☐ Bicycle Safety: Myths and Facts

☐ The Child as Passenger on an Adult's Bicycle

☐ Choosing the Right Size Bicycle for Your Child

☐ Safe Bicycling Starts Early

☐ Tips for Getting Your Child to Wear Bicycle Helmets

Immunization Information

☐ The Chickenpox Vaccine: What Parents Need to Know

☐ Chickenpox Vaccine: What You Need to Know—Vaccine Information Statement

☐ Diphtheria, Tetanus, and Pertussis Vaccines: What You Need to Know—Vaccine Information Statement

☐ *Haemophilus influenzae* type b

☐ *Haemophilus influenzae* type b (Hib) Vaccine: What You Need to Know—Vaccine Information Statement

☐ Hepatitis B

☐ Hepatitis B Vaccine: What You Need to Know—Vaccine Information Statement

☐ Immunizations and Your Child

☐ Influenza Vaccine: What You Need to Know—Vaccine Information Statement

☐ Measles, Mumps, and Rubella Vaccines: What You Need to Know—Vaccine Information Statement

☐ Meningococcal Vaccine: What You Need to Know—Vaccine Information Statement

☐ Pneumococcal Infection and Vaccine

☐ Pneumococcal Vaccine Information Sheet

☐ Polio Vaccine: What You Need to Know—Vaccine Information Statement

☐ Tetanus and Diphtheria (Td): What You Need to Know Before You or Your Child Gets the Vaccine—Vaccine Information Statement

Promoting Pediatric Care

☐ How Special is Your Child?

☐ What is a Pediatric Allergist/Immunologist?

☐ What is a Pediatric Anesthesiologist?

☐ What is a Pediatric Neurosurgeon?

☐ What is a Pediatric Ophthalmologist?

☐ What is a Pediatric Orthopedic Surgeon?

☐ What is a Pediatric Otolaryngologist?

☐ What is a Pediatric Plastic Surgeon?

☐ What is a Pediatric Surgeon?

☐ What is a Pediatric Surgical Specialist?

☐ What is a Pediatric Urologist?

☐ You and Your Pediatrician

Table of Contents

Table of Contents

SECTION THREE

Common Illnesses and Conditions

SECTION FOUR

Feeding and Nutrition

SECTION FIVE

Behavior and Psychosocial Issues

SECTION SIX

Developmental Issues

SECTION SEVEN

Safety and Prevention

Table of Contents

SECTION EIGHT

TIPP® Bicycle Safety

SECTION NINE

Immunization Information

Promoting Pediatric Care

SECTION ONE

Infants and Toddlers

Baby Bottle Tooth Decay—
How to Prevent It

Proper dental care is a lifelong commitment that starts even before your baby's first tooth forms. While daily cleanings and fluoride are important, they alone may not prevent Baby Bottle Tooth Decay (BBTD), a major cause of tooth decay in infants. Baby Bottle Tooth Decay is costly to treat. If left untreated, however, it can quickly destroy the teeth involved. It also can lead to pain, infection, early loss of baby teeth, crooked permanent teeth, and an increased risk of decay in permanent teeth. When you consider the possible dental problems that can result from BBTD and the cost of treating those problems, it is best to prevent BBTD from developing in the first place.

How Does Baby Bottle Tooth Decay Develop?

Baby Bottle Tooth Decay can develop if your child's teeth and gums are in prolonged contact with almost any liquid other than water. This can happen from putting your child to bed with a bottle of formula, milk, juice, soft drinks, sugar water, sugared drinks, etc. Allowing your baby to suck on a bottle or breastfeed for longer than a mealtime, either when awake or asleep, also can cause BBTD.

When liquid from a baby bottle builds up in the mouth, the natural or added sugars found in the liquid are changed to acid by germs in the mouth. This acid then starts to dissolve the teeth (mainly the upper front teeth), causing them to decay. Baby Bottle Tooth Decay can lead to severe damage to your child's baby teeth and also can cause dental problems that affect your child's permanent teeth.

Why Are Baby Teeth Important?

Many parents assume that decay does not matter in baby teeth because the teeth will fall out anyway, but decay in baby teeth poses risks. If your child loses his baby teeth too early because of decay or infection, the permanent teeth will not be ready to replace them yet. Baby teeth act as a guide for the permanent teeth. If baby teeth are lost too early, the teeth that are left may shift position to fill in the gaps. This may not leave any room for the permanent teeth to come in.

What Can I Do to Prevent Baby Bottle Tooth Decay?

Take the following steps to prevent Baby Bottle Tooth Decay:
- Never put your child to bed with a bottle. By 7 or 8 months of age, most children no longer need feedings during the night. Children who drink bottles while lying down also may be more prone to getting ear infections.

- Only give your baby a bottle during meals. Do not use the bottle as a pacifier; do not allow your child to walk around with it or to drink it for extended periods. These practices not only may lead to BBTD, but children can suffer tooth injuries if they fall while sucking on a bottle.
- Teach your child to drink from a cup as soon as possible, usually by 1 year of age. Drinking from a cup does not cause the liquid to collect around the teeth, and a cup cannot be taken to bed. If you are concerned that a cup may be messier than a bottle, especially when you are away from home, use one that has a snap-on lid with a straw or a special valve to prevent spilling.
- If your child must have a bottle for long periods, fill it only with water.

Keeping your baby's mouth clean is also important in preventing tooth decay. After feedings, gently brush your baby's gums and any baby teeth with a soft infant toothbrush.

Start using water and a soft child-sized toothbrush for daily cleanings once your child has seven to eight teeth. By the time your toddler is 2 years of age, you should be brushing her teeth once or twice a day, preferably after breakfast and before bedtime.

Begin using a fluoride toothpaste when you are sure the toothpaste will not be swallowed (usually when your child is around 3 years of age). Use a pea-sized amount of toothpaste to limit the amount your child can swallow. Too much fluoride can be harmful to a child.

Detect Decay Early

Baby Bottle Tooth Decay first shows up as white spots on the upper front teeth. These spots are hard to see at first—even for a pediatrician or dentist—without proper equipment. A child with tooth decay needs to get treatment early to stop the decay from spreading and to prevent lasting damage to the teeth.

If you are concerned that your child may have BBTD, your pediatrician can refer you to a pediatric dentist who will carefully examine your child's teeth for signs of decay.

With the right balance of proper home and professional dental care, your child can grow up to have healthy teeth for a lifetime of smiles.

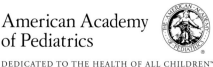

American Academy of Pediatrics

DEDICATED TO THE HEALTH OF ALL CHILDREN™

The American Academy of Pediatrics is an organization of 55,000 primary care pediatricians, pediatric medical subspecialists, and pediatric surgical specialists dedicated to the health, safety, and well-being of infants, children, adolescents, and young adults.

American Academy of Pediatrics
PO Box 747
Elk Grove Village, IL 60009-0747
Web site — http://www.aap.org

Baby walkers

- Baby walkers sent an estimated 8,800 children younger than 15 months to the hospital in 1999.
- Thirty-four children died during the years of 1973 through 1998 because of baby walkers.

Children in baby walkers can:

- Roll down the stairs — which often causes broken bones and severe head injuries. This is how most children get hurt in baby walkers.
- Get burned — a child can reach higher when in a walker. A cup of hot coffee on the table, pot handles on the stove, a radiator, a fireplace, or a space heater are all now in baby's reach.
- Drown — a child can fall into a pool, bathtub, or toilet while in a walker.
- Be poisoned — reaching high objects is easier in a walker.

There are no benefits to baby walkers

You may think a walker can help your child learn to walk. But walkers do not help children walk sooner. In fact, walkers can delay normal muscle control and mental development.

Most walker injuries happen while adults are watching. Parents or caregivers simply cannot respond quickly enough. A child in a walker can move more than 3 feet in 1 second! Therefore, walkers are never safe to use, even with close adult supervision. Make sure there are no walkers at home or wherever your child is being cared for. Child care facilities should not allow the use of baby walkers. If your child is in child care at a center or at someone else's home, make sure there are no walkers.

Throw out your baby walkers!

Try something just as enjoyable but safer, such as the following:
- "Stationary walkers" — have no wheels but have seats that rotate, tip, and bounce.
- Playpens — great safety zones for children as they learn to sit, crawl, or walk.
- High chairs — older children often enjoy sitting up in a high chair and playing with toys on the tray.

On July 1, 1997, new safety standards were implemented for baby walkers. Walkers are now made wider so they cannot fit through most doorways, or are made with a braking mechanism to stop them at the edge of a step. But these new walker designs will not prevent all injuries from walkers. They still have wheels, so children can still move fast and reach higher.

The American Academy of Pediatrics and the National Association of Children's Hospitals and Related Institutions have called for a ban on the manufacture and sale of baby walkers with wheels. *Keep your child safe…throw away your baby walker.*

The information contained in this publication should not be used as a substitute for the medical care and advice of your pediatrician. There may be variations in treatment that your pediatrician may recommend based on individual facts and circumstances.

From your doctor

The American Academy of Pediatrics is an organization of 55,000 primary care pediatricians, pediatric medical subspecialists, and pediatric surgical specialists dedicated to the health, safety, and well-being of infants, children, adolescents, and young adults.

American Academy of Pediatrics
PO Box 747
Elk Grove Village, IL 60009-0747
Web site — http://www.aap.org

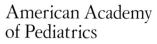

American Academy of Pediatrics

DEDICATED TO THE HEALTH OF ALL CHILDREN™

Bed-wetting

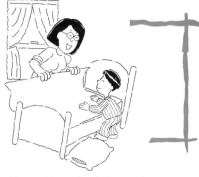

Toilet training a child takes a lot of patience, time, and understanding. Most children do not become fully toilet trained until they are between 2 and 4 years of age. While many children at this age are able to stay dry during the day, others may not be able to stay dry during the night until they are older.

Causes of bed-wetting

Although all of the causes of bed-wetting (enuresis) are not fully understood, following are some that are possible:

- Your child's bladder is not yet developed enough to hold urine for a full night.
- Your child is not yet able to recognize when his bladder is full, wake up, and use the toilet.
- Your child is responding to changes or stresses going on at home such as a new baby, moving, or divorce.

All young children occasionally wet their beds while going through nighttime toilet training. Even after your preschooler is able to stay dry at night for a number of days or weeks, she may start wetting at night again. When this happens, don't make an issue out of it. Simply put her back in training pants at night for a while until she is ready to try again. The problem will probably disappear as your child gets older.

Most school-aged children who wet their beds have primary enuresis. This means they have never developed nighttime bladder control. Instead, they have had this condition since birth and often have a family history of the problem. Children who are older when they develop nighttime bladder control often have at least one parent who had the same problem.

If you are concerned about your child's bed-wetting, talk to your pediatrician. He or she may ask you the following questions in order to find the cause of your child's bed-wetting:

- Is there a family history of bed-wetting?
- How often does your child urinate, and at what times of the day?
- When does your child wet the bed? Is your child very active, upset, or under unusual stress when it happens?
- Does your child tend to wet the bed after drinking carbonated beverages, caffeine, citrus juices, or a lot of water?
- Is there anything unusual about how your child urinates or the way his urine looks?

Signs of a problem

If your child has been completely toilet trained for 6 months or longer and suddenly begins wetting the bed again, talk to your pediatrician. It may be a sign of a medical problem such as:

- Bladder or kidney infections
- Diabetes
- Defects in the child's urinary system

However, keep in mind that less than 1% of bed-wetting cases are related to diseases or defects.

If your child has a medical problem that is causing the bed-wetting, there are usually other signs including:

- Changes in how much and how often your child urinates during the day
- Discomfort while urinating
- Unusual straining during urination
- A very small or narrow stream of urine, or dribbling that is constant or happens just after urination
- Cloudy or pink urine, or bloodstains on underpants or nightclothes
- Daytime as well as nighttime wetting
- Burning during urination

If there are signs that wetting is due to more than just delayed development of bladder control, and your child is older than 5 years of age, your pediatrician may order additional tests, such as an ultrasound of the kidneys or bladder. If necessary, your pediatrician will recommend that your child see a pediatric urologist, who is specially trained to treat children's urinary problems.

Tips to manage bed-wetting

It is important for parents to be sensitive to the child's feelings about bed-wetting. For instance, children may not want to spend the night at a friend's house or go to summer camp. They may be embarrassed or scared that their friends will find out they wet the bed.

Make sure your child understands that bed-wetting is not his fault and that it will get better in time. Remember, your child does not have control over the problem and would like it to stop, too! Until that happens, the following steps might help:

Protect the bed. Until your child can stay dry during the night, put a rubber or plastic cover between the sheet and mattress. This protects the bed from getting wet and smelling like urine.

Let your child help. Encourage your child to help change the wet sheets and covers. This teaches responsibility. At the same time it can relieve your child of any embarrassment from having family members know every time she wets the bed. If your child sees this as punishment, it is not recommended.

Set a no-teasing rule in your family. Do not let family members, especially siblings, tease a child who wets the bed. Explain to them that their brother or sister does not wet the bed on purpose. Do not make an issue of the bed-wetting every time it occurs.

Take steps before bedtime. Have your child use the toilet and avoid drinking large amounts of fluid just before bedtime.

Try to wake him up to use the toilet again right before you go to bed if he's been asleep for an hour or more.

Reward him for "dry" nights, but do not punish him for "wet" ones.

Use a bed-wetting alarm device. If your child is still not able to stay dry during the night after using the above steps for 1 to 3 months, your pediatrician may recommend using a bed-wetting alarm. When the device senses urine, it sets off an alarm so that the child can wake up to use the toilet. When used exactly as directed, it will detect the wetness right away and sound the alarm. Be sure your child resets the alarm before going back to sleep.

These alarms are available at most pharmacies and cost about $50 to $70. They produce a 50% to 75% cure rate, although some children occasionally relapse once they stop using them. Alarms tend to be most helpful when children are starting to have some dry nights and already have some bladder control on their own.

Medications. If the bed-wetting alarm does not solve the problem after 4 or 6 months, your pediatrician may prescribe an oral medication. Different medications are available. Medications usually are a last resort and are not recommended for preschool-aged children. Although it can be helpful for older children, some medications can have side effects. About four to five out of 10 children are helped by these medications. Your pediatrician will discuss medication options with you, if necessary.

Avoid unproven treatments. Because bed-wetting is such a common problem, many mail-order treatment programs and devices advertise that they are the cure. Use caution; many of these products make false claims and promises and may be very expensive. Your pediatrician is the best source for advice, and you should ask for it before your child starts any treatment program.

If none of the treatments work

A small number of children who wet the bed do not respond to any treatment. Fortunately, as each year passes, bed-wetting will decrease as the child's body matures. By the teen years almost all children will have outgrown the problem. Only 1 in 100 adults is troubled by persistent bed-wetting.

Until your older child outgrows bed-wetting, he will need a lot of emotional support from the family. Support from a pediatrician or a mental health professional also can help.

Parents need to provide support

Try not to pressure your child to develop nighttime bladder control before his or her body is ready to do so. As hard as your child might try, the bed-wetting is beyond control, and your child may get frustrated or depressed because he or she cannot stop it.

If your child has enuresis, discussing it with your pediatrician can help you to understand it better. Your pediatrician can also reassure you that your child is normal, and will eventually outgrow bed-wetting.

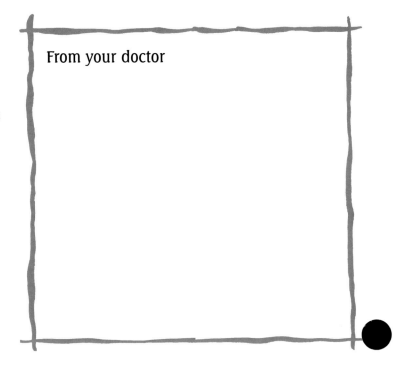

From your doctor

The American Academy of Pediatrics is an organization of 55,000 primary care pediatricians, pediatric medical subspecialists, and pediatric surgical specialists dedicated to the health, safety, and well-being of infants, children, adolescents, and young adults.

American Academy of Pediatrics
PO Box 747
Elk Grove Village, IL 60009-0747
Web site — http://www.aap.org

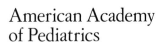

American Academy
of Pediatrics

DEDICATED TO THE HEALTH OF ALL CHILDREN™

Car Safety Seats:
A Guide for Families
2002

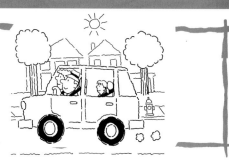

Every state requires that infants and children ride buckled up. However, state laws do not always require the safest way to transport a child. More children are still killed as passengers in car crashes than from any other type of injury. Using a car safety seat correctly can help prevent injuries to young children, but it is not as easy as you think. Just a little mistake in how the seat is used could cause serious injury to your child.

Which is the "best" car safety seat?

- No one seat is "safest" or "best." The "best" car safety seat is one that fits your child's size and weight, and can be installed correctly in your car.
- Price does not always make a difference. Higher prices can mean added features that may or may not make the seat easier to use.
- When you find a seat you like, try it out! Put your child in the seat and adjust the harnesses and buckles. Make sure it fits in your car.
- Keep in mind that displays or illustrations of seats in stores do not always show them being used correctly.

Types of car safety seats

Infant-only seats

- Only can be used rear-facing
- Are used for babies who weigh up to 20 pounds (or more, depending on the model)
- Are small and portable and fit newborns best
- Come with a 3-point harness or a 5-point harness

Infant-only seat

Infant-only seat features

Detachable base. Several infant-only seat models come with detachable bases. The base attaches to the car and the car safety seat easily snaps into the base. This way, you can carry your baby in and out of the car without needing to re-install the seat. After buckling your baby into the seat, you simply lock the seat into the installed base. Some bases are adjustable to make it easier to correctly recline newborns. These seats also can be used without the base or you can buy additional bases for other cars. However, this feature is only helpful if the base fits tightly into your car. In some cases, the seat may fit better without the base.

Higher weight and height limits. Several infant-only seats are available for use up to 22 pounds, and at least one is available for use up to 35 pounds. Many convertible seats also now have higher weight and height limits in the rear-facing position for heavier or taller babies. Keep in mind that some babies may reach the top height limits of the seat before they reach the top weight limits. If your infant's weight or height exceeds the limits of the seat before a year, use an infant-only seat or a rear-facing convertible seat that has a higher limit.

Harness slots. Infant-only seats that come with more than one harness slot give more room for growing babies. In the rear-facing position, the harness slots usually should be at or below your baby's shoulders. Check the car safety seat manufacturer's instructions to be sure.

Handles. Carrying handles on car safety seats vary greatly in style and ease of use. Check the instructions for how to adjust the handle during travel.

Other features. Angle indicators, built-in angle adjusters, harness adjusters, and head support systems are other features that may make correct installation easier to achieve.

Convertible seats

- Are bigger and heavier than infant-only seats, but can be used longer and for larger children.
- May not fit newborns as well as some infant-only seats. Make sure that your baby can recline comfortably in the seat. Check the car safety seat manufacturer's instructions to be sure that harnesses can be adjusted properly.
- Are used rear-facing for infants until they have reached at least 1 year of age *and* weigh at least 20 pounds (or more depending on model). The American Academy of Pediatrics (AAP) recommends that babies be kept in rear-facing seats until they reach the maximum weight allowed, as long as the top of the head is below the top of the seat back.
- Can be used forward-facing for toddlers who are at least 1 year of age *and* weigh at least 20 pounds and not more than 40 pounds. When your child is older than 1 year of age *and* has reached the highest weight or height allowed by the seat for use rear-facing, you may turn the seat forward-facing and make the following 3 adjustments:
  —Move the shoulder straps to the slots at or above your child's shoulders (usually the top slots, but check your instructions to make sure).
  —Move the seat into the upright position. (Check the car safety seat manufacturer's instructions for the recline angle allowed when forward-facing.)
  —Route the seat belt through the forward-facing belt path.
- Have the following 3 types of harnesses:
  —**5-point harness** — 5 straps: 2 at the shoulders, 2 at the hips, 1 at the crotch
  —**Overhead shield** — A padded tray-like shield that swings down around the child
  —**T-shield** — A padded T-shaped or triangular shield attached to shoulder straps
  Note: If using a convertible seat for a small infant, the best choice for a more secure fit is the 5-point harness. A small baby's face can hit a shield in a crash.

5-point harness

Overhead shield

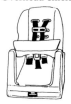

Convertible seat features

Adjustable buckles and shields. Many convertible seats have 2 or more buckle positions to give you extra room for a growing child or bulky clothing. Many overhead shields can be adjusted as well.

Higher weight limits. Several convertible seats are now available with higher rear-facing weight limits for bigger babies. For larger babies, look for a seat that can be used rear-facing up to 30 or 35 pounds.

T-shield

Car seats and shopping carts

Do not place a child of any age in a shopping cart. Many infant-only car seats lock into shopping carts. Although infant seats may help prevent falls from shopping carts, injuries can still occur if the cart tips over. The weight of an infant in an infant seat placed high in a shopping cart may make the cart more top-heavy and more likely to tip over. This is true even for shopping carts with built-in infant seats. Thousands of children are hurt every year from falling from shopping carts or from the carts tipping over. Instead, use a backpack, front pack, or stroller while shopping.

Combination seats

- Cannot be used rear-facing.
- Are only for children who are at least 1 year of age *and* weigh at least 20 pounds.
- Have an internal harness system for children who weigh 40 pounds or less.
- Convert to belt-positioning boosters (by removing the harnesses) for children who weigh more than 40 pounds. This allows the seat to be used longer.

Forward-facing seats/restraints

- Cannot be used rear-facing
- Are only for children who are at least 1 year of age *and* weigh at least 20 pounds
- Can be used with lap only belt or lap/shoulder belt

Booster seats

When your child reaches the top weight allowed for his car safety seat or his ears have reached the top of his car safety seat, your child needs a booster seat. Booster seats should be used until your child can correctly use a lap/shoulder seat belt. Following are 2 types of booster seats:

- **Belt-positioning boosters** are used with lap/ shoulder belts. The booster raises your child so that the lap/shoulder belt fits properly. This helps protect your child's upper body and head. Both high-backed and backless models are available.

High-backed belt-positioning booster

- **Shield boosters:** Based on Federal Motor Vehicle Safety Standards established by the National Highway Transportation Safety Administration (NHTSA), shield boosters have not been certified by their manufacturers for use by children who weigh more than 40 pounds. For these children, or for children who are too heavy or too tall to fit in a seat with a full harness, the shield may be removed and the seat used with a lap/shoulder belt as a belt-positioning booster.

Children who weigh 40 pounds or less are best protected in a seat with a full harness. Significant injuries have occurred to children in shield boosters in crashes due to ejection, excessive head movement, and shield contact. Although boosters with shields may meet current Federal Motor Vehicle Safety Standards for use by children who weigh 30–40 pounds, on the basis of current published peer-reviewed data, the AAP does not recommend their use. Children should remain in a convertible, forward-facing, or combination seat with a full harness until they reach the top weight or height allowed by the seat.

Travel vests

A travel vest may be an option if your car has only lap belts.

Built-in seats (integrated seats)

Built-in seats are available in some cars and vans. They may be used for children who are at least 1 year of age *and* weigh at least 20 pounds. Built-in seats eliminate installation problems. However, weight and height limits vary. Check with vehicle manufacturers for details about built-in seats that are currently available.

Basics of car safety seat use

- Always use a car safety seat, starting with your baby's first ride home from the hospital. Help your child form a lifelong habit of buckling up.
- Read the car safety seat manufacturer's instructions and always keep them with the car safety seat.
- Read your vehicle owner's manual for important information on how to install the car safety seat correctly in your vehicle.
- The safest place for all children to ride is in the back seat.
- Never place a child in a rear-facing car safety seat in the front seat of a vehicle that has a passenger air bag.
- The harness system holds your child in the car safety seat and the seat belt or an anchor system holds the seat in the car. Attach both snugly to protect your child.

Using car safety seats correctly

Read the car safety seat manufacturer's instructions and the child restraint section of your vehicle owner's manual carefully to be sure you are installing and using the car safety seat correctly. When you install the seat in your car, check the following:

Is your child buckled into the car safety seat correctly?

- Be sure to use the correct harness slots for the child.
- Keep the harnesses snug. Place the plastic harness clip, if provided, at armpit level to hold shoulder straps in place.
- Make sure the straps lie flat and are not twisted.
- Dress your baby in clothes that allow the straps to go between the legs. Adjust the straps to allow for the thickness of your child's clothes, making sure that the harness still holds the child securely.
- In cold weather, tuck blankets around your baby after adjusting the harness straps snugly.
- To keep your newborn from slouching, pad the sides of the seat and between the crotch with rolled up diapers or receiving blankets.

Is the car safety seat buckled into your vehicle correctly?

- Place the seat facing the correct direction for the size and age of your child. Route the seat belt through the correct path on the car safety seat (check your instructions to make sure) and pull it tight. Before each trip, check to make sure the car safety seat is installed tightly enough by pulling on the car safety seat where the seat belt passes through. It should not move easily side to side or toward the front of the car.
- If your infant's head flops forward, the seat may not be reclined enough. Tilt the seat back until it is reclined as close as possible to a 45-degree angle (according to manufacturer's instructions). Your seat may have a built-in recline adjuster for this purpose. If not, you may wedge firm padding, such as a rolled towel, under the front of the base of the seat.

- Check the seat belt buckle. Make sure it does not lie just at the point where the belt bends around the car safety seat. If it does, you will not be able to get the belt tight enough. If you cannot get the belt tight, check the car safety seat and vehicle manufacturers' instructions for recommendations. You may need to use another set of belts in the car that can be tightened properly.
- Many lap/shoulder belts allow passengers to move freely even when they are buckled. Read your car owner's manual to see if your seat belts can be locked into position or if you will need to use a locking clip. Locking clips come with all new car safety seats (some have them built in). Read your instructions for information on how to use the locking clip.
- Some lap belts need a special, heavy-duty locking clip, available from the vehicle manufacturer. Check your car owner's manual for more information.

What is LATCH?

A new car safety seat attachment system has been developed to make car safety seats easier to use and safer. The system is called LATCH, which stands for Lower Anchors and Tethers for Children. This new anchor system will make correct installation much easier because you will no longer need to use seat belts to secure the car safety seat. Starting in model year 2002, most new vehicles and new safety seats will be equipped with these lower anchors and attachments. However, unless both the vehicle and the car safety seat have this new anchor system, seat belts will still be needed to secure the car safety seat.

Why are tethers important?

Most new car safety seats that can be used facing forward come with top tethers. A tether is a strap that hooks the top of the car safety seat to a special permanent anchor in the vehicle. Most anchors are located on the rear window ledge, the back of the vehicle seat, or the floor or ceiling of the vehicle. Tethers give extra protection by keeping the car safety seat from being thrown forward in a crash.

Tether kits are available for most older car safety seats. Check with the car safety seat manufacturer to find out how to get a top tether for your seat. Be sure to install it according to instructions. The tether strap may help make some seats that are difficult to install fit more tightly.

All new cars, minivans, and light trucks have been required to have upper tether anchors for securing the tops of car safety seats since September 2000.

Is your child ready for a regular seat belt?

Keep your child in a car safety seat for as long as possible. When your child is big enough, make sure the seat belts in your vehicle fit your child correctly. The shoulder belt should lie across the chest, not the neck or throat. The lap belt must be low and snug across the thighs, not the stomach. The child should sit against the vehicle seat back with her feet hanging down when the legs are bent at the knee. Seat belts are made for adults. If the seat belt does not fit your child correctly, she should stay in a booster seat until the belt fits. This is usually when the child reaches about 4' 9" in height and is between 8–12 years of age.

Other points to keep in mind when using seat belts include the following:

- Never tuck the shoulder belt under the child's arm or behind the child's back.
- If only a lap belt is available, make sure it is snug and low on the child's thighs, not across the stomach. Try to get a lap/shoulder belt installed in your car.

For specific information about installing your car safety seat, you may consult a certified Child Passenger Safety (CPS) Technician. CPS Technicians are certified by the American Automobile Association (AAA). A list of certified CPS Technicians is available by state or ZIP code on the NHTSA Web site at **http://www.nhtsa.dot.gov/people/injury/childps/Contacts/index.cfm**.

A list of inspection stations staffed by certified CPS Technicians is available at **http://www.nhtsa.dot.gov/people/injury/childps/CPSFitting/Index.cfm**.

The information is available by telephone on the NHTSA Auto Safety Hot Line at 888/DASH-2-DOT (888/327-4236), from 8 am to 10 pm ET, Monday through Friday.

There are a number of add-on products on the market that claim to solve the problem of poorly fitting seat belts. However, these products may actually interfere with proper lap and shoulder belt fit by causing the lap belt to ride too high on the abdomen and making the shoulder belt too loose. Until the NHTSA develops standards for these products, the AAP recommends they not be used.

Are you using a secondhand seat? Double-check everything!

A new car safety seat is best. However, if you must get a used seat, shop very carefully. Keep the following points in mind:

Do not use a car safety seat that

- **Is too old.** Look on the label for the date it was made. If it is more than 10 years old, it should not be used. Some manufacturers recommend that seats only be used for 5–6 years. Check with the manufacturer to find out when the company recommends getting a new seat.
- **Was in a crash.** It may have been weakened and should not be used, even if it looks fine. Do not use a seat if you do not know its full history.
- **Does not have a label with the date of manufacture and seat name or model number.** Without these, you cannot check on recalls.
- **Does not come with instructions.** You need them to know how to use the car safety seat. Do not rely on the former owner's directions. Get a copy of the instruction manual from the manufacturer before you use the seat.
- **Has any cracks in the frame of the seat.**
- **Is missing parts.** Used seats often come without important parts. Check with the manufacturer to make sure you can get the right parts.

Has the car safety seat been recalled?

You can find out by calling the manufacturer or the Auto Safety Hot Line at 888/DASH-2-DOT (888/327-4236), from 8 am to 10 pm ET, Monday through Friday. This information is also available on the NHTSA Web site at http://www.nhtsa.dot.gov/cars/problems/recalls/index.cfm.

If the seat has been recalled, be sure to follow instructions to fix it or get the necessary parts. You also may get a registration card for future recall notices from the hot line.

Common questions about car safety seats

"What if my baby is premature?"

Use a car safety seat without a shield. Shields often are too high and too far from the body to fit correctly. A small baby's face could hit a shield in a crash. While still in the hospital, your baby should be observed in her car safety seat to make sure the semi-reclined position does not cause low heart rate, low oxygen, or other breathing problems. If your baby needs to lie flat during travel, use a crash-tested car bed. If possible, an adult should ride in the back seat next to your baby to watch him closely.

"What if my baby weighs more than 20 pounds but is not 1 year of age yet?"

There are now several infant-only and convertible seats that can be used rear-facing for children weighing more than 20 pounds.

"What if my child has special health care needs?"

Children with special health problems may need other restraint systems. Discuss this with your pediatrician. Easter Seals, Inc offers programs about car safety seat safety for children with special health care needs in the following states: California, Colorado, Florida, Georgia, Hawaii, Louisiana, Kentucky, New Mexico, Michigan, Missouri, Ohio, Pennsylvania, and West Virginia. More information is available from Easter Seals, Inc at 800/221-6827.

"What if my car has air bags?"

Most new cars have air bags. When used with seat belts, air bags work very well to protect older children and adults. However, air bags are very dangerous when used with rear-facing car safety seats. If your car has a passenger air bag, infants in rear-facing seats must ride in the back seat. Even in a low-speed crash, the air bag can inflate, strike the car safety seat, and cause serious brain injury and death.

Toddlers who ride in forward-facing car safety seats also are at risk from air bag injuries. All children, even through school age, are safest in the back seat. If you must put an older child in the front seat, slide the vehicle seat back as far as it will go. Make sure your child is buckled and stays in the proper position at all times. This will help prevent the air bag from striking your child.

For most families, air bag on/off switches are not necessary. Air bags that are turned off cannot protect other passengers riding in the front seat. Air bag on/off switches only should be used if *all* of the following are true:

- Your child has special heath care needs.
- Your pediatrician recommends constant supervision of your child during travel.
- No other adult is available to ride in the back seat with your child. On/off switches also must be used if you have a vehicle with no back seat or a back seat that is not made for passengers.

"What if my car has side air bags?"

Side air bags improve safety for adults in side impact crashes. However, children who are seated near a front or rear side air bag can be at risk for serious injury. Refer to your vehicle owner's manual for recommendations that apply to your vehicle.

"What if my car only has lap belts in the back seat?"

Lap belts work fine with infant-only, convertible, and forward-facing seats. They cannot be used with belt-positioning boosters (which are safest for children who weigh more than 40 pounds and who are not big enough to fit in adult seat belts). If your car only has lap belts, use a forward-facing seat with a harness approved for use to higher weights, use a forward-facing restraint, or check with your dealer or the manufacturer of your car to see if shoulder harnesses can be installed. Some travel vests can be used with lap belts. Another thing you can do is buy another car with lap/shoulder belts in the back seat.

"What if I drive more children than can be buckled safely in the back seat?"

Avoid this situation, especially if your car has passenger air bags. However, in an emergency, place the child most likely to sit in the proper forward-facing position in the front seat, with the vehicle seat moved as far back as possible. A child in a forward-facing car safety seat may be the best choice because a child who is in a booster seat or using a regular seat belt can more easily move out of position and be at greater risk for injuries from the air bag.

"What if I lose my instructions to my car safety seat?"

Call or write the manufacturer and ask for a new set of instructions.

"What if my car safety seat was in a crash?"

A seat that was in a crash may have been weakened and should not be used even if it looks fine. Call the car safety seat manufacturer if you have questions about the safety of your seat.

"Can I use a car safety seat on an airplane?"

The Federal Aviation Administration (FAA) and the AAP recommend that children be securely fastened in child safety seats until 4 years of age, then be secured with the airplane seat belts. This will help keep them safe during takeoff and landing, or in case of turbulence. Most infant, convertible, and forward-facing seats are certified to be used on airplanes. Booster seats and travel vests are not. Check the label on your seat and call the airline before you travel to be sure your seat meets current FAA regulations.

ALWAYS READ AND FOLLOW MANUFACTURER'S INSTRUCTIONS.

If you do not have the car safety seat manufacturer's instructions, write or call the company's consumer relations department, identifying the model number, name of seat, and date of manufacture. The manufacturer's address and phone number may be on the label on the seat. Before purchasing a car safety seat, check the manufacturer's instructions for important safety information about proper fitting and use.

Although the American Academy of Pediatrics (AAP) is not a testing or standard setting organization, this guide sets forth the Academy's recommendations based upon the peer reviewed literature available at the time of its publication and sets forth some of the factors that parents should consider before selecting and using a car safety seat.

The information contained in this publication should not be used as a substitute for the medical care and advice of your pediatrician. There may be variations in treatment that your pediatrician may recommend based on individual facts and circumstances.

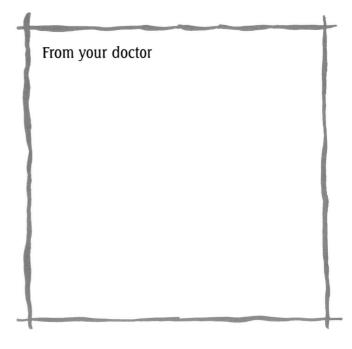

From your doctor

American Academy of Pediatrics

DEDICATED TO THE HEALTH OF ALL CHILDREN™

The American Academy of Pediatrics is an organization of 55,000 primary care pediatricians, pediatric medical subspecialists, and pediatric surgical specialists dedicated to the health, safety, and well-being of infants, children, adolescents, and young adults.

American Academy of Pediatrics
PO Box 747
Elk Grove Village, IL 60009-0747
Web site — http://www.aap.org

Care of the Uncircumcised Penis

One of the first decisions you will make for your new baby boy is whether or not to have him circumcised. If you have chosen not to have your son circumcised, there are some things you should be aware of and teach your son as he gets older.

What is foreskin retraction?

Sometime during the first several years of your son's life, his foreskin, which covers the head of the penis, will separate from the glans. Some foreskins separate soon after birth or even before birth, but this is rare. When it happens is different for every child. It may take a few weeks, months, or years.

After the foreskin separates from the glans, it can be pulled back away from the glans toward the abdomen. This is called *foreskin retraction*.

Most boys will be able to retract their foreskins by the time they are 5 years old, yet others will not be able to until the teenage years. As a boy becomes more aware of his body, he will most likely discover how to retract his own foreskin. But *foreskin retraction should never be forced*. Until separation occurs, do not try to pull the foreskin back — especially an infant's. Forcing the foreskin to retract before it is ready may severely harm the penis and cause pain, bleeding, and tears in the skin.

What is smegma?

When the foreskin separates from the glans, skin cells are shed. These skin cells may look like whitish lumps, resembling pearls, under the foreskin. These are called *smegma*. Smegma is normal and nothing to worry about.

Does my son's foreskin need special cleaning?

Your son's intact or uncircumcised penis requires no special care and is easy to keep clean. When your son is an infant, bathe or sponge him regularly and wash all body parts, including the genitals. Simply wash the penis with soap and warm water. Remember, do not try to forcibly retract the foreskin.

If your son's foreskin is separated and retractable before he reaches puberty, an occasional retraction with cleansing beneath will do. Once your son starts puberty, he should retract the foreskin and clean beneath it on a regular basis. It should become a part of your son's total body hygiene, just like shampooing his hair and brushing his teeth. Teach your son to clean his foreskin in the following way:
- Gently pull the foreskin back away from the glans.
- Rinse the glans and inside fold of the foreskin with soap and warm water.
- Pull the foreskin back over the head of the penis.

Is there anything else I should watch for?

While your son is still a baby, you should make sure the hole in the foreskin is large enough to allow a normal stream when he urinates. Talk to your pediatrician if any of the following occurs:
- The stream of urine is never heavier than a trickle.
- Your baby seems to have some discomfort while urinating.
- The foreskin becomes considerably red or swollen.

The information contained in this publication should not be used as a substitute for the medical care and advice of your pediatrician. There may be variations in treatment that your pediatrician may recommend based on individual facts and circumstances.

From your doctor

American Academy
of Pediatrics

DEDICATED TO THE HEALTH OF ALL CHILDREN™

The American Academy of Pediatrics is an organization of 55,000 primary care pediatricians, pediatric medical subspecialists, and pediatric surgical specialists dedicated to the health, safety, and well-being of infants, children, adolescents, and young adults.

American Academy of Pediatrics
PO Box 747
Elk Grove Village, IL 60009-0747
Web site — http://www.aap.org

Circumcision:
Information for Parents

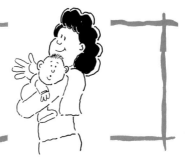

Circumcision is a surgical procedure in which the skin covering the end of the penis is removed. Scientific studies show some medical benefits of circumcision. However, these benefits are not sufficient for the American Academy of Pediatrics to recommend that all infant boys be circumcised. Parents may want their sons circumcised for religious, social, and cultural reasons. Since circumcision is not essential to a child's health, parents should choose what is best for their child by looking at the benefits and risks. This brochure answers common questions you may have about circumcision. Use this as a guide to help you decide what is best for your baby boy.

What is circumcision?

At birth, boys have skin that covers the end of the penis, called the foreskin. Circumcision surgically removes the foreskin, exposing the tip of the penis. Circumcision is usually performed by a doctor in the first few days of life. An infant must be stable and healthy to safely be circumcised.

Many parents choose to have their sons circumcised because "all the other men in the family were circumcised" or because they do not want their sons to feel "different." Others feel that circumcision is unnecessary and choose not to have it done. Some groups such as followers of the Jewish and Islamic faiths, practice circumcision for religious and cultural reasons. Since circumcision may be more risky if done later in life, parents may want to decide before or soon after their son is born if they want their son circumcised.

Common questions about circumcision

Is circumcision painful?

When done without pain medicine, circumcision is painful. There are pain medicines available that are safe and effective. The American Academy of Pediatrics recommends that they be used to reduce pain from circumcision. Local anesthetics can be injected into the penis to lower pain and stress in infants. There are also topical creams that can help. Talk to your pediatrician about which pain medicine is best for your son. Problems with using pain medicine are rare and usually not serious.

What should I expect for my son after circumcision?

After the circumcision, the tip of the penis may seem raw or yellowish. If there is a bandage, it should be changed with each diapering to reduce the risk of the penis becoming infected. Petroleum jelly should be used to keep the bandage from sticking. Sometimes a plastic ring is used instead of a bandage. The plastic ring that is left on the tip of the penis usually drops off within 5 to 8 days. It takes about 1 week to 10 days for the penis to fully heal after circumcision.

Reasons parents may choose circumcision

Research studies suggest that there may be some medical benefits to circumcision. These include the following:

- A slightly lower risk of urinary tract infections (UTIs). A circumcised infant boy has about a 1 in 1,000 chance of developing a UTI in the first year of life; an uncircumcised infant boy has about a 1 in 100 chance of developing a UTI in the first year of life.
- A lower risk of getting cancer of the penis. However, this type of cancer is very rare in both circumcised and uncircumcised males.
- A slightly lower risk of getting sexually transmitted diseases (STDs), including HIV, the AIDS virus.
- Prevention of foreskin infections.
- Prevention of phimosis, a condition in uncircumcised males that makes foreskin retraction impossible.
- Easier genital hygiene.

Reasons parents may choose not to circumcise

The following are reasons why parents may choose NOT to have their son circumcised:

- Possible risks. As with any surgery, circumcision has some risks. Complications from circumcision are rare and usually minor. They may include bleeding, infection, cutting the foreskin too short or too long, and improper healing.
- The belief that the foreskin is necessary to protect the tip of the penis. When removed, the tip of the penis may become irritated and cause the opening of the penis to become too small. This can cause urination problems that may need to be surgically corrected.
- The belief that circumcision makes the tip of the penis less sensitive, causing a decrease in sexual pleasure later in life.
- Almost all uncircumcised boys can be taught proper hygiene that can lower their chances of getting infections, cancer of the penis, and sexually transmitted diseases.

Are there any problems that can happen after circumcision?

Problems after a circumcision are very rare. However, call your pediatrician right away if

- Your baby does not urinate normally within 6 to 8 hours after the circumcision.
- There is persistent bleeding.
- There is redness around the tip of the penis that gets worse after 3 to 5 days.

It is normal to have a little yellow discharge or coating around the head of the penis, but this should not last longer than a week.

What if I choose not to have my son circumcised?

If you choose not to have your son circumcised, talk to your pediatrician about how to keep your son's penis clean. When your son is old enough, he can learn how to keep his penis clean just as he will learn to keep other parts of his body clean.

The foreskin usually does not fully retract for several years and should *never* be forced. The uncircumcised penis is easy to keep clean by gently washing the genital area while bathing. You do not need to do any special cleansing, such as with cotton swabs or antiseptics.

Later, when the foreskin fully retracts, boys should be taught how to wash underneath the foreskin every day. Teach your son to clean his foreskin by

- Gently pulling it back away from the head of the penis
- Rinsing the head of the penis and inside fold of the foreskin with soap and warm water
- Pulling the foreskin back over the head of the penis

See the AAP brochure *Newborns: Care of the Uncircumcised Penis* for more details. See your pediatrician if you notice any signs of infection such as redness, swelling, or foul-smelling drainage.

Female "circumcision"

Female genital mutilation, sometimes called female circumcision, is common in many cultures. It involves removing part or all of a female's clitoris. It may also involve sewing up the opening of the vagina. It is often done without any pain medicine. The purpose of this practice is to prove that a female is a virgin before she gets married, reduce her ability to experience sexual pleasure after marriage, and promote marital fidelity. There are many serious side effects, including the following:

- Pelvic and urinary tract infections
- Negative effects on self-esteem and sexuality
- Inability to deliver a baby vaginally

The Academy is absolutely opposed to this practice in all forms as it is disfiguring and has no medical benefits.

The information contained in this publication should not be used as a substitute for the medical care and advice of your pediatrician. There may be variations in treatment that your pediatrician may recommend based on individual facts and circumstances.

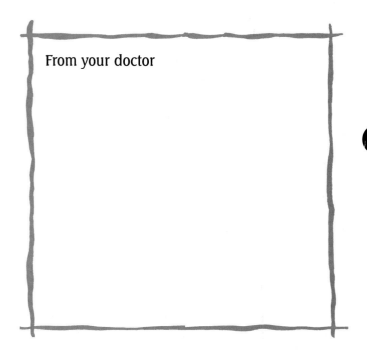

From your doctor

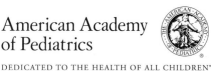

American Academy of Pediatrics

DEDICATED TO THE HEALTH OF ALL CHILDREN™

The American Academy of Pediatrics is an organization of 55,000 primary care pediatricians, pediatric medical subspecialists, and pediatric surgical specialists dedicated to the health, safety, and well-being of infants, children, adolescents, and young adults.

American Academy of Pediatrics
PO Box 747
Elk Grove Village, IL 60009-0747
Web site — http://www.aap.org

Copyright ©1995, Updated 3/00
American Academy of Pediatrics

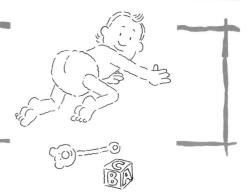

Diaper Rash

Diaper rash affects most babies, but it is usually not serious. Below we explain the causes of diaper rash, steps you can take to help prevent it, and how to treat it if it develops.

What is diaper rash?

Diaper rash can be any rash that develops inside the diaper area. In mild cases, the skin might be red. In more severe cases, there may be painful open sores. You will usually see a rash around the abdomen, genitalia, and inside the skin folds of the thighs and buttocks. Mild cases clear up within 3 to 4 days without any treatment. If a rash persists or develops again after treatment, consult your pediatrician.

What causes diaper rash?

Over the years diaper rash has been blamed on various causes, such as teething, diet, and ammonia in the urine. However, medical experts now believe it is caused by any of the following:

- Too much moisture
- Chafing or rubbing
- Prolonged contact of the skin with urine, feces, or both
- Yeast infection
- Bacterial infection
- Allergic reaction to diaper material

When skin stays wet for too long, the layers that protect it start to break down. When wet skin is rubbed, it also damages more easily. Moisture from a soiled diaper can harm your baby's skin and make it more prone to chafing. When this happens, a diaper rash may develop.

Further rubbing between the moist folds of the skin only makes the rash worse. This is why diaper rash often forms in the skin folds of the groin and upper thighs.

More than half of babies between 4 months and 15 months of age develop diaper rash at least once in a 2-month period. Diaper rash occurs more often in the following instances:

- As infants get older—mostly between 8 to 10 months of age
- If babies are not kept clean and dry
- In babies who have frequent stools, especially when the stools stay in their diapers overnight
- When babies begin to eat solid foods
- When babies are taking antibiotics, or in nursing babies whose mothers are taking antibiotics

Infants taking antibiotics are more likely to get diaper rashes caused by yeast infections. Yeast infects the weakened skin and causes a bright red rash with red spots at its edges. You can treat this with over-the-counter antifungal medications. If you see these symptoms, you may wish to consult with your pediatrician.

What can I do to prevent diaper rash?

To help prevent diaper rash from developing, you should:

- Change the diaper promptly after your child wets or has a bowel movement. This limits moisture on the skin.
- Do not put the diaper on airtight, especially overnight. Keep the diaper loose so that the wet and soiled parts do not rub against the skin as much.
- Gently clean the diaper area with water. You do not need to use soap with every diaper change or after every bowel movement. (Breastfed infants may stool as many as 8 times a day.) Use soap only when the stool does not come off easily.
- Do not use talcum or baby powder because they could cause breathing problems in your infant.
- Avoid over-cleansing with wipes that can dry out the skin. The alcohol or perfume in these products may irritate some babies' skin.

What can I do if my baby gets diaper rash?

If diaper rash develops despite your best efforts to prevent it, try the following:

- Change wet or soiled diapers often.
- Use clear water to cleanse the diaper area with each diaper change.
- Using water in a squirt bottle lets you clean and rinse without rubbing.
- Pat dry; do not rub. Allow the area to air dry fully.
- Apply a thick layer of protective ointment or cream (such as one that contains zinc oxide or petrolatum) to form a protective coating on the skin. These ointments are usually thick and pasty and do not have to be completely removed at the next diaper change. Remember, heavy scrubbing or rubbing will only damage the skin more.
- Check with your pediatrician if the rash:
  - Has blisters or pus-filled sores
  - Does not so away within 48 to 72 hours
  - Gets worse
- Use creams with steroids only if your pediatrician recommends them. They are rarely needed and may be harmful.

Which type of diaper should I use?

There are many different brands of diapers. Diapers are made of cloth or disposable materials. After they get soiled, you can wash cloth diapers and use them again and you throw away disposable diapers.

Research suggests that diaper rash is less common with the use of disposable diapers. In child care settings, children who wear super-absorbent disposable diapers tend to have lower rates of diaper rash. Regardless of which type of diaper you use, diaper rash occurs less often and is less severe when you change diapers often. If you use a cloth diaper, you can use a stay-dry liner inside it to keep your baby drier.

If you choose not to wash cloth diapers yourself, you can have a diaper service clean them. If you do your own washing, you will need to presoak heavily soiled diapers. Keep and wash soiled diapers separate from other clothes. Use hot water and double-rinse each wash. Do not use fabric softeners or antistatic products on the diapers because they may cause rashes in young, sensitive skin.

Whether you use cloth diapers, disposables, or both, always change diapers as needed to keep your baby clean, dry, and healthy.

Remember—never leave your baby alone on the changing table or on any other surface above the floor. Even a newborn can make a sudden turn and fall to the floor.

Diaper rash is usually not serious, but it can cause your child discomfort. Follow the steps listed above to help prevent and treat diaper rash. Discuss any questions you have about these steps with your pediatrician.

The information contained in this publication should not be used as a substitute for the medical care and advice of your pediatrician. There may be variations in treatment that your pediatrician may recommend based on individual facts and circumstances.

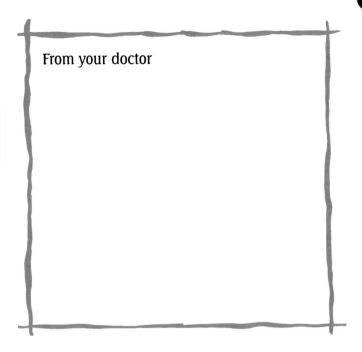

From your doctor

American Academy of Pediatrics

DEDICATED TO THE HEALTH OF ALL CHILDREN™

The American Academy of Pediatrics is an organization of 55,000 primary care pediatricians, pediatric medical subspecialists, and pediatric surgical specialists dedicated to the health, safety, and well-being of infants, children, adolescents, and young adults.

American Academy of Pediatrics
PO Box 747
Elk Grove Village, IL 60009-0747
Web site — http://www.aap.org

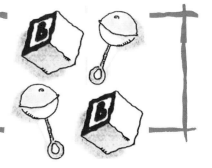

Early Arrival:
Information for Parents of Premature Infants

Your Very Special Delivery

Congratulations! You have welcomed a new baby to your family! While every child brings his own joys and challenges, you may be worried because your baby was born earlier than expected. But as you will see, while premature infants may need extra care at first, they have bright futures.

Premature Birth Is Common

Every year, about 11% of babies are born prematurely. But, thanks to medical advances, children born after 28 weeks and weighing more than 2 lb 3 oz, have a 95% or better chance of survival. They usually catch up in height and weight with their peers by age 2. In fact, 80% of babies born after the 30th week of pregnancy have no long-term health or developmental problems.

Premature Babies Need Special Care

At the Hospital

Because premature babies are born before they are physically ready to leave the womb, they require extra medical attention immediately after delivery. Your child may need special tests as well as medical help that is different from that needed by full-term babies. It may be a few days or weeks before his lungs fully develop, before he begins to breathe and feed on his own, and before he is able to maintain his own body temperature.

Your baby will probably be admitted to a *neonatal intensive care unit* or a *neonatal intermediate care unit*. There, a specially educated team of doctors and nurses can give your child the care he needs.

At Home

Like any child, your premature baby needs your love and attention in order to thrive. There are many things you can do at home to make sure your baby has a healthy start. This booklet will help you care for your child so that you can help him stay healthy and grow strong.

Answers to Parents' Common Questions

Q: Why was my baby premature? Is it my fault?

A: Many mothers of premature infants worry that they might have done something during pregnancy that caused their babies to be born early. Smoking, drinking alcohol, and using drugs during pregnancy can contribute to prematurity; however, no one knows for sure why most premature babies are born early. If you smoke, have a drinking problem, or use drugs, get help right away. These behaviors can harm your baby after she is born, too. Your new baby needs you to be as healthy as possible.

Q: Will I be able to hold my baby?

A: All babies need to be touched, held, snuggled, and talked to. This can reduce stress and help their brains develop. Although your baby may look fragile, you should gently touch, hold, and cradle her if your doctor says it is OK.

Q: Why does my baby look different?

A: Babies who are born early do not look like full-term infants. Your baby's head may seem larger compared to the rest of her body. Her body will have less fat and her skin may look thin. Her blood vessels may show underneath. Also, your baby's facial features may appear sharper. But don't worry, she will begin to look like a typical newborn as she grows.

Q: What will happen to my baby when I leave the hospital without her?

A: Leaving your baby, even for a short time, can be difficult, but your baby is in good hands. You can visit often to spend time with your child. Use the time away from the hospital to rest and get ready for your baby's homecoming.

Q: Will my child always have problems because she was born early?

A: Though premature babies are at higher risk for some problems, most of them grow into healthy children. Early diagnosis, treatment, and ongoing care can give your child a brighter future.

Some Helpful Definitions

- **Apgar Score:** This exam measures your baby's heart rate, breathing, muscle tone, reflex response, and color at birth. The Apgar score helps the hospital staff know how your baby is doing as he gets used to life outside the womb. Because of their early birth, premature babies are more likely to have lower scores.
- **Cardiorespiratory Monitor:** Because your baby's lungs are still immature, he may have trouble breathing. His breathing and heart rate can be watched using special equipment called a cardiorespiratory monitor. If he needs help breathing, the doctors may give him extra oxygen or use other equipment to help him breathe.
- **Warmer/Incubator:** Because your baby has less body fat, he can get cold in normal room temperatures. For that reason, he will be placed in a warmer bed or an incubator. These special beds have built-in heaters to help keep your baby warm.

Your Baby's Nutrition Needs

Because premature infants are small, they have a great need for food to gain strength and build resistance to disease. At first they may need to receive fluids intravenously (through an IV) or through a feeding tube.

Breast milk is the best nutrition for your baby. However, if your baby is not able to nurse at first, you can pump your milk and it can be given to her. Express your milk at the times when your baby would usually feed, so that your body becomes used to the schedule (usually about 8 times per day at the start). Most hospitals have breastfeeding experts to help you get started. Once you start to breastfeed, let your baby nurse often to build up your milk supply.

Breastfeeding is best for most infants, however, for medical or personal reasons, your baby may need infant formula. You and your pediatrician should discuss this decision.

Special Health Issues

Premature infants are not as fully developed as full-term babies. That is why they have a somewhat higher risk for certain health problems.

- **Respiratory Distress Syndrome (RDS)**
  <u>What It Is:</u> RDS is a breathing problem caused by immature lungs. Premature infants' lungs may lack a liquid substance called surfactant that gives fully developed lungs the elastic qualities required for easy breathing. Without surfactant, the lungs tend to collapse, forcing a tiny baby to work harder to breathe.
  <u>Treatment:</u> Many infants will require a ventilator, or respirator, to breathe for them. Artificial surfactants are now available and are very effective in treating RDS. Many babies respond very well to this treatment. Lung problems in premature infants usually improve within several days to several weeks.

- **Chronic Lung Disease/Bronchopulmonary Dysplasia (BPD)**
  <u>What It Is:</u> Babies who need oxygen for more than a month are described as having *bronchopulmonary dysplasia* (BPD) or chronic lung disease. They may need oxygen and other treatments for several weeks or months.
  <u>Treatment:</u> Babies often outgrow BPD as their lungs mature and grow, although some premature infants continue to require oxygen when they go home.

- **Respiratory Syncytial Virus (RSV)**
  <u>What It Is:</u> RSV is the leading cause of lower respiratory tract illness in infants and children. In the United States, RSV outbreaks usually occur between October and May. Infants who get RSV may develop apnea (pauses in a baby's breathing that last more than 15 seconds); *bronchiolitis* (an infection of the small breathing tubes of the lungs); or long-term lung problems. Premature infants and babies with BPD are at highest risk for complications from RSV infection.
  <u>Prevention and Treatment:</u> RSV is very contagious. It can be spread in the hospital or after babies are sent home. Make sure that family and friends who visit your new baby do not have colds or other infections. Ask them to wash their hands before touching your baby. There is no proven effective treatment for RSV infection. As a result, your pediatrician may recommend medication to prevent RSV infection if your baby is at very high risk for serious complications.

- **Retinopathy of Prematurity (ROP)**
  <u>What It Is:</u> ROP is an eye disease that occurs when part of the eye, called the retina, has not fully developed.
  <u>Treatment:</u> Most cases of ROP are mild and will resolve without treatment. However, in some cases ROP can result in serious vision problems. Severe cases of ROP are often treated with surgery. Your pediatrician will talk to you about this treatment if it is needed.

- **Apnea and Bradycardia**
  <u>What It Is:</u> Apnea refers to pauses in your baby's breathing that last more than 15 seconds. This is common in preterm babies. When apnea occurs, the heart rate will often decrease as well. This is called *bradycardia*.
  <u>Treatment:</u> If your baby has apnea spells, your pediatrician may prescribe a medicine to help regulate breathing. Your baby's heart and breathing will also be watched by monitors. Most premature babies outgrow this before they go home. If your baby does not, he may need a home apnea monitor.

- **Jaundice**
  <u>What It Is:</u> Jaundice happens because a baby's liver has not matured enough to completely filter a yellowish substance called bilirubin from the blood. Newborns often produce more *bilirubin* than their livers can handle.
  <u>Treatment:</u> Most cases can be treated effectively by placing the baby under special lights. During the treatment, most of the baby's skin is exposed and his eyes are covered to protect them from the light.

- **Other Health Problems**
  Premature infants may also develop other conditions such as *anemia of prematurity* (low blood cell count) and *heart murmurs*. Heart murmurs are sounds that the flow of blood makes as it goes through the heart. Your pediatrician and the other health care professionals caring for your baby will keep you informed about your baby's condition and progress.

Choosing a Pediatrician

Because your baby arrived early, you may not have had time to choose a pediatrician for your child. Your baby's doctor or nurse at the hospital may be able to recommend a pediatrician. You can also write the American Academy of Pediatrics for the names of pediatricians in your area. See the "Helpful Organizations" section at the end of this booklet for the address.

A Happy Homecoming

The OK to Go

You finally get to bring your baby home! Your pediatrician will approve the discharge of your baby from the hospital, based on the following guidelines. Your baby should be:

- breathing on her own,
- able to maintain body temperature,
- able to be fed by breast or bottle, and
- gaining weight steadily at time of discharge.

Other medical problems should also be resolved, or home care should be set up before your baby leaves the hospital.

Questions to Ask Before You Leave the Hospital

Your pediatrician will talk with you before your baby leaves the hospital. Be sure that he or she explains the following:

- How to care for your baby at home
- When to call his or her office or go to the hospital
- How to know if your baby is eating properly, getting enough sleep and gaining enough weight
- What medicines to give, if any are needed
- How often you will need to bring your baby in for an exam. Regular contact with your pediatrician is very important to your child's health. Be sure to discuss any worries that you have about your baby.

Safe Traveling With Your Baby

It is not only unsafe, but also illegal for any baby to ride in a car without being secured in a car safety seat. Premature infants should be observed in a car seat before discharge from the hospital to see if the semireclined position adds to or causes breathing problems. If your pediatrician recommends that your baby lie flat during travel, a crash-tested car bed may be used for a short period.

The back seat is the only safe place for babies. Whenever possible, an adult should ride in the back seat next to your baby to watch her closely. Depending on your baby's condition, you may want to limit her amount of car travel for the first month or two at home. You can check this with your pediatrician.

If You Must Bring the Hospital Home With You

Some premature babies need monitors and other equipment at home. For example, if apnea is a problem, monitoring may be done at home. Some babies may also need to go home with oxygen or other treatments. You and other caregivers will be trained on how to take care of your child's special needs before you take her home. You will also be taught how to perform *infant cardiopulmonary resuscitation* (CPR).

Settling in at Home

Premature babies need to be fed more often, and it will take a little while for them to adjust to being at home. Accept any offers of help around the house during the first few weeks, so you can take time to get used to having a new baby in the house.

A Good Night's Rest for Both of You

Your baby needs plenty of sleep in order to grow and develop. He will rest easier—and you will, too—if you follow a few simple rules when you put your baby down for a nap or for the night.

Sleeping Position: Back to Sleep

The American Academy of Pediatrics recommends that healthy infants be placed on their backs to sleep. Babies who are placed on their stomachs to sleep are at higher risk for sudden infant death syndrome (SIDS).

Placing babies on their backs to sleep does not increase the risk of other problems (for example, choking, flat head, or poor sleep). However, premature infants with certain medical problems (such as lung problems) may need to sleep on their side. Whether your baby sleeps on his back or side, a certain amount of "tummy time" is needed when he is awake. Ask your pediatrician about the best sleeping position for your baby.

In addition to proper sleeping position, you can reduce the risk of SIDS by:

- keeping blankets, pillows, soft bedding, and large stuffed toys out of your baby's crib;
- making sure your baby's room is not too hot or too cold;

- not smoking in your home;
- getting regular health care for your child; and
- breastfeeding.

Your Child's Growth and Development

Your baby's first year is a time of great change, just as it would be if she had been born on or near her due date. A child's development is complex, ongoing process. No two children mature at the same rate or in the same way. Development even varies from day to day and week to week. Over time, you will get to know your baby as an individual.

Timing Is Everything

Because your child was born early, you should think of her progress in terms of "adjusted age." For example, if your baby was 8 weeks early, adjust your expectations by 2 months. Therefore, a 4-month-old premature baby may act like a full-term 2 month old. Try not to compare your child with full-term babies or focus too much on developmental charts. Your pediatrician will follow your child's developmental progress.

Early Intervention Can Help

If there are any developmental problems, the important thing is to catch them early, so that your child can be helped to adapt.

Some problems can show up right away; others do not show up for some time. You are in the best position to monitor your child's development. Become familiar with your child's general pattern of development, and if you think your child is showing signs of a hearing, vision, speech, muscle, or learning delay, see your pediatrician as soon as possible. Early intervention programs that work with children from birth to 3 years may do a lot to lessen any long-term effect on your child's learning.

Keeping Your Child Healthy

One of the most important things you can do to keep your child healthy is to make sure he receives all recommended check-ups and immunizations. Check-ups will help make sure your baby's growth is on track, give your pediatrician a chance to catch any health problems early, and help you get your questions answered. If your baby has trouble gaining weight, has breathing problems, or any other problems that are of concern, your pediatrician may wish to see your child more often.

Immunizations can make sure your child's health is not put at risk by serious childhood diseases, such as whooping cough, hepatitis, and meningitis. These diseases can cause death or leave your child with long-term health problems.

When to Begin Immunizations

Some parents think their children do not need immunizations until they enter school. Actually, they should start when they are infants. Children should receive most of their immunizations during their first 2 years.

Most premature infants need to receive their immunizations at the same age as full-term infants, unless your pediatrician feels that this is not appropriate. Your pediatrician can help you make sure your child's immunizations are given on time and are up-to-date.

Immunizations Your Child Needs

Your child needs all of these immunizations to stay healthy:

- Hepatitis B
- Diphtheria, Tetanus, Pertussis (DTaP/DTP)
- *Haemophilus influenzae* type b (Hib)
- Polio
- Measles, Mumps, Rubella (MMR)
- Varicella (Chicken Pox)

Talk to your pediatrician about when your baby should have these immunizations.

If You Need Support

Sometimes parents need help taking care of a premature baby. Or they may need a shoulder to lean on when facing the stresses of being a new parent. If this is the case:

- Talk to your pediatrician, he or she can be a great source of support.
- Take a parenting class or join a parent support group. Your local hospital may offer these or can refer you to counselors or other professionals who can help.
- If you need more information or support, contact the other organizations listed below.

Helpful Organizations

For parents of PREMATURE BABIES:

Association for the Care of Children's Health
7910 Woodmont Ave, Suite 300
Bethesda, MD 20814
609/224-1742

The National Perinatal Association
3500 E Fletcher Ave, Suite 209
Tampa, FL 33613
813/971-1008

La Leche League
1400 N Meacham
PO Box 4079
Schaumburg, IL 60168-4079
847/519-7730 or
800/LaLeche

Healthy Mothers/Healthy Babies Coalition
409 12th St, SW
Washington, DC 20024-8811
202/863-2458

March of Dimes
1275 Mamaroneck Ave
White Plains, NY 10605
888/663-4637

For a referral to a pediatrician in your area, send the name of the area where you live and a self-addressed, stamped envelope to:

American Academy of Pediatrics
Pediatrician Referral Source
PO Box 927
Elk Grove Village, IL 60009-0927

Look Forward to the Future

Because your child was born early and may have some health problems, you may be afraid to plan too far ahead. But it is never too early to start bonding with your child. Today, premature babies have a good chance of doing well, thanks to medical advancements and early intervention.

Pediatrician's Name: _____

_____

Address: _____

_____

Phone Number: _____

Immunization Record
Record month/day/year below

DTaP/DTP	Hepatitis B	Td
_____	_____	_____
_____	_____	**Other**
_____	_____	_____
_____	**Polio**	_____
Hib	_____	_____
_____	_____	_____
_____	_____	_____
_____	**Varicella**	_____
MMR	_____	
_____		

The information contained in this publication should not be used as a substitute for the medical care and advice of your pediatrician. There may be variations in treatment that your pediatrician may recommend based on individual facts and circumstances.

American Academy of Pediatrics

DEDICATED TO THE HEALTH OF ALL CHILDREN™

The American Academy of Pediatrics is an organization of 55,000 primary care pediatricians, pediatric medical subspecialists, and pediatric surgical specialists dedicated to the health, safety, and well-being of infants, children, adolescents, and young adults.

American Academy of Pediatrics
PO Box 747
Elk Grove Village, IL 60009-0747
Web site — http://www.aap.org

Fun in the Sun: Keep Your Baby Safe

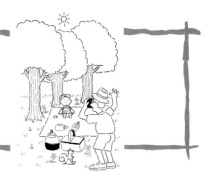

Warm, sunny days are wonderful. The sun feels good on your skin. But what feels good can be very bad for you, your family, and especially your baby. Before you take your baby to the park, beach, or even out into the backyard, please read this. It will help you learn how to protect your entire family and develop safe sun habits that can last a lifetime.

Skin cancer and the sun

The sun provides energy to all living things on earth. But it can also harm us. Its ultraviolet (UV) rays can cause sunburn and skin cancer.

The sun is the main cause of skin cancer, the most common form of cancer in the United States. There will be a million new cases of skin cancer this year. Skin cancer can and does occur in children and young adults, but most of the people who get skin cancer are older. Older people get skin cancer because they have already received too much of the sun's damaging rays. Your skin remembers each sunburn and each suntan year after year.

All skin cancers are harmful and some, especially malignant melanoma, can be deadly if left untreated. Malignant melanoma is the second most common form of cancer in women 25 to 34 years of age. Sun exposure in early childhood and adolescence contributes to skin cancer.

The sun and your baby's skin

Your baby's skin is very delicate and it's up to you to protect it. Sunburns hurt. Sunburns can also cause dehydration and fever. Too many sunburns and too much sun exposure over the years can cause not only skin cancer, but also wrinkles and cataracts of the eye.

Most of our sun exposure—between 60% and 80%—happens before we turn 18 years of age. That's because children spend more time outdoors than most adults, especially in the summer.

The dangers of sunburns

Research has shown that two or more blistering sunburns as a child or teen increase the risk of developing skin cancer later in life. It is very important, therefore, to protect babies and children from sunburn.

- A baby's sensitive skin is thinner than adult skin and a baby will sunburn more easily than an adult. Even babies with naturally darker skin need protection.
- It's up to you to protect your baby. A baby can't tell you when he is too hot or beginning to sunburn. Your baby can't move out of the sun and into the shade without your help.

Protecting your baby

Follow these simple rules to protect your baby from sunburns now and from skin cancer later in life:

- Babies under 6 months of age should be kept out of direct sunlight. Move your baby to the shade or under a tree, umbrella, or the stroller canopy.
- Dress your baby in clothing that covers the body, such as comfortable lightweight long pants, long-sleeved shirts, and hats with brims that shade the face and cover the ears.
- Select clothes made of tightly woven fabrics. Clothes that have a tighter weave—the way a fabric is constructed—generally protect better than clothes with a broader weave. If you're not sure about how tight a fabric's weave is, hold the clothing up to a lamp or window and see how much light shines through. The less light, the better. Clothing made of cotton is both cool and protective.
- When using a cap with a bill, make sure the bill is facing forward to shield the baby's face. Child-sized sunglasses with UV protection are also a good idea for protecting your child's eyes.

Remember...

- The sun's rays are the strongest between 10:00 am and 4:00 pm. Try to keep your baby out of the sun during these hours.
- The sun's damaging UV rays can bounce back from sand, snow, or concrete; so be particularly careful in these areas.
- Most of the sun's rays can come through the clouds on an overcast day; so use sun protection *even on cloudy days.*

Sunscreen for your baby

Choose a sunscreen made for children. For babies *under* 6 months of age, sunscreen may be used on small areas of the body such as the face and the backs of the hands if adequate clothing and shade are not available. For babies over 6 months of age, test the sunscreen on your baby's back for a reaction before applying it all over. Apply carefully around the eyes, avoiding the eyelids. If your baby rubs sunscreen into her eyes, wipe the eyes and hands clean with a damp cloth. If the sunscreen irritates her eyes, try a different brand or try a sunscreen stick or sunblock with titanium dioxide or zinc oxide. If a rash develops, talk to your pediatrician.

When choosing a sunscreen, look for the words "broad-spectrum" on the label—it means that the sunscreen will screen out both ultraviolet B (UVB) and ultraviolet A (UVA) rays. A sunscreen with a sun protection factor (SPF) of 15 should be adequate in most cases.

Use enough sunscreen and rub it in well, making sure to cover all exposed areas, especially your baby's face, nose, ears, feet, and hands and even the backs of the knees. Put it on 30 minutes before going outdoors. The sunscreen needs time to work on the skin. Reapply the sunscreen frequently, especially if your baby is playing in the water. Zinc oxide, a very effective sunblock, can be used as extra protection on the nose, cheeks, tops of the ears, and the shoulders.

Remember...

- Sunscreens should be used for sun protection and not as a reason to stay in the sun longer.

Sunburn can be dangerous

If your baby gets a sunburn and is under 1 year of age, contact your pediatrician at once—a severe sunburn is an emergency. For babies over the age of 1 year, tell your pediatrician if there is blistering, pain, or fever.

Remember...

- Avoid sunburns—they can be very dangerous to a baby.
- If your baby gets a sunburn, give juice or water to your baby to replace lost fluids.
- Cool water soaks may help your baby's skin feel better.
- *Do not use* any medicated lotions on your baby's skin unless your pediatrician recommends it.
- Keep your baby completely out of the sun until the sunburn is totally healed.

Set a good example

Make sun protection a regular family event. Your baby needs you for protection from the sun and from sunburns. Since babies learn by imitation, you can be the best teacher by practicing sun protection yourself. Teach all members of your family how to protect their skin.

Sun myths

Myth: A suntan is good for your baby.
Fact: A tan is a sign of skin damage.

Myth: Babies can't get sunburned on a cloudy day.
Fact: Most of the sun's rays can come through clouds and cause sunburns.

Myth: Baby oil is good sun lotion.
Fact: Baby oil causes the skin to burn faster and offers no protection at all.

Myth: Your baby needs the vitamins that the sun provides.
Fact: A proper well-balanced diet and minimum sunlight will give your baby all the necessary vitamins.

The information contained in this publication should not be used as a substitute for the medical care and advice of your pediatrician. There may be variations in treatment that your pediatrician may recommend based on individual facts and circumstances.

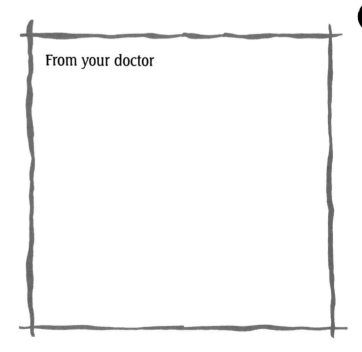

From your doctor

American Academy
of Pediatrics

DEDICATED TO THE HEALTH OF ALL CHILDREN™

The American Academy of Pediatrics is an organization of 55,000 primary care pediatricians, pediatric medical subspecialists, and pediatric surgical specialists dedicated to the health, safety, and well-being of infants, children, adolescents, and young adults.

American Academy of Pediatrics
PO Box 747
Elk Grove Village, IL 60009-0747
Web site — http://www.aap.org

Copyright ©1995, Updated 1/00
American Academy of Pediatrics

Infant Sleep Positioning and SIDS

Parents and caregivers should now consider placing healthy infants on their backs when putting them down to sleep. This is because recent studies have shown an increased incidence of Sudden Infant Death Syndrome (SIDS) in infants who sleep on their stomachs. There is no evidence that sleeping on the back is harmful to healthy infants.

Keep the following points in mind:

- Placing a child to sleep on the back has the lowest risk and is preferred. Sleeping on the side, however, is a reasonable alternative and is safer than sleeping on the stomach.
- Do not place your infant to sleep on soft surfaces or with pillows or stuffed toys. They could cover your child's airway.
- This recommendation is for healthy infants. Some infants with certain medical conditions or malformations may need to be placed on their stomachs to sleep. Talk to your pediatrician about which sleeping position is best for your child.
- This recommendation is for *sleeping* infants. A certain amount of "tummy time," while the baby is awake and observed, is recommended.

The information contained in this publication should not be used as a substitute for the medical care and advice of your pediatrician. There may be variations in treatment that your pediatrician may recommend based on individual facts and circumstances.

From your doctor

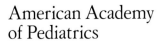

American Academy of Pediatrics

DEDICATED TO THE HEALTH OF ALL CHILDREN™

The American Academy of Pediatrics is an organization of 55,000 primary care pediatricians, pediatric medical subspecialists, and pediatric surgical specialists dedicated to the health, safety, and well-being of infants, children, adolescents, and young adults.

American Academy of Pediatrics
PO Box 747
Elk Grove Village, IL 60009-0747
Web site — http://www.aap.org

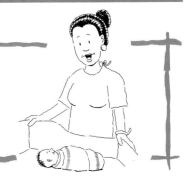

Newborn Hearing Screening and Your Baby

Before you bring your newborn home from the hospital, your baby needs to have a hearing screening. Although most babies can hear normally, 2 to 3 of every 1,000 babies are born with some degree of hearing loss. Without newborn hearing screening, it can be difficult to detect hearing loss in the important first months and years of your baby's life. About half of the children with hearing loss have no risk factors for it.

Newborn hearing screening can detect possible hearing loss in the first days of a baby's life. If a possible hearing loss is found, further tests will be done to confirm the results. If a hearing loss is confirmed, treatment and early intervention can start promptly. Early intervention helps babies with hearing loss and their families learn important communication skills.

That is why the American Academy of Pediatrics (AAP) recommends that all babies receive newborn hearing screening before they go home from the hospital.

What is hearing loss?

Hearing loss is the decreased ability to hear sounds. It may be mild to profound (severe), temporary or permanent, and can make it difficult to hear different kinds of sounds (especially consonants), which are essential in learning to talk.

It can affect one or both ears, and can occur anywhere along the hearing channel, including the following:

- **Outer ear** (eg, because of too much wax or a block in the outside ear canal)
- **Middle ear** (eg, because of an infection or fluid in the middle ear)
- **Cochlea** (inner ear), where sound waves are detected and passed on to the hearing nerve
- **Hearing nerve,** which connects to the brain
- **The hearing center in the brain**

Why do newborns need hearing screening?

Babies learn from the time they are born. One of the ways they learn is through hearing. If they have problems with hearing and do not receive the right treatment and early intervention services, babies will have trouble with language development. For some babies early intervention services may include the use of sign language and/or hearing aids. Studies show that children with hearing loss who receive appropriate early intervention services by age 6 months usually develop good language and learning skills.

Some parents think they would be able to tell if their baby could not hear. This is not always the case. Babies may respond to noise by startling or turning their heads toward the sound. This does not mean they have normal hearing. Most babies with hearing loss can hear some sounds but still not hear enough to develop full speaking ability.

Timing is everything. Your baby will have the best chance for normal language development if any hearing loss is discovered and treated by the age of 6 months—and the earlier, the better.

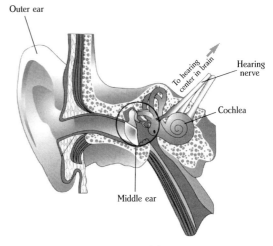

Cross-section of the ear

Illustration adapted from *Middle Ear Fluid in Young Children* brochure from the US Department of Health and Human Services (1994).

How is newborn hearing screening done?

There are 2 screening tests that may be used.

Auditory brainstem response (ABR)—This test measures how the brain responds to sound. Clicks or tones are played through soft earphones into the baby's ears. Three electrodes placed on the baby's head measure the brain's response.

Otoacoustic emissions (OAE)—This test measures sound waves produced in the inner ear. A tiny probe is placed just inside the baby's ear canal. It measures the response (echo) when clicks or tones are played into the baby's ears.

Both tests are quick (about 5 to 10 minutes), painless, and may be done while your baby is sleeping or lying still. Either or both tests may be used.

Can I assume that my hospital will screen my newborn's hearing?

It is best to ask. Most hospitals do hearing screening for all newborns. Some only screen newborns who are considered high risk, such as those with a family history of hearing loss.

Most states now have Early Hearing Detection and Intervention (EHDI) programs. Such programs try to ensure that all newborns in the state are screened for hearing loss and that those who need help get it.

What if my baby passes the hearing screening?

If your baby does not have any risk factors for hearing loss Toddlers has passed the newborn screening test, then your baby's pediatrician still will look at your baby's hearing and speech/language development along with other milestones at each of your baby's regular visits. Keep in mind that some forms of hearing loss develop as a child gets older.

If your baby has certain risk factors (eg, family history of hearing loss, premature birth, face/skull deformities), your baby's pediatrician should arrange for regular hearing tests to make sure that your baby continues to hear well.

What if my baby does not pass the hearing screening?

If your baby does not pass the hearing screening at birth, it does not mean that your baby has hearing loss. In fact, most babies who do not pass the screening test have normal hearing. But to be sure, it is extremely important to have further testing. This should include a more thorough hearing evaluation and a medical evaluation. These tests should be done as soon as possible, but definitely before your baby is 3 months old. These tests can confirm whether hearing is normal or not.

If hearing loss is found, what can be done?

This depends on the type of hearing loss that your baby has. Every baby with hearing loss should be seen by a hearing specialist (audiologist) experienced in testing babies and a pediatric ear/nose/throat doctor (otolaryngologist).

Special hearing tests can be performed by the audiologist who, together with the otolaryngologist, can tell you the degree of hearing loss and what can be done to help.

If the hearing loss is permanent, hearing aids and speech and language services may be recommended for your baby. The Individuals with Disabilities Education Act (IDEA) requires that free early intervention programs be offered to children with hearing loss, beginning at the time the child's hearing loss is identified.

The outlook is good for children with hearing loss who begin an early intervention program before the age of 6 months. Research shows these children usually develop language skills on par with those of their peers.

What if I do not receive my baby's hearing screening results?

Usually parents receive the results of their babies' hearing screening before mother and baby leave the hospital. If you did not get the results of your baby's hearing screening, call your baby's pediatrician to confirm the results.

How will I pay for newborn hearing screening and early intervention services?

Hearing screening tests usually cost between $25 and $40. Check with your health insurance company to see if it will cover the cost of newborn hearing screening and follow-up services. In some cases, your local school system, state programs, or local service clubs may cover the cost.

What if my baby did not receive hearing screening as a newborn?

If your baby did not receive hearing screening as a newborn in the hospital, call your baby's pediatrician and ask to have your baby screened (with ABR and/or OAE) as soon as possible. It is important to know that hearing can be tested at any age. Talk to your baby's pediatrician if you are concerned at any time about your baby's hearing or speech development.

Resources

Alexander Graham Bell Association for the Deaf and Hard of Hearing
202/337-5220
www.agbell.org

American Society for Deaf Children
Voice/TTY: 800/942-2732
www.deafchildren.org

American Speech-Language-Hearing Association
Voice/TTY: 800/638-8255
www.asha.org

Family Voices
888/835-5669
www.familyvoices.org

Medem (an e-health network)
www.medem.com

National Association of the Deaf
Voice: 301/587-1788
TTY: 301/587-1789
www.nad.org

National Center for Hearing Assessment and Management
Voice/TTY: 435/797-3584
www.infanthearing.org

National Institute on Deafness and Other Communication Disorders
Voice: 800/241-1044
TTY: 800/241-1055
www.nidcd.nih.gov

Please note: Inclusion on this list does not imply an endorsement by the American Academy of Pediatrics. The AAP is not responsible for the content of the resources mentioned above. Addresses, phone numbers, and Web site addresses are as current as possible, but may change at any time.

The information contained in this publication should not be used as a substitute for the medical care and advice of your pediatrician. There may be variations in treatment that your pediatrician may recommend based on individual facts and circumstances.

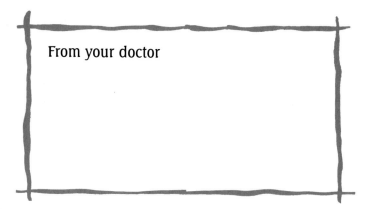

From your doctor

American Academy of Pediatrics

DEDICATED TO THE HEALTH OF ALL CHILDREN™

The American Academy of Pediatrics is an organization of 55,000 primary care pediatricians, pediatric medical subspecialists, and pediatric surgical specialists dedicated to the health, safety, and well-being of infants, children, adolescents, and young adults.

American Academy of Pediatrics
PO Box 747
Elk Grove Village, IL 60009-0747
Web site — http://www.aap.org

Copyright ©2002   American Academy of Pediatrics

One-Minute Car Seat Safety Check-up

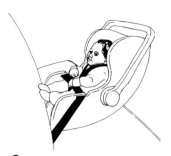

A. Infant-only seat

Using a car seat correctly makes a big difference. Even the "safest" seat may not protect your child in a crash unless it is used correctly. So take a minute to check to be sure…

» Does your car have a passenger air bag?

- An infant in a rear-facing seat should NEVER be placed in the front seat of a vehicle that has a passenger air bag.
- The safest place for all children to ride is in the back seat.
- If an older child must ride in the front seat, move the vehicle seat as far back from the air bag as possible and buckle the child properly.

» Is your child facing the right way for both weight and age?

- Infants should ride facing the back of the car until they have reached at least 1 year of age **AND** weigh at least 20 pounds (A and B).
- A child who weighs over 20 pounds **AND** is older than 1 year of age may face forward (C). However, it is safest for a child to ride rear-facing until she reaches the highest weight limit of the seat.
- A child who weighs 20 pounds before he reaches 1 year of age should ride rear-facing in a convertible seat approved for use at higher weights.

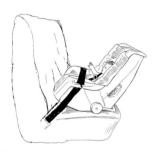

B. Rear-facing convertible seat

» Has your child grown too tall or reached the top weight limit (usually 40 pounds) for the convertible or forward-facing seat?

- Use a belt-positioning booster seat to help protect your child until she is big enough to use a seat belt properly.
- A belt-positioning booster seat is used with a lap and shoulder belt (D).
- Shield boosters should only be used without the shield and with a lap/shoulder belt, as belt-positioning boosters for children over 40 pounds. Shield boosters, used only with lap belts, are not safe for children over 40 pounds. Children under 40 pounds should use a convertible or forward-facing seat.
- A seat belt fits properly when the shoulder belt crosses the chest, the lap belt fits flat across the hips while the child's seat bottom is against the back of the seat, and his knees bend over the edge of the seat.

» Have you tried the car seat in your vehicle?

- Not all car seats fit in all vehicles.
- When the car seat is installed, be sure it does not move side-to-side or toward the front of the car.
- Be sure to read the section on car seats in the owner's manual for your car.

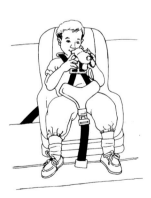

C. Convertible seat turned to face forward

» Is the seat belt in the right place and pulled tight?

- Route the seat belt through the correct path (check your instructions to make sure), kneel in the seat to press it down, and pull the belt *tight*.
- A convertible seat has two different belt paths, one for infants and one for toddlers.
- Check the owner's manual for your car to see if you need to use a locking clip and read the car seat instructions to see if you need a tether to keep the safety seat secure.

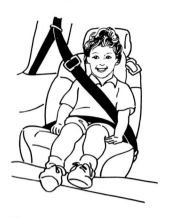

D. Belt-positioning
    booster seat

›› Is the harness snug; does it stay on your child's shoulders?

- The shoulder straps of the car seat usually go in the lowest slots for infants riding backward, and in the highest slots for children facing forward. (Check the car seat manufacturer's instructions to be sure.)
- The chest clip should be placed at armpit level (C) to keep the harness straps on the shoulders.
- Harnesses should fit snugly against your child's body. Check the instructions on how to adjust the straps.

›› Do you have the instructions for the car seat?

- Follow them and keep them with the car seat. You will need them as your child gets bigger.
- Be sure to send in the registration card that comes with the car seat. It will be important in case your car seat is recalled.

›› Has your child's car seat been recalled?

- Call the Auto Safety Hotline (number below) for a list of recalled seats that need repair.
- Be sure to make any necessary repairs to your car seat.

›› Has your child's car seat been in a crash?

- If so, it may have been weakened and should not be used, even if it looks all right.
- Call the car seat manufacturer if you have questions about the safety of your seat.

Questions?

Ask your pediatrician, local safety group, or call the US Department of Transportation Auto Safety Hotline, 888/327-4236 (8:00 am – 10:00 pm ET, Monday – Friday).

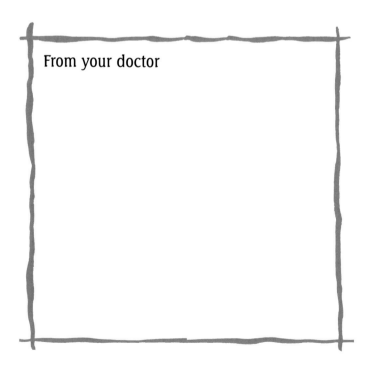

From your doctor

The American Academy of Pediatrics is an organization of 55,000 primary care pediatricians, pediatric medical subspecialists, and pediatric surgical specialists dedicated to the health, safety, and well-being of infants, children, adolescents, and young adults.

American Academy of Pediatrics
PO Box 747
Elk Grove Village, IL 60009-0747
Web site — http://www.aap.org

**American Academy
of Pediatrics**

DEDICATED TO THE HEALTH OF ALL CHILDREN™

Prevent Shaken Baby Syndrome

Shaken baby syndrome describes the serious injuries that can occur when an infant or toddler is severely or violently shaken. These children, especially babies, have very weak neck muscles and do not yet have full support for their heavy heads. When they are shaken, their fragile brains move back and forth within their skulls. This can cause serious injuries such as:

- blindness or eye damage
- delay in normal development
- seizures
- damage to the spinal cord (paralysis)
- brain damage
- death

Shaken baby syndrome usually occurs when a parent or other caregiver shakes a baby because of anger or frustration, often because the baby would not stop crying. Shaken baby syndrome is a serious form of child abuse. Parents should be aware of the severe injuries that shaking can cause. Remember, it is never okay to shake a baby.

If you or your caregiver severely or violently shakes your baby because of anger or frustration, the most important step is to get medical care right away. Immediately take your child to the pediatrician or emergency room. Don't let embarrassment, guilt, or fear get in the way of your child's health or life.

If your baby's brain is damaged or bleeding inside from severe shaking, it will only get worse without treatment. Getting medical care right away may save your child's life and prevent serious health problems from developing.

Be sure to tell your pediatrician or other doctor if you know or suspect that your child was shaken. A doctor who is not aware that a child has been shaken may assume the baby is vomiting or having trouble breathing because of an illness. Mild symptoms of shaken baby syndrome are very much like those of infant colic, feeding problems, and fussiness. Your pediatrician should have complete information so that he or she can treat your child properly.

When Your Child Cries, Take a Break— Don't Shake!

Taking care of an infant can be challenging, especially when an end to the crying seems nowhere in sight. If you have tried to calm your crying child but nothing seems to work, it's important to stay in control of your temper. Remember, it's never okay to shake, throw, or hit your child. If you feel as though you could lose control:

- Take a deep breath and count to 10.
- Take time out and let your baby cry alone.
- Call someone close to you for emotional support.
- Call your pediatrician. There may be a medical reason why your child is crying.

The information contained in this publication should not be used as a substitute for the medical care and advice of your pediatrician. There may be variations in treatment that your pediatrician may recommend based on individual facts and circumstances.

From your doctor

The American Academy of Pediatrics is an organization of 55,000 primary care pediatricians, pediatric medical subspecialists, and pediatric surgical specialists dedicated to the health, safety, and well-being of infants, children, adolescents, and young adults.

American Academy of Pediatrics
PO Box 747
Elk Grove Village, IL 60009-0747
Web site — http://www.aap.org

American Academy of Pediatrics

DEDICATED TO THE HEALTH OF ALL CHILDREN™

Thumbs, Fingers, and Pacifiers
Guidelines for Parents

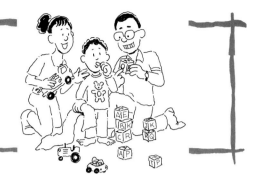

Does your baby suck his thumb or use a pacifier? Don't worry, these habits are very common and have a soothing and calming effect. The need to suck is present in all infants. Some infants suck their thumbs even before they are born, and some will do it right after being born. This brochure has been developed by the American Academy of Pediatrics to inform parents about thumb and finger sucking, and the use of pacifiers. The information in this brochure is based on the Academy's parenting manual, *Caring for Your Baby and Young Child: Birth to Age 5.*

Thumb and finger sucking

Thumb and finger sucking is normal for young children. Most children suck their thumbs or fingers at some time in their early life. Many thumb or finger suckers stop by age 6 or 7 months. The only time it might cause you concern is if it goes on beyond 6 to 8 years of age or affects the shape of your child's mouth or teeth. If you see changes in the roof of your child's mouth (palate) or in the way the teeth are lining up, talk to your pediatrician or pediatric dentist.

Children who suck their thumbs past 6 to 8 years often get teased by friends, brothers, sisters, and relatives. Sometimes these comments are enough to get the child to stop. If not, talk to your pediatrician about other ways to help your child stop.

Pacifiers

Many parents have strong feelings about pacifiers. Some oppose their use because of the way they look. Some resent the idea of "pacifying" a baby with an object. Others believe that using a pacifier can harm a baby. This is not true. Pacifiers do not cause any medical or psychological problems. If your baby wants to suck beyond what nursing or bottle-feeding provides, a pacifier will satisfy that need.

A pacifier should not be used to replace or delay meals. Offer a pacifier only after or between feedings, when you are sure your baby is not hungry. If your child is hungry, and you offer a pacifier as a substitute, he may become so upset that it interferes with feeding. It may be tempting to offer your child the pacifier when it is easy for you. However, it is best to let your child decide whether and when to use it.

Some babies use a pacifier to fall asleep. The trouble is, they often wake up when it falls out of their mouths. Once your baby is older and has the skill to find and replace it, there is no problem. Until then, your child may cry for you to find the pacifier. **Do not attempt to solve this problem by tying a pacifier to your child's crib, or around your child's neck or hand. This is very dangerous and could cause serious injury or even death.** Babies who suck their fingers or hands have a real advantage here, because their hands are always readily available.

Shopping for a pacifier

When buying a pacifier, keep the following points in mind:

- Look for a one-piece model that has a soft nipple (some models can break into two pieces).
- The shield should be at least 1½ inches across, so a baby cannot put the entire pacifier into her mouth. Also, the shield should be made of firm plastic with air holes.
- Make sure the pacifier is dishwasher-safe. Follow the instructions on the pacifier and either boil it or run it through the dishwasher before your baby uses it. Clean it this way frequently until your baby is 6 months old so that your child is not exposed to germs. After that, your baby is less likely to get an infection in that way, so you can just wash it with soap and rinse it in clear water.
- Pacifiers come in two sizes, one for the first 6 months and another for children after that age. For your baby's comfort, make sure the pacifier is the right size.
- You will also find a variety of nipple shapes, from squarish "orthodontic" versions to the standard bottle type. Try different shapes until you find the one your baby prefers.
- Buy some extras. Pacifiers have a way of getting lost or falling on the floor or street when you need them most.
- *Never* tie a pacifier around your baby's neck or hand, or to your child's crib. The danger of serious injury or even death is too great.
- Do not use the nipple from a baby bottle as a pacifier. If the baby sucks hard, the nipple may pop out of the ring and choke her.
- Pacifiers fall apart over time. Inspect them every once in a while to see whether the rubber has changed color or torn. If so, replace them.

How to help your child stop

As children grow and develop, their need to suck usually goes away, most often by the time they are 6 to 8 years old. Also, with increases in peer pressure, children are more able to control their behavior.

As a first step in dealing with your child's sucking habits, ignore them! Most often, they will disappear with time. Harsh words, teasing, or punishment may upset your child, and the habit will get worse. Punishment is not an effective way to get rid of habits.

Older children (more than 3 years of age) may use sucking to relieve boredom. Try getting your child's attention with an activity that she finds fun. Rewarding good behavior is the best way to produce a change. Praise and reward your child when she does not suck her thumb or use the pacifier. Star charts, daily rewards, and gentle reminders, especially during the daytime hours, are also very helpful.

If these measures do not work and your child wants to stop, your pediatrician might recommend trying a reminder such as covering the thumb with a plastic strip or "thumb guard" (an adjustable plastic cap that is taped to the thumb).

Your child should be directly involved with the treatment chosen. Before using these methods, be sure to explain them to your child. If they make your child afraid or tense, stop them at once. If your child's teeth are affected by the behavior and you have tried all the methods described above, talk to a pediatric dentist. Some dentists will install a device in the mouth that prevents the fingers or thumb from putting pressure on the palate or teeth. In fact, this device usually makes it so unpleasant to place the thumb or finger into the mouth that your child removes his thumb or finger.

Severe emotional upsets or stress-related problems might cause your child to suck his thumb or use a pacifier for a long time. It is also possible that your child may be one of the very few who cannot seem to stop. However, most children stop daytime sucking habits before they get very far in school. This is because of peer pressure. These same children might still use sucking as a way of going to sleep or calming themselves when they are upset. This is usually done in private and causes no harm either emotionally or physically. Putting too much pressure on your child to stop this type of behavior may cause more harm than good. Even these children eventually stop the habit on their own.

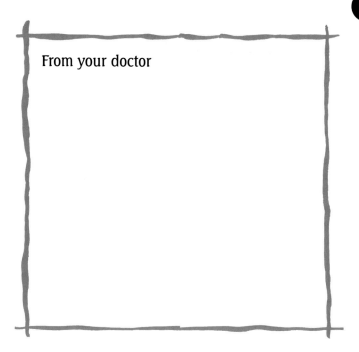

From your doctor

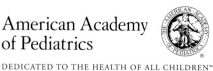

American Academy of Pediatrics
DEDICATED TO THE HEALTH OF ALL CHILDREN™

The American Academy of Pediatrics is an organization of 55,000 primary care pediatricians, pediatric medical subspecialists, and pediatric surgical specialists dedicated to the health, safety, and well-being of infants, children, adolescents, and young adults.

American Academy of Pediatrics
PO Box 747
Elk Grove Village, IL 60009-0747
Web site — http://www.aap.org

Copyright ©1997 American Academy of Pediatrics

©2002 American Academy of Pediatrics

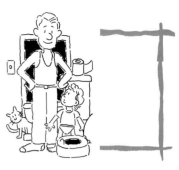

Toilet Training

Bowel and bladder control is a necessary social skill. Teaching your child to use the toilet takes time, understanding, and patience. The important thing to remember is that you cannot rush your child into using the toilet. The American Academy of Pediatrics has developed this brochure to help you guide your child through this important stage of social development.

When is a child ready for toilet training?

There is no set age at which toilet training should begin. The right time depends on your child's physical and psychological development. Children younger than 12 months have no control over bladder or bowel movements and little control for 6 months or so after that. Between 18 and 24 months, children often start to show signs of being ready, but some children may not be ready until 30 months or older.

Your child must also be emotionally ready. He needs to be willing, not fighting or showing signs of fear. If your child resists strongly, it is best to wait for a while.

It is best to be relaxed about toilet training and avoid becoming upset. Remember that no one can control when and where a child urinates or has a bowel movement except the child. Try to avoid a power struggle. Children at the toilet-training age are becoming aware of their individuality. They look for ways to test their limits. Some children may do this by holding back bowel movements.

Look for any of the following signs that your child is ready:

- Your child stays dry at least 2 hours at a time during the day or is dry after naps.
- Bowel movements become regular and predictable.
- Facial expressions, posture, or words reveal that your child is about to urinate or have a bowel movement.
- Your child can follow simple instructions.

Stress in the home may make learning this important new skill more difficult. Sometimes it is a good idea to delay toilet training in the following situations:

- Your family has just moved or will move in the near future.
- You are expecting a baby or you have recently had a new baby.
- There is a major illness, a recent death, or some other family crisis.

However, if your child is learning how to use the toilet without problems, there is no need to stop because of these situations.

- Your child can walk to and from the bathroom and help undress.
- Your child seems uncomfortable with soiled diapers and wants to be changed.
- Your child asks to use the toilet or potty chair.
- Your child asks to wear grown-up underwear.

How to teach your child to use the toilet

Decide what words to use

You should decide carefully what words you use to describe body parts, urine, and bowel movements. Remember that friends, neighbors, teachers, and other caregivers also will hear these words. It is best to use proper terms that will not offend, confuse, or embarrass your child or others.

Avoid using words like "dirty," "naughty," or "stinky" to describe waste products. These negative terms can make your child feel ashamed and self-conscious. Treat bowel movements and urination in a simple, matter-of-fact manner.

Your child may be curious and try to play with the feces. You can prevent this without making him or her feel upset by simply saying, "This is not something to be played with."

Pick a potty chair

Once your child is ready, you should choose a potty chair. A potty chair is easier for a small child to use, because there is no problem getting on to it and a child's feet can reach the floor.

Children are often interested in their family's bathroom activities. It is sometimes helpful to let children watch parents when they go to the bathroom. Seeing grown-ups use the toilet makes children want to do the same. If possible, mothers should show the correct skills to their daughters, and fathers to their sons. Children can also learn these skills from older brothers and sisters, friends, and relatives.

Help your child recognize signs of needing to use the potty

Encourage your child to tell you when he or she is about to urinate or have a bowel movement. Your child will often tell you about a wet diaper or a bowel movement *after* the fact. This is a sign that your child is beginning to recognize these bodily functions. Praise your child for telling you, and suggest that "next time" she let you know in advance.

Before having a bowel movement, your child may grunt or make other straining noises, squat, or stop playing for a moment. When pushing, his or her face may turn red. Explain to your child that these signs mean that a bowel movement is about to come, and it's time to try the toilet.

It often takes longer for a child to recognize the need to urinate than the need to move bowels. Some children do not gain complete bladder control for many months after they have learned to control bowel movements. Some children achieve bladder control first. Most, but not all, boys learn to urinate sitting down first, and then change to standing up. Remember that all children are different!

Make trips to the potty routine

When your child seems to need to urinate or have a bowel movement, go to the potty. Keep your child seated on the potty for only a few minutes at a time. Explain what you want to happen. Be cheerful and casual. If he protests strongly, don't insist. Such resistance may mean that it is not the right time to start training.

It may be helpful to make trips to the potty a regular part of your child's daily routine, such as first thing in the morning when your child wakes up, after meals, or before naps. Remember that you cannot control when your child urinates or has a bowel movement.

Success at toilet training depends on teaching at a pace that suits your child. You must support your child's efforts. Do not try to force quick results. Encourage your child with lots of hugs and praise when success occurs. When a mistake happens, treat it lightly and try not to get upset. Punishment and scolding will often make children feel bad and may make toilet training take longer.

Teach your child proper hygiene habits. Show your child how to wipe carefully. (Girls should wipe thoroughly from front to back to prevent bringing germs from the rectum to the vagina or bladder.) Make sure both boys and girls learn to wash their hands well after urinating or a bowel movement.

Some children believe that their wastes are part of their bodies; seeing their stools flushed away may be frightening and hard for them to understand. Some also fear they will be sucked into the toilet if it is flushed while they are sitting on it. Parents should explain the purpose of body wastes. To give your child a feeling of control, let him or her flush pieces of toilet paper. This will lessen the fear of the sound of rushing water and the sight of things disappearing.

Encourage the use of training pants

Once your child has repeated successes, encourage the use of training pants. This moment will be special. Your child will feel proud of this sign of trust and growing up. However, be prepared for "accidents." It may take weeks, even months, before toilet training is completed. It may be helpful to continue to have your child sit on the potty at specified times during the day. If your child uses the potty successfully, it's an opportunity for praise. If not, it's still good practice.

In the beginning, many children will have a bowel movement or will urinate right after being taken off the toilet. It may take time for your child to learn how to relax the muscles that control the bowel and bladder. If these "accidents" happen a lot, it may mean your child is not really ready for training.

Sometimes your child will ask for a diaper when a bowel movement is expected and stand in a special place to defecate. Instead of considering this a failure, praise your child for recognizing the bowel signals. Suggest that he or she have the bowel movement in the bathroom while wearing a diaper. Encourage improvements and work toward sitting on the potty without the diaper.

Stooling patterns vary. Some children move their bowels 2 or 3 times a day. Others may go 2 or 3 days between movements. Soft, comfortable stools brought about by a well-balanced diet make training easier for both child and parent. Trying too hard to toilet train your child before she is ready can result in long-term problems with bowel movements.

Talk with your pediatrician if there is a change in the nature of the bowel movements or if your child becomes uncomfortable. Don't use laxatives, suppositories, or enemas unless your pediatrician advises these for your child.

Most children achieve bowel control and daytime urine control by 3 to 4 years of age. Even after your child is able to stay dry during the day, it may take months or years before he achieves the same success at night. Most girls and more than 75% of boys will be able to stay dry at night after age 5.

Most of the time, your child will let you know when he is ready to move from the potty chair to the "big toilet." Make sure your child is tall enough, and practice the actual steps with him.

Your pediatrician can help

If any concerns come up before, during, or after toilet training, talk with your pediatrician. Often the problem is minor and can be resolved quickly, but sometimes physical or emotional causes will require treatment. Your pediatrician's help, advice, and encouragement can help make toilet training easier. Also, your pediatrician is trained to identify and manage problems that are more serious.

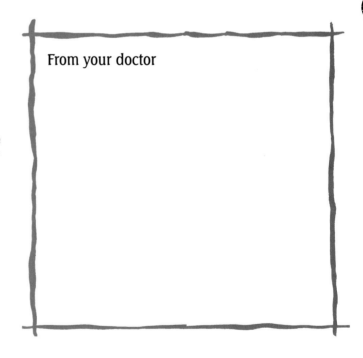

From your doctor

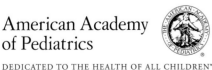

American Academy of Pediatrics

DEDICATED TO THE HEALTH OF ALL CHILDREN™

The American Academy of Pediatrics is an organization of 55,000 primary care pediatricians, pediatric medical subspecialists, and pediatric surgical specialists dedicated to the health, safety, and well-being of infants, children, adolescents, and young adults.

American Academy of Pediatrics
PO Box 747
Elk Grove Village, IL 60009-0747
Web site — http://www.aap.org

SECTION TWO

Adolescents and School-age Children

Acne Treatment and Control

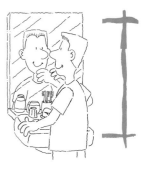

Almost all teenagers get acne at one time or another. Whether your case is mild or severe, the information here can help you keep your acne under control.

What causes acne?

You haven't done anything to cause your acne. It's not your fault if you have it. Pimples are caused when oil ducts in the skin get plugged up and then burst, causing redness and swelling. Although there are many myths about acne, the following are the three main factors that cause it.

1. Hormones

When you begin puberty, certain hormones, called **androgens,** increase in both males and females. These hormones trigger oil ducts on the face, back, and upper chest to begin producing oil. This can cause acne in some people.

2. Heredity

If other members of your family had acne as teenagers, there may be a chance that you've inherited a tendency toward getting acne as well.

3. Plugged oil ducts

If you are prone to acne, the cells that line the oil ducts in your skin tend to get larger and produce more oil, and the ducts get plugged. This traps the oil and leads to the formation of blackheads or whiteheads. The plugged ducts allow germs in the skin to multiply and produce chemicals that cause redness and swelling. This is why simple blackheads and whiteheads may turn red and bumpy and turn into the pimples of acne.

There is not much you can do about heredity, so your best control efforts are those that keep the oil ducts unplugged.

What makes acne worse?

- Pinching (or "popping") pimples, which forces oil from the oil ducts into the surrounding normal skin, causing redness and swelling
- Harsh scrubbing, which irritates the skin
- Things that rub on the skin, such as headbands, hats, hair, and chin straps, which also cause irritation
- Certain cosmetics (makeup), such as creams and oily hair products, which can block oil ducts and aggravate acne
- Some medications
- For young women, changes in hormone levels brought on by menstrual periods
- Emotional stress and nervous tension

What doesn't cause acne?

- Acne is not caused by foods you eat. Despite what you may have heard, there is no proof that soft drinks, chocolate, and greasy foods cause acne.
- It's *not* caused by dirt. The black plug in a blackhead is caused by a chemical reaction. It's not dirt. No matter how carefully you wash your face, you can still have acne.
- It's *not* something you can "catch" or "give" to another person.
- It's *not* caused by sexual thoughts or masturbation.

Treating acne

It's important to know that there is no true cure for acne. If untreated, it can last for many years, though acne usually clears up as you get older. The following treatments, however, generally can keep acne under control.

1. Use topical benzoyl peroxide lotion or gel.

Benzoyl peroxide helps kill skin bacteria, unplug the oil ducts, and heal acne pimples. It is the most effective acne treatment you can get without a doctor's prescription. Many brands are available in different levels of strength (2.5%, 5%, or 10%). Read the labels or ask your pediatrician or pharmacist about it.

- Start slowly with a 2.5% or 5% lotion or gel once a day. After a week, increase use to twice a day (morning and night) if your skin isn't too red or isn't peeling.
- Apply a thin film to the entire area where pimples may occur. Don't just dab it on current blemishes. Avoid the delicate skin around the eyes, mouth, and corner of the nose.
- If your acne isn't better after 4 to 6 weeks, you may increase to a 10% strength lotion or gel. Start with one application each day and increase to two daily applications if your skin tolerates it.

2. If you don't see results, see your pediatrician.

Your doctor can prescribe stronger treatments, if needed, and will teach you how to use them properly. Three kinds of medications may be recommended:

- **Tretinoin (Retin-A) cream or gel** helps unplug oil ducts but must be used exactly as directed. Be aware that exposure to the sun (or tanning parlors) can cause increased redness in some people who are using the medication.
- **Topical antibiotic solutions** may be used in addition to other medications for a type of acne called pustular acne.
- **Oral antibiotic pills** may be used in addition to creams, lotions, or gels if your acne doesn't respond to topical treatments alone.

3. What about the "miracle drug" Accutane?

Isotretinoin (Accutane) is a very strong chemical taken in pill form. It is used only for severe cystic acne that hasn't responded to any other treatment. Accutane must never be taken just before or during pregnancy. There is a danger of severe or even fatal deformities to unborn babies whose mothers have taken Accutane while pregnant or who become pregnant soon after taking Accutane. You should *never* have unprotected sexual intercourse while taking Accutane. Patients who take Accutane must be carefully supervised by a doctor knowledgeable about its usage, such as a pediatric dermatologist or other expert on treating acne. Your pediatrician may require a negative pregnancy test and a signed consent form before prescribing Accutane to females.

Important things to remember

Be patient. It takes 3 to 6 weeks to see any improvement. Give each treatment enough time to work.

Be faithful. Follow your program every day. Don't stop and start each time your skin changes. Remember, sometimes your skin may appear to worsen early in the program before you begin to see improvement.

Follow directions. Not using the treatment as directed is the most common reason the treatment fails.

Don't use medication prescribed for someone else. This holds true for all medications, especially Accutane. Doctors prescribe medication specifically for particular patients. What's good for a friend may be harmful for you. Never take Accutane that's prescribed for another person.

Don't overdo it. Too much scrubbing makes skin worse. Too much benzoyl peroxide or Retin-A cream makes your face red and scaly. Too much oral antibiotic may cause side effects.

Finally, many people don't understand acne and may say hurtful things about it. Although acne may bother you, keep in mind it's only temporary. With present-day treatment, it usually can be controlled.

A word about...acne and birth control pills

In 1996, the Food and Drug Administration (FDA) approved a low-dose birth control pill to be used as an effective treatment for acne in women over 15 years of age. Research has shown that certain birth control pills lower the levels of hormones that cause acne.

However, taking birth control pills along with other medications for the prevention of acne may reduce the effectiveness of both medications. If you are taking birth control pills, talk to your pediatrician about their effect on acne.

The information contained in this publication should not be used as a substitute for the medical care and advice of your pediatrician. There may be variations in treatment that your pediatrician may recommend based on individual facts and circumstances.

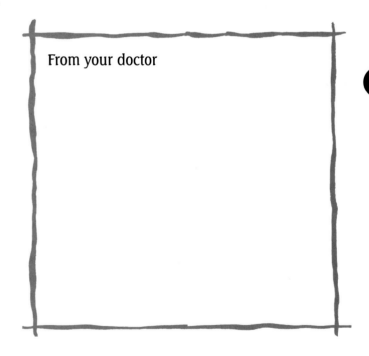

From your doctor

American Academy of Pediatrics

DEDICATED TO THE HEALTH OF ALL CHILDREN™

The American Academy of Pediatrics is an organization of 55,000 primary care pediatricians, pediatric medical subspecialists, and pediatric surgical specialists dedicated to the health, safety, and well-being of infants, children, adolescents, and young adults.

American Academy of Pediatrics
PO Box 747
Elk Grove Village, IL 60009-0747
Web site — http://www.aap.org

ADHD and Your School-Aged Child

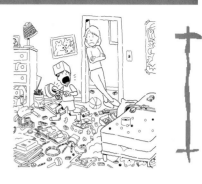

Attention-deficit/hyperactivity disorder (ADHD) is a condition of the brain that makes it hard for children to control their behavior. It is one of the most common chronic conditions of childhood. All children have behavior problems at times. Children with ADHD have frequent, severe problems that interfere with their ability to live normal lives.

A child with ADHD may have one or more of the following behavior symptoms:

- **Inattention** — Has a hard time paying attention, daydreams, is easily distracted, is disorganized, loses a lot of things.
- **Hyperactivity** — Seems to be in constant motion, has difficulty staying seated, squirms, talks too much.
- **Impulsivity** — Acts and speaks without thinking, unable to wait, interrupts others.

How can I tell if my child has ADHD?

Your pediatrician will assess whether your child has ADHD using standard guidelines developed by the American Academy of Pediatrics. Keep in mind the following:

- These guidelines are for children 6 to 12 years of age. It is difficult to diagnose ADHD in children who are younger than this age group.
- The diagnosis is a process that involves several steps. It requires information about your child's behavior from you, your child's school, and/or other caregivers.
- Your pediatrician also will look for other conditions that have the same types of symptoms as ADHD. Some children have ADHD and another (coexisting) condition, e.g., conduct disorder, depression, anxiety, or a learning disability.
- There is no proven test for ADHD at this time.

If your child has ADHD, the symptoms will

- Occur in more than one setting, such as home, school, and social settings.
- Be more severe than in other children the same age.
- Start before your child reaches 7 years of age.
- Continue for more than six months.
- Make it difficult to function at school, at home, and/or in social settings.

What does treatment for ADHD involve?

As with other chronic conditions, families must manage the treatment of ADHD on an ongoing basis. In most cases, treatment for ADHD includes the following:

1. **A long-term management plan.** This will have:
   - **Target outcomes** (behavior goals, e.g., better school work)
   - **Follow-up activities** (e.g., medication, making changes that affect behavior at school and at home)
   - **Monitoring** (checking the child's progress with the target outcomes)
2. **Medication.** For most children, stimulant medications are a safe and effective way to relieve ADHD symptoms.
3. **Behavior Therapy.** This focuses on changing the child's environment to help improve behavior.
4. **Parent Training.** Training can give parents specific skills to deal with ADHD behaviors in a positive way.
5. **Education.** All involved need to understand what ADHD is.
6. **Teamwork.** Treatment works best when doctors, parents, teachers, caregivers, other health care professionals, and the child work together.

   It may take some time to tailor your child's treatment plan to meet his needs. Treatment may not fully eliminate the ADHD-type behaviors. However, most school-aged children with ADHD respond well when their treatment plan includes both stimulant medications and behavior therapy.

Is there a cure for ADHD?

There is no proven cure for ADHD at this time. The cause of ADHD is unclear. Research is ongoing to learn more about the role of the brain in ADHD and the best ways to treat the disorder. Many good treatment options are available. The outlook for children who receive treatment for ADHD is encouraging.

As a parent, you play a very important part in providing effective treatment for your child.

For further information *ask your pediatrician about* "Understanding ADHD: Information for Parents About Attention-Deficit/Hyperactivity Disorder," *a new booklet from the American Academy of Pediatrics.*

This information is based on the American Academy of Pediatrics' policy statements *Diagnosis and Evaluation of the Child with Attention-Deficit/Hyperactivity Disorder,* published in the May 2000 issue of *Pediatrics,* and *Treatment of the School-Aged Child with Attention-Deficit/Hyperactivity Disorder,* published in the October 2001 issue of *Pediatrics. Parent Pages* offer parents relevant facts that explain current policies about children's health.

The information contained in this publication should not be used as a substitute for the medical care and advice of your pediatrician. There may be variations in treatment that your pediatrician may recommend based on individual facts and circumstances.

American Academy of Pediatrics

DEDICATED TO THE HEALTH OF ALL CHILDREN™

The American Academy of Pediatrics is an organization of 55,000 primary care pediatricians, pediatric medical subspecialists, and pediatric surgical specialists dedicated to the health, safety, and well-being of infants, children, adolescents, and young adults.

American Academy of Pediatrics
PO Box 747
Elk Grove Village, IL 60009-0747
Web site — http://www.aap.org

©Copyright October 2001 American Academy of Pediatrics

Better Health and Fitness Through Physical Activity
Guidelines for Teens

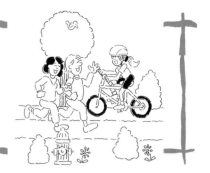

What exactly is physical fitness? Being fit means you have more energy to do daily tasks, can be more active, and do not tire as easily during the day. Being fit also helps you build a positive self-image and feel better about yourself.

You do not have to spend hours in a gym to be physically active. Every time you throw a softball, swim a lap, or climb up a flight of stairs, you are improving your health and fitness level.

The American Academy of Pediatrics has developed this brochure to help you understand what physical fitness is and to give you ideas on how you can become more physically active.

Benefits of physical activity

Physical activity has many proven benefits. When you are physically fit, you feel and look better, and you stay healthier. Physical activity can help you to:
- Prevent high blood pressure
- Strengthen your bones
- Ward off heart disease and other medical problems
- Relieve stress
- Stay active as an adult
- Maintain or achieve an appropriate weight for your height and body build

A major benefit of physical activity is that it helps reduce stress. Learning to cope with stress is an important part of healthy living. Family problems, conflicts with friends, and school pressures can cause stress. Major changes in your life, such as moving to a new home or breaking up with someone, are also sources of stress. Exercise helps you relax by causing physical changes inside your body that help it react to and handle stress.

Physical activity also has many other health benefits, such as helping to ward off heart disease. Coronary heart disease is the leading cause of death in the United States. Research has shown that your risk factors as an adult for developing heart disease start during your childhood. A lack of physical activity is one of the major risk factors influencing heart disease, such as high blood pressure, and other medical illnesses.

Physical fitness is a balance of many areas

To be physically fit, you must work on all aspects of fitness, including the following:

Cardiorespiratory endurance (aerobic fitness)—This is the ability of the heart, lungs, and circulatory system to deliver oxygen and nutrients to all areas of your body. When you are active, you breathe harder and your heart beats faster so that your body is able to get the oxygen it needs. If you are not fit, your heart and lungs have to work extra hard during physical activity.

Body composition (body fat)—This is the percentage of body weight that is fat. Overweight people have more body fat in relation to the amount of bone and muscle in their bodies than do people who are physically fit. Overeating, not exercising enough, or both often lead to more body fat. Being overweight increases your risk of diabetes, high blood pressure, and heart attacks.

Muscle strength and endurance—This is the amount of work and the amount of time that your muscles are able to do a certain activity before they get tired, such as lifting heavy objects or in-line skating.

Flexibility—Flexibility is the ability to move joints and stretch muscles through a full range of motion. For example, people who are very flexible can bend over and touch the floor easily. A person with poor flexibility is more likely to get hurt during physical activity.

What can I do to become more fit?

First, you have to make the commitment to become more physically active. Try to do some physical activity every day, whether it is through physical education classes in school or an activity on your own. Exercise should be a routine part of your day, just like brushing your teeth, eating, and sleeping. It may help to plan a physical activity with a friend or family member. Most people find that it is more fun to exercise with someone else. More importantly, though, is that you like the exercise or activity. You are more apt to stay in the habit of doing whatever activity you choose if it is one that you enjoy.

Now is a good time to pick a "life sport" that you enjoy. Unlike a competitive team sport like football or baseball, a life sport is any kind of physical exercise or activity that you can do throughout your life. Examples of life sports are:
- Swimming
- Golf
- Bicycling
- Jogging
- Tennis
- Walking
- Skating

Regular exercise should include aerobic activity. Aerobic activity is continuous. It makes you breathe harder and increases your heart rate. This type of exercise increases your fitness level and makes your heart and lungs work more efficiently. It also helps you maintain a normal weight by burning off excess fat. Examples of aerobic activities are brisk walking, basketball, bicycling, swimming, in-line or ice skating, soccer, jogging, and taking an aerobics or step class. Baseball and football do not involve as much continuous exercise because you are not active the whole time.

In general, the more aerobic an activity, the more calories—and eventually fat—you will burn. The chart at the end of this brochure gives you an estimate of the aerobic level of many different activities. You will notice that all physical activities burn more calories than sitting does.

Choose any activity you enjoy. If you like the exercise, you will want to keep doing it. Anything that involves movement qualifies as exercise. You do not have to be on a sports team, have expensive athletic clothes or shoes, or be good at sports to become more fit. Any type of regular, physical activity is good for your body. Household chores, such as mowing the lawn, vacuuming, or scrubbing, involve exercise and may have fitness benefits, depending on how vigorously you do the chores. The most important thing is that you keep moving.

Be sure to include stretching exercises in your daily routine. Before you do any physical activity, you should stretch out your muscles. This warms them up and helps protect against injury. Stretching makes your muscles and joints more flexible, too. It is also important to stretch out after you exercise to cool down your muscles. Exercise videotapes, programs on television, and magazines can show you examples of how to stretch out different muscle groups, as well as different exercises you can do.

Just about any physical activity will improve fitness. For example, walking is better than riding in a car, and using the stairs is better than taking an elevator. Making small changes like these in your everyday life can make you more physically fit.

Whenever possible, eat three healthy meals a day, including at least two to four servings of fruit and three to five servings of vegetables each day. Limit your intake of fat, cholesterol, salt, and sugar. Also, get enough sleep and take time to do things you enjoy. For even better health, don't smoke, drink alcohol, or do other drugs.

Physical activity is just one important part of preventive health care, which should be a part of your daily lifestyle. The activities you decide to do should be enjoyable, use a variety of muscle groups, and include some weight-bearing exercises. If you are not exercising much now, increase your level of activity gradually and have fun! Exercise for a better today and a healthier tomorrow!

Is it safe to train with weights?

You may want to include strength training as part of your regimen of physical activity, along with some form of aerobic exercise. Strength training, also called "weight training" or "resistance training," is where you use free weights and/or weight machines to increase muscle strength and muscle endurance.

When you strength train, it is more important to focus on proper technique and number of repetitions than on the amount of weight you are lifting. If you decide to strength train or weight train, make sure you use the proper safety measures. You should always have a trained adult supervise you.

You should avoid weight lifting, power lifting, and body building until your body has reached full adult development (usually between the ages of 15 and 18) because these sports can result in serious injury. Your pediatrician can help determine your stage of development.

How Often Should I Exercise?

Make exercise a part of your lifestyle. Your goal should be to do some type of exercise every day, or at the very least, three to four times a week. Try to do some kind of aerobic activity that requires continuous physical activity without stopping for at least 20 to 30 minutes each time. Do the activity as often as possible, but do not exercise to the point of pain because this can lead to injury.

Like all things, exercise can be overdone. You may be exercising too much if:

- Your weight falls below what is normal for your age, height, and build
- It starts to interfere with your normal school and other activities
- Your muscles become so sore that you risk injuring yourself

If you notice any of these signs, talk with your parents or pediatrician before health problems occur.

Exercise is only one part of living healthy

Besides the physical and mental health benefits, regular physical activity can also help you become more self-confident, organize your time better, learn new skills, and meet people with similar interests. To make more time for exercise, limit the amount of time you watch television or play computer or video games.

Fitness Activity Chart

Activity	Calories Burned During 10 Minutes of Continuous Activity	
	77-lb Person (35 kg)	132-lb Person (60 kg)
Basketball (game)	60	102
Cross Country Skiing	23	72
Bicycling (9.3mph or 15 km/h)	36	60
Judo	69	118
Running (5 mph or 8 km/h)	60	90
Sitting (complete rest)	9	12
Soccer (game)	63	108
Swimming (30 m/min or 33 yd)		
Breaststroke	34	58
Freestyle	43	74
Tennis	39	66
Volleyball (game)	35	60
Walking (2.5 mph or 4 km/h)	23	34
3.7 mph or 6km/h	30	43

kg = kilogram; mph = miles per hour

km = kilometer; m = meter

Modified from Bar-Or O. Pediatric Sports Medicine for the Practitioner. New York, NY: Springer-Verlag; 1983: 349-350.

Ferguson JM. Habits, Not Diets. Palo Alto, CA: Bull Publishing Co; 1998.

The information contained in this publication should not be used as a substitute for the medical care and advice of your pediatrician. There may be variations in treatment that your pediatrician may recommend based on individual facts and circumstances.

American Academy of Pediatrics

DEDICATED TO THE HEALTH OF ALL CHILDREN™

The American Academy of Pediatrics is an organization of 55,000 primary care pediatricians, pediatric medical subspecialists, and pediatric surgical specialists dedicated to the health, safety, and well-being of infants, children, adolescents, and young adults.

American Academy of Pediatrics
PO Box 747
Elk Grove Village, IL 60009-0747
Web site — http://www.aap.org

Breast Self-Exam

Once a month, right after your period, you should examine your breasts. Although breast cancer is rare in young women, it usually can be cured if found early, and a breast self-exam is the best way to find it.

Do the following to examine your breasts:

1. Stand in front of your mirror with your arms at your sides and see if there are any changes in the size or shape of your breasts. Look for any puckers or dimples, and press each nipple to see if any fluid comes out. Raise your arm above your head and look for changes in your breasts from this position.

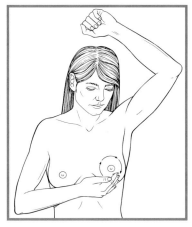

2. Lie down and place a towel or pillow under your right shoulder. Place your right hand under your head. Hold your left hand flat and feel your right breast with little, pressing circles. Think of each breast as a pie divided into 4 pieces. Feel each piece and then feel the center of the "pie" (the nipple area).

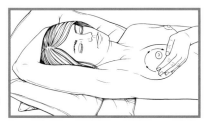

3. Now put your right arm down at your side, and do the same thing on the outside of the breast, starting under the armpit.
4. Repeat steps 2 and 3 for the other breast.

Most women have some lumpiness or texture to their breasts; breasts are not just soft tissue. Get to know your breasts, then be alert for any lumps or other changes should they ever appear. Remember, most lumps and changes are not cancerous. However, if you think you have found a lump or notice any other changes, don't press or squeeze it; see your pediatrician.

The information contained in this publication should not be used as a substitute for the medical care and advice of your pediatrician. There may be variations in treatment that your pediatrician may recommend based on individual facts and circumstances.

Illustrations by Lauren Shavell

American Academy
of Pediatrics

DEDICATED TO THE HEALTH OF ALL CHILDREN™

The American Academy of Pediatrics is an organization of 55,000 primary care pediatricians, pediatric medical subspecialists, and pediatric surgical specialists dedicated to the health, safety, and well-being of infants, children, adolescents, and young adults.

American Academy of Pediatrics
PO Box 747
Elk Grove Village, IL 60009-0747
Web site — http://www.aap.org

The Correct Use of Condoms
A Message to Teens

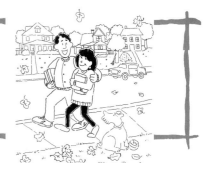

As a teen, you are faced with many challenges and decisions that will affect the rest of your life. Deciding when to begin having sex is one of the most important decisions you will ever make. It is perfectly normal not to have sex until marriage.

Sexually transmitted diseases (STDs) and unplanned pregnancies are at all-time highs for people your age. Not having sex (abstinence) is the only sure way to prevent pregnancy and STDs. It's also the only way to avoid getting sexually transmitted HIV, the AIDS virus. However, if you do decide to have sex, correct use of latex condoms will help you protect yourself and your partner against these risks. The American Academy of Pediatrics has designed this brochure to help you understand the importance of always using latex condoms and how to use them correctly.

Why use condoms?

A condom acts like a barrier or wall to keep semen, fluid from the vagina, and blood from passing from one person to the other during sex. These fluids can carry germs. If no condom is used, the germs can pass from the infected person to the uninfected person. Use of a condom also prevents unwanted pregnancies by keeping sperm out of the vagina.

Other good reasons to use condoms:
- They are cheap.
- They are easy to get (you don't need a prescription to buy them).
- They rarely have side effects.
- They are easy to use.

Some people have excuses for not using condoms, such as they are not comfortable, they lessen their enjoyment of sex, or they are unnatural. However, using a condom can make sex more enjoyable becauseboth partners are more relaxed and secure. Besides, the risks involved with **not** using condoms make any excuses seem pretty weak.

How to buy condoms

When buying condoms, be sure the ones you choose:
- are latex—some condoms are made of natural membranes (lambskin) and not latex. Only *latex* condoms have been proved to work against STDs because they prevent the passage of harmful germs.
- have a reservoir (nipple) at the tip to catch semen.
- are lubricated with *nonoxynol-9*, which is a spermicide (chemical) that has been proved to give additionalprotection against STDs, including the AIDS virus.

Condoms come in different colors, textures, and sometimes sizes. A good-quality condom is the most important feature for safer sex. Other points to keep in mind when buying condoms:
- Be sure to check the expiration date on the package. Do not buy or use them if they have expired.

- Condoms should be stored in a cool, dry place. You can carry a condom with you at all times, but do not store them where they will get hot (like in the glove box of a car). Heat can damage the condom. Also, carrying them in a purse or wallet is okay as long as it is not for long periods of time—this shortens their life.

Try not to feel embarrassed about buying condoms. By using condoms, you are proving that you are being responsible and there is nothing embarrassing about that.

How to put condoms on

Condoms are easy to use. However, they only work it they are used correctly. Follow these easy steps to make sure you are using them the right way (see illustration):

1. Carefully remove the condom from the package.
2. Put the condom on the end of the penis when the penis is *erect* ("hard").
3. Hold the condom by the tip and carefully roll the condom all the way to the base of the penis.
4. Leave extra space (1/4 to 1/2 inch) at tip of the condom to catch the semen.

If you do not have much experience with condoms, you should practice putting a condom on and taking it off **by yourself**, before you use it for sex with another person.

Be sure to put the condom on when an erection first occurs. Do not wait until you are ready to have sex—it may be too late. Drops of semen may leak from the uncovered penis. These small drops are enough to pass STDs to the other person or to cause a woman to get pregnant.

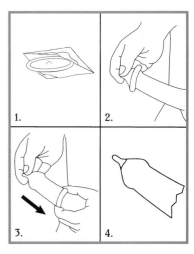

For added protection against STDs and pregnancy, use a spermicidal foam, cream, or jelly **along with** the condom. Make sure the spermicide you use contains nonoxynol-9.
- Before unrolling the condom, place a small amount of the spermicidal foam, cream, or jelly inside its tip.
- After unrolling the condom over the erect penis, place some more of the foam, cream, or jelly on the outside of the condom. Females can also use the spermicide inside the vagina for extra protection in case the condom breaks. Follow the directions on the spermicide package.

How to take condoms off

Withdraw the penis from the vagina right after ejaculation, while it is still erect or "hard." Hold on to the condom at the rim while the penis is withdrawn. Be careful as you slide it off the penis. Do not tug to pull condom off—it may tear. Throw away used condoms immediately. Never use a condom more than once. Be sure to keep used condoms away from your partner's genitals and other areas of the body as well. This will prevent semen from getting on hands or other body parts. If this happens, wash any areas of the body that have been touched by the semen.

Always insist that a condom be used *every* time you have sex. It is the only way to be sure that you are protected from infection. You should say **NO** to sex if you don't have a condom or if your partner refuses to use one.

Special points to remember

- Whenever possible, buy lubricated condoms.
- If you buy condoms that are not lubricated, you also may need a lubricant to help prevent the condom from breaking. Lubricants may also prevent irritation, which could increase the chances of infection.Use only **water-based** lubricants (like K-Y jelly). Do not use oil-based lubricants such as petroleum jelly (like Vaseline), hand or body lotions, or vegetable oil with latex condoms, since they can damage the condom.
- Other forms of birth control like the pill, diaphragm, or IUD **do not** prevent the spread of STDs—only condoms do. If another form of birth control is being used, a latex condom must also be used to make sure both partners are protected from STDs.

Why should I use a condom?

To prevent the spread of AIDS and other diseases
To prevent pregnancy

When should I use a condom?

Every time you have sex

How do I use a condom?

- Roll the condom all the way to the base of the erect penis.
- Leave space at the tip.
- After intercourse, carefully withdraw the penis and then slide the condom off.
- Throw away the used condom - condoms can only be used once.

- If you have had sex and you did not use a latex condom, you could have an infection and not know it. Some STDs take several months to show symptoms and some have no symptoms. See your pediatrician if you or your partner have any of the following:
  - discharge from the vagina, penis, or rectum
  - pain or burning during urination or sex
  - pain in the abdomen, testes, buttocks, and legs
  - blisters, open sores, warts, rash, or swelling in the genital area or mouth
  - flu-like symptoms, including fever, headache, aching muscles, or swollen glands
  - miss a period and think you might be pregnant

Condoms do not make sex 100% safe, but if used properly, they will reduce the risk of STDs, including AIDS. Know the facts so that you can protect yourself and others from getting infected. Not having sex is the safest. However, if you are having sex, be sure to always use a latex condom. It is the best way for you and your partner to stay healthy. For more information about condoms and how to prevent STDs and pregnancy, talk with your pediatrician.

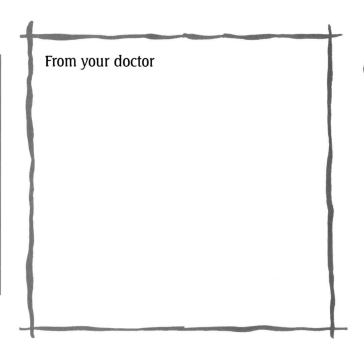

From your doctor

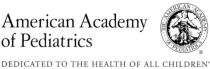

American Academy of Pediatrics

DEDICATED TO THE HEALTH OF ALL CHILDREN™

The American Academy of Pediatrics is an organization of 55,000 primary care pediatricians, pediatric medical subspecialists, and pediatric surgical specialists dedicated to the health, safety, and well-being of infants, children, adolescents, and young adults.

American Academy of Pediatrics
PO Box 747
Elk Grove Village, IL 60009-0747
Web site — http://www.aap.org

Copyright ©1996 American Academy of Pediatrics

Deciding to Wait

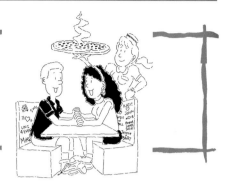

Guidelines for Teens

Becoming a teen is exciting. Because you're becoming an adult, you'll experience new physical changes. It's a time when you'll try new things and make new friends. You also may think more about dating.

Dating can lead to sharing private thoughts, becoming very good friends, or just having fun with your new friend. Becoming close with someone may be confusing, and it could feel awkward at first. Don't worry, just be yourself.

As you get to know each other better, you may think about being more than just friends. You may get the urge to kiss and touch someone you're dating. But what happens if your date wants to have sex? Would you understand your feelings? How would you react?

Pressure to have sex

You hear about sex in songs, on television and in the movies. Some of your friends may talk about it, too. They may even tell you sex is fun or that "everyone is doing it."

No matter what you've heard, not everyone your age has had sexual intercourse. In fact, most young people your age choose not to have sexual intercourse.

Teenagers you know may talk a lot about having sex. There are several reasons for this. These young people may be curious about sex or may just want attention. Talking about sex also may mean that your friends feel lonely or that they simply want someone to care.

New feelings

During a date, you may find that you become physically attracted to a person. These new feelings may excite and confuse you. It's normal.

If you decide to kiss and hug your partner, he or she may ask you to have sex. At that moment, you may be tempted to give in to your feelings right away. But before you make a quick decision, stop and ask yourself the following questions:

- Is this person pressuring me to have sex?
- What will happen after I have sex with this person?
- Am I ready to have sex?

If somebody you're dating wants to have sex, it doesn't mean you have to want it, too. Before you act on your feelings, remember that you can be sexual with someone **without** actually having sexual intercourse.

Waiting to have sexual intercourse is one of the most important decisions you'll ever make. Why not take your time and think it through?

What does it mean to be sexual?

When you are sexual, it can mean:

- Making up romantic and sexy stories
- Touching yourself in places that feel good
- Getting the urge to kiss and touch someone you like

Sexual intercourse is very different than these things. When you choose to have intercourse with someone, you are making a choice that could affect the rest of your life.

Your decision to have intercourse with your partner could lead to a pregnancy. Having intercourse also can lead to a sexually transmitted disease (STD), such as AIDS.

Know what the risks are

Did you know that having intercourse increases your risk of catching many diseases? Would your family and friends understand if you caught a sexually transmitted disease or if you became a parent? Would the person you're having intercourse with help you raise a child? Are you willing to get married at your age? If marriage isn't for you, could you raise a child on your own?

These are just a few of the questions you should ask yourself before you have sexual intercourse. Whether you have intercourse is up to you. But before you make a decision, make sure you know all the facts.

The medical and physical reasons why you should not have sexual intercourse at a young age are:

- Having an unwanted pregnancy
- Getting sexually transmitted diseases (STDs) like gonorrhea, syphilis, chlamydia, herpes or genital warts
- Catching the HIV virus that causes AIDS

There also are emotional risks to having sexual intercourse, such as:

- Regretting it when you are older and after you've met someone you "truly love"
- Being hurt by a relationship that is based only on sex
- Feeling guilty and scared
- Getting a bad name or reputation

Some of your friends may decide that they want to have intercourse. That's their business. But don't let them force you into a decision. You know what's best for you.

What are your limits?

Once you start dating, it's important to know what you want from a relationship.

- Think about what you want from a relationship before you make a split-second decision during a date.
- Talk to your parents or your date about your feelings and limits *before* you get too serious.
- Know your limits, and never let someone else talk you into doing something you don't want to do.

Some boys think that girls should set the limits. Girls also may think that boys will know when to stop. A boy or a girl may try to pressure their date to have intercourse. You both need to understand that forcing someone to have intercourse is not right. If your partner really cares, he or she will respect your feelings and your choice not to have intercourse.

Stick by your decision

Saying NO isn't always easy. But it's better to say NO than to be pressured into doing something you'll regret later. Sometimes it's twice as hard to say STOP to someone you care about, because you don't want to hurt your date's feelings. But if neither one of you stops, you both may regret what can happen next.

You can say NO without hurting your date's feelings. For example, you might say:

- I like you a lot, but I'm just not ready to have sex.
- You're really fun to be with, and I wouldn't want to ruin our relationship with sex.
- You're a great person, but sex isn't how I prove I like someone.
- I'd like to wait until I'm married before I have sex.

If you choose to wait to have intercourse, try to avoid situations where you'll be forced into a decision. Try not to spend all of your time with someone you're dating, and avoid being alone with your date too often. It's also not a good idea for you and your friend to "make out together" if you don't really want intercourse. Be fair to your partner; don't be a "tease." It could give your date the wrong idea.

Acquaintance (date) rape is a serious problem for children and teens. This means a person threatens to hurt (assault) you if you don't have intercourse with them. **No matter who threatens you, make sure you tell your parents, your pediatrician, or your teachers if you think you've been assaulted or put in danger.**

Using alcohol or drugs also can cause problems during a date. Both of these affect your judgment, which may make it hard to stick to your decision **not** to have intercourse.

Don't pay attention to the sexual bragging and the dares of your friends or classmates. Decide for yourself. Being liked by your friends may seem more important than what you know is right. You may be tempted to keep up with the crowd, but usually these stories are just made up.

If you're having a hard time with your decision, talk to your parents, clergy or your pediatrician.

Young people can wait

People who wait until marriage to have sexual intercourse usually find out that it is:

- Less risky to health
- Easier to act responsibly and take precautions to avoid infections and pregnancy
- More special
- More satisfying
- More accepted by others

Be patient. At some point, you will be ready for sexual intercourse. Move at your own pace, not someone else's. Talk with your parents about their values. Your pediatrician can explain how intercourse affects your body, and why you should wait until you are older. To avoid the risks—and to make intercourse really special in the future—why not just wait for now?

Remember to ask your pediatrician if you have any questions about growing up. Your doctor is there to help. If you feel uncomfortable about discussing certain private things with your parents, you can always trust your pediatrician to help. Don't be afraid to ask.

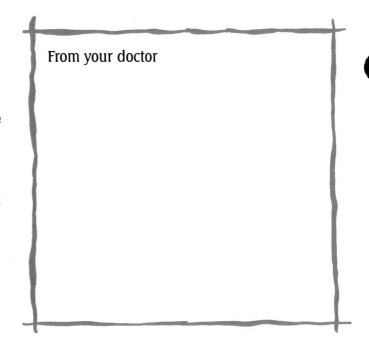

From your doctor

American Academy of Pediatrics

DEDICATED TO THE HEALTH OF ALL CHILDREN™

The American Academy of Pediatrics is an organization of 55,000 primary care pediatricians, pediatric medical subspecialists, and pediatric surgical specialists dedicated to the health, safety, and well-being of infants, children, adolescents, and young adults.

American Academy of Pediatrics
PO Box 747
Elk Grove Village, IL 60009-0747
Web site — http://www.aap.org

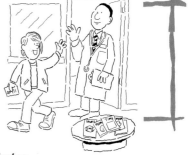

For Today's Teens:
A Message From Your Pediatrician

Your pediatrician may have cared for you since you were a small child. As you continue to grow and change, you will have new health needs. Even though you are becoming an adult, your pediatrician can still help you stay healthy.

When you are 11 or 12 years old, most pediatricians will speak with you and your parent or guardian at your checkup and suggest that you spend some time alone with him or her during future health care visits. What you talk about during these visits will remain confidential. This way you will begin to learn how to take care of your own health.

Growing up is often confusing. Your body is changing and you may feel differently than you did a few years ago. The changes you feel now may leave you wondering what's happening to your mind and body. You may have questions about these changes and how you should take care of yourself. Your pediatrician can answer questions about the following:

- eating right
- your height and weight
- exercise and sports
- acne
- dating
- body changes
- school performance
- alcohol and other drugs
- other concerns you may have

Why do teens need a pediatrician?

Some teenagers only visit their pediatrician when they are sick or hurt, but staying healthy means more than just seeing a doctor when something is wrong. As you become an adult, you need to take charge of your own health. This means preventing problems before they start. A first step might be to see your pediatrician once a year, just to make sure everything is OK and any problems are prevented from becoming serious.

You should also see your pediatrician when you are sick or concerned about what is happening to your body. Most likely, your concerns are normal. Growing up may also trigger changes in how you think and feel. You may feel sad, angry, or nervous at times. You should feel free to talk to your pediatrician about these things. After all, these emotions are a part of being healthy too.

What health services do pediatricians offer?

The following is a partial list of different things that you can talk about with your pediatrician:

Sports or school physicals:

Many schools ask students to get a physical before joining a team sport. It's important for you to talk about your health with your pediatrician before you participate in any sport. Your pediatrician can help you avoid injuries and stay healthy and fit.

Treatment of illnesses or injuries:

It is important for you to tell your pediatrician about any illnesses or injuries you have. Let your pediatrician know about pain you have or changes in the way you feel, even if you think they aren't serious. This is the only way your pediatrician can help you stay healthy.

A word about...privacy

Talking about personal things with your family and friends can sometimes be difficult. When you feel uncomfortable talking about certain things with your parents, you can always ask your pediatrician. Getting answers about how your body works, how you can take care of yourself, how to handle your emotions, and how to stay healthy, will help you make the right decisions about your health.

Your pediatrician will respect you as a patient. Because the pediatrician is your doctor, he or she will keep your discussions private whenever possible. However, your parents are obviously very concerned about your health and well-being, and your pediatrician will want to keep them informed of extreme situations; for example, if your life, or someone else's, is in danger. In most cases though, the information you share with your pediatrician will stay between you and your pediatrician.

Growth and development:

Your body is probably changing fast and you might want to talk to your pediatrician about what to expect as you grow. For example, you may be wondering about the following:

- Will you be as tall as your parents?
- Is your sexual development normal?
- Will your acne clear up?
- Will your body fill out more?
- Should you be worried about your weight?

These are all things you can discuss openly and freely with your pediatrician. Just ask.

Personal and/or family problems:

Sometimes you might have a hard time dealing with problems with friends or family. Feeling like your parents don't understand you, losing a best friend, getting teased at school, pressure from friends- all these things can get the best of you once in a while. If you don't know where to turn, remember that your pediatrician is there to help.

School problems:

As a student, you may worry sometimes about your grades and your future. No matter what you try, it may be hard to keep up with school, a job, sports, or other activities. Maybe you find it difficult to get along with others at school or to concentrate on your studies. Your pediatrician may be able to help you through this busy time of your life.

Alcohol and drug use:

You may be tempted to take risks as you make new friends. You may also get a lot of pressure from your friends. Remember, what's right for them might not always be right for you. Becoming an adult means more than just physical growth. It also means determining what is right for you. This is especially important since many people you know may be using cigarettes, alcohol, or other drugs. Instead of going along with the crowd, you need to decide what is the best choice for you. Your pediatrician can explain how smoking, drinking, or taking other drugs can affect you.

Sexual relationships:

During visits with your pediatrician, you'll have a chance to ask questions about dating, sexual activity, and infections. Your pediatrician also can talk to you confidentially about postponing sex and how to protect yourself against sexually transmitted diseases (STDs) and pregnancy. It's important to make smart choices about sex now. The wrong choice could affect the rest of your life.

Conflicts with parents:

At times, It might be hard to get along with your family and this could lead to problems at home. Maybe it seems like no one understands you or respects your ideas. You're not alone. If you have a problem that your parents may not understand, talk with your pediatrician. Sometimes an outside person can give a better view of these difficult situations.

Referrals to other doctors for special health needs:

You may have a medical problem that will require you to see another doctor or specialist. In that case, your pediatrician can refer you to another doctor who can take care of your needs. A referral may involve an ophthalmologist (eye doctor) for vision, a psychologist or psychiatrist for stress or depression, or other doctors that handle specific medical needs. Even though you may need to see a specialist for a special problem, you should continue to see your pediatrician for regular checkups or illnesses. After all, he or she is still your doctor and will want to keep up with your general needs.

Educational brochures, magazines, or videos on health topics:

In addition to talking about your health with your pediatrician, you also may be able to learn more about how to take better care of yourself by reading brochures or by watching videos. The American Academy of Pediatrics offers free material covering health topics that might interest you, such as acne, sports and fitness, sexuality, substance abuse, eating disorders, and more. Ask your pediatrician for more information.

What you can do to stay healthy

Use the following list to take care of yourself and stay healthy:

- **Eat right and get plenty of sleep.**
- **Know how to handle minor injuries,** such as cuts and bruises, as well as minor illnesses like colds.
- **Know how to seek medical attention** for problems such as vomiting, headache, high fever, earache, sore throat, diarrhea, or abdominal pain.
- **Take care of your mental health** and ask for help if you have sleep problems, sadness, family stress, school problems, problems with alcohol or other drugs, or trouble relating to friends, family, or teachers.
- **Avoid alcohol, cigarettes, smokeless tobacco (chew), and other drugs.**
- **Delay having sexual relations** or use protection if you choose to have sex.
- **Exercise regularly,** with help from an adult who knows what is right for your body.
- *Always* **wear your seat belt** when you are in a car or truck.

As you become an adult, you'll face many challenges. With help from your pediatrician, you'll learn how to make the right decisions that will help you grow up healthy.

The information contained in this publication should not be used as a substitute for the medical care and advice of your pediatrician. There may be variations in treatment that your pediatrician may recommend based on individual facts and circumstances.

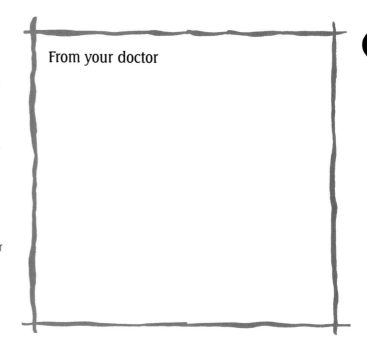

From your doctor

American Academy of Pediatrics

DEDICATED TO THE HEALTH OF ALL CHILDREN™

The American Academy of Pediatrics is an organization of 55,000 primary care pediatricians, pediatric medical subspecialists, and pediatric surgical specialists dedicated to the health, safety, and well-being of infants, children, adolescents, and young adults.

American Academy of Pediatrics
PO Box 747
Elk Grove Village, IL 60009-0747
Web site — http://www.aap.org

Copyright ©1994, Updated 11/98
American Academy of Pediatrics

©2002 American Academy of Pediatrics

Gay, Lesbian, and Bisexual Teens:
FACTS FOR TEENS AND THEIR PARENTS

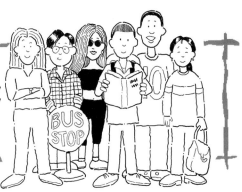

The teenage years are filled with new experiences, changes, and a growing sense of who you are. But for teenagers who feel "different" from their peers, these years can be confusing, frustrating, and even scary.

It is important for everyone to understand more about the diversity in people's sexual orientation. If you are a teenager, this brochure provides information to help as you discover more about yourself, your friends, and your place in the world. There also is information that may help your parents understand you better.

"Am I gay?"

Many gay and lesbian adults remember their late childhood or early teenage years as the time when they first began to wonder about their sexual orientation. Unfortunately, because we live in a society that is not always accepting of gay, lesbian, and bisexual people, dealing with the possibility that they may be gay can be a very difficult thing for teens.

How do you know if you are gay? Many young people go through an anxious stage during which they wonder, "Am I gay?" It is normal to feel this way as your sexual identity is taking shape. Maybe you feel attracted to someone of the same gender or you have had some same-sex activity. This is normal and does not necessarily mean that you are gay, lesbian, or bisexual.

Sexual *behavior* is not always the same as sexual *orientation*. Many people have had same-sex experiences but do not consider themselves gay, lesbian, or bisexual. Others call themselves gay without having had any sexual experience.

Sexual orientation develops as you grow and experience new things. It may take time to figure it all out. Do not worry if you are not sure. If over time you find you feel romantic attraction to members of the same sex, and these feelings continue to grow stronger as you get older, you probably are gay or bisexual. It is not a bad thing, it is just who you are.

Definitions

Gay (or *homosexual*): People who have sexual and/or romantic feelings for people of the same gender. Men are attracted to men and women are attracted to women.

Lesbian: Gay woman.

Straight (or *heterosexual*): People who have sexual and/or romantic feelings for people of the opposite gender. Men are attracted to women and women are attracted to men.

Bisexual (or *bi*): People who have sexual and/or romantic feelings for both men and women.

Sexual orientation: How an individual is physically and emotionally attracted to other males and females.

You are not alone

Some estimates say that about 10% of the population is gay. You cannot tell by looking at people whether they are gay. Gay people are all shapes, sizes, and ages. They have many types of racial and ethnic backgrounds.

Pay no attention to stereotypes. Just because a boy has some feminine qualities or a girl acts somewhat masculine does not mean that he or she is gay. Most gay males and females look and act just like their straight peers.

"Am I normal?"

First, homosexuality is not a mental disorder. The American Psychiatric Association confirmed this in 1974. The American Psychological Association and the American Academy of Pediatrics agree that homosexuality is not an illness or disorder, but a form of sexual expression.

No one knows what causes a person to be gay, bisexual, or straight. There probably are a number of factors. Some may be biological. Others may be psychological. The reasons can vary from one person to another. The fact is, you do not choose to be gay, bisexual, or straight.

Talking about it

Most people find that it is hard to start talking about their sexual feelings and attractions, but in the long run it feels better if you do not keep these important feelings a secret. You do not have to *know* that you are lesbian, gay, or bisexual before you talk to people about your feelings. Remember that the process of sharing what you are feeling is different for every person. Start with people you trust the most. This may include the following:

- Close friends
- Gay, lesbian, or bisexual friends
- Parents
- Close family members
- Your pediatrician
- A teacher, school counselor, coach, or other adult mentor
- A minister, priest, rabbi, or spiritual advisor
- A local gay, lesbian, and bisexual support group

The important thing is to find someone you trust with whom you can talk about your thoughts and worries.

Coming out

Because of the negative feelings some people have about homosexuality, "coming out of the closet," or revealing your sexual orientation, can be difficult. Some people wrestle with revealing their identity for years before finally deciding to do so. Others keep their sexual orientation a secret for their entire lives.

Talk to other gay friends about their "coming out" experiences. This may help you know what to expect. Gay youth organizations also can be a great source of support. See the end of this brochure for a list of such groups.

If you do know that you are gay, lesbian, or bisexual, do not feel pressured to "come out" before you are ready. On the other hand, keeping your identity a secret can be a burden. It is up to you to decide the best time to share your sexual orientation with your family and friends.

Telling your family and friends that you are gay probably will not be easy. Your family may respond well. But most parents picture a traditional future for their child. News that their child is gay may require them to rethink a whole new future.

Choose a good time and place to tell your family. If this information comes out during a family conflict or crisis, it may be even harder for your parents to accept it.

Be prepared for a variety of reactions including shock, denial, anger, guilt, sadness, and even rejection. Remember, you have had time to accept your identity. Give your family and friends time, too. Keep in mind that you can help them by being open, honest, and patient.

Often family and friends will be relieved that you have helped them to understand you better. Whether right away, or after some time, they may be happy to help you sort out your sexual orientation and how it affects your life.

Health concerns for gay and lesbian youth

Gay, lesbian, and bisexual teens are not the only ones who need to be concerned about their health. All teens need to be aware of what can happen if they are sexually active, use drugs, or engage in other risky behaviors.

Sexual activity: You do not have to have sex to be aware of your sexual identity. Most teenagers, whether they are gay, lesbian, bisexual, or straight, are not sexually active. In fact, not having sex is the *only* way to protect yourself completely against sexually transmitted diseases (STDs). But if you choose to have sex, make sure you know the risks and how to protect yourself.

- Gay and bisexual males must be particularly careful and always use latex condoms. Using condoms is the only way to protect against human immunodeficiency virus (HIV)/acquired immune deficiency syndrome (AIDS) and many other diseases that are spread during anal, vaginal, or oral intercourse. Condoms also help to prevent pregnancy during vaginal intercourse.
- Lesbians and bisexual females also must *always* use protection such as latex dental dams and condoms to avoid sexually transmitted diseases and unplanned pregnancies.
- Avoid risky sexual practices like using alcohol and drugs before or during sex, having unknown sexual partners, or having sex in unfamiliar or public places.
- Regular health examinations are crucial. Ask your pediatrician if you have questions or concerns about STDs or other health issues.
- Make sure all of your immunizations are up-to-date. Check that you have had three doses of the hepatitis B vaccine. Hepatitis B is a virus that can make you very sick. It can be spread through contact with infected blood or other body fluids. This can happen during sexual intercourse or when drug users share needles.

Substance use: Being a gay or lesbian teen in our society can be very difficult. Avoid using drugs or alcohol to relieve depression, anxiety, and low self-esteem. Doing so can lead to addiction.

In many communities, bars are popular places for gay and lesbian people to socialize. This increases the pressure to drink and use other drugs. Drug and alcohol use can lead to unsafe sex. Adopt a drug-free lifestyle and look for other ways to socialize and meet new people.

Mental health: Isolation, peer rejection, ridicule, harassment, depression, and thoughts of suicide — any teen may feel these things at some time. However, gay and lesbian youth are more than twice as likely to attempt suicide than straight teenagers. About 30% of those who try to kill themselves actually die.

A message to parents: when your teenager is gay, lesbian, or bisexual

Each year some parents learn that their son or daughter is gay, lesbian, or bisexual. This news is sometimes difficult. Most parents dream that their child's future will include a traditional marriage and grandchildren. Keep in mind that your son or daughter still can find lifelong companionship and become a parent.

Parents also often have to deal with their own guilt. They may ask themselves questions like, "Did I do anything to cause this?" "Should we have done something differently when he was a child?" "Is it my fault?" Questions like these are common, but do not help.

Rejecting your child also is not a good response. When gay, lesbian, and bisexual teens make their sexual orientation known, some families reject them. Perhaps that is how you think you would react. But that is the wrong response. It may be very difficult for your teenager to come to terms with her or his sexuality. Your child may find it devastating if you reject her or him at the same time. Your child needs you very much!

So take a deep breath and think. Take a little time to come to grips with your child's sexual orientation. You may need to readjust your dreams for your child's future. You may have to deal with your own negative stereotypes of gay, lesbian, and bisexual people. But you must not reject your teenager for his or her sexual orientation. He or she is still your child and needs your love and support.

Many parents find that it helps to talk to other parents whose children are lesbian, gay, or bisexual. Check the end of this brochure for information about support groups for parents.

Your teenager did not choose to be gay, lesbian, or bisexual. Accept her or him and be there to help with any problems that arise. Your pediatrician may be able to help you with this new challenge or suggest a referral for counseling.

Gay and lesbian youth who fear rejection or discovery may not know whom to turn to for support. Try your pediatrician, parents, a trusted teacher, or a counselor. Members of the gay, lesbian, and bisexual community, or gay and lesbian youth groups, also can be helpful. They can be a real source of support and a place to find healthy role models.

Counseling may be helpful for you if you feel confused about your sexual identity. Avoid any treatments that claim to be able to change a person's sexual orientation, or treatment ideas that see homosexuality as a sickness.

Discrimination and violence: Gay and lesbian youth are at high risk for becoming victims of violence. Studies have found that 30% to 70% of gay youth have experienced verbal or physical assaults in school. They also may be called names, harassed by others, or rejected by friends and family.

There are things you can do to avoid becoming a victim of violence, especially at school.

- Talk to a trusted school counselor, administrator, or teacher about any harassment or violence you have experienced at school. You have the right to attend a safe school that is free from discrimination, harassment, violence, and abuse.
- Get involved in gay/straight alliances at your school (or help form one). These groups can help promote better understanding between gay, lesbian, and bisexual youth, and other students and teachers.
- Join a gay youth support group in your community.
- Encourage your parents to join a support group for parents and family members of gay and lesbian teenagers.

Resources

Hetrick-Martin Institute for the Protection of Gay and Lesbian Youth
2 Astor Pl
New York, NY 10003
212/674-2400
www.hmi.org

Lambda Youth OUTreach
www.lambda.org

National Gay and Lesbian Task Force
1700 Kalorama Rd NW
Washington, DC 20009-2624
202/332-6483
www.ngltf.org

National Youth Advocacy Coalition
1638 R St NW
Suite 300
Washington, DC 20009
202/319-7596
Fax: 202/319-7365
www.nyacyouth.org

OutProud, the National Coalition for Gay, Lesbian, Bisexual and
    Transgender Youth
369 Third St
Suite B-362
San Rafael, CA 94901-3581
www.outproud.org

Parents, Families and Friends of Lesbiansand Gays (PFLAG)
1726 M St NW
Suite 400
Washington, DC 20036
202/467-8180
www.pflag.org

Youth Guardian Services, Inc
8665 Sudley Rd
#304
Manassas, VA 20110-4588
877/270-5152
www.youth-guard.org

Youth Resource
A Project of Advocates for Youth
1025 Vermont Ave NW
Suite 200
Washington, DC 20005
202/347–5700
www.youthresource.com

The information contained in this publication should not be used as a substitute for the medical care and advice of your pediatrician. There may be variations in treatment that your pediatrician may recommend based on individual facts and circumstances.

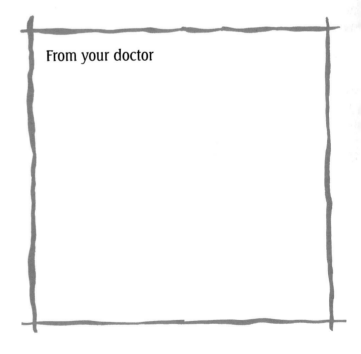

From your doctor

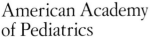

American Academy
of Pediatrics

DEDICATED TO THE HEALTH OF ALL CHILDREN™

The American Academy of Pediatrics is an organization of 55,000 primary care pediatricians, pediatric medical subspecialists, and pediatric surgical specialists dedicated to the health, safety, and well-being of infants, children, adolescents, and young adults.

American Academy of Pediatrics
PO Box 747
Elk Grove Village, IL 60009-0747
Web site — http://www.aap.org

Health Care for College Students
What Your Pediatrician Wants You to Know

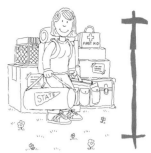

Starting college is an exciting time in your life. New worlds are opening up to you, and there are many choices to make: what classes to take, what to major in, what kind of work you want to do when you graduate. All of these choices are now yours. This is both a great freedom and a huge responsibility.

In much the same way, you are now largely in charge of your health and well-being. You probably have a lot of questions about keeping healthy while in college. This brochure will answer some of your questions about how to take care of yourself.

Your pediatrician and the student health service

Your pediatrician will not abandon you just because you are starting college. He or she may give you a physical before you start school (some colleges require you to have a physical before you can attend classes). Your pediatrician will also make sure all your immunizations are up-to-date, and that all your medical records are complete. You will still be able to call him or her if you have any questions. If you continue to live near your pediatrician, you may still want to see him or her for your care. But if you are going to live on campus, and the school provides a student health service, it may be the first place you go for health care. If one is not available, most schools will provide you with a list of health services in the community.

What is a student health service?

The student health service is an important part of the college or university you are about to attend. It is there for you when you need medical care, advice, information, or counseling. Student health services are not Band-Aid stations. Their medical, nursing, and counseling staffs are familiar with the problems and needs of college students. They also know pediatricians and other physicians in the community in case you need additional care.

Yet, if you are used to going to your pediatrician for your health care, the student health service may seem a bit strange at first. You may see a team of health care providers, which may include doctors, nurse practitioners, therapists, and health educators. This system will work best if you keep open the lines of communication between yourself, your parents, the student health service, and your pediatrician.

Things to do before you go

Get your medical and immunization records. Make sure the student health service has the following information about your medical history:

1. A complete list of every medication you take, including its dosage and strength
2. A list of your allergies, significant past medical problems (including surgeries and hospitalizations), and special needs (such as chronic conditions and disabilities)
3. A record of any mental health problems
4. Relevant family medical history

Make sure you have health insurance. If you will still be on your parents' policy, take a copy of the insurance card with you. Find out what type of plan you have (HMO, PPO, etc), what the policy covers, how to file claims, and what to do in case of an emergency. Talk this over with your parents. Remember that if you are on your parents' insurance policy, they will be notified each time the insurance company is billed for something.

Take extras of any prescription medications you need. Also, find out the name of a pharmacy near your school and how to obtain prescription refills when you need them.

Get a book. Everyone should own a book on personal health care.

Things to take with you

A good first aid kit is a useful thing to have in case you don't feel well or you have a small emergency. Your first aid kit should contain:
- bandages for small cuts and scrapes
- gauze and adhesive tape
- an elastic bandage for wrapping sprains
- liquid soap
- antibacterial/antibiotic ointment (such as bacitracin)
- a thermometer
- an ice pack or chemical cold pack
- medicine for upset stomach
- acetaminophen or ibuprofen for aches, pains, and fever
- medicine for diarrhea
- medicine for allergies
- cough and cold medicine
- sore throat lozenges or spray

The basics of staying healthy

There are many things you can do on your own to keep yourself healthy.

Rest

College students often skimp on rest because there is so much to do. However, trying to get by on too little sleep can cause some serious problems. What happens when you do not get enough sleep?
- You may be more likely to catch colds and other minor illnesses. Your body cannot fight off germs as well when you are tired and run-down.
- You are more likely to feel stressed or become depressed.
- You may have a hard time staying awake in class.
- You may have trouble concentrating on papers and exams.

Young adults often need a bit more sleep than older adults—sleeping about 8 to 9 hours a night is necessary for most 18 year olds.

Nutrition

Eating well is just as important as getting enough rest. This means eating enough fruits and vegetables every day; eating lean meats, fish, and poultry; and limiting fried and processed foods. Watching your intake of junk food, fatty foods, sugar, and salt is important. Also, women must be careful to consume enough low-fat dairy products high in calcium to help maintain bone mass and strength.

It is also possible to eat a healthy vegetarian diet at college. However, this may require some additional planning to make sure you get all the nutrients you need.

Exercise

Another important part of staying healthy is getting enough exercise.

There are three basic types of exercise, and ideally everyone should do all three:

- **Aerobic** exercise strengthens your heart and lungs (good examples are biking, running, fast walking, swimming, aerobic dancing, and rowing). Three times a week you should get some type of aerobic exercise for at least 20 minutes.
- **Strengthening** exercise tones and builds muscles and bone mass (you can do this by doing sit-ups, push-ups, and leg lifts, or by working out with weights or resis-tance bands).
- **Stretching** exercise, like yoga, improves your flexibility or range of motion.

There are a number of ways to sneak more exercise into your day. Instead of driving or taking a bus to run errands, walk or ride a bike (wear a helmet when biking). Walking to class can be good exercise, too. Even rollerblading around campus can be a good workout (but make sure you wear a helmet, wrist guards, and knee pads). If you are not used to exercising or if you have a chronic health problem, you may want to talk with your pediatrician at the student health service before starting an exercise program.

Sexual health

College is often a time when young people begin to explore their sexuality. This does not mean that all college students are sexually active. In fact, many are not. If you have decided to wait to have sex, you are not alone. Remember, the decision as to when to have sex is yours and yours alone. Do not let yourself be pressured into having sex if you do not want to.

If you are sexually active or are thinking about it, you owe it to yourself to make responsible decisions about sex. Make sure you can talk to your partner about the quality of your relationship and about sexual issues. Discuss whether or not you will date other people. Find out his or her sexual history, including exposure to sexually transmitted diseases (STDs). If you are in a heterosexual relationship, talk about birth control and what you would do if it failed. If you cannot talk about these issues with your partner, you should think about whether you should have a sexual relationship with him or her.

College may also be a time for sorting out your sexual identity. If you are questioning your sexual identity, talking with a counselor may help. Many colleges have support and social groups for gay, lesbian, and bisexual students. These groups can help students feel less isolated.

Sexual relationships expose you to the risk of STDs and viruses that can cause cancer and AIDS. The more sexual partners you have, the greater your risk. There are over 25 diseases that are spread through sexual contact. Some of them are easy to treat, but when left untreated they can cause serious health problems. Others, like herpes, have no cure. AIDS, also sexually transmitted, can kill you. Not having sex is the only sure way to prevent STDs. If you do have sex, the safest way is to have sex with only one person who has no STDs and no other sex partners. Use a latex condom *every time* you have sex.

Common health problems

There are times when you should contact the student health service immediately. Call the health service if you:

- have a fever of 102.5°F or higher
- have a headache accompanied by a stiff neck
- have pain with urination
- have an unusual discharge from your penis or vagina
- have a change in your menstrual cycle
- have pain in the abdomen that will not go away
- have a persistent cough, chest pain, or trouble breathing
- have pain or any other symptoms that worry you or last longer than you think they should

Respiratory infections

Illnesses like colds, the flu, and sore throats are hard to escape while in college. With students living together in dorms and apartments, eating together in large cafeterias, and sitting together in classrooms, these respiratory infections spread easily. Washing your hands often will help you avoid these illnesses. Dust allergy and exposure to cigarette smoke will make you more likely to get cold symptoms.

> ## The truth about mononucleosis ("mono")
>
> College students often worry about a disease called **"mono"**—also known as "the kissing disease." Mono, a viral infection, is not as common or usually as serious as most people think. Symptoms include fever, sore throat, headache, swollen glands, and extreme tiredness. If you seem to have a sore throat or bad flu that does not go away in a week to 10 days, the problem might be mono. See your doctor. Mono is diagnosed by a blood test called the "mono spot." Even if the test confirms that you have mono, there is no specific treatment, except to get plenty of rest and eat a healthy diet. The good news is that most people are better within a month. If you have had a documented case of mono, you cannot get it again.

How you treat a respiratory infection will depend on whether it is caused by bacteria or a virus. **Colds and flu** are caused by viruses. There is really nothing you can do to get rid of them quickly—the most you can do is rest, drink a lot of fluids, and treat the symptoms. How can you tell a cold from the flu? Colds usually cause milder symptoms than the flu. Coughing, sneezing, watery eyes, and mild fevers are common cold symptoms. The flu, on the other hand, is more serious. You will probably have a fairly high fever, body aches, and a dry cough with the flu. You may also have an upset stomach or vomit. If you are vomiting, eat only very bland foods like cereal or dry toast, and drink clear liquids such as sports drinks, water, or tea. Otherwise, the only thing you can do is rest and wait it out.

Over-the-counter cold and flu medications may help relieve your symptoms. Read labels when buying medications for colds and flu to make sure you are getting the right medicine for your symptoms.

Strep throat and most sinus and ear infections are caused by bacteria. These are treated with antibiotics. If you have a very sore throat, pain in your ears or sinuses, or a persistent fever, go to the student health service. They will be able to tell you what the problem is and give you antibiotics if you need them. If your doctor does give you antibiotics, *take them exactly as you are told*, and *be sure to take all of them*. If you do not, bacteria can become resistant to the antibiotics and result in a more serious infection.

Bruises, sprains, and strains

Bruises, sprains, and strains are very common, and usually are not very serious.

- **Bruises** are injuries to the skin that cause the surface of the skin to turn purple, brown, or red in color.
- **Strains** are injuries to the muscles and tendons that result from too much or sudden stretching
- **Sprains** are injuries to the ligaments, the connecting tissue between bones.

Bruises, strains, and sprains should be treated with:
- **Rest**—especially for the first 24 hours
- **Ice**—put ice packs or cold gel packs on the injury for 20 minutes every 4 hours
- **Compression**—wrap the injured body part in an elastic bandage
- **Elevation**—for example, if you have sprained your ankle, prop your foot up on pillows to keep it at a level higher than your heart

Visit the student health service if your pain or swelling does not get better in a day or two.

Taking care of your mental health

Starting college brings with it many new stresses. You may be away from home for the first time in your life, and may miss your family and friends. You will have more schoolwork to do, and it may take more time and effort than in high school. It may take you a while to find people with whom you have things in common. All these things can make you feel alone, overworked, and stressed out.

Friends

Friends usually become your main support system while in college. In fact, college friends often become close friends for life.

You may be worried about how you will make new friends. You will probably meet some people you like in the first few days of school, and you will meet more in your classes, in clubs or sports, and through other friends. If it takes a while to find people you click with, don't worry—it will happen.

Roommates can be terrific friends or great sources of stress. Even roommates who like each other will have conflicts over things like cleaning, bedtimes, and music. Talk these things over early on, and you will be less likely to have problems later. If you and your roommate just cannot get along, talk to a resident counselor. He or she can offer advice on how to handle your roommate problem.

Homesickness

Homesickness is very common among students away from home—even those who had previously been away at overnight camp or traveled far away. There is a difference between being away from home for 8 weeks and being gone for 8 months. There is also a difference between leaving home for a while (knowing you will be going back) and the start of leaving for good (knowing your returns may never be the same again). Feeling homesick does not make you less mature or mean you are not ready to be on your own. If you feel homesick, talk to your friends at school about it. Chances are they are feeling the same way. Keep in touch with family and friends back home, but make sure you develop new relationships at school. If your homesickness will just not go away and does not seem to be getting better after a few months at school, speaking with a counselor might help. Also, remember that going home for the first visit may be difficult because of changes in yourself or your family. Old conflicts do not just disappear once you go to college, and new ones may surface. Again, if things are too stressful for you to handle alone, talk to a counselor.

Depression

There will be days when you feel down, when the pressures of college life really get to you. Those feelings are normal and will pass in time. When you feel down, take some time out for yourself and do something that makes you feel good. Spend time with friends. Exercise. Read a good book.

Sometimes, though, feeling down can turn into depression. Depression is a serious illness that can be treated. If you have had any of the following symptoms for 2 weeks or more, see a counselor right away:
- sad mood
- hopeless, helpless, worthless, or guilty feelings
- loss of pleasure in things you usually enjoy
- sleep problems
- eating problems
- low energy, extreme tiredness, lack of concentration
- thoughts of death or suicide
- physical symptoms such as headaches, stomach aches, or body aches that do not respond to treatment

Do not think you can handle depression on your own. If one of your friends seems depressed, suggest that he or she see a counselor as soon as possible.

Drinking and violence

Drinking is a huge problem on most college campuses. The majority of college students drink, and a large number drink to excess. More than half of all male college students are binge drinkers (those who have five or more drinks at one sitting), and over a third of female students are binge drinkers. Heavy or binge drinking can lead to physical illness (or death), long-term drinking problems, and aggression and violence. Drinking is known to increase sexual aggressiveness, which can lead to sexual harassment and date rape. Drinking also clouds your judgment, and may make you more likely to engage in unsafe sexual practices, which in turn may lead to STDs and unintended pregnancies.

The legal drinking age in the United States is 21. The best way to prevent drinking-related problems is to avoid drinking altogether. If you are of legal age and choose to drink, be responsible. Stop after one or two drinks. *Do not* drink and drive, *do not* let friends drink and drive, and *do not* ride with someone who has been drinking. Follow the designated driver rule. *Do not* drink with people you do not know. If you feel you need to cut down on your drinking, if friends comment on the amount of drinking you do, or if you ever feel guilty about something you have done while drinking, see a counselor at school.

Just some friendly advice...

- Poor study habits are the primary reason students do poorly in college. College means increased freedom, with less time spent in the classroom and more time spent studying independently. Learn to budget your time and use it wisely.

- Violence, crime, racism, sexism, and cults are alive and well on every college campus. A college campus is no safer than your home town. Lock your doors and take care of yourself.

- Sorority and fraternity life can offer many advantages, but it can also isolate students from the rest of the college experience. Make sure you thoroughly investigate any sorority or fraternity you are interested in.

College life will present many opportunities and challenges. Take care of yourself, and enjoy your college years.

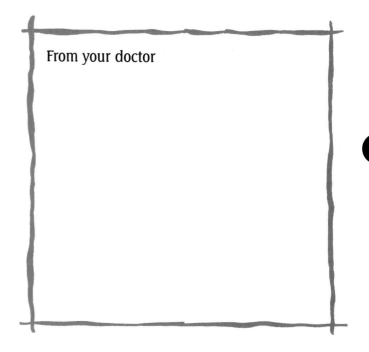

Health Record Card   Use this card to keep track of important health information.

Name:

Address:

Phone:

Date of Birth:

Pediatrician's Name:

Office Address:

Telephone/Fax:

Immunization Record

	Date Given		Date Given
DTaP/DTP		Others	
Hib		Allergies:	
Polio		Chronic Medical Conditions:	
Hepatitis B			
MMR			
Td		Blood Type:	
Varicella			

The information contained in this publication should not be used as a substitute for the medical care and advice of your pediatrician. There may be variations in treatment that your pediatrician may recommend based on individual facts and circumstances.

From your doctor

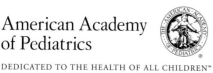

American Academy of Pediatrics

DEDICATED TO THE HEALTH OF ALL CHILDREN™

The American Academy of Pediatrics is an organization of 55,000 primary care pediatricians, pediatric medical subspecialists, and pediatric surgical specialists dedicated to the health, safety, and well-being of infants, children, adolescents, and young adults.

American Academy of Pediatrics
PO Box 747
Elk Grove Village, IL 60009-0747
Web site — http://www.aap.org

Important Information for Teens Who Get Headaches
Guidelines for Teens

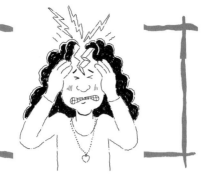

A headache is not a disease, but it may indicate that something is wrong. Headaches are common among teenagers and generally are not serious. In fact, 50% to 75% of all teens report having at least one headache per month. However, more frequent headaches can be upsetting and worrisome for you and your family. The most common headaches for teenagers are tension headaches and migraines. Sometimes these problems may be associated with health concerns that require a visit to your pediatrician.

What causes headaches?

Headaches are most commonly caused by:

Illness—Headaches often are a symptom of other illnesses. Viral infections, strep throat, allergies, sinus infections, and urinary tract infections can be accompanied by headaches. Fever may also be associated with headaches.

Skipping meals—Even if you're trying to lose weight, you still need to eat regularly. Fad diets can make you hungry and also can give you a headache. Not getting enough fluids—which leads to dehydration—also may cause a headache.

Drugs—Alcohol, cocaine, amphetamines, diet pills, and other drugs may give you a headache.

Often headaches are triggered by sleep problems, minor head injuries, or certain foods (dairy products, chocolate, food additives like nitrates, nitrites, and monosodium glutamate).

Sometimes, headaches can also be caused by prescribed medication, such as birth control pills, tetracycline for acne, and high doses of vitamin A.

Less commonly, headaches can be caused by a dental infection or abscess, and jaw alignment problems (TMJ syndrome). Although headaches are only rarely caused by eye problems, pain around the eyes—which can feel like a headache—can be caused by eye muscle imbalance or not wearing glasses that have been prescribed for you.

Only in **very** rare cases are headaches a symptom of a brain tumor, high blood pressure, or other serious problem.

Types of headaches

Tension headaches often feel like a tight band is around your head. The pain is dull and aching and usually will be felt on both sides of your head, but may be in front and back as well.

Pressure at school or at home, arguments with parents or friends, having too much to do, and feeling anxious or depressed can all cause a headache.

Migraines often are described as throbbing and usually are felt on only one side of your head, but may be felt on both. A migraine may make you feel light-headed or dizzy, and/or make your stomach upset. You may see spots or be sensitive to light, sounds, and smells. If you get migraines, chances are one of your parents or other family members also have had this problem.

A third, less common, type of headache is called a **psychogenic** headache. Psychogenic headaches are similar to tension headaches, but the cause is an emotional problem such as depression. Signs of depression include loss of energy, poor appetite or overeating, loss of interest in usual activities, change in sleeping patterns (trouble falling asleep, waking in the middle of the night or too early in the morning), and difficulty thinking or concentrating.

When should I see the pediatrician?

If you are worried about your headaches—or if this problem begins to disrupt your school, home, or social life—see your pediatrician. Other signs that may mean you should visit your pediatrician include:

Head injury—Headaches from a recent head injury should be checked right away—especially if you were knocked out by the injury.

Seizures/convulsions—Any headaches associated with seizures or fainting require immediate attention.

Frequency—You get more than one headache a week.

Degree of pain—Headache pain is severe and prevents you from doing activities you want to do.

Time of attack—Headaches that wake you from sleep or occur in early morning.

Visual difficulties—Headaches that cause blurred vision, eye spots, or other visual changes.

Other associated symptoms—If fever, vomiting, stiff neck, toothache, or jaw pain accompany your headache, you may require an examination—including laboratory or x-ray tests.

How are headaches treated?

Whichever type of headache you get, and whatever the cause, your pediatrician can explain why you get headaches and how they can be controlled. Be sure to ask any questions you may have.

If you get tension headaches or mild migraines, your pediatrician may suggest an aspirin or an aspirin substitute, such as acetaminophen or ibuprofen, and rest. If you get more severe headaches or classic migraines (when you have a visual disturbance called an "aura"), prescription medicine may be required. Your pediatrician may suggest that you keep a **headache diary** to help pinpoint information about what is causing the headaches. A headache diary helps you keep track of the following: when headaches occur, how long they last, what you were doing when the headaches start, what you had eaten, how much sleep you have had, and what seems to make the headaches better or worse.

If what you eat seems to trigger your headaches, your pediatrician will suggest that you eliminate certain foods from your diet. If stress is the culprit, your doctor can help you cope by suggesting special treatments such as relaxation exercises. Headaches that are caused by an emotional or psychological problem may require additional visits to your pediatrician or to other health care professionals to get to the cause of the problem. Sometimes entire families need counseling to eliminate the stress that is causing headaches.

It's important to know that, whatever the cause, headache pain is real. More importantly, with your pediatrician's help, you can identify the source of your headaches and get this problem under control.

The information contained in this publication should not be used as a substitute for the medical care and advice of your pediatrician. There may be variations in treatment that your pediatrician may recommend based on individual facts and circumstances.

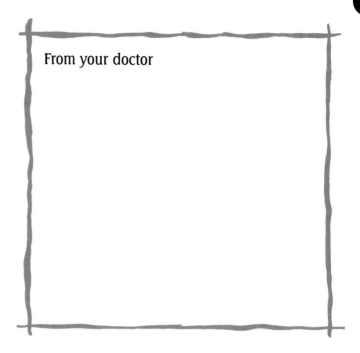

From your doctor

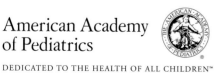

American Academy of Pediatrics

DEDICATED TO THE HEALTH OF ALL CHILDREN™

The American Academy of Pediatrics is an organization of 55,000 primary care pediatricians, pediatric medical subspecialists, and pediatric surgical specialists dedicated to the health, safety, and well-being of infants, children, adolescents, and young adults.

American Academy of Pediatrics
PO Box 747
Elk Grove Village, IL 60009-0747
Web site — http://www.aap.org

Know the Facts About HIV and AIDS

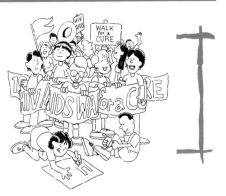

AIDS, which stands for **acquired immune deficiency syndrome,** is a very serious disease that affects children, teens, and adults. It is caused by a virus called the human immunodeficiency virus (HIV). The virus is **acquired** and causes a **deficiency** in the body's **immune** system. AIDS has rapidly become a leading cause of death in young adults and children in many areas in the United States. Although there is treatment available, there is no cure for AIDS. The disease can be prevented by educating yourself and your children about AIDS and HIV, including the behaviors that can increase the risk of getting AIDS.

What are HIV and AIDS?

HIV is the virus that causes AIDS. When someone is infected with HIV, it means the virus is attacking the immune system. The immune system is the body's way of fighting infections and helping to prevent some types of cancer. Damage to the immune system from HIV can occur over months, as sometimes happens in infants. Sometimes it occurs slowly over years, as more often happens in adults. AIDS is diagnosed in an HIV-infected person when the immune system is severely damaged or when certain other serious infections or cancer occurs.

Many people do not know they are infected with HIV because it can take many years for serious symptoms to develop. However, even if an infected person shows no symptoms, the infection can be spread to others. Many people with HIV infection look and act healthy. You cannot tell just by looking at people whether they are infected with HIV. A blood test for HIV is the only way to be sure.

How is HIV spread?

HIV is spread from one person to another through certain body fluids. These fluids include blood and blood products, semen (sperm), fluid from the vagina, and breast milk. The following are ways HIV can be spread:

- **By sexual intercourse (vaginal, anal, or oral) with a person who is infected with HIV.** Both males and females can spread HIV. Latex condoms can help prevent the spread of HIV and other sexually transmitted diseases (STDs). The safest way to prevent these diseases is to abstain from all forms of sexual intercourse until married or in a long-term mature relationship with an uninfected partner.
- **Through contact with an infected person's blood.** Sharing syringes or needles for drug use or for other activities such as tattooing or ear piercing can spread HIV. Accidental injuries from contaminated needles can also cause HIV infection. This can happen if a person comes into contact with used needles that have been thrown away. Rarely, HIV has been spread by an infected person's blood directly contacting the mucous membranes, cuts, scrapes, or open sores of another person.

- **To a baby by an HIV-infected mother** during pregnancy, labor, delivery, or breastfeeding.
- **Through blood or blood products from blood transfusions, organ transplants, or artificial insemination.** This occurs very rarely because donors of blood, sperm, tissue, and organs in the United States are tested routinely for HIV.

How is HIV not spread?

It is very important to know how HIV is **not** spread. Fear and wrong information about HIV and AIDS cause suffering to those who have been infected with HIV. Make sure you and your children understand that HIV **cannot** be spread through casual contact with someone who has AIDS or is infected with HIV. You cannot get HIV in the following ways:
- Shaking hands
- Hugging
- Sitting next to someone
- Sharing bathrooms
- Eating food prepared by an HIV-infected person

Also, you **cannot** get HIV from the following:
- The air
- Insect bites
- Giving blood
- Swimming pools

Teaching your young child about HIV and AIDS

Children need to learn about HIV and AIDS at a very early age. By the time your children are 3 or 4 years old, make sure you have clearly explained the following to them:
- They should never touch anyone else's blood or open sores.
- They should never touch needles or syringes. If they see someone who is bleeding or if they find a needle or syringe, they should tell an adult. Remind your children never to touch a needle or syringe if they find one in the garbage or on the ground.
- AIDS cannot be caught by playing with HIV-infected children.

By grade-school age, your child should begin to have a better understanding of illness and body parts. Your child should begin to learn more about how HIV can and cannot be spread.

©2002 American Academy of Pediatrics

Teaching your preteen or teenager about HIV and AIDS

To avoid being infected with HIV through sexual contact, preteens and teenagers need to know that the best way to protect themselves against HIV and AIDS is to refrain from having any type of sexual intercourse. Urge your teenager to postpone sexual intercourse until married or in a long-term, mature relationship with an uninfected partner. Neither person should have any other sexual partners.

If teenagers do not postpone having sexual intercourse, then proper use of latex condoms and limiting the relationship to one partner will help them avoid HIV infection. This will also lower the risk of getting other sexually transmitted diseases (STDs) such as syphilis, gonorrhea, Chlamydia infection, and genital warts. Adolescents should also know about other types of birth control. However, it should be emphasized that other forms of birth control do **not** prevent HIV infection or other STDs.

For more information for you and your adolescent, ask your pediatrician about the following brochures from the American Academy of Pediatrics:

- *Making the Right Choice: Facts for Teens on Preventing Pregnancy*
- *Deciding to Wait*
- *The Correct Use of Condoms: A Message to Teens*

HIV and drug use

Adolescents also need to know about the extremely high risk of being infected with HIV if they use drugs, especially intravenous (IV) drugs that are injected with needles. Sharing a needle or syringe spreads blood from one person to another. People who do not use drugs themselves but are having sexual intercourse with an HIV-infected drug user can also be infected with HIV. Sharing needles for non-drug use, such as for tattoos, ear piercing, intentional scarring or cutting with a razor or needle, or injecting drugs like steroids, can also spread HIV.

When talking to your adolescent about drugs, make sure your adolescent understands that using drugs is very dangerous. The risk of getting HIV increases even when non-IV drugs like alcohol or cocaine are used. This is because drugs affect a person's judgment and can lead to risky behaviors, such as having sex without a latex condom or having sex with multiple partners.

See the following brochures from the American Academy of Pediatrics for more information on drug use (including alcohol and tobacco) and children:

- *Marijuana: Your Child and Drugs*
- *Cocaine: Your Child and Drugs*
- *Alcohol: Your Child and Drugs*
- *The Risks of Tobacco Use: A Message to Parents and Teens*
- *Smoking: Straight Talk for Teens*

If your preteen or teenager is using drugs or alcohol or is involved in risky sexual behaviors, he is at higher risk of HIV infection. If you think your adolescent or child is at risk of becoming infected with HIV, it is very important to discuss this with your pediatrician.

Who should be tested for HIV?

Anyone involved in the risky behaviors mentioned previously *should* get an HIV test. Anyone who wants to know whether or not they have HIV can be tested. However, a negative test does not mean a person is uninfected if the risky behaviors took place only a few months before the test.

The following symptoms may suggest a need for HIV testing:

- Persistent fevers
- Loss of appetite
- Frequent diarrhea
- Poor weight gain or rapid weight loss
- Chronic lymph node swelling
- Persistent or recurring extreme tiredness or lethargy
- White spots in the mouth
- Recurring or unusual infections

While there is no cure for HIV or AIDS, there are medications that can help delay symptoms, help prevent the spread of HIV to an unborn baby, and help prevent additional infections in HIV-infected people.

HIV and AIDS are important issues to think about and discuss. Educating yourself and your family about HIV and AIDS is the best way to keep your family healthy. If you need more information, talk to your pediatrician. Most importantly, talk to your child or adolescent. Make sure she knows the facts about this serious yet preventable disease.

The information contained in this publication should not be used as a substitute for the medical care and advice of your pediatrician. There may be variations in treatment that your pediatrician may recommend based on individual facts and circumstances.

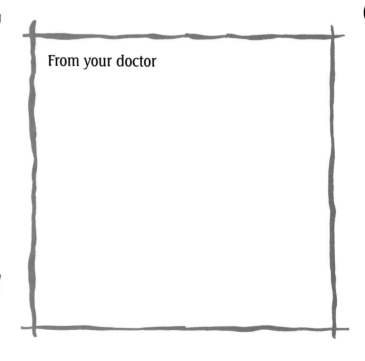

From your doctor

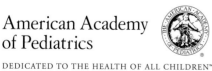

American Academy of Pediatrics

DEDICATED TO THE HEALTH OF ALL CHILDREN™

The American Academy of Pediatrics is an organization of 55,000 primary care pediatricians, pediatric medical subspecialists, and pediatric surgical specialists dedicated to the health, safety, and well-being of infants, children, adolescents, and young adults.

American Academy of Pediatrics
PO Box 747
Elk Grove Village, IL 60009-0747
Web site — http://www.aap.org

Making the Right Choice

Facts for Teens on Preventing Pregnancy
Guidelines for Teens

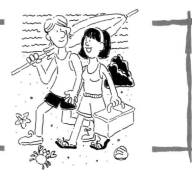

This brochure contains facts to help you make choices about your health and preventing pregnancy. Many people your age find it hard to talk about things like whether or not to have sex or types of birth control methods. The facts in this brochure will help you make informed choices that are right for you.

You can abstain from sex

You may be feeling a lot of pressure to have sex. Maybe the person you are dating, your friends, or other kids are pushing you to do it. Maybe it seems like "everyone is doing it."

Fact: There is nothing strange about waiting to have sex. Half of all teens say "no" to sex.

Fact: Before you find yourself in a situation that could lead to sex, make up your mind to say "no." Then stick with your decision. Many young women get pregnant from having unplanned sex.

Fact: Many young people have sex without meaning to when they drink alcohol or use drugs. Not using alcohol and drugs will help you make clearer choices about sex.

Fact: Sex has health risks. Sexually transmitted diseases (STDs) like chlamydia, herpes, and AIDS can affect males and females for life. Also, teens have a higher risk of medical problems when they are pregnant and give birth.

Fact: Teen parents may find it hard to finish school. This can limit the types of jobs they can get and may affect their income.

Sexually active teens should know the following facts about the condom:

Fact: The condom is the **only** birth control method that protects against STDs.

Fact: Because condoms protect against STDs, you should use a latex condom every time you have sex-no matter what other type of birth control you and your partner might also use.

Fact: The condom is the only effective method of birth control for males.

Fact: If you use a condom the right way, it has a 90% chance of preventing pregnancy.

Fact: Withdrawal (when the male "pulls out" of the female before he ejaculates) does not prevent pregnancy. Even if a small amount of sperm enters a woman, pregnancy can occur.

Sexually active teens should know the following facts about female contraceptives:

Fact: "The pill" is the most popular type of birth control used by women. There are many brands of the birth control pill. For the pill to work, a woman must take it everyday. There are higher risks for heavy smokers who take the pill.

Fact: Of those women who use the pill properly, 99 of 100 will not get pregnant.

Fact: Depo-Provera is a popular choice of birth control for women who sometimes forget to take the pill everyday. It is also a good choice for females with special medical problems. This type of birth control is given as a shot every 3 months. It prevents pregnancy during that whole time.

Fact: The pill and Depo-Provera may cause a few minor side effects. You could have mild irregular bleeding, tender breasts, or a slight weight gain. On the upside, your periods may be shorter and lighter, and you may have few or no cramps.

Fact: Another type of birth control is Norplant. Norplant is made up of six capsules the size of matchsticks, which are put into a woman's arm. Each capsule contains a chemically made hormone that is released into the blood over a period of 5 years to prevent pregnancy. Norplant will protect against pregnancy for 5 years, you can have the capsules removed at any time. A common side effect of Norplant is irregular bleeding.

There are other types of birth control that are not recommended for young people.

Fact: Other birth control methods such as diaphragms and spermicides require some planning. The teenage pregnancy rate using these methods is very high.

Fact: Natural family planning, sometimes called the "rhythm method," also has a high failure rate for young people. Using this method means you cannot have sex during certain times of a woman's monthly cycle.

It is important to discuss different birth control methods with a health professional. Your pediatrician can let you know how safe and effective these methods are, what side effects they can cause, and how much they cost.

The choice is yours

The choice to become sexually involved is yours to make. Remember that even though some people your age decide to have sex, just as many people decide not to. Choosing not to have sex is the only way to avoid all STDs and getting pregnant.

If you do choose to have sex, you need to make plans to prevent pregnancy and avoid catching an STD. Whether you are male or female, **a latex condom should be used every time you have sex to protect yourself from STDs.** However, not having sex is the best way to protect against STDs.

Birth control methods that work best for young women include:

- the birth control pill taken everyday
- a shot of Depo-Provera every 3 months
- Norplant capsules placed under the skin, which last for 5 years

For more information on preventing pregnancy, see your pediatrician or health clinic.

The information contained in this publication should not be used as a substitute for the medical care and advice of your pediatrician. There may be variations in treatment that your pediatrician may recommend based on individual facts and circumstances.

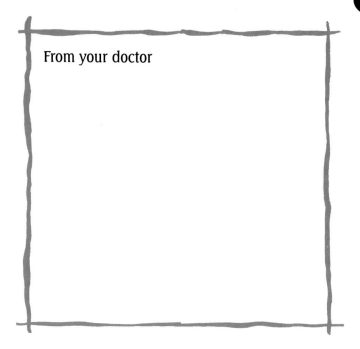

From your doctor

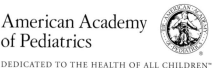

American Academy of Pediatrics

DEDICATED TO THE HEALTH OF ALL CHILDREN™

The American Academy of Pediatrics is an organization of 55,000 primary care pediatricians, pediatric medical subspecialists, and pediatric surgical specialists dedicated to the health, safety, and well-being of infants, children, adolescents, and young adults.

American Academy of Pediatrics
PO Box 747
Elk Grove Village, IL 60009-0747
Web site — http://www.aap.org

Copyright ©1990, Updated 2/96
American Academy of Pediatrics

©2002 American Academy of Pediatrics

The Pelvic Exam
Guidelines for Teens

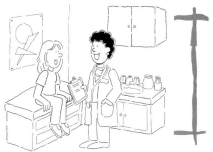

As a young woman, your body has gone through a number of changes over the past few years. An important part of growing up is taking responsibility for keeping yourself healthy. This includes establishing a partnership with your pediatrician regarding your health. Pelvic exams can be an important way to take care of your health. Most women have questions and concerns about their first pelvic exam, but knowing what to expect can help you to feel more at ease. This brochure has been developed by the American Academy of Pediatrics to help young women understand the pelvic exam.

Why do I need a pelvic exam?

A pelvic exam is the best way for your pediatrician to examine your reproductive system, which includes the vagina, cervix, ovaries, fallopian tubes, and uterus (see illustration). This visit is also a great time to talk to your pediatrician about important health issues such as:

- your growth and development
- breast health
- menstruation ("periods")
- sexuality
- pregnancy and birth control
- infection risk or to simply get advice about your health.

The exam also includes lab tests for common problems that can be easily treated if found early.

Most young women should have a pelvic exam by the end of high school. It should be done earlier than this if the woman is sexually active or has a problem with her reproductive system.

The Female Reproductive System

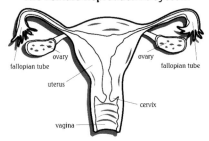

ovary
ovary
fallopian tube
fallopian tube
uterus
cervix
vagina

The interview

Before the pelvic exam, your pediatrician will ask you a number of questions to find out whether you are having problems or are at risk for problems. For example, your pediatrician may ask about your menstrual periods. Questions about your periods may include:

- When did you have your first period? When did your last period start?
- Do you have your periods regularly? How often?
- How long do your periods last?
- Do you have any discomfort (pain, cramping, headaches, mood swings) with your periods?

- Do you use tampons, pads, or both?
- Have you ever had vaginal itching, discharge, or problems urinating?

Your answers to these questions tell your pediatrician if your periods are normal. He or she may give advice about menstrual discomfort, tampon use, and other issues.

Your pediatrician may also ask you about your sexual experiences. This is so your doctor can get to know you and help you to protect your health, so giving honest answers is important.

The information you give to your pediatrician is confidential and will not be discussed with anyone else without your permission (unless it is something life threatening). The questions may include:

- Have you ever had sexual intercourse?
- How old were you the first time you had sex?
- How many sexual partners have you had?
- What do you use to prevent pregnancy and infection?

Your answers to these questions help your pediatrician decide what services you need. He or she can give you advice on decision making, abstinence, and prevention of pregnancy and infection.

The exam

Your pediatrician will tell you what he or she is going to do at each step of the exam. If you have any questions or feel uncomfortable, just let your pediatrician know. If you have a male doctor, a female nurse or chaperone will normally be present during the exam. You may request that your mother, older sister, or friend join you if it makes you more at ease. You may also request that no one, other than the doctor, be in the room during the exam.

Before the exam, your height, weight, blood pressure, lungs, heart, and neck may be checked. You may be asked to give a small sample of urine and to empty your bladder to make the exam more comfortable.

You will then be left alone to completely undress and put on a gown. A sheet will be given for extra coverage. When your pediatrician comes into the room, he or she will ask you to lie down on the examining table for the breast examination. He or she will feel each breast for lumps, sores, or swelling. Be sure to tell your pediatrician if your breasts are sore in any way or if you have had any fluid leaking from your breasts.

Your pediatrician will teach you "breast self-exam," an important part of keeping yourself healthy. You should do a breast self-exam each month. This will alert you to any changes or problems in your breasts and help you to be more familiar with your body. Practicing breast self-exam as a young woman prepares you for later on, when breast cancer is more common and regular breast self-exams are so important.

 69

How to do a breast self-exam

Once a month, right after your period, you should examine your breasts. Although breast cancer is rare in young people, it usually can be cured if found early, and a breast self-exam is the best way to find it.

1. Stand in front of your mirror with your arms at your sides and see if there are any changes in the size or shape of your breasts. Look for any puckers or dimples, and press each nipple to see if any fluid comes out. Raise your arm above your head and look for changes in your breasts from this position as well.
2. Lie down and place your left hand under your head. Hold your right hand flat and feel your left breast with little, pressing circles. Think of each breast as a pie divided into four pieces. Feel each piece and then feel the center of the "pie" (the nipple area).
3. Now put your left arm down at your side, and do the same thing on the outside of the breast, starting under the armpit.
4. Repeat steps 2 and 3 for the other side.

Most women have some lumpiness or texture to their breasts; breasts are not just soft tissue. Get to know your breasts__then be alert for any lumps or other changes if they should ever appear. Remember, most lumps and changes are not cancer. However, if you think you have found a lump or notice any other changes, don't press or squeeze it; see your pediatrician.

Usually after the breast examination, your pediatrician will check your abdomen and then do the pelvic exam. The entire pelvic exam only takes about 5 minutes. It can be done even if you have never had sexual intercourse, because the opening that allows your period blood out is large enough to allow examination. Some young women who have not had intercourse worry that having a pelvic exam will mean they are no longer virgins. You should not worry about this; the pelvic exam does not change whether or not you are a virgin. Also, the pelvic exam is not a "test" to see if you are a virgin.

The pelvic examination has three parts. In the *first* part, the pediatrician will use a light to look at the outside of your vagina and surrounding areas to make sure everything looks normal.

During the *second* part, the pediatrician will look inside your vagina. Your pediatrician will use an instrument called a speculum to see inside. It will be made of disposable plastic or sterilized metal. The speculum will be gently inserted into your vagina. You will feel some pressure, but it should not hurt. Taking deep breaths and trying not to tense up will help relax your vagina muscles and make this part of the test easier. While the speculum is in place, your pediatrician will take a sample of cells from the cervix. This is called a Pap smear. The Pap smear is a test for infections or abnormalities of the cervix, and you should not even feel it. The speculum will then be removed.

In the *third* part of the pelvic exam, the pediatrician feels your uterus and ovaries to check their size and see if they are tender. This is done by the pediatrician gently inserting one or two gloved fingers into your vagina and pressing on the outside of your abdomen with the other hand.

That's it! Most patients are surprised when their first pelvic exam is over, it really is quick.

If your pediatrician finds that you have an infection or other problems with your reproductive system, he or she may refer you to an OB/GYN (obstetrician/gynecologist). This type of doctor specializes in women's reproductive health.

Take care of yourself

Your first pelvic exam is one of the many steps you will take as part of taking care of yourself as a young adult. It is easiest to do this when you are well, before any problems occur. If you are having sex, you should have a pelvic exam at least once a year. Even if you are not having sex, you should begin having regular pelvic exams before you finish high school or if you have any concerns about your vagina, uterus, and periods.

Along with eating right, getting enough exercise, not smoking, and wearing seat belts, regular visits to your pediatrician for checkups are important. Your pediatrician cares about your health. Even as you get older, seeing your pediatrician regularly will help you learn the best ways to take care of yourself.

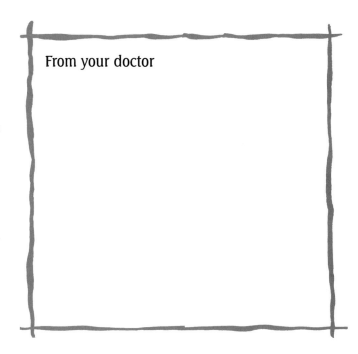

From your doctor

American Academy of Pediatrics

DEDICATED TO THE HEALTH OF ALL CHILDREN™

The American Academy of Pediatrics is an organization of 55,000 primary care pediatricians, pediatric medical subspecialists, and pediatric surgical specialists dedicated to the health, safety, and well-being of infants, children, adolescents, and young adults.

American Academy of Pediatrics
PO Box 747
Elk Grove Village, IL 60009-0747
Web site — http://www.aap.org

Copyright ©1996   American Academy of Pediatrics

Puberty
Information for Girls

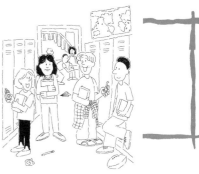

As part of growing up, you will go through puberty. Puberty is the time in your life when your body changes from that of a child to that of an adult. These changes are caused by chemicals in the body called hormones. Because there are so many changes that happen during puberty, you may feel like your body is out of control. In time, your hormones will balance out and your body will catch up.

Not only does your body change, but your emotions change too. How you think and feel about yourself, your family and friends, and your whole world, may seem different. As you go through puberty, you will begin to make important decisions for yourself, take on more responsibilities, and become more independent.

If you are already going through some of these changes, you may be asking yourself, "Am I normal?" or "Do other people my age feel the way I do?" Don't worry. Lots of changes happen during puberty and, although it can be a confusing time of life, it can be exciting.

This brochure was written to help you understand and deal with the changes puberty brings.

Information for Girls

Puberty is the time in a girl's life when her body changes from that of a young girl to that of a woman. It is also the time when a girl becomes physically able to have babies. Although there is no "right" time for puberty to begin, it generally starts earlier for a girl than it does for a boy—usually between 9 and 13 years of age. This is why many girls are taller and may act more mature than boys for a few years until the boys catch up.

How will my body change?

Following are some of the changes your body will go through during puberty:

Breasts: In most girls, puberty starts with breast growth. When your breasts start to develop, you may notice small, tender lumps under one or both nipples that will get bigger over the next few years. When breasts first begin to develop, it is not unusual for one breast to be larger than the other. However, as they develop, they will most likely even out before they reach their final size and shape.

As your breasts develop, you may need a bra. Some girls feel that wearing a bra for the first time is exciting—it is the first step toward becoming a woman! However, some girls feel embarrassed, especially if they are among the first of their friends to need a bra. If the people around you make a bigger deal of your first bra than you would like, try to remember that they do not mean to embarrass you, they are just proud of how much you have grown.

Hair: Soft hair will start to grow in the pubic area (the area between your legs). This hair will eventually become thick and very curly. You may also notice hair under your arms and on your legs. Many women shave this hair. There is no medical reason to shave, it is simply a personal choice. If you decide to shave, be sure to use a lot of soap and water and a clean razor made for women. It is a good idea to use your own personal razor or electric shaver and not to share one with your family or friends.

Body shape: Hips get wider and your waist will get smaller. Your body will also begin to build up fat in the stomach, buttocks, and legs. This is normal and gives your body the curvier shape of a woman.

Body size: Arms, legs, hands, and feet may grow faster than the rest of your body. Until the rest of your body catches up, you may feel a little clumsier than usual.

Skin: Skin may get more oily and you may notice you sweat more. This is because your glands are growing too. It is important to wash every day to keep your skin clean and to use a deodorant or antiperspirant to keep odor and wetness under control. Despite your best efforts to keep your face clean, you still may get pimples. This is called acne and is normal during this time when your hormone levels are high. Almost all teenagers get acne at one time or another. Whether your case is mild or severe, there are things you can do to keep it under control. For more information on controlling acne, talk to your pediatrician or see the brochure "Acne Treatment and Control" from the American Academy of Pediatrics.

Menstruation: Your menstrual cycle, or "period," begins. Most girls get their periods between 9 and 16 years of age.

What happens during my period?

During puberty, your ovaries begin to release eggs. If an egg is fertilized by sperm from a man's penis, it will grow inside your uterus and develop into a baby. To prepare for this, a thick layer of tissue and blood cells builds up in your uterus. If the egg does not meet with a sperm, these tissues and cells are not needed by the body. They turn into a blood-like fluid and flow out of the vagina. The menstrual period is the monthly discharge of this fluid out of the body. When a girl first begins to have her periods, she is able to get pregnant.

During your period, you will need to wear some kind of sanitary pad and/or tampon to absorb this fluid and keep it from getting on your clothes. Pads have adhesive strips and are worn inside the panties. Tampons are placed inside the vagina.

The decision to use pads or tampons is your choice. Some girls prefer tampons because they do not like the feeling of wetness or the odor that may accompany pads. Some girls prefer pads because they are not comfortable inserting tampons into their vaginas.

When using a tampon for the first time, take your time, relax, and insert the tampon slowly into your vagina. This will allow the muscles in your vagina to relax and the tampon to go in easily. Make sure the string remains on the outside of your vagina so that you can remove the tampon. To avoid infection, change tampons often and do not wear them overnight.

Pads are often called "maxi" pads or "mini" pads and can be thick or thin. These are good for when the flow of your period is heaviest. Panty liners, which are very thin, can be used for the end of your period when there is usually very little discharge. Tampons come in different levels of thickness for when your period is heavy or light. Try out different brands and find the ones you like the best.

Most periods last from 3 to 7 days. After your period you may have a day or two of light bleeding, called spotting. This is normal. If you start bleeding regularly between periods, however, see your pediatrician.

Having your period does not mean you have to avoid any of your normal activities like swimming, horseback riding, or gym class. Exercise can even help get rid of cramps and other discomforts that you may feel during your period.

Beginning with their first period, many girls expect their menstrual cycles to occur exactly on schedule. But that rarely happens. During the first year (and sometimes longer) some girls have periods that seem to have no schedule. Cycles can be as short as 3 weeks; others as long as 6 weeks—or sometimes even longer. It may take a while for your periods to become regular (every 3 to 5 weeks). Even after they do become regular, it is not unusual for a girl to miss a period if she is sick, under a lot of stress, exercising heavily, has a poor diet, or is nervous about something. Of course, more than any other reason, pregnancy can cause a girl's period to stop.

Some girls bleed heavier than others during their periods. But don't worry, you won't bleed too much. You have about 5 quarts of blood in your body and you only lose 1 to 3 ounces of it during your period. However, if your period is really heavy (you soak more than 6 to 8 pads or tampons in a single day), talk to your pediatrician.

You may also feel some discomfort before, during, or after your period. Some common symptoms include:

- cramps
- bloating
- soreness or swelling in your breasts
- headaches
- sudden mood changes, such as sadness or irritability
- depression

If you feel your symptoms are severe, talk to your pediatrician. Most of the time, cramping and other symptoms are mild and easy to control. Your pediatrician may suggest some medications or exercises to help you feel better. There are other menstrual problems that require a visit to your pediatrician. If you have any of the following symptoms, contact your pediatrician:

- a sudden change in your period that does not have an obvious cause (like an illness)
- very heavy menstrual bleeding that lasts more than 7 to 10 days
- bleeding between periods
- severe abdominal pain that lasts for more than 2 days and is not early in your period

- you think you might be pregnant
- any other concern you may have that something is wrong with your menstrual cycle

If your pediatrician finds that you have an infection or other problems with your reproductive system, he or she may refer you to a doctor who specializes in women's reproductive health. This type of doctor is called an obstetrician/gynecologist.

Emotional changes during puberty

In addition to the many physical changes you will go through during puberty, there are many emotional changes as well. You may start to care more about what other people think about you. You want to be accepted and liked. At this time in your life, your relationships with others may begin to change. Some become more important and some less so. You start to separate more from your parents and identify with others your age. You may begin to make decisions that could affect the rest of your life.

Many people your age feel self-conscious about their changing bodies—too tall, too short, too fat, too skinny. Because puberty causes so many changes, it is hard not to compare what is going on with your body with what is happening to your friends' bodies. Try to keep in mind that everyone goes through puberty differently. Eventually, everyone catches up.

Sex and growing up

During this time, you also become more aware of your sexuality. A look, touch, or just thinking about someone may make your heart beat faster and produce a warm, tingling feeling all over. This is completely normal. You may be asking yourself the following questions:

- "Is it okay to masturbate (touch your genitals for sexual pleasure)?"
- "When should I start dating?"
- "When is it okay to kiss?"
- "How far is too far?"
- "When will I be ready to have sexual intercourse?"
- "Will having sex help my relationship?"

Masturbation is normal and will not harm you. Many boys and girls masturbate, many do not.

Deciding to become sexually active can be very confusing. On one hand, you hear so many warnings and dangers about having sex. On the other hand, movies, TV, magazines, even billboards seem to be telling you that having sex is okay. The fact is, sex is a part of life and, like many parts of life, it can be good or bad. It all depends on you and the choices you make.

As you continue through puberty, you may experience pressure from many sources to have sex. Knowing where the pressures come from will make them much easier to deal with. Pressure to have sex may come from:

- **The media:** Because there are so many images in the media about sex, it is easy to get the idea that having sex is the right thing to do. Sex in movies, TV shows, magazines, and in music is often shown as not having any risks. Do not let these messages fool you. In real life, having sex can be very risky.
- **Your own body:** It is perfectly normal to be interested in sex. After all, growing sexually is what puberty is all about. The sexual urges you feel during puberty can be very powerful. What is most important is to stay in control of these feelings and not let them control you. Keep in mind that sex is not the only way to express how you feel about someone. Taking walks, talking, holding hands, hugging, and touching are great ways to be close to someone you have strong feelings for.

- **Your friends:** It may seem like "everybody's doing it" or that people who have sex are "cool." Maybe you feel like you should have sex to be popular and fit in with the group. However, people like to talk about sex and some may want others to believe that they are having sex even when they are not. Someone who does not want to be your friend just because you are not having sex is probably someone who is not worth being friends with anyway. Do not let friends—or anyone—talk you into having sex. This is a decision you make when it is right for you, not for your friends.

Deciding whether or not to have sexual intercourse is one of the most important decisions you will ever make. Why not take your time and think it through? Talk with your parents about their values. Waiting to have sexual intercourse until you are older, in a serious relationship, and able to accept the responsibilities that come along with it is a great idea! You should enjoy being young without having to worry about things like pregnancy and deadly diseases.

However, if you decide to have sex, talk with your pediatrician about which type of birth control is best for you. When using condoms, *always* use latex condoms to prevent sexually transmitted diseases like chlamydia, herpes, and HIV (the AIDS virus). For more information on preventing pregnancy, ask your pediatrician about the AAP brochures "Deciding to Wait" and "Making the Right Choice: Facts for Teens on Preventing Pregnancy."

Learning to take care of yourself

As you get older, there will be many decisions that you will need to make to ensure that you stay healthy. Eating right, exercising, and getting enough rest are important during puberty because of all the changes your body is going through. It is also important to feel good about yourself and the decisions you make. You have to learn to care for your own body, work hard and maintain good health, and to like yourself as you are.

The information contained in this publication should not be used as a substitute for the medical care and advice of your pediatrician. There may be variations in treatment that your pediatrician may recommend based on individual facts and circumstances.

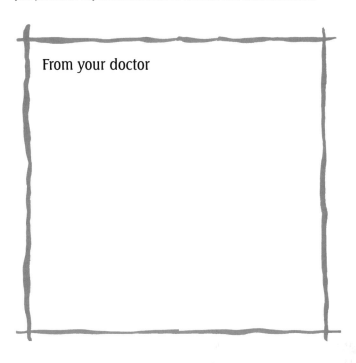

From your doctor

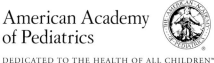

American Academy
of Pediatrics

DEDICATED TO THE HEALTH OF ALL CHILDREN™

The American Academy of Pediatrics is an organization of 55,000 primary care pediatricians, pediatric medical subspecialists, and pediatric surgical specialists dedicated to the health, safety, and well-being of infants, children, adolescents, and young adults.

American Academy of Pediatrics
PO Box 747
Elk Grove Village, IL 60009-0747
Web site — http://www.aap.org

Puberty
Information for Boys

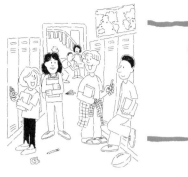

As part of growing up, you will go through puberty. Puberty is the time in your life when your body changes from that of a child to that of an adult. These changes are caused by chemicals in the body called hormones. Because there are so many changes that happen during puberty, you may feel like your body is out of control. In time, your hormones will balance out and your body will catch up.

Not only does your body change, but your emotions change too. How you think and feel about yourself, your family and friends, and your whole world, may seem different. As you go through puberty, you will begin to make important decisions for yourself, take on more responsibilities, and become more independent.

If you are already going through some of these changes, you may be asking yourself, "Am I normal?" or "Do other people my age feel the way I do?" Don't worry. Lots of changes happen during puberty and, although it can be a confusing time of life, it can be exciting.

This brochure was written to help you understand and deal with the changes puberty brings.

Information for Boys

Puberty for boys usually starts with a growth spurt at about 10 to 16 years of age. You may notice that you grow out of your clothes or shoes a lot faster than you used to. Don't worry, your hormones will balance out and your body will catch up.

How will my body change?

Following are some other changes you will notice during puberty:

Body size: Arms, legs, hands, and feet may grow faster than the rest of your body. Until the rest of your body catches up, you may feel a little clumsy.

Body shape: You will get taller and your shoulders will get broader. You will gain a lot of weight. During this time, many boys experience swelling under their nipples. This may cause them to worry that they are growing breasts. If you experience this, don't worry. It is common among boys your age and is a temporary condition. If you are worried about it, talk to your pediatrician.

During puberty, your muscles will also get bigger. Try not to rush this part of your growth. You may have friends who work out with weights and equipment to build up muscles, and you may want to begin this type of training yourself—often before your body is ready for it. If you are interested in these activities, talk to your pediatrician about a safe time for you to begin weight training.

Voice: Your voice will get deeper. This may start with voice cracking. As you continue to grow, the cracking will stop and your voice will stay at the lower range.

Hair: Hair will appear under your arms, on your legs and face, and above your penis. Chest hair may appear during puberty or years after, although not all men have chest hair. Some men shave the hair on their faces. There is no medical reason to shave, it is simply a personal choice. If you decide to shave, be sure to use shaving cream and a clean razor made for men. It is a good idea to use your own personal razor or electric shaver and not to share one with your family or friends.

Skin: Skin may get more oily and you may notice you sweat more. This is because your glands are growing too. It is important to wash every day to keep your skin clean and to use a deodorant or antiperspirant to keep odor and wetness under control. Despite your best efforts to keep your face clean, you still may get pimples. This is called acne and is normal during this time when your hormone levels are high. Almost all teenage boys get acne at one time or another. Whether your case is mild or severe, there are things you can do to keep it under control. For more information on controlling acne, talk to your pediatrician or see the AAP brochure "Acne Treatment and Control."

Penis: Your penis and testes will get larger. You may have erections more often due to an increase in sex hormones. Erections occur when the penis gets stiff and hard—sometimes for no reason. This is normal. Even though you may feel embarrassed, try to remember that most people will not even notice your erection unless you draw attention to it. Many boys become concerned about their penis size; a boy may compare his own penis size with that of his friends. It is important to remember that the size of a man's penis has nothing to do with his manliness or sexual functioning.

Your body will also begin to produce sperm during puberty. This means that during an erection, you may also experience ejaculation. This occurs when semen (made up of sperm and other fluids) is released through the penis. This could happen while you are sleeping. You might wake up to find your sheets or pajamas are wet. This is called a nocturnal emission or "wet dream." This is normal and will stop as you get older.

Emotional changes during puberty

In addition to the many physical changes you will go through during puberty, there are many emotional changes as well. You may start to care more about what other people think about you. You want to be accepted and liked. At this time in your life, your relationships with others may begin to change. Some become more important and some less so. You start to separate more from your parents and identify with others your age. You may begin to make decisions that could affect the rest of your life.

Many people your age feel self-conscious about their changing bodies— too tall, too short, too fat, too skinny. Because puberty causes so many changes, it is hard not to compare what is going on with your body with what is happening to your friends' bodies. Try to keep in mind that everyone goes through puberty differently. Eventually, everyone catches up.

Sex and growing up

During this time, you also become more aware of your sexuality. A look, touch, or just thinking about someone may make your heart beat faster and produce a warm, tingling feeling all over. This is completely normal. You may be asking yourself the following questions:

- "Is it okay to masturbate (touch your genitals for sexual pleasure)?"
- "When should I start dating?"
- "When is it okay to kiss?"
- "How far is too far?"
- "When will I be ready to have sexual intercourse?"
- "Will having sex help my relationship?"

Masturbation is normal and will not harm you. Many boys and girls masturbate, many do not.

Deciding to become sexually active can be very confusing. On one hand, you hear so many warnings and dangers about having sex. On the other hand, movies, TV, magazines, even billboards seem to be telling you that having sex is okay. The fact is, sex is a part of life and, like many parts of life, it can be good or bad. It all depends on you and the choices you make.

As you continue through puberty, you may experience pressure from many sources to have sex. Knowing where the pressures come from will make them much easier to deal with. Pressure to have sex may come from:

- **The media:** Because there are so many images in the media about sex, it is easy to get the idea that having sex is the right thing to do. Sex in movies, TV shows, magazines, and in music is often shown as not having any risks. Do not let these messages fool you. In real life, having sex can be very risky.
- **Your own body:** It is perfectly normal to be interested in sex. After all, growing sexually is what puberty is all about. The sexual urges you feel during puberty can be very powerful. What is most important is to stay in control of these feelings and not let them control you. Keep in mind that sex is not the only way to express how you feel about someone. Taking walks, talking, holding hands, hugging, and touching are great ways to be close to someone you have strong feelings for.
- **Your friends:** It may seem like "everybody's doing it" or that people who have sex are "cool." Maybe you feel like you should have sex to be popular and fit in with the group. However, people like to talk about sex and some may want others to believe that they are having sex even when they are not. Someone who does not want to be your friend just because you are not having sex is probably someone who is not worth being friends with any-way. Do not let friends—or anyone—talk you into having sex. This is a decision you make when it is right for you, not for your friends.

Deciding whether or not to have sexual intercourse is one of the most important decisions you will ever make. Why not take your time and think it through? Talk with your parents about their values. Waiting to have sexual intercourse until you are older, in a serious relationship, and able to accept the responsibilities that come along with it is a great idea! You should enjoy being young without having to worry about things like pregnancy and deadly diseases.

However, if you decide to have sex, talk with your pediatrician about which type of birth control is best for you. When using condoms, *always* use latex condoms to prevent sexually transmitted diseases like chlamydia, herpes, and HIV (the AIDS virus). For more information on preventing pregnancy, ask your pediatrician about the AAP brochures "Deciding to Wait" and "Making the Right Choice: Facts for Teens on Preventing Pregnancy."

Learning to take care of yourself

As you get older, there will be many decisions that you will need to make to ensure that you stay healthy. Eating right, exercising, and getting enough rest are important during puberty because of all the changes your body is going through. It is also important to feel good about yourself and the decisions you make. You have to learn to care for your own body, work hard and maintain good health, and to like yourself as you are.

The information contained in this publication should not be used as a substitute for the medical care and advice of your pediatrician. There may be variations in treatment that your pediatrician may recommend based on individual facts and circumstances.

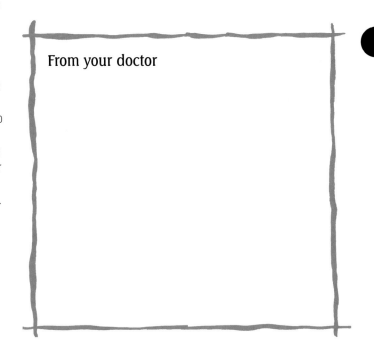

From your doctor

American Academy of Pediatrics

DEDICATED TO THE HEALTH OF ALL CHILDREN™

The American Academy of Pediatrics is an organization of 55,000 primary care pediatricians, pediatric medical subspecialists, and pediatric surgical specialists dedicated to the health, safety, and well-being of infants, children, adolescents, and young adults.

American Academy of Pediatrics
PO Box 747
Elk Grove Village, IL 60009-0747
Web site — http://www.aap.org

Copyright ©1996   American Academy of Pediatrics

The Risks of Tobacco Use:
A Message to Parents and Teens

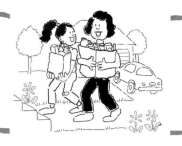

Many people think tobacco-related health problems affect only adults after a lifetime of smoking or tobacco use. Yet, children and teens suffer from tobacco-related health problems as well. The fact is tobacco use can affect every member of the family.

Infants and children

As a parent, you would never knowingly harm your child. Yet, if you are a smoker, the smoke from your cigarette, cigar, or pipe may be putting your child's health in danger. Environmental tobacco smoke, or ETS, is the smoke that is breathed out by a smoker. ETS also includes the smoke that comes from a burning cigarette, cigar, or pipe.

Exposure to ETS is a serious health threat to children. Children exposed to ETS have a greater risk of many health problems including:
- upper respiratory tract infections
- ear infections
- pneumonia
- bronchitis
- asthma
- long-term lung damage

Smoking and ETS are also dangerous to pregnant women and their unborn babies. They have been linked to low birth weight, delayed growth, miscarriage, and stillbirth. Recent studies have found that infants are at greater risk of dying from SIDS (sudden infant death syndrome) if exposed to ETS or if their mother was exposed to ETS during pregnancy.

For more information on ETS, ask your pediatrician about the brochure, *Environmental Tobacco Smoke: A Danger to Children* from the American Academy of Pediatrics.

Teenagers

Ninety percent of all smokers begin the habit during their teens. Over the past 10 years, the number of smokers has decreased in every age-group except teenagers. Among teens, the number of young women smokers has actually increased. Teenage smokers suffer from:
- addiction to nicotine
- long-term cough
- faster heart rate
- decreased lung function
- increased blood pressure
- decreased stamina
- increased risk of developing lung cancer
- increased respiratory tract infection

Smoking is a lifelong addiction that is often hard to break. It may also lead to other addictions and a poorer quality of life. Fighting the influence of the tobacco companies and convincing children not to use tobacco products is a tough task. Parents need to give teenagers the facts about the negative effects of smoking.

Smoking and the media

A big influence on a teen's decision to smoke is the media. Young people today are surrounded by images in the media that smoking is normal, desirable, and harmless. Tobacco companies spend billions of dollars every year promoting their products on TV, in movies and magazines, on billboards, and at sporting events. In fact, tobacco products are among the most advertised products in the nation. The tobacco companies hope to get back the profits they lose as older smokers die and as more and more adults quit smoking. As a result, young people are the primary targets of many of these ads.

Tobacco companies and advertisers never mention the harmful effects of smoking, such as bad breath, stained teeth, heart disease, and cancer. Most ads show smokers as healthy, energetic, sexy, and successful. Help your teenager understand the difference between these misleading messages in advertising and the truth about the dangers of smoking.

What parents can do:
- If you smoke or use tobacco, quit. Your actions will influence your child's behavior too.
- Talk about ads with your children. Help them to understand the real messages being conveyed.
- Teach your kids to be wary consumers.
- Make sure the TV shows and movies your child watches do not normalize or glamorize the use of tobacco.
- Do not allow your child to wear T-shirts, jackets, or hats that promote tobacco products.
- Talk to administrators at your teen's school about starting a media education program.

Adults

Smoking is the most preventable cause of death and disability in the United States. Consider the following facts:
- In this country, 350,000 deaths a year are related to tobacco use.
- One third of all deaths from cancer and heart disease are caused by smoking, chewing tobacco, or snuff.
- Three fourths of the deaths from chronic lung disease are related to tobacco.
- A nonsmoking spouse of a smoker has a 30% greater risk of lung cancer. This alone accounts for 2,000 deaths a year.
- Teenagers whose parents smoke are twice as likely to start smoking than children of nonsmokers.
- In 1964, 55% of adult Americans smoked cigarettes. By 1993, this percentage decreased to 25%. This shows that thousands of Americans have found a way to stop smoking. By doing so, they will live longer, feel better, and improve the health of their families.

Smokeless tobacco: not a safe choice!

The term "smokeless tobacco" refers to both chewing tobacco and snuff (also called "dip"). Chewing tobacco is a form of leaf tobacco. Snuff is finely ground tobacco. Both products lead to nicotine addiction because the nicotine is absorbed into the bloodstream. Smokeless tobacco products damage the lining of the mouth and throat and may cause mouth cancer, throat cancer, and gum disease.

Use of smokeless tobacco products also results in:

- stained teeth
- bad breath
- slow healing of mouth wounds
- lowered sense of taste and smell.

Tobacco companies have increased their advertising programs to promote smokeless tobacco products. Famous athletes often endorse these products, making them seem even more appealing to teenagers. As a result, the number of teenagers and young adults who are chewing tobacco is increasing. Parents need to oppose the use of smokeless tobacco. Inform your children of the serious side effects of its use. The facts on the health risks from smokeless tobacco make one thing very clear: IT IS NOT A SAFE CHOICE!

Break the habit

Would you like to join the growing numbers who have quit using tobacco? Have you tried in the past and failed, but would now like to try again? Why not ask your doctor for help? Your doctor may be just the person to help you find an effective stop-smoking program. For more information, contact any of the following organizations:

American Cancer Society:
1-800/ACS-2345
Web site: www.cancer.org

American Heart Association:
1-800/242-8721
Web site: www.americanheart.org

American Lung Association:
1-800/586-4872
Web site: www.lungusa.org

Your pediatrician understands that good communication between parents and children is one of the best ways to prevent drug use. If talking with your child about tobacco use is difficult, your pediatrician may be able to help open the lines of communication. If you suspect your child is smoking cigarettes or cigars, chewing tobacco, or using any other drug, rely on your pediatrician for advice and help.

The information contained in this publication should not be used as a substitute for the medical care and advice of your pediatrician. There may be variations in treatment that your pediatrician may recommend based on individual facts and circumstances.

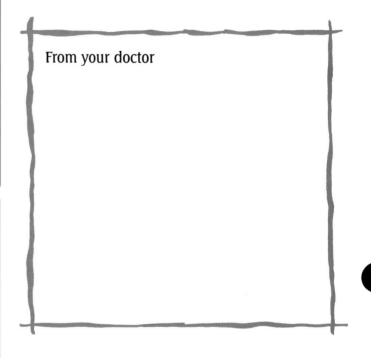

From your doctor

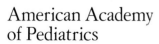

American Academy of Pediatrics

DEDICATED TO THE HEALTH OF ALL CHILDREN™

The American Academy of Pediatrics is an organization of 55,000 primary care pediatricians, pediatric medical subspecialists, and pediatric surgical specialists dedicated to the health, safety, and well-being of infants, children, adolescents, and young adults.

American Academy of Pediatrics
PO Box 747
Elk Grove Village, IL 60009-0747
Web site — http://www.aap.org

School Health Centers and Your Child

School health centers are becoming more and more common. Most handle medical emergencies, provide health screenings and refer students to doctors for health problems. A growing number of these centers also offer health services such as immunizations and physical examinations. Therapies for children with special needs may also be available.

School health centers can provide important health care to students who need it. However, it is important that your child's pediatrician stay involved in that care. While school-based centers are convenient, your child's own pediatrician remains his or her best source for health supervision and medical care.

Many parents assume that because a school health clinic and the regular school health office exist side-by-side, that they communicate and work together well. Unfortunately this is not always what occurs. Parents need to stay involved.

What you can do:

- Make sure that your child's school nurse, counselor or health center staff routinely contact your pediatrician about his medical care.
- Check with your school's regular health office and your school's clinic to be sure that they work together. Give them permission to exchange health information that is important for keeping your child healthy in school. Be certain that they keep you informed.
- Continue to take your child to his pediatrician for regular preventive health care. This is important even if he or she has many of his or her health needs met at school.
- Stay involved in the health education, the health services and the supervision that your child receives at school.

Your Child Needs A Medical Home

All children and teens need a "medical home." This means health care that is available 24 hours a day, 7 days a week. This care is coordinated by one team of pediatric health care professionals.

A medical home is family centered. Your pediatrician knows you and your child. Mutual trust develops.

When your child or teen has a medical home, she or he receives ongoing medical care. Care is provided based on your child's medical history. If she or he graduates or transfers to another school, her or his medical home remains the same.

Signs of a Good School Health Program

- The staff works in partnership with other community health and social service programs.
- Students and parents sit on its administrative board. This board makes group decisions about the health care that is provided.
- The center helps students who do not have a medical home find one.
- The center assists in arranging health insurance for students who need it.
- It is easily accessible for all students.
- It provides quality health care that focuses on the long-term needs of each student.

This information is based on the American Academy of Pediatrics' policy statement School Health Centers and Other Integrated School Health Services, published in January 2001. Parent Pages offers parents relevant facts that explain current policies about children's health.

The information contained in this publication should not be used as a substitute for the medical care and advice of your pediatrician. There may be variations in treatment that your pediatrician may recommend based on individual facts and circumstances.

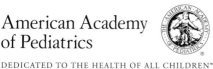

American Academy of Pediatrics

DEDICATED TO THE HEALTH OF ALL CHILDREN™

The American Academy of Pediatrics is an organization of 55,000 primary care pediatricians, pediatric medical subspecialists, and pediatric surgical specialists dedicated to the health, safety, and well-being of infants, children, adolescents, and young adults.

American Academy of Pediatrics
PO Box 747
Elk Grove Village, IL 60009-0747
Web site — http://www.aap.org

Smokeless Tobacco
Guidelines for Teens

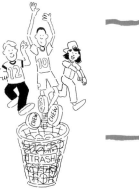

What is smokeless tobacco?

There are two forms of smokeless tobacco: chewing tobacco and snuff. Chewing tobacco is usually sold as leaf tobacco (packaged in a pouch) or plug tobacco (in brick form) that is put between the cheek and gum. Users keep chewing tobacco in their mouths for several hours to get a continuous buzz from the nicotine in the tobacco.

Snuff is a powdered tobacco (usually sold in cans) that is put between the lower lip and gum. Just a pinch is all that is needed to release the nicotine, which is then swiftly absorbed into the bloodstream, resulting in a quick high. Sounds harmless, right? Keep reading . . .

What is in smokeless tobacco?

Chemicals. Keep in mind that the smokeless tobacco you or your friends are using contains many chemicals that can be harmful to your health. Here are a few of the ingredients found in smokeless tobacco:
- Nicotine (addictive drug)
- Polonium 210 (nuclear waste)
- Cadmium (used in car batteries)
- N-Nitrosamines (cancer-causing)
- Lead (poison)
- Formaldehyde (embalming fluid)

The nicotine contained in smokeless tobacco is what gives the user a buzz. It also makes it very hard to quit. Why? Because every time you use smokeless tobacco your body gets used to the nicotine; it actually starts to crave it. Craving is one of the signs of addiction, or dependence.

Your body also adjusts to the amount of tobacco you need to chew to get a buzz. Pretty soon you will need a little more tobacco to get the same feeling. This process is called tolerance, which is another sign of addiction.

Some people say smokeless tobacco is okay because there is no smoke like a cigarette has. Do not believe them. It is not a safe alternative to smoking. You just move health problems from your lungs to your mouth.

Physical and mental effects of smokeless tobacco

If you use smokeless tobacco, here is what you might have to look forward to:
- **Cancer.** Cancer of the mouth (including the lip, tongue, and cheek) and throat. Cancers usually occur at the spot in the mouth where the tobacco is held. The surgery for cancer of the mouth could lead to removal of parts of your face, tongue, cheek, or lip.
- **Leukoplakia.** When you hold tobacco in one place in your mouth, your mouth becomes irritated by the tobacco juice. This causes a white, leathery-like patch to form, and this is called leukoplakia. These patches can be different in size, shape, and appearance. They are also considered precancerous: If you find one in your mouth, see your doctor immediately.

- **Heart Disease.** The constant flow of nicotine into your body causes many side effects including increased heart rate, increased blood pressure, and sometimes irregular heart beats. Nicotine in the body also causes constricted blood vessels that can slow down reaction time and cause dizziness—not a good move if you play sports.
- **Gum and Tooth Disease.** Smokeless tobacco permanently discolors teeth. Chewing tobacco causes halitosis (BAD BREATH). Its direct and repeated contact with the gums cause them to recede, which can cause your teeth to become loose. Smokeless tobacco contains a lot of sugar which, when mixed with the plaque on your teeth, forms acid that eats away at tooth enamel and causes cavities and chronic painful sores.
- **Social Effects.** Having really bad breath, discolored teeth, and gunk stuck in your teeth and constant spitting can have a very negative effect on your social life.

What if I want to quit?

You have just read the bad news, but here is the good news. Even though it is very difficult to quit chewing tobacco, it can be done. Read the following Tips to Quit for some helpful ideas to kick the habit. Remember, most people do not start chewing on their own, so do not try quitting on your own. Ask for help and positive reinforcement from your doctor, friends, parents, coaches, teachers, whomever . . .

Check for early warning signs of oral cancer

Check your mouth often, looking closely at the places where you hold the tobacco. See your doctor right away if you have any of the following:
- a sore that bleeds easily and does not heal
- a lump or thickening anywhere in your mouth or neck
- soreness or swelling that does not go away
- a red or white patch that does not go away
- trouble chewing, swallowing, or moving your tongue or jaw

Even if you do not find a problem today, if you are still using smokeless tobacco be sure to have your mouth checked at every routine doctor or dentist visit. Your chances for a cure are higher if oral cancer is found early.

Tips to Quit

Many smokeless tobacco users say it is even harder to quit smokeless tobacco than cigarettes. Chewing tobacco and snuff contain nicotine and are addictive. A recent study showed that the amount of nicotine in the bloodstream was actually twice as great for smokeless tobacco as for cigarettes. Trying to quit can be difficult, but not impossible. Here are some tips to spit it out and keep it out!

1. **Think of reasons why you want to quit.** You may want to quit because:
   - You do not like having bad breath after chewing and dipping.
   - You do not want stained teeth.
   - You do not want to risk getting cancer.
   - You do not like being addicted to nicotine.
   - You want to start leading a healthier life.
   - The people around you find it offensive.
   - You do not want to waste your money.

2. **Pick a quit date and throw out all your chewing tobacco and snuff.**

3. **Ask your friends, family, teachers, and coaches to help you kick the habit by giving you support and encouragement.** Tell friends not to offer you smokeless tobacco. You may want to ask a friend to quit with you.

4. **Ask your doctor about a tobacco quitting program.** These include nicotine chewing gum, a nicotine patch you wear on your arm (if you are old enough), and special support groups.

5. **Find alternatives to smokeless tobacco.** A few good examples are sugarless gum, pumpkin or sunflower seeds, or apple slices.

6. **Find activities to keep your mind off of smokeless tobacco.** You could work on a hobby, listen to music, or talk to a friend. Getting into exercise, such as bike riding, running, in-line skating, or cross-country skiing, also can help relieve any tension caused by quitting.

7. **Remember that everyone is different, so develop a personalized plan that works best for you.** Set realistic goals so you will be more likely to achieve them.

8. **Reward yourself.** You could save the money that would have been spent on smokeless tobacco and buy something nice for yourself.

The information contained in this publication should not be used as a substitute for the medical care and advice of your pediatrician. There may be variations in treatment that your pediatrician may recommend based on individual facts and circumstances.

From your doctor

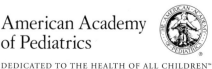
American Academy of Pediatrics

DEDICATED TO THE HEALTH OF ALL CHILDREN™

The American Academy of Pediatrics is an organization of 55,000 primary care pediatricians, pediatric medical subspecialists, and pediatric surgical specialists dedicated to the health, safety, and well-being of infants, children, adolescents, and young adults.

American Academy of Pediatrics
PO Box 747
Elk Grove Village, IL 60009-0747
Web site — http://www.aap.org

Smoking:
Straight Talk for Teens

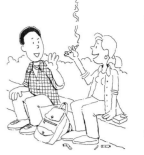

Have you ever tried smoking? Maybe your friends who smoke gave you a cigarette or cigar.Maybe you thought it would be cool. Yet your first puff was probably not pleasant. You coughed and your throat burned. You might have felt sick to your stomach or dizzy. These reactions make sense when you think about what smoking does to your body.

Most Teens Don't Smoke

The good news is that about 80% of teenagers in the United States don't smoke. They have made a healthy choice. However, consider the following facts:

- Nearly 90% of all smokers started when they were teenagers.
- Today, 4.5 million young people, aged 12-17, smoke. Another 3,000 start smoking every day—more than 1 million teens each year.
- One third of these new smokers will eventually die of smoking-related diseases.
- Young people are more likely to smoke if they live with someone who smokes.
- Today, the smoking rates for high school seniors is at a 17-year high. Though the numbers are surprising, perhaps the most important fact is that most American teenagers choose not to smoke.

Smoking Harms the Body

The chemicals in cigarettes and cigars can cause a lot of damage to the body. They reduce the amount of oxygen delivered to your body. They harm the lungs by damaging the tiny hairs (called cilia) that help sweep out dirt and waste products. This leads to that annoying "smoker's" cough. Depending on how much you smoke, your lungs become gray and "dirty," instead of pink and healthy.

Nicotine, a drug contained in tobacco, causes the heart to beat faster and work less effectively. This is not only bad for your health, but can also lead to poor athletic performance. This is why coaches tell athletes not to smoke. Athletes who smoke cannot run or swim as well as nonsmoking athletes because the carbon monoxide in tobacco smoke robs the body of oxygen.

Early warning signs that smoking is harming you include:

- dizziness
- coughing
- burning of the eyes, nose, and throat

Tobacco Is a Killer

The nicotine in tobacco is extremely toxic. A few drops of pure nicotine, if taken all at once, are enough to kill the average person. Smokers take nicotine in small amounts, allowing the body time to break down the nicotine and get rid of it, which is why cigarettes don't kill instantly.

Each time you take a puff on a cigarette, you also inhale over 4,000 other chemicals. Of these chemicals, 400 are toxic and about 40 are known to cause cancer. Some of the chemicals found in cigarette smoke include:

- cyanide (a deadly poison)
- benzene (used in making paints, dyes, and plastics)
- formaldehyde (embalming fluid)
- acetylene (fuel used in torches)
- ammonia (used in fertilizers)
- carbon monoxide (poisonous gas)

In the long run, your body pays a heavy price for smoking:

- Smokers get **cancer**. Smokers are more than 10 times as likely to die of lung cancer than nonsmokers. The odds are higher for people who smoke a lot, smoke for many years, and/or inhale deeply.
- Smoking doubles the chances of **heart disease.**
- Smoking is the main cause of **chronic bronchitis,** a serious disease of the airways to the lung, and **emphysema,** a crippling disease of the lung. The earlier a person starts smoking, the greater the risk of these diseases.
- Smoking by pregnant women increases the **risks of premature birth, underweight babies, and infant deaths.**
- Smoking **harms nonsmokers** as well as smokers. When nonsmokers are around people who smoke, they absorb nicotine, carbon monoxide, and other ingredients of tobacco smoke just as smokers do. This is called "passive smoking."

Young children who are exposed to smoking are more likely to suffer from upper respiratory tract problems, *otitis media* (chronic inflammation of the middle ear), and asthma. Adult nonsmokers who are exposed can suffer from a variety of problems. They are more likely than other people to develop upper respiratory tract and lung infections, heart disease, and cancer.

Smoking Is Addictive

It takes only a short time for users of cigarettes and cigars to become addicted to nicotine. If you are a smoker, you will know you are addicted when you find yourself craving cigarettes and feeling nervous without them. You will really know you are addicted when you try to quit smoking and have trouble doing it.

Quitting can be hard and it can take a long time. Often people try several times before they succeed. The longer you smoke, the harder it is to stop.

Smoking Is Ugly

Studies show that smoking is harmful to health. You know that. But did you ever think about how smoking affects your looks and how people relate to you? Think about this:

- Smoking causes bad breath and stained teeth.
- Smoking often makes other people not want to be around you.
- Even if you don't smoke, you might smell like smoke after being near someone who does.
- In one study, 78% of boys, aged 12 to 17, said they don't want to date someone who smokes. In the same study, 69% of girls said they would rather date someone who doesn't smoke.

As one teenage girl put it, "Kissing a boy who smokes is like kissing a dirty ashtray."

Smoking Is Expensive

The cost of smoking adds up. Do the math: if a pack of cigarettes costs $2.50 and you smoke a pack a day, you are spending over $900 a year just on cigarettes instead of on CDs, clothes, or saving for a car.

Smoking also costs you a lot in other ways—getting sick, missing school or work, and having increased medical bills. That's a high price to pay for something that isn't good for you in the first place.

Chewing Tobacco and Snuff Are Also Harmful

Tobacco is not only found in cigarettes and cigars. Chewing tobacco and snuff ("dip") are also dangerous to health. Smokeless tobacco can cause cancer, especially in the cheeks, gums, and throat. These substances also lead to a decreased sense of taste and smell. Users run the risk of getting gum disease, which can lead to loss of teeth.

Immediately after using smokeless tobacco, the gums and lips can sting, crack, bleed, and wrinkle. Sores and white patches may appear. Mouth wounds in people who use smokeless tobacco take longer to heal.

Smoking and the Media

Young people today are surrounded by messages in the media that smoking is normal, desirable, and harmless. Tobacco companies spend billions of dollars every year promoting their products on TV, in movies and magazines, on billboards, and at sporting events. In fact, tobacco products are among the most advertised products in the nation. If you are a teenager, you are one of the primary targets of many of these ads.

Tobacco companies and advertisers never mention the harmful effects of smoking, such as bad breath, stained teeth, heart disease, and cancer. Most ads falsely show smokers as healthy, energetic, sexy, and successful. It's important to understand the difference between the misleading messages in advertising and the truth about the dangers of smoking.

The fact is, tobacco companies need 3,000 new smokers every day to make up for the 400,000 people who die each year from tobacco-related diseases. Don't fall for the tobacco companies' tricks.

There Is Help

Quitting is possible, and is a must if you want the best for yourself and those around you. Many young people think they are not at risk from smoking. They tell themselves, "I won't smoke forever" or "I can quit any time." However, if you ignore warning signs and continue to smoke, your body will change. It will get used to the smoke. You won't cough or feel sick every time you puff on a cigarette. Yet the damage to your body continues and worsens each time you smoke.

In order to quit, you'll need support from your family and friends. Try again if you don't succeed the first time. Deciding to stop is up to you. Once you make that commitment, you can get help from your pediatrician or school health office. For more information, visit the Web site of the American Academy of Pediatrics at **www.aap.org** or contact any of the following organizations:

American Cancer Society:
1-800-ACS-2345/Web site: www.cancer.org

American Heart Association:
1-800-242-8721/Web site: www.americanheart.org

American Lung Association:
1-800-586-4872/Web site: www.lungusa.org

Campaign for Tobacco-Free Kids:
1-800-284-KIDS/Web site: www.tobaccofreekids.org

The information contained in this publication should not be used as a substitute for the medical care and advice of your pediatrician. There may be variations in treatment that your pediatrician may recommend based on individual facts and circumstances.

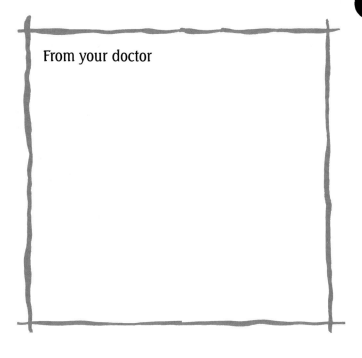

From your doctor

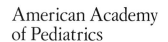

American Academy of Pediatrics

DEDICATED TO THE HEALTH OF ALL CHILDREN™

The American Academy of Pediatrics is an organization of 55,000 primary care pediatricians, pediatric medical subspecialists, and pediatric surgical specialists dedicated to the health, safety, and well-being of infants, children, adolescents, and young adults.

American Academy of Pediatrics
PO Box 747
Elk Grove Village, IL 60009-0747
Web site — http://www.aap.org

Steroids:
Play Safe, Play Fair

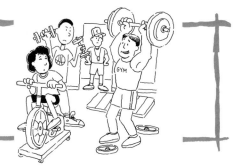

Athletes, whether they are young or old, professional or amateur, are always looking to gain an advantage over their opponents. The desire for an "edge" exists in all sports, at all levels of play. Successful athletes rely on practice and hard work to increase their skill, speed, power, and ability. However, some athletes resort to drugs to improve their performance on the field or the court.

Some high school and even middle school students are using steroids to gain an edge, improve their skill level, or become more athletic. Steroid use is not limited to males. More and more females are putting themselves at risk by using these drugs. It is important to know that using anabolic steroids not only is illegal, but it also can have serious side effects.

What are steroids?

You may have heard them called 'roids, juice, hype, or pump. Anabolic steroids are powerful drugs that many people take in high doses to boost athletic performance. Anabolic means "building body tissue." *Anabolic* steroids help build muscle tissue and increase body mass by acting like the body's natural male hormone, testosterone.

Lower doses of anabolic steroids sometimes are used to treat a handful of very serious medical conditions. They should not be confused with corticosteroids, which are used to treat common medical conditions such as asthma and arthritis. *Corticosteroids* are strong medications, but do not have muscle-building effects. Anabolic steroids are the ones abused by athletes and others who want a shortcut to becoming bigger and stronger.

Who uses steroids?

In the past, steroid use was seen mostly in college, Olympic, and professional sports. Today, steroids are being used by athletes as well as nonathletes, in high schools and middle schools. Most major professional and amateur athletic organizations have banned steroids for use by their athletes. These organizations include the International Olympic Committee, National Collegiate Athletic Association (NCAA), and the National Football League (NFL).

Most commonly, steroid use can be found among the following groups:
- Athletes involved in sports that rely on strength and size, like football, wrestling, or baseball
- Endurance athletes, such as those involved in track-and-field and swimming
- Athletes involved in weight training or bodybuilding
- Anyone interested in building and defining muscles

How are steroids used?

Steroids can be taken in the following two ways:
- By mouth (pills)
- Injected with a needle (Athletes who share needles to inject steroids also are at risk for serious infections including Hepatitis B and HIV, the AIDS virus.)

Some athletes take even higher doses, called "megadoses," to produce faster results. Others gradually increase the amount they take over time, which is called "pyramiding." Taking different kinds of anabolic steroids, possibly along with other drugs, is a particularly dangerous practice known as "stacking."

Will steroids make me a better athlete?

No. Steroids *cannot* improve an athlete's agility or skill. Many factors help determine athletic ability, including genetics, body size, age, sex, diet, and how hard the athlete trains. It is clear that the medical dangers of steroid use far outweigh the advantage of gains in strength or muscle mass.

What are the side effects of steroids?

Steroids can cause serious health problems. Many changes take place inside the body and may not be noticed until it is too late. Some of the effects will go away when steroid use stops, but some may not.

For both sexes

Possible side effects for males and females include the following:
- High blood pressure and heart disease
- Liver damage and cancers
- Stroke and blood clots
- Urinary and bowel problems, such as diarrhea
- Headaches, aching joints, and muscle cramps
- Nausea and vomiting
- Sleep problems
- Increased risk of ligament and tendon injuries
- Severe acne, especially on face and back
- Baldness

A special danger to adolescents

High school and middle school students and athletes need to be aware of the effect steroids have on growth. Anabolic steroids, even in small doses, have been shown to stop growth too soon. Adolescents also may be at risk for becoming dependent on steroids. Adolescents who use steroids are also more likely to use other addictive drugs and alcohol.

Males

One of the more disturbing effects of steroid use for males is that the body begins to produce less of its own testosterone. As a result, the testicles may begin to shrink. Following is a list of some of the other effects of steroid use for males:

- Reduced sperm count
- Impotence
- Increase in nipple and breast size (gynecomastia)
- Enlarged prostate (gland that mixes fluid with sperm to form semen)

Females

Since steroids act as a male hormone, females may experience the following side effects:

- Reduced breast size
- Enlarged clitoris (a very sensitive part of the genitals)
- Increase in facial and body hair
- Deepened voice
- Menstrual problems

A word about...supplements

Over-the-counter supplements such as creatine and androstenedione ("andro") are gaining popularity. Though these supplements are not steroids, manufacturers claim they can build muscles, and improve strength and stamina, without the side effects of steroids.

It is important to know that these substances are not regulated by the Food and Drug Administration (FDA) and are not held to the same strict standards as drugs. Like steroids, they are also banned by the NFL, NCAA, and International Olympic Committee.

Although both creatine and androstenedione occur naturally in foods, there are serious concerns about the long-term effects of using them as supplements. These products may be unsafe. Remember, there is no replacement for a healthy diet, proper training, and practice.

Emotional effects

Steroids also can have the following effects on the mind and behavior:

- "Roid rage"—severe, aggressive behavior that may result in violence, such as fighting or destroying property
- Severe mood swings
- Hallucinations—seeing or hearing things that are not really there
- Paranoia—extreme feelings of mistrust and fear
- Anxiety and panic attacks
- Depression and thoughts of suicide
- An angry, hostile, or irritable mood

Play safe, play fair

Success in sports takes talent, skill, and most of all, practice and hard work. Using steroids is a form of cheating and interferes with fair competition. More importantly, they are dangerous to your health. There are many healthy ways to increase your strength or improve your appearance. If you are serious about your sport and your health, keep the following tips in mind:

- Train safely, without using drugs.
- Eat a healthy diet.
- Get plenty of rest.
- Set realistic goals and be proud of yourself when you reach them.
- Seek out training supervision, coaching,and advice from a reliable professional.
- Avoid injuries by playing safely and using protective gear.
- Talk to your pediatrician about nutrition, your health, preventing injury, and safe ways to gain strength.

If you, your friends, or teammates are using steroids, get help. Share this information with friends and teammates. Take a stand against the use of steroids and other drugs. Truly successful athletes combine their natural abilities with hard work to win. There is no quick and easy way to become the best.

For more information, contact the following organizations:

National Institute on Drug Abuse (NIDA)
888/644-6432
Web site: http://www.nida.nih.gov/

National Clearinghouse for Alcohol and Drug Information (NCADI)
800/729-6686
Web site: http://www.health.org

The information contained in this publication should not be used as a substitute for the medical care and advice of your pediatrician. There may be variations in treatment that your pediatrician may recommend based on individual facts and circumstances.

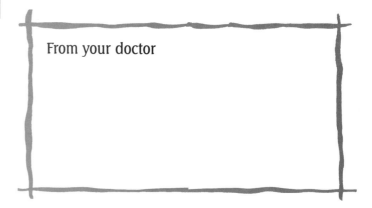

From your doctor

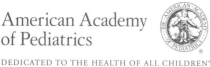

American Academy of Pediatrics

DEDICATED TO THE HEALTH OF ALL CHILDREN™

The American Academy of Pediatrics is an organization of 55,000 primary care pediatricians, pediatric medical subspecialists, and pediatric surgical specialists dedicated to the health, safety, and well-being of infants, children, adolescents, and young adults.

American Academy of Pediatrics
PO Box 747
Elk Grove Village, IL 60009-0747
Web site — http://www.aap.org

Substance Abuse Prevention

Part I What Every Parent Needs to Know

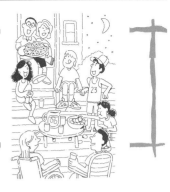

The use of tobacco, alcohol, and other drugs is one of the biggest problems facing young people today. This brochure is designed to help parents prevent some of these problems. Your pediatrician cares very much about your family, and wants to help if there are problems in any area—especially if you have concerns about substance abuse.

Prevention starts with parents

There are no guarantees that your child will not choose to use drugs, but as a parent, you can influence that decision by:

- not using drugs yourself
- providing guidance and clear rules about not using drugs
- spending time with your child sharing the good and the bad times

All of these are necessary to help your child grow up free from the problems of drug use.

Ask yourself a few questions

Much of what children learn about drugs comes from parents. Take a few minutes to answer the following questions about your feelings and behaviors about tobacco, alcohol, and other drugs.

- Do you usually offer alcoholic drinks to friends and family when they come to your home?
- Do you frequently take medicine for minor aches and pains or if you are feeling sad or nervous?
- Do you take sleeping pills to fall asleep?
- Do you use alcohol or any other drug in a way that you would not want your child to?
- Do you smoke cigarettes?
- Are you proud about how much you can drink?
- Do you make jokes about getting drunk or using drugs?
- Do you go to parties that involve a lot of drinking?
- Do you drink and drive or ride with drivers who have been drinking?
- Has your child ever seen you drunk?
- Do you let minors drink alcohol in your home?

Teach your child to say no

Tell your child exactly how you expect her to respond if someone offers her drugs:

- Ask questions ("What is it?" "Where did you get it?")
- Say no firmly.
- Give reasons ("No thanks, I'm not into that.")
- Suggest other things to do (go to a movie, the mall, or play a game)
- Leave (go home, go to class, join other friends)

Parents can also help their children choose not to use tobacco, alcohol, and other drugs in these ways:

- Build your child's self-esteem with praise and support for decisions. A strong sense of self-worth will help your child to say no to tobacco, alcohol, and other drugs and mean it.
- Gradually allow your child to make more decisions alone. Making a few mistakes is a normal part of growing up, so try not to be too critical when your child makes a mistake.
- Listen to what your child says. Pay attention, and be helpful during periods of loneliness or doubt.
- Offer advice about handling strong emotions and feelings. Help your child cope with emotions by letting her know that feelings will change. Explain that mood swings are not really bad, and they won't last forever. Model how to control mental pain or tension without the use of tobacco, alcohol, or other drugs.
- Plan to discuss a wide variety of topics with your child including alcohol, tobacco, and other drugs and the need for peer-group acceptance. Young people who don't know the facts about tobacco, alcohol, and other drugs are at greater risk of trying them.
- Encourage fun and worthwhile outside things to do; avoid turning too much of your child's leisure time into chores.
- Be a good role model by avoiding tobacco, alcohol, or other drugs yourself. You're the best role model for your child. Make a stand against drug issues—your child will listen.

Your pediatrician understands that good communication between parents and children is one of the best ways to prevent drug use. If talking to your child becomes a problem, your pediatrician may provide the key to opening the lines of communication.

Parents guide to teenage parties

If your teen is giving a party:

- **Plan in advance.** Go over party plans with your teen. Encourage your teen to plan some organized group activities or games.
- **Keep parties small.** 10 to 15 teens for each adult. Make sure at least one adult is present at all times. Ask other parents to come over to help you if you need it.
- **Set a guest list.** The party should be for invited guests only. No "crashers" allowed. This will help avoid the "open party" situation.
- **Set a time limit.** Set starting and ending times for the party. Check local curfew laws to determine an ending time.

- **Set party "rules."** Discuss them with your teen before the party. Rules should include the following:
  - ✓ No tobacco, alcohol, or other drugs.
  - ✓ No one can leave the party and then return.
  - ✓ Lights are left on at all times.
  - ✓ Certain rooms of the house are off-limits.
- **Know your responsibilities.** Remember, you are legally responsible for anything that happens to a minor who has been served alcohol or other drugs in your home. Help your child feel responsible for this as well. Guests who bring tobacco, alcohol, or other drugs to the party should be asked to leave. Be ready to call the parents of anyone who comes to the party intoxicated to make sure they get safely home.
- **Be there, but not square.** Pick out a spot where you can see what is going on without being in the way. You can also help serve snacks and beverages.

If your teen is going to a party:

- **Call the host's parent** to verify the party and offer any help. Make sure a parent will be at the party and that tobacco, alcohol, and other drugs will not be allowed.
- **Know where your child is going.** Have the phone number and address of the party. Ask your teen to call you if the location of the party changes. Be sure to let your child know where you will be during the party.
- **Make sure your teen has a way to get home from the party**. Make it easy for your child to leave a party by making it clear that he can call at any time for a ride home. Discuss why he might need to make such a call. Remind your teen NEVER to ride home with a driver who has been drinking.
- **Be up to greet your child when he comes home.** This can be a good way to check the time and talk about the evening.

Talk to your teen about safe partying

Maybe your teen has been to parties where there were tobacco, alcohol, and other drugs. Maybe he tried them. Maybe after using them your teen did something stupid, something he wouldn't normally do.

It's hard for people to stay safe when they aren't thinking clearly. How can teens keep a clear head and still have fun? Give them the following suggestions for staying safe while having a good time:

- Hang out with people who don't smoke, drink, or use other drugs.
- Plan not to smoke, drink, or use other drugs. Do whatever it takes to help you remember.
- Use the "buddy system"—team up with a friend. Use a code word to remind each other when it's time to leave a party.
- If your teen likes to meet new people, suggest trying some of the following activities instead of parties:

free concerts	dances
espresso bars	museums
extra-curricular "anythings"	community centers
libraries	sports events
religious activities	film festivals
athletic clubs	volunteer work

How can I tell if my child is doing drugs?

Despite your best efforts, your teen may still abuse drugs. Some warning signs of drug use are:

- Smell of alcohol, smoke, or other chemicals on your child's breath or clothing
- Obvious intoxication, dizziness, or bizarre behavior
- Change in dress, appearance, and grooming
- Change in choice of friends
- Frequent arguments, sudden mood changes, and unexplained violent actions
- Change in eating and sleeping patterns
- Skipping school
- Failing grades
- Runaway and delinquent behavior
- Suicide attempts

How parents can help

As you read this brochure, you may be worried that your child is using tobacco, alcohol, or other drugs. Before you confront your child, consider talking to friends, relatives, teachers, employers, and others who know your child. Get their impressions as to how she is doing. If others are concerned, this may make you more comfortable in your decision to talk to your child. Always choose a time when your child is awake, alert, and receptive to talking. Avoid interruptions, maintain privacy, and keep your wits about you. Go over the checklist with your child, highlighting those concerns that have you worried.

Send loving messages, for example:

- "I love you too much to let you hurt yourself."
- "I know other people your age use drugs, but I can't let you continue to behave this way."
- "We'll do anything we can to help you. If tobacco, alcohol, or other drugs are part of the problem, we must talk about it right away."
- "If you are sad, upset, or mad, we want to help you. But our family will not permit any use of tobacco, alcohol, or other drugs."

Don't be critical (avoid these statements):

- "There's only one reason you could be acting this way—you must be on drugs."
- "Don't think you are fooling me. I know what you are doing."
- "How could you be so stupid as to start using drugs and alcohol?"
- "How could you do this to our family?"
- "Where did I go wrong? What did I do to make you start using tobacco, alcohol, and other drugs?"

Remember, if your child is using drugs, she needs your help. Don't be afraid to be a strong parent! However, the problem could become too much for you to handle alone. Don't hesitate to seek professional help, such as your pediatrician, a counselor, support group, or treatment program.

The information contained in this publication should not be used as a substitute for the medical care and advice of your pediatrician. There may be variations in treatment that your pediatrician may recommend based on individual facts and circumstances.

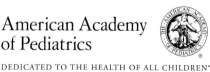

American Academy of Pediatrics

DEDICATED TO THE HEALTH OF ALL CHILDREN™

The American Academy of Pediatrics is an organization of 55,000 primary care pediatricians, pediatric medical subspecialists, and pediatric surgical specialists dedicated to the health, safety, and well-being of infants, children, adolescents, and young adults.

American Academy of Pediatrics
PO Box 747
Elk Grove Village, IL 60009-0747
Web site — http://www.aap.org

Substance Abuse Prevention

Part II Additional Information

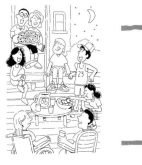

First a child needs roots to grow...then wings to fly

As a parent you can do a lot to prevent your child from using drugs. Use the following tips to help guide your child's thoughts and behaviors about drugs:

1. **Talk with your child honestly.** Don't wait to have "the drug talk" with your child. Make discussions about tobacco, alcohol, and other drugs part of your daily conversation. Know the facts about how drugs can harm your child. Clear up any wrong information, such as "everybody drinks" or "marijuana won't hurt you." Be clear about family rules for use of tobacco, alcohol, and other drugs.

2. **Really listen to your child.** Encourage your child to share questions and concerns about tobacco, alcohol, and other drugs. Do not do all the talking or give long lectures.

3. **Help your child develop self-confidence.** Look for all the good things in your child—and then tell your child how proud you are. If you need to correct your child, criticize the action, not your child. Praise your child's efforts as well as successes.

4. **Help your child develop strong values.** Talk about your family values. Teach your child how to make decisions based on these standards of right and wrong. Explain that these are the standards for your family, no matter what other families might decide.

5. **Be a good example.** Look at your own habits and thoughts about tobacco, alcohol, and other drugs. Your actions speak louder than words.

6. **Help your child deal with peer pressure and acceptance.** Discuss the importance of being an individual and the meaning of real friendships. Help your child to understand that he does not have to do something wrong just to feel accepted. Remind your child that a real friend won't care if he does not use tobacco, alcohol, and other drugs.

7. **Make family rules that help your child say "no."** Talk with your child about your expectation that he will say "no" to drugs. Spell out what will happen if he breaks these rules. (For example, "My parents said I can't use the car if I drink.") Be prepared to follow through, if necessary.

8. **Encourage healthy, creative activities.** Look for ways to get your child involved in athletics, hobbies, school clubs, and other activities that reduce boredom and excess free time. Encourage positive friendships and interests. Look for activities that you and your child can do together.

9. **Team up with other parents.** Work with other parents to build a drug-free environment for children. When parents join together against drug use, they are much more effective than when they act alone. One way is to form a parent group with the parents of your child's friends. The best way to stop a child from using drugs is to stop his friends from using them too.

10. **Know what to do if your child has a drug problem.** Realize that no child is immune to drugs. Learn the signs of drug use. Take seriously any concerns you hear from friends, teachers, or other kids about your child's possible drug use. Trust your instincts. If you truly feel that something is wrong with your child, it probably is. If there's a problem, seek professional help.

Tobacco, alcohol, and the media

A big influence on a teen's decision to use tobacco or alcohol is the media. Young people today are surrounded by messages in the media that smoking cigarettes, using smokeless tobacco, and drinking alcohol are normal, desirable, and harmless. Alcohol and tobacco companies spend billions of dollars every year promoting their products on TV, in movies and magazines, on billboards, and at sporting events. In fact, tobacco and alcohol products are among the most advertised products in the nation. Young people are the primary targets of many of these ads.

Ads for these products appeal to young people by suggesting that drinking alcohol and smoking cigarettes will make them more popular, sexy, and successful. Help your teenager understand the difference between the misleading messages in advertising and the truth about the dangers of using alcohol and tobacco products.

What parents can do:

- Talk about ads with your child. Help your child understand the real messages being conveyed.
- Teach your child to be a wary consumer.
- Make sure the TV shows and movies your child watches do not glamorize the use of tobacco, alcohol, and other drugs.
- Do not allow your child to wear T-shirts, jackets, or hats that promote alcohol or tobacco products.
- Talk to administrators at your teen's school about starting a media education program.

The information contained in this publication should not be used as a substitute for the medical care and advice of your pediatrician. There may be variations in treatment that your pediatrician may recommend based on individual facts and circumstances.

American Academy
of Pediatrics

DEDICATED TO THE HEALTH OF ALL CHILDREN™

The American Academy of Pediatrics is an organization of 55,000 primary care pediatricians, pediatric medical subspecialists, and pediatric surgical specialists dedicated to the health, safety, and well-being of infants, children, adolescents, and young adults.

American Academy of Pediatrics
PO Box 747
Elk Grove Village, IL 60009-0747
Web site — http://www.aap.org

Surviving: Coping With Adolescent Depression and Suicide
Guidelines for Parents

A 19-year-old college sophomore finished his term paper, asked his roommate to hand it in, and then drove himself to a park and rigged his car's exhaust pipe with a hose to the inside of his car. He died of carbon monoxide poisoning, leaving a note that asked his family for forgiveness because he "could not go on."

Like many other teens he seemed happy, well-adjusted, and high achieving. But inside him was an unhappiness and depression so great that the only solution he could see was suicide.

This is not an isolated incident. Children, teenagers, and young adults are killing themselves at rising rates.Suicide is the third leading cause of death among young people 15 to 24 years old, and it appears to be on the rise. According to a 1991 Centers for Disease Control and Prevention study, 27% of high school students thought about suicide, 16% had a plan, and 8% made an attempt. The Alcohol, Drug Abuse and Mental Health Administration has declared adolescent suicide as a national mental health problem.

Why do teens kill themselves? Experts cite divorce, family violence, the breakdown of the family unit, stress to perform and achieve, and even the threat of AIDS as factors that contribute to the higher suicide rate. More than 50% of teens who commit suicide also have a history of alcohol and drug use. Stressful life events, such as the loss of a significant person or school failure, often trigger suicides among teens.

Depression plays a role

To better understand the cause of adolescent suicide, one must look past the surface to figure out what is going on inside the suicidal teen's head. Many teens who are considering suicide suffer from depression. People who work with depressed teens see a common theme of unhappiness, as well as feelings of inner turmoil, chaos, and low self-worth. Also hopelessness and anger often contribute to adolescent suicide.

One study found that 90% of suicidal adolescents believed that their families did not understand them. These teens felt alone and anonymous. They also believed that their parents either denied or ignored their attempts to communicate feelings of unhappiness, frustration, or failure. Some parents view depression and complaining as weaknesses, so they encourage their children to be strong and not to show their emotions. Suicidal teens often feel that their emotions are played down, not taken seriously, or met with hostility by the people around them.

One pediatrician who counsels suicidal adolescents said they often talk about how hopeless everything seems. They often feel that they are not in control, as an example, not in control over the direction of their lives.

Depressed teens may be drawn to others who feel as they do forming a bond of hopelessness and despair. Some popular music reflects these feelings of alienation, self-destructive rage, and thoughts about suicide.

Adolescents need to learn that with treatment, depression ends. However, a teen who is experiencing deep depression for the first time may not be able to focus on that. Something that may seem trivial to a parent or teacher may crush an adolescent who is already in a fragile emotional state—so much so that he or she is unable to think clearly and see a way out of the problem. The teen may then see suicide as the only choice.

Adolescent suicide is treatable and preventable

People who are depressed and thinking about suicide often show changes in their behavior. These changes in behavior are usually an outgrowth of depression and are warning signs. If your teen shows these warning signs, please talk to her about her concerns and have her get help if the warning signs continue.

- Noticeable changes in eating or sleeping habits
- Unexplained, or unusually severe, violent or rebellious behavior
- Withdrawal from family or friends
- Running away
- Persistent boredom and/or difficulty concentrating
- Drug and/or alcohol abuse
- Unexplained drop in the quality of schoolwork
- Unusual neglect of appearance
- Drastic personality change
- Complaints of physical problems that are not real
- A focus on themes of death
- Giving away prized possessions
- Talking about suicide or making plans, even jokingly
- Threatening or attempting to kill oneself

Before committing suicide, people often threaten to kill themselves. These threats should always be taken seriously, as should previous suicide attempts. Most people who commit suicide have made at least one previous attempt.

Asking your teen whether he is depressed or is thinking about suicide lets him know that someone cares. You're not putting thoughts of suicide into his head. Instead you're giving your teen the chance to talk about his problems.

Remember that depression and suicidal feelings are treatable mental disorders. The first step is to listen to your adolescent. A professional must then diagnose your teen's illness and determine a proper treatment plan. Your teen needs to share her feelings, and many suicidal teens are pleading for help in their own way. Your teen needs to feel that there is hope-that people will listen, that things will get better, and that she can overcome her problems.

Parents and friends can help a depressed teen through the following strategies:
1. Talk, ask questions, and be willing to really listen. Don't dismiss your teen's problems as unimportant. Parents and other influential adults should never make fun of or ignore an adolescent's concerns, especially if they matter a great deal to her and are making her unhappy.
2. Be honest. It you're worried about your teen, say so. You will not spark thoughts of suicide just by asking about it.

3. Share your feelings. Let your teen know he's not alone. Everyone feels sad or depressed at times.

4. Get help for your teen and yourself. Talk to your pediatrician, teacher, counselor, clergy, or other trained professional. Don't wait for the problem to "go away." Although feelings of sadness and depression can disappear as quickly as they came, they can also build to the point that an adolescent thinks of suicide as the only way out. Be careful not to assume that your teen's problems have been so easily solved.

A teen attempting suicide should immediately be taken to a hospital emergency room for a psychiatric evaluation. If a depressed adolescent is assessed to be safe to go home, it's a good idea to remove from your home any lethal, accessible means to commit suicide, such as medications, firearms, razors, knives, etc.

Sources of help

There are many sources of information to help troubled teens and their families. Often a pediatrician, who has charted the adolescent's physical and emotional progress since infancy, is in the best position to detect and help treat adolescent depression. Your teen may, however, need additional counseling.

Check the *Yellow Pages* in your city for the phone numbers of local suicide hot lines, crisis centers, and mental health centers.

The following organizations can also supply information on suicide prevention:

American Academy of Child and Adolescent Psychiatry
3615 Wisconsin Ave, NW,
Washington, DC 20016
202/966-7300

American Association of Suicidology
4201 Connecticut Ave, NW, Suite 310,
Washington, DC 20008
202/237-2280

American Psychiatric Association
1400 K St, NW, Suite 501,
Washington, DC 20005
202/682-6000

American Psychological Association
750 1st St, NE,
Washington, DC 20002
202/336-5700

National Mental Health Association
1021 Prince St,
Alexandria, VA 22314-2971
800/969-6642

With professional treatment and support from family and friends, teens who are suicidal can become healthy again.

The information contained in this publication should not be used as a substitute for the medical care and advice of your pediatrician. There may be variations in treatment that your pediatrician may recommend based on individual facts and circumstances.

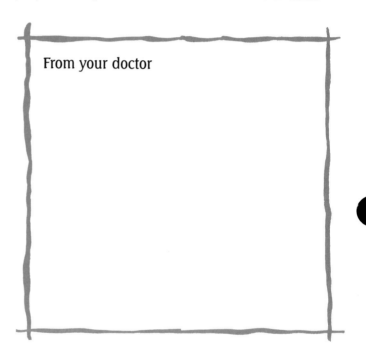

From your doctor

American Academy
of Pediatrics

DEDICATED TO THE HEALTH OF ALL CHILDREN™

The American Academy of Pediatrics is an organization of 55,000 primary care pediatricians, pediatric medical subspecialists, and pediatric surgical specialists dedicated to the health, safety, and well-being of infants, children, adolescents, and young adults.

American Academy of Pediatrics
PO Box 747
Elk Grove Village, IL 60009-0747
Web site — http://www.aap.org

Talking With Your Young Child About Sex

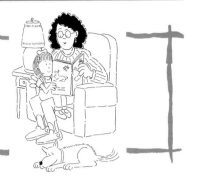

As a parent, you know it's coming—that dreaded moment when your adorable, innocent little boy or girl suddenly glances up and asks, "Where do babies come from?"

Learning about sex begins as soon as your child is able to view, listen, and sense the world around her. Sexuality is part of every person's life, no matter what the age. As your child grows and develops, she may giggle with friends about "private parts," share "dirty" jokes, and scan through dictionaries looking up taboo words. Her curiosity is natural, and children of all ages have questions. When she is ready to ask you, as a parent you should be ready to answer.

Talking about sex and sexuality gives you a chance to share your values and beliefs with your child. Sometimes the topic or the questions may seem embarrassing, but your child needs to know there is always a reliable, honest source she can turn to for answers—you.

The best teacher

Your child will learn many things about the world from friends, movies, television, music, the Internet, and even advertisements. When it comes to something as important as sexuality, nothing can replace the influence of a parent. The best place for your child to learn about relationships, love, commitment, and respect is from you. When your child feels loved and respected by you, he is more likely to turn to you for answers and advice. Giving advice and teaching your child to make wise choices is one of your most important jobs as a parent.

Where to begin

Everyday events will give you plenty of chances to teach your child about topics related to sex. These are called *teachable moments*. For example, talking about body parts during bath time will be much more effective than talking about body parts during dinner. A pregnancy or birth in the family is a good time to discuss how babies are conceived and born. Watching television with your child may also be a good time to discuss sexuality issues.

Teachable moments can happen anywhere—while shopping, at the movies, or even at the park. Use them when they happen. You won't need to make a speech. First, find out what your child already knows. Let your child guide the talk with her questions. Some children may not ask for information if they think you might be uneasy with it. Others might test you by asking embarrassing questions. Talk openly, and let your child know she can ask you about anything.

When your child begins to ask questions, the following might make it easier for both of you:

- **Don't laugh or giggle,** even if the question is cute. Your child shouldn't be made to feel ashamed for her curiosity.
- **Try not to appear overly embarrassed or serious** about the matter.
- **Be brief.** Don't go into a long explanation. Answer in simple terms. Your 4-year old doesn't need to know the details of intercourse.

- **Be honest.** Use proper names for all body parts.
- **See if your child wants or needs to know more.** Follow up your answers with, "Does that answer your question?"
- **Listen** to your child's responses and reactions.
- **Be prepared to repeat yourself.**

If you are uneasy talking about sex or answering certain questions, be honest about that too. Consider asking a relative, close family friend, or your pediatrician to help talk to your child.

Questions, questions, questions

The questions your child asks and the answers that are appropriate to give will depend on your child's age and ability to understand. Following are some of the issues your child may ask about and what he should know at each stage:

Preschool children

"How did I get in your tummy?"
"Where was I before I got in your tummy?"
"How did I get out?"
"Where do babies come from?"
"How come girls don't have a penis?"

18 months to 3 years of age—Your child will begin to learn about his own body. It is important to teach your child the proper names for body parts. Making up names for body parts may give the idea that there is something bad about the proper name. Also, teach your child which parts are private (parts covered by a bathing suit).

4 to 5 years of age—Your child may begin to show an interest in basic sexuality, both her own and that of the opposite sex. She may ask where babies come from. She may want to know why boys' and girls' bodies are different. She may also touch her own genitals and may even show an interest in the genitals of other children. These are not adult sexual activities, but signs of normal interest. However, your child needs to learn what is all right to do and what is not. Setting limits to exploration is really a family matter. You may decide to teach your child the following:

- Interest in genital organs is healthy and natural.
- Nudity and sexual play in public are not all right.
- No other person, including even close friends and relatives, may touch her "private parts." The exceptions are doctors and nurses during physical exams and her own parents when they are trying to find the cause of any pain in the genital area.

As your child approaches school-age, she should know the following:
- Proper names of body parts
- Functions of each
- Physical differences between boys and girls

School-age children

"How old do girls have to be before they can have a baby?"
"Why do boys get erections?"
"What is a period?"
"How do people have sexual intercourse?"
"Why do some men like other men?"

5 to 7 years of age—Your child is learning much more about how people get along with each other. He may become interested in what takes place sexually between adults. His questions will become more complex as he tries to understand the connection between sexuality and making babies. He may come up with his own explanations about how the body works or where babies come from. He may also turn to his friends for answers.

It is important to help your child understand sexuality in a healthy way. Lessons and values he learns at this age will stay with him as an adult. It will encourage meaningful adult relationships later.

8 to 9 years of age—Your child probably already has developed a sense of right and wrong. She is able to understand that sex is something that happens between two people who love each other. She may begin to become interested in how mom and dad met and fell in love. As questions about romance, love, and marriage arise, she may also ask about homosexual relationships. Use this time to discuss your family's thoughts about homosexuality. Explain that liking or loving someone does not depend on the person's gender and is different from liking someone sexually.

Media Matters

Most children can mimic a movie or TV character, sing an advertising jingle, or give other examples of what they have learned from media. Sadly, these examples may include naming a popular brand of beer, striking a "sexy" pose, or play fighting. Media offer entertainment, culture, news, sports, and education and are an important part of our lives. But some of what they teach may not be what we want children to learn.

American media today (TV, movies, videos, ads, computer games, as well as music lyrics and music videos), often contain sexual images and suggestive content. In fact, the average young viewer is exposed to over 14,000 sexual references each year. Only a small amount of what is seen in the media shows responsible sexual behavior or gives accurate information about birth control, abstinence, or the risks of pregnancy and sexually transmitted disease.

Whatever the form of media, messages can have a positive or negative effect on your child. Just as you would limit certain foods in your child's diet that may be unhealthy, you also should limit your child's media diet of messages.

At this age, your child will be going through many changes that will prepare her for puberty. As she becomes more and more aware of her sexuality, it is important that you talk to her about delaying sexual intercourse until she is older. You should also talk about contraception and sexually transmitted diseases (STDs), especially AIDS. Be sure she understands how these

diseases can spread and how she can protect herself from them and from pregnancy. Teaching your child to be sexually responsible is one of the most important lessons in her life.

A word about...masturbation

Masturbation is a part of childhood sexuality that many parents find difficult to discuss. Up to the age of 5 or 6, it is quite common. Around age 6, children become more socially aware and may feel embarrassed about touching themselves in public. Make sure your child understands that masturbation is a private activity, not a public one. Masturbation in private may continue and is normal.

There are times when frequent masturbation can point to a problem. It could be a sign that the child is under a lot of stress or not receiving enough attention at home. In rare cases, it could even be a tip-off to sexual abuse. Some sexually abused children become overly interested in their sexuality. If masturbation becomes a problem, talk to your pediatrician. For most children, masturbation is nothing to worry about. It is normal.

As your child approaches puberty, she should know about the following:

- The body parts related to sex and their functions
- How babies are conceived and born
- Puberty and how the body will change
- Menstruation (Both boys and girls can benefit from this information.)
- Sexual intercourse
- Birth control
- Sexually transmitted diseases (STDs) and how they are spread, including HIV and AIDS
- Masturbation
- Homosexuality
- Family and personal guidelines

For more information, visit the American Academy of Pediatrics (AAP) on the Web at www.aap.org or ask your pediatrician about other AAP brochures on sexuality. You also may want to look for books on talking to your child about sexuality from your local library or bookstore.

The information contained in this publication should not be used as a substitute for the medical care and advice of your pediatrician. There may be variations in treatment that your pediatrician may recommend based on individual facts and circumstances.

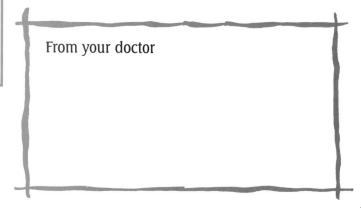

From your doctor

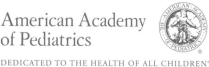

American Academy of Pediatrics

DEDICATED TO THE HEALTH OF ALL CHILDREN™

The American Academy of Pediatrics is an organization of 55,000 primary care pediatricians, pediatric medical subspecialists, and pediatric surgical specialists dedicated to the health, safety, and well-being of infants, children, adolescents, and young adults.

American Academy of Pediatrics
PO Box /4/
Elk Grove Village, IL 60009-0747
Web site — http://www.aap.org

Copyright ©2000   American Academy of Pediatrics

Talking to Your Young Teen About Sex and Sexuality
Guidelines for Parents

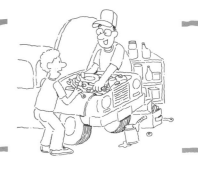

Sex seems to be everywhere these days—on television, in the movies, and in popular songs. Sex in the media is so common that you might think that your young teenager already knows everything he or she needs to know about sex. In fact, your teenager may claim that he or she already knows everything about sex, but this is not true. Teens today need information about sex more than ever, and you are still the best source for that information. The American Academy of Pediatrics offers the following tips to help you talk to your teen about this important and sensitive subject.

Why should I talk to my teen about sex?

Talks about sex should begin when your child first asks a question like "where do babies come from?". Children usually start asking such questions at age 3 or 4. Waiting until your child is a teenager to have "the big talk" means your child will probably learn his first lessons about sex from someone other than you. Studies show that children who learn about sex from friends instead of their parents are more likely to have sex before marriage. They are also more likely to have sex at a young age, and to have more than one sexual partner before marriage. You can have a great effect on your child by talking to him about sex even at a young age.

What should I tell my teen about sex?

Well before they reach their early teens, both boys and girls should already know:

- The basics of sexual "plumbing," that is, the names and functions of male and female sex organs
- The purpose and meaning of puberty (moving into young womanhood or young manhood)
- The function of the menstrual cycle (period)
- What sexual intercourse is and how women become pregnant

Once your child becomes a teenager, the focus of your talks about sex should shift. You should begin to talk to your teen about the social and emotional aspects of sex, and about your values. You will want to deal with issues that help your teenager answer questions like these:

- "When should I start dating?"
- "When is it okay to kiss a boy (or a girl)?"
- "How far is too far?"
- "How will I know when I'm ready to have sex?"
- "Won't having sex help me keep my boyfriend (or girlfriend)?"

You should answer your teen's questions based on your own value system — even if you think your values are old-fashioned by today's standards. If you feel strongly that sex before marriage is wrong, you should tell your teenager that, but be sure to explain why you feel that way. If you explain the reasons for your beliefs, your teen is more likely to understand and adopt your values.

You also need to listen to what your teenager is saying. Find out what she knows about sex and try to answer her questions as clearly and directly as possible.

Other important topics to address are:

- **Resisting pressure to have sex:** Teens face a lot of peer pressure to have sex. If your teenager is not ready to have sex, she may feel left out. Help her understand that many teenagers decide to wait to have sex.

- **Sexually transmitted diseases (STDs) and how to prevent them:** Teenagers need to know that having sex exposes them to the risk of sexually transmitted diseases. Your teen should also know that AIDS is a leading cause of death in young people, aged 15 to 24. These young people were probably infected with HIV when they were teenagers. The only sure way to prevent STDs is not to have sex. Explain to your teen that if she chooses to have sex, using a latex condom every time is the only proven way to lower the risk of getting STDs. Be sure to explain that even condoms do not eliminate the risk.

- **Birth Control:** Even if you have made it clear that you would prefer that your teenager wait to have sex, your teen still needs basic information about birth control. (Both girls and boys need to know about birth control.) Your teen may decide to have sex despite your wishes. Without birth control information, an unplanned pregnancy might result. Be sure to explain that birth control pills, shots (Depo-Provera), and implants (Norplant) only prevent pregnancy. They do not protect against sexually transmitted diseases. Only latex condoms protect against STDs, including HIV/AIDS. Both condoms and another reliable birth control method need to be used each time.

- **Acquaintance (date) rape:** Acquaintance rape is a serious problem for teens. It happens when a person your teenager knows (for example, a date, friend, or neighbor) forces her (or him) to have sex. Make sure your teenager understands that "no always means no." Discuss with your teen that avoiding drugs and alcohol may make date rape less likely to happen.

- **Forms of sexuality (heterosexuality, homosexuality, bisexuality):** This is a difficult topic for many parents. However, your teen probably has many questions about the different forms human sexuality can take. Many young people go through a stage when they wonder, "Am I gay?" It often happens when a teenager realizes that he is attracted to a friend of the same sex, or that he has a crush on a teacher of the same sex. This is normal and does not mean your teenager is gay or bisexual. Sexual identity may not be firmly set until adulthood. You should also let your teen know that if he is gay or bisexual, you will not reject him.

- **Masturbation:** Masturbation is a topic few people feel comfortable discussing. But it is a normal and healthy part of human sexuality. Discuss this in terms of your values.

When talking about sex with your teen is difficult

Talking about sex with your teenager may be a hard thing to do. Perhaps you find it embarrassing to talk about sex. Maybe you think talking about it will make your teen want to have sex. Maybe your teen does not seem to want to talk to you about sex.

Don't worry. Many parents find talking about sex with their children hard. Sex is a very personal and private matter. If talking about sex is hard for you, try these tips:

- Be honest. Explain your discomfort to your teenager. Let her know that talking about sex is not easy for you—perhaps because of your own background—but that you think it is important for her to get her information about sex from you.
- If certain subjects make you uncomfortable, try speaking slowly, calmly, and coolly.
- Practice with your spouse or partner, a friend, or another parent. Knowing what you want to say and going over the words may make it easier to talk about sex with your teen when the time comes.
- If you just cannot talk to your teen about sex, ask your pediatrician to provide her with sex-related information. A trusted aunt or uncle, or a minister, priest, or rabbi may also be able to help. Finally, many parents find it useful to give their teenagers a book on human sexuality.

"Won't talking about sex with my son make him want to have sex?"

Parents often fear that even talking about sex may make it seem exciting to their children and make them want to try it. Teenagers are curious about sex, whether you talk to them about it or not. Studies show that teens whose parents talk openly about sex are actually more responsible in their sexual behavior.

Your guidance is important. It will help your teen make difficult decisions about sex, and it may make it less likely that he or she will be exposed to STDs or have an unplanned pregnancy. Teenagers who have poor information about sex (usually those who learn about sex from friends) or who have no information at all are the most likely to get into trouble.

"I want to talk to my teenager about sex, but every time I try to start a conversation, she just stares at me."

It is not always easy to talk to your teenager about anything, let alone something as private and difficult as sex. Your teen may be embarrassed to talk to you about sex. She may fear that if she opens up to you about sex, you might use what she says against her later. She may also feel that what she thinks about sex is none of your business.

Teenagers do need privacy. However, they also need information and guidance from parents. Try to strike a balance. Let your teen know that while you would prefer that she would accept your values, she will have to make her own sexual decisions. Give your teenager a chance to share what she thinks and to ask questions. If your teen does not say anything when you try to talk about

sex, say what you have to say anyway. Your message will get through. If your teen disagrees with what you have to say or gets angry, take heart. This means that she has at least heard what you have said. These talks will help your teenager learn to think about her actions. They will also help her develop a solid value system, even if it is different from your own.

For more information, see the following American Academy of Pediatrics Publications:

The Correct Use of Condoms: A Message to Teens

Deciding to Wait: Guidelines for Teens

Know the Facts About HIV and AIDS: Guidelines for Parents

Making the Right Choice: Facts for Teens on Avoiding Pregnancy

Puberty: Information for Girls and Boys

The Pelvic Exam: Guidelines for Teens

Sex Education: A Bibliography for Children, Adolescents, and Their Parents

---

Television and sex

Television exposes children and teens to adult behaviors by showing these actions as being normal and risk-free. Being sexually active is often shown on TV as a popular thing to do. Because sexual activity happens so often on TV, the message that is sent is "everybody does it" with no harmful results. In addition, young teens may think that these behaviors will make them more grown-up.

Ten percent of adolescent girls in the United States get pregnant each year. Although TV viewing is not the only way that your teen learns about sexuality, the risks and results of sexual activity are not given equal time on TV. Programs on many cable TV channels are often even more extreme in the way they portray sex. This makes it even more important for you to talk about these issues with your young teen.

The information contained in this publication should not be used as a substitute for the medical care and advice of your pediatrician. There may be variations in treatment that your pediatrician may recommend based on individual facts and circumstances.

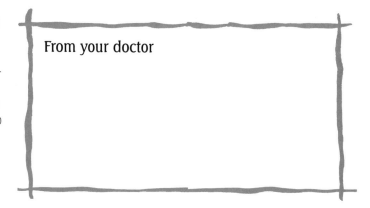

From your doctor

American Academy of Pediatrics

DEDICATED TO THE HEALTH OF ALL CHILDREN™

The American Academy of Pediatrics is an organization of 55,000 primary care pediatricians, pediatric medical subspecialists, and pediatric surgical specialists dedicated to the health, safety, and well-being of infants, children, adolescents, and young adults.

American Academy of Pediatrics
PO Box 747
Elk Grove Village, IL 60009-0747
Web site — http://www.aap.org

The Teen Driver
Guidelines for Parents

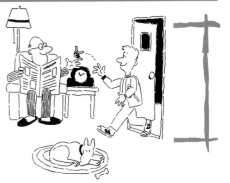

Traffic crashes are the leading cause of death for teens and young adults. More than 5,000 young people die every year in car crashes and thousands more are injured. Drivers who are 16 years old are more than 20 times as likely to have a crash as are other drivers. State and local laws, safe driving programs, and driver's education classes all help keep teens safe on the roads. Parents can also play an important role in keeping young drivers safe. This information has been developed by the American Academy of Pediatrics to inform parents about the risks that teen drivers face and how parents can help keep them safe on the roads.

Why teens are at risk

There are two main reasons why teens are at a higher risk for being in a car crash: lack of driving experience and their tendency to take risks while driving.

- **Lack of experience.** Teens drive faster and do not control the car as well as more experienced drivers. Their judgment in traffic is often insufficient to avoid a crash. In addition, teens do most of their driving at night, which can be even more difficult. Standard driver's education classes include 30 hours of classroom teaching and 6 hours of behind-the-wheel training. This is not enough time to fully train a new driver.
- **Risk taking.** Teen drivers are more likely to be influenced by peers and other stresses and distractions. This can lead to reckless driving behaviors such as speeding, driving while under the influence of drugs or alcohol, and not wearing safety belts.

Programs that help

Graduated licensing laws. Most teens get their driver's licenses in two stages: a learner's permit followed a few months later by a regular driver's license. The US Department of Transportation recommends "graduated licensing" so that learning to drive is spread over three stages. Each stage gives teens more driving privileges. Teen drivers have to meet certain restrictions for at least 6 months in each stage in order to move to the next stage. Driver's education classes would cover more and more complex decision-making and skills training during each stage. Twelve states have some form of graduated licensing laws.

Minimum drinking age and zero tolerance laws. Drunk and drugged driving are major problems for American teens. In one study, an estimated 6% to 14% of drivers younger than 21 years who were stopped at roadside sobriety checkpoints had been drinking. The misuse of alcohol and other drugs can severely hurt teenagers in many ways—especially on the road. A teen driver with a blood alcohol level (BAC) above 0.05% is more likely to be involved in a crash than is a sober teen driver.

Two types of laws exist to help lower the number of teens who drive after drinking alcohol. These are *minimum drinking* age laws and zero tolerance laws. Minimum drinking age laws prohibit the sale of alcohol to anyone under 21 years of age. These laws have helped reduce the number of alcohol-related crashes by 40%. But in some states, these laws have many loopholes and are hard to enforce. Many states have or will soon adopt zero tolerance laws that lower the allowable BAC limits for minors. Some states also require that licenses be suspended, sometimes for up to 1 year, after drivers younger than 21 years of age are arrested for driving drunk. These laws work. In Maryland, alcohol-related crashes decreased by at least 11% as a result of zero tolerance laws.

Safety belt laws. Even though all states have laws that require the use of safety belts, these laws may not apply to all passengers or all seats in a vehicle. In addition, studies show that teens do not use safety belts as often as older drivers do. Young people between 10 and 20 years old use safety belts only about 35% of the time—the lowest usage rate of any group. Strictly enforced safety belt laws, along with air bags, could greatly reduce the number of teens who are injured and killed in car crashes. In addition, teen drivers need to learn to take the responsibility of making sure all passengers are buckled up.

Curfew laws. Curfew laws ban teen driving during certain hours at night, such as midnight to 5 am. States with nighttime driving curfews for young drivers have lower crash rates than other states. The more strict the law, the fewer fatal crashes occur.

Educational efforts. Various state and national groups have programs to educate teens about unsafe driving practices, such as not wearing a safety belt and drunk driving. Pediatricians also play a role in such efforts.

There are several groups that encourage alternatives to drinking and driving by hosting social events for teens such as alcohol-free proms and parties. They also help teens and parents communicate. For example, SADD (Students Against Driving Drunk) encourages parents and teens to sign a contract in which both parties agree to avoid using alcohol or other drugs before driving and avoid riding with those who have. The contract also states that if a teen has been drinking he or she will call home for a ride. The group also encourages young people to help other teens change drinking habits and save lives on the roadways.

Safe ride programs. In some areas, "safe ride" programs help parents get involved by volunteering to drive to proms and other parties. Other programs give rides to teens who might otherwise have to drive home after drinking or ride with someone who has been drinking. A California program, for example, combines an educational program about alcohol abuse and an escort service for "stranded" teens on weekend nights. Teens can use this service in confidence. Teens volunteer to be drivers, but adults are also on-call in case questions or problems come up. Volunteer drivers stay in the car when they drop teens at home. They watch the teens enter their homes but do not talk with parents. Adults on-call handle any questions from parents.

How parents can help

Establish and discuss "house rules" about driving even before your teen gets a license. Remind your teen that these rules are in place because you care about his or her safety. If your teen complains about the rules, stand firm. You might say something like, "I don't care what other parents are doing—I care about you and don't want you to get in a crash." Remember, you control the car keys. Don't hesitate to take away driving privileges if your teen breaks any rules. Resist the urge to break the house rules yourself and let your teen drive because it is too much trouble for you to drive. Instead, try to arrange a car pool of parents and take turns driving.

You do not need to wait for graduated licensing laws to be passed in your state to adopt your own graduated driving rules. By slowly increasing driving privileges, you can help your teen get the experience needed to drive safely and responsibly. Here are some suggestions on how you can create a graduated licensing program for your teen driver. It may not be necessary to use all of the following restrictions; choose the ones that make the most sense for you and your teen.

Stage one

- teen must be at least 15½ years old or have a legal learner's permit
- teen must drive with a licensed adult driver at all times, the parent if possible
- no driving between 10 pm and 5 am or no driving after sunset
- driver and all passengers must wear safety belts
- no use of tobacco, alcohol, or other drugs
- teen must remain ticket-free and crash-free for 6 months before moving up to the next stage

Stage two

- teen must be at least 16 years old or have driven with a learner's permit for at least 6 months
- teen must drive with a licensed adult driver during nighttime hours, the parent if possible
- teen allowed to drive unsupervised during daytime hours
- passengers restricted to one nonfamily member during daytime hours

- no use of tobacco, alcohol, or other drugs
- driver and all passengers must wear safety belts
- teen must remain ticket-free and crash-free for 12 months before moving up to the next stage

Stage three

- teen must be at least 18 years old or have driven at least 2 years at the previous stage
- no restrictions on driving as long as the teen driver remains ticket-free and crash-free for 6 months
- no use of tobacco, alcohol, or other drugs
- all passengers must wear safety belts
  Other ways parents can help:
- Require that your teen maintain good grades in school before he or she can drive. Check with your auto insurance company to see if any "good student" discounts are available.
- Set a good driving example (no use of alcohol or other drugs, no speeding, always wear your safety belt, and require that safety belts be worn by all passengers).
- Remind your teen how important it is to stay focused on driving, not getting distracted by excessively loud music or talking on a cellular phone.
- Let your teen know that driving after drinking or using other drugs will not be tolerated. Tell your teen to always call you or someone else for a ride any time he or she or any other driver has been drinking or using drugs. Let your teen know that you will pick him or her up. However, if you find he or she was drinking, it may be better to wait until the next day before you discuss the incident.
- Be alert to any signs that your teen has a drinking or other substance abuse problem. If you suspect a problem, urge your teen to talk with his or her pediatrician or school counselor. Such trusted adults can refer your teen for other help, if needed.
- Support efforts to protect teens. These might include "safe ride" programs or Mothers Against Drunk Driving (MADD). Encourage alcohol-free community events.
- Encourage schools to teach about the dangers of driving after drinking or using drugs.
- Support showing safety films in schools. Also support efforts to promote safety belt use in all vehicles that take children and teens to and from school.

Driving is a privilege and a big responsibility. Teen drivers, because of their age and inexperience, are at a higher risk for car crashes. Licensing programs, rules of the road, and safe ride programs are designed to help teen drivers stay safe. Along with support and encouragement from parents, these programs are the best way to help teens learn to become responsible drivers.

The information contained in this publication should not be used as a substitute for the medical care and advice of your pediatrician. There may be variations in treatment that your pediatrician may recommend based on individual facts and circumstances.

American Academy of Pediatrics

DEDICATED TO THE HEALTH OF ALL CHILDREN™

The American Academy of Pediatrics is an organization of 55,000 primary care pediatricians, pediatric medical subspecialists, and pediatric surgical specialists dedicated to the health, safety, and well-being of infants, children, adolescents, and young adults.

American Academy of Pediatrics
PO Box /4/
Elk Grove Village, IL 60009-0747
Web site — http://www.aap.org

Copyright ©1996   American Academy of Pediatrics

Testicular Self-Exam

Most people think that cancer is a disease that only old people get. Cancer of the testicles — the male reproductive glands — is different. It is one of the most common types of cancer in men 15 to 34 years old.

Most testicular cancers are found by young men themselves. By doing a regular exam of your testicles, you greatly increase your chance of finding testicular cancer early if it does occur. It takes only 3 minutes a month to do a simple check for lumps on your testicles.

Here's How:

1. Do the exam once a month, after a warm bath or shower when the scrotal skin is most relaxed.
2. Roll each testicle gently between the thumb and first two fingers of both hands. The testicles should be smooth, with the consistency of a hard-boiled egg without the shell.

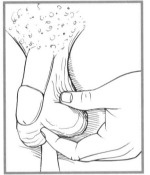

3. Feel for the small, comma-shaped cord, about the size of a pea, that is attached at the back of each testicle. This is a natural part of your testicles, and is called the epididymis. Learn what it feels like, so you will not confuse it with an abnormal lump.
4. Check each testicle for lumps. If you find a lump, tell your doctor about it right away. Not all lumps are cancerous, but only your doctor will be able to tell the difference. Don't let fear keep you from getting the medical help you need.

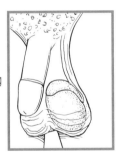

What Is Normal?

- Testicles hang in the scrotum, and are about the same size.
- The left testicle usually hangs down a little more in the scrotum than the right testicle.
- A rope-like structure called the spermatic cord runs from your scrotum up into your groin.

What Are Possible Signs of Cancer?

- A lump on one of the testicles, which usually doesn't hurt.
- One testicle that gets larger than the other.
- A dull ache in your groin that doesn't go away.
- Your testicles feel heavy, like they are dragging.

The information contained in this publication should not be used as a substitute for the medical care and advice of your pediatrician. There may be variations in treatment that your pediatrician may recommend based on individual facts and circumstances.

Illustrations by Lauren Shavell

American Academy
of Pediatrics

DEDICATED TO THE HEALTH OF ALL CHILDREN™

The American Academy of Pediatrics is an organization of 55,000 primary care pediatricians, pediatric medical subspecialists, and pediatric surgical specialists dedicated to the health, safety, and well-being of infants, children, adolescents, and young adults.

American Academy of Pediatrics
PO Box 747
Elk Grove Village, IL 60009-0747
Web site — http://www.aap.org

©Copyright 1999 American Academy of Pediatrics

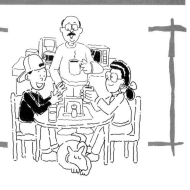

Tips for Parents of Adolescents

Adolescence is a time of change and challenge for your preteen or teenager. The changes that occur during adolescence are often confusing not only for your son or daughter, but for you as well. Though these years can be difficult, the reward is watching your child become an independent, caring, and responsible adult. The American Academy of Pediatrics (AAP) offers the following tips to help you face the challenges of your child's adolescence:

1. **Spend family time with your adolescent.** Although many preteens and teens may seem more interested in friends, this does not mean they are not interested in family.

2. **Spend time alone with your adolescent.** Even if your teen does not want time alone with you, take a moment here and there to remind him that your "door is always open," and you are always there if he needs to talk. Remind him often.

3. **When your adolescent talks**
   - Pay attention.
   - Watch, as well as listen.
   - Try not to interrupt.
   - Ask him to explain things further if you don't understand.
   - If you don't have time to listen when your child wants to talk, set a time that will be good for both of you.

4. **Respect your adolescent's feelings.** It's okay to disagree with your child, but disagree respectfully, not insultingly. Don't dismiss her feelings or opinions as silly or senseless. You may not always be able to help when your child is upset about something, but it is important to say, "I want to understand" or "Help me understand."

5. **When rules are needed, set and enforce them.** Don't be afraid to be unpopular for a day or two. Believe it or not, adolescents see setting limits as a form of caring.

6. **Try not to get upset if your adolescent makes mistakes.** This will help him take responsibility for his own actions. Remember to offer guidance when necessary. Direct the discussion toward solutions.

   > "I get upset when I find clothes all over the floor," is much better than, "You're a slob."

   Be willing to negotiate and compromise. This will teach problem solving in a healthy way. Remember to choose your battles. Some little annoying things that adolescents do may not be worth a big fight—let them go.

7. **Criticize a behavior, not an attitude.** For example, instead of saying,

   > "You're late. That's so irresponsible. And I don't like your attitude,"

   try saying,

   > "I worry about your safety when you're late. I trust you, but when I don't hear from you and don't know where you are, I wonder whether something bad has happened to you. What can we do together to help you get home on time and make sure I know where you are or when you're going to be late?"

8. **Mix criticism with praise.** While your teen needs to know how you feel when she is not doing what you want her to do, she also needs to know that you appreciate the positive things she is doing. For example,

   > "I'm proud that you are able to hold a job and get your homework done. I would like to see you use some of that energy to help do the dishes after meals."

9. **Let your child be the adolescent he wants to be, not the one you wish he was.** Also, try not to pressure your adolescent to be like you were or wish you had been at that age. Give your teen some leeway with regard to clothes, hairstyle, etc. Many teens go through a rebellious period in which they want to express themselves in ways that are different from their parents. However, be aware of the messages and ratings of the music, movies, and video games to which your child is exposed.

10. **Be a parent first, not a pal.** Your adolescent's separation from you as a parent is a normal part of development. Don't take it personally.

11. **Don't be afraid to share with your adolescent that you have made mistakes as a parent.** A few parenting mistakes are not crucial. Also, try to share with your teen mistakes you made as an adolescent.

12. **Talk to your pediatrician if you are having trouble with your adolescent.** He or she may be able to help you and your child find ways to get along.

The following is additional information you may find helpful in understanding some of the life changes and pressures your adolescent may be experiencing.

Dieting and body image

"My daughter is always trying new diets.
How can I help her lose weight safely?"

We live in a society that is focused on thinness. Adolescents see many role models in fashion magazines, on television, and in the movies that emphasize the importance of being thin. This concern about weight and body image leads many adolescents, especially girls, to resort to extreme measures to lose weight. Be aware of any diet or exercise program with which your child is involved. Be watchful of how much weight your child loses, and make sure the diet program is healthy. Eating disorders such as anorexia nervosa and bulimia nervosa can be very dangerous. If you suspect your child has an eating disorder, talk to your pediatrician right away. Ask about the brochure from the AAP called *Eating Disorders: What You Should Know About Anorexia and Bulimia.*

Many diets are unhealthy for adolescents because they do not have the nutritional value that bodies need during puberty. If your teen wants to lose weight, urge her to increase physical activity and to take weight off slowly. Let her eat according to her own appetite, but make sure she gets enough fats, carbohydrates, protein, and calcium.

Make sure your teen is not confusing a "low-fat" diet with a "no fat" diet. Teens need 30% of their calories from fat, and cutting fat out of the diet altogether is not healthy. A low-fat diet should still include 30 to 50 grams of fat daily. Many teens choose vegetarian diets. If your child decides to become a vegetarian, make certain she reads about it and becomes an educated vegetarian. She may need to see her pediatrician or a nutritionist to ensure that she is getting enough fat, calories, protein, and calcium.

Many adolescents are uncomfortable with their bodies. If your adolescent is unhappy with the way she looks, encourage her to start a physical activity program. Physical activity will stop hunger pangs, create a positive self-image, and take away the "blahs". Unfortunately, some teens may try to change their bodies by dangerous means such as unhealthy dieting (as discussed previously) or with drugs such as anabolic steroids. Encourage healthy exercise. If your child wants to train with weights, she should check with her pediatrician, as well as a trainer, coach, or physical education teacher. Help create a positive self-image by praising your child about her appearance. Set a good example by practicing what you preach. Make exercise and eating right a part of your daily routine also.

Nutrition

The growth rate during adolescence is one of the most dramatic changes the body ever goes through. It is very important for your adolescent to have a proper diet. Follow these suggestions to help keep your teen's diet a healthy one

- Limit fast food meals. Discuss the options available at fast food restaurants, and help your teen find a good balance in her diet. Fat should not come from junk food but from healthier foods such as cheese or yogurt. Vegetables and fruit are also important.
- Keep the household supply of "junk food" such as candy, cookies, and potato chips to a minimum.
- Stock up on low-fat healthy items for snacking such as fruit, raw vegetables, whole-grain crackers, and yogurt.
- Check with your pediatrician about the proper amounts of calories, fat, protein, and carbohydrates for your child.
- As a parent, model good eating habits.

Dating and sex education

"With all the sex on television, how can I teach
my son to 'wait' until he is ready?"

There are constant pressures for your adolescent to have sex. These pressures may come from the movies, television, music, friends, and peers. Teens are naturally curious about sex. This is completely normal and healthy. Talk to your adolescent to understand his feelings and views about sex. Start early and provide your teen with access to information that is accurate and appropriate. Delaying sexual involvement could be the most important decision your child can make. Talk to your teen or preteen about the following things he needs to think about before becoming sexually active:

Medical and physical risks, like unwanted pregnancy and STDs (sexually transmitted diseases) such as

- Gonorrhea
- Syphilis
- Chlamydia
- Herpes
- Hepatitis B
- HIV, the virus that causes AIDS

Emotional risks—that go along with an adolescent having sex before he is ready. The adolescent may regret the decision when he is older or feel guilty, frightened, or ashamed from the experience. Have your adolescent ask himself, "Am I ready to have sex?" "What will happen after I have sex?"

Methods of contraception—Anyone who is sexually active needs to be aware of the various methods of contraception that help prevent unintended pregnancies, as well as ways to protect against sexually transmitted diseases. Remember to tell your teen that latex condoms should always be used along with a second method of contraception to prevent pregnancy and STDs.

Setting limits—Make sure your adolescent has thought about what his limits are before dating begins.

Most importantly, let your adolescent know that he can talk to you and his pediatrician about dating and relationships. Offer your guidance throughout this important stage in your teen's life.

The following AAP brochures may help your teen in dealing with these difficult issues: *Deciding to Wait and Making the Right Choice: Facts For Teens on Preventing Pregnancy.*

If you smoke... quit

If you or someone else in the household smokes, now is a good time to quit. Watching a parent struggle through the process of quitting can be a powerful message for a teen or preteen who is thinking about starting. It also shows that you care about your health, as well as your child's.

Smoking and tobacco

"My daughter smokes behind my back. How do I convince her to quit?"

Smoking can turn into a lifelong addiction that can be extremely hard to break. Discuss with your adolescent some of the more undesirable effects of smoking, including bad breath, stained teeth, wrinkles, a long-term cough, and decreased athletic performance. Addiction can also lead to serious health problems like emphysema and cancer.

"Chew" or "snuff" can also lead to nicotine addiction and causes the same health problems as smoking cigarettes. Mouth wounds or sores also form and may not heal easily. Smokeless tobacco can also lead to cancer.

If you suspect your teen or preteen is smoking or using smokeless tobacco, talk to your pediatrician. Arrange for your child to visit the pediatrician, who will want to discuss the risks associated with smoking and the best ways to quit before it becomes a lifelong habit. Smokers young and old often are more likely to listen to advice from their doctor than from others.

Alcohol

"I know my son drinks once in a while, but it's just beer. Why should I worry?"

Alcohol is the most socially accepted drug in our society, and also one of the most abused and destructive. Even small amounts of alcohol can impair judgment, provoke risky and violent behavior, and slow down reaction time. An intoxicated teenager (or anyone else) behind the wheel of a car is a lethal weapon. Alcohol-related car crashes are the leading cause of death for young adults, aged 15 to 24 years.

Though it's illegal for people under age 21 to drink, we all know that most teenagers are no strangers to alcohol. Many of them are introduced to alcohol during childhood. If you choose to use alcohol in your home, be aware of the example you set for your teen. The following suggestions may help:

- Having a drink should never be shown as a way to cope with problems.
- Don't drink in unsafe conditions—driving the car, mowing the lawn, using the stove, etc.
- Don't encourage your child to drink or to join you in having a drink.
- Never make jokes about getting drunk; make sure that your children understand that it is neither funny nor acceptable.
- Show your children that there are many ways to have fun without alcohol. Happy occasions and special events don't have to include drinking.
- Do not allow your children to drink alcohol before they reach the legal age and teach them never, ever to drink and drive.
- Always wear your seatbelt (and ask your children to do the same.)

Drugs

"I am afraid some of my daughter's friends have offered her drugs. How can I help her make the right decision?"

Your child may be interested in using drugs other than tobacco and alcohol, including marijuana and cocaine, to fit in or as a way to deal with the pressures of adolescence. Try to help your adolescent build her self-confidence or self-esteem. This will help your child resist the pressure to use drugs. Encourage your adolescent to "vent" emotions and troubles through conversations and physical activity rather than by getting "high."

Set examples at home. Encourage your adolescent to participate in leisure and outside activities to stay away from the peer pressure of drinking and drugs. Talk with your children about healthy choices.

For more information on tobacco, alcohol, and other drugs, visit the AAP Web site at www.aap.org, or ask your pediatrician about the following AAP brochures:

Alcohol: Your Child and Drugs
Cocaine: Your Child and Drugs
Marijuana: Your Child and Drugs
Smoking: Straight Talk for Teens
Steroids: Play Safe, Play Fair
The Risks of Tobacco Use: A Message to Parents and Teens

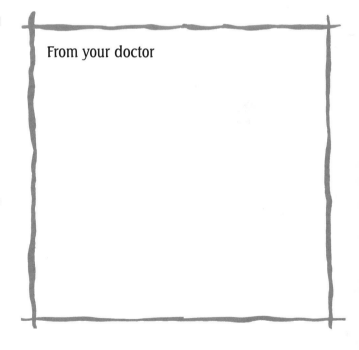

From your doctor

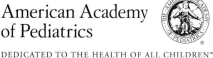

American Academy of Pediatrics

DEDICATED TO THE HEALTH OF ALL CHILDREN™

The American Academy of Pediatrics is an organization of 55,000 primary care pediatricians, pediatric medical subspecialists, and pediatric surgical specialists dedicated to the health, safety, and well-being of infants, children, adolescents, and young adults.

American Academy of Pediatrics
PO Box 747
Elk Grove Village, IL 60009-0747
Web site — http://www.aap.org

Common Illnesses and Conditions

Allergies in Children

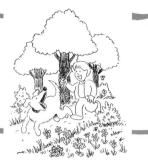

You probably know a child who has asthma or allergies. Perhaps it is your own child. Asthma, hay fever, hives, and eczema are familiar words for most of us. In fact, in the United States over 35 million adults and children have these allergy-related problems.

Allergies can be as minor as sneezing and itching. For some children, however, allergies can become very serious or even life-threatening. Whether minor or serious, allergies can be prevented and controlled. The more you understand about allergies and asthma—the symptoms, causes, and treatments—the better prepared you will be to help improve the quality of life for you and your child.

What is an allergy?

An allergy happens when the human body's natural defense system (the immune system) overreacts to an otherwise harmless substance (like pollen). There are many ways in which an allergy can exhibit itself:

- **Asthma** is when airways swell and air passages in the lungs become narrow. This may be triggered by an allergic reaction, although nonallergic triggers can be involved.
- **Allergic rhinitis** is an allergic reaction mainly in the nasal passages. It can occur in one or more "seasons" (seasonal allergic rhinitis or **"hay-fever"**) or all year long (perennial allergic rhinitis).
- **Eczema** (atopic dermatitis) is a chronic, itchy rash, most commonly found in young children. It may be made worse by certain allergies.
- **Hives** (urticaria) are itchy welts that may be due to allergies, viral infections, or unknown causes. Certain foods, viral infections, and medications are most likely to cause hives.
- **Contact dermatitis** can be just a skin irritation or an allergic reaction. The allergic type is an itchy skin rash caused by touching, rubbing, or coming into contact with things like poison ivy, chemicals, or household detergents.
- **Food allergy** is an allergic reaction to food that can range from stomachache, to skin rash, to a serious respiratory and medical emergency.

What causes allergies?

The causes of allergies are not fully understood. Children get allergies from coming into contact with allergens. Allergens can be inhaled, eaten, injected (from stings or medicine), or they can come into contact with the skin. Some of the more common allergens are:

- pollens
- molds
- house dust mites
- animal dander and saliva (cat, dog, horse, rabbit)
- chemicals used in industry
- some foods and medicines
- venom from insect stings

The tendency to have allergies is often passed on in families. For example, if a parent has an allergy problem, there is a higher than normal chance that his or her child also will have allergies. This risk increases if both parents are allergic.

How can I tell an allergy from a cold?

The symptoms of an allergy include:

- an itchy runny nose, with thin, clear nasal discharge and/or a stuffy nose
- itchy watery eyes
- repeated attacks of sneezing and itching of the nose, eyes, or skin that last for weeks or months
- no fever
- often seasonal (spring, summer, fall before frost)

Cold symptoms include:

- stuffy nose
- nasal discharge that is usually clear initially but can turn colored and thick
- a duration of 3 to 10 days, with or without fever
- occasional sneezing
- absence of itching

When do allergies in children first show up?

A few children show signs of allergic reactions during infancy. Other children experience their first problems during adolescence. The first signs of eczema often occur in the first few years of life. Children with asthma and hay fever usually start to show signs during preschool or at least by early grade school. For some children, allergies lessen around the time of puberty. Others will continue to have problems into adult years.

Do drug treatments help?

There are many good medicines to treat allergies and asthma. Some, like antihistamines, are available over-the-counter. They may help relieve many of the symptoms of hay fever and eczema, especially itching, sneezing, and runny nose. Other kinds of medications must be prescribed by your pediatrician. Both allergy and asthma medicines may have side effects. Some antihistamines may cause sleepiness, sometimes interfering with mental tasks. Decongestants (like pseudoephedrine) and oral asthma medications (like albuterol) may make your child irritable. Before using any medication you should talk to your pediatrician and carefully read the warnings listed on the label. If any of these medicines fail to relieve the symptoms, or if side effects interfere with rest, school, or play, you should call your pediatrician. Your child may need a different medication or dose.

When does my child need to see an allergist?

In some cases, avoiding the cause of the allergy or using medicines may not control allergic symptoms. If this happens, your pediatrician may recommend that you see a *pediatric allergist,* a doctor who specializes in hay fever, asthma, eczema, and other allergy-related diseases. The allergist will most likely:

- look for unsuspected triggers for your child's allergic disease
- suggest ways to avoid the cause of your child's allergic symptoms
- give you a specific medication plan to follow

Allergy shots may be recommended. These shots contain small but gradually increasing amounts of the substances to which your child is allergic. This binds the antibodies that cause the allergic symptoms so your child is less sensitive to these substances. Allergy shots are not effective for food allergies. Staying away from the substance that causes trouble is best. Only a small number of children require allergy shots.

How can I help my child?

If you know your child has an allergy, you can try to prevent a problem with the following measures:

- Keeping windows closed during the pollen season, especially on windy days when dust and pollen blow around and in the morning when some pollen counts are highest
- Keeping the house clean and dry to reduce mold and dust mites
- Keeping the household free of pets and indoor plants
- Avoiding foods or other substances known to cause allergic reactions in your child
- Preventing anyone from smoking anywhere near your child, especially in your home and car

You can help your child live a happy, healthy life by working closely with your pediatrician to prevent problems and by using recommended medications. Your pediatrician also can tell you about simple environmental precautions to take and help you decide if your child needs to see an allergy specialist.

Milk allergy

Everyone has heard of children who are allergic to ordinary cow's milk. However, milk allergy is rare. Only 1 child in 100 is truly allergic to cow's milk.

If you suspect your baby has a milk allergy, talk to your pediatrician. Be sure to mention if there is a family history of allergy. Contact your pediatrician or go to the emergency room *right* away if your child:

- Has difficulty with breathing
- Turns blue
- Is pale or weak
- Has swelling in the head and neck area
- Has bloody diarrhea

The best way to prevent a milk allergy is to breastfeed your baby for as long as possible. Very few breastfed babies develop milk allergy. This is especially important if anyone in the immediate family is allergy-prone. When you introduce other foods to your baby, do it gradually (a new one at 1- or 2-week intervals). Watch for the signs of allergy.

If you cannot breastfeed, you may need to use a milk substitute. Talk to your pediatrician about the best milk substitute for your child.

Common allergies

Condition	Triggers	Symptoms
Asthma	A wide range of things can trigger an asthma attack. These include cigarette smoke, viral infections, pollen, dust mites, furry animals, cold air, changing weather conditions, exercise, and even stress.	Coughing, wheezing, difficult breathing; coughing with activity or exertion; chest tightness.
Hay Fever	Pollen from trees, grasses, or weeds.	Stuffy nose, sneezing, and a runny nose; breathing through the mouth because of stuffy nose; rubbing or wrinkling the nose and facial grimacing to relieve nasal itch; watery, itchy eyes; redness or swelling in and under the eyes.
Food allergies	Any foods, but the most common are eggs, peanuts, milk (see information on milk allergies), nuts, soy, fish, wheat, peas, and shellfish.	Vomiting, diarrhea, hives, eczema, difficult breathing, and possibly a drop in blood pressure (shock).
Eczema (atopic dermatitis)	Sometimes made worse by food allergies, contact with allergens (pollen, dust mites, furry animals), irritants, sweating.	A patchy, dry, red, itchy rash that often occurs in the creases of the arms, legs, and neck; however, in infants it often starts on the cheeks, behind the ears, and on the thighs.
Hives	Viral infections, food allergies, and drugs (such as aspirin, penicillin, or sulfa) but cause is often unknown.	Itchy, mosquito-bite-like skin patches that are more red or pale than the surrounding skin. Hives may be found on different parts of the body and do not stay at the same spot for more than a few hours.
Contact dermatitis	Contact with a plant substance such as poison ivy or oak, household detergents and cleansers, and chemicals in some cosmetics and perfumes.	Itchy, red, raised patches that may blister if severe. Most of these patches are confined to the areas of direct contact with the allergen.

American Academy of Pediatrics

DEDICATED TO THE HEALTH OF ALL CHILDREN™

The American Academy of Pediatrics is an organization of 55,000 primary care pediatricians, pediatric medical subspecialists, and pediatric surgical specialists dedicated to the health, safety, and well-being of infants, children, adolescents, and young adults.

American Academy of Pediatrics
PO Box 747
Elk Grove Village, IL 60009-0747
Web site — http://www.aap.org

Anemia and Your Young Child

Guidelines for Parents

Adapted from *Caring for Your Baby and Young Child: Birth to Age 5.*

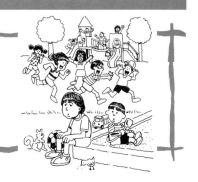

Anemia is a condition that is sometimes found in young children. It can make your child feel cranky, tired, and weak. Though these symptoms may worry you, most cases of anemia are easily treated. This brochure explains the different types of anemia and its causes, symptoms, and treatments.

What is anemia?

Anemia is a condition that occurs when there are not enough red blood cells or hemoglobin to carry oxygen to the other cells in the body. The body's cells need oxygen to survive. Your child may become anemic for any of the following reasons:

- Her body does not produce enough red blood cells.
- Her body destroys or loses (through bleeding) too many red blood cells.
- There is not enough hemoglobin in her red blood cells. *Hemoglobin* is a special pigment that makes it possible for the red blood cells to carry oxygen to all the cells of the body, and to carry waste material (carbon dioxide) away.

Types of anemia

Iron-deficiency anemia is the most common type of anemia in young children. It is caused by a lack of iron in the diet. The body needs iron to produce hemoglobin. If there is too little iron, there will not be enough hemoglobin in the red blood cells. Infants who are given cow's milk too early (before 1 year of age) often develop anemia because there is very little iron in cow's milk. Also, it is hard for young infants to digest cow's milk. Cow's milk can irritate a young infant's bowel and cause slight bleeding. This bleeding lowers the number of red blood cells, and can result in anemia.

A lack of other nutrients in the diet can also cause anemia. Too little folic acid can lead to anemia, though this is very rare. It is most often seen in children fed on goat's milk, which contains very little folic acid. Rarely, too little vitamin B12, vitamin E, or copper can also cause anemia.

Blood loss can also cause anemia. Blood loss can be caused by illness or injury. In rare cases, the blood does not clot properly. This can cause a newborn infant to bleed heavily from his circumcision or a minor injury. Because newborns often lack vitamin K, which helps the blood clot, infants generally get a vitamin K injection right after birth.

Hemolytic anemia occurs when the red blood cells are easily destroyed. *Sickle-cell anemia*, a very severe hemolytic anemia, is most common in children of African heritage. Sickle-cell anemia is caused by an abnormal hemoglobin. Children with sickle-cell anemia may suffer many "crises" or periods of great pain, and need to be hospitalized. *Thalassemia*, another hemolytic anemia, is most common in children of Mediterranean or East Asian origin. If you have a history of sickle-cell anemia or thalassemia in your family, make sure you tell your pediatrician so that your child is tested for it.

Signs and symptoms of anemia

Anemia causes the following signs and symptoms:

- Pale, gray, or "ashy" skin (also, the lining of the eyelids and the nail beds may look less pink than normal)
- Irritability
- Mild weakness
- Tiring easily

Children with severe anemia may have the following additional signs and symptoms:

- Shortness of breath
- Rapid heart rate
- Swollen hands and feet

Also, a newborn with hemolytic anemia may become jaundiced (turn yellow), although many newborns are mildly jaundiced and do not become anemic.

Children who lack iron in their diets may also eat strange things such as ice, dirt, clay, and cornstarch. This behavior is called "pica." It is not harmful unless your child eats something toxic, such as lead paint chips. Usually the pica stops after the anemia is treated and as the child grows older.

If your child shows any of these symptoms or signs, see your pediatrician. A simple blood count can diagnose anemia in most cases.

Treatment for anemia

Since there are so many different types of anemia, it is very important to identify the cause before beginning any treatment. Do not try to treat your child with vitamins, iron, or other nutrients or over-the-counter medications unless your pediatrician recommends it. This is important because such treatment may mask the real cause of the problem. This could delay a proper diagnosis.

If the anemia is due to a lack of iron, your child will be given an iron-containing medication. This comes in a drop form for infants, and liquid or tablet forms for older children. Your pediatrician will determine how long your child should take the iron medication by checking her blood regularly. Do not stop giving the medication until your pediatrician tells you it is no longer needed.

Iron medications are extremely poisonous if too much is taken. Iron is one of the most common causes of poisoning in children under 5 years of age. Keep this and all medication out of the reach of small children.

Following are a few tips concerning iron medication:

- Do not give iron with milk. Milk blocks the absorption of iron.
- Vitamin C increases iron absorption. You might want to follow the dose of iron with a glass of orange juice.
- Liquid iron can turn the teeth a grayish-black color. Have your child swallow it quickly and then rinse her mouth with water. You also may want to brush your child's teeth after every dose of iron. Tooth-staining by iron looks bad, but it is not permanent.
- Iron can cause the stools to become a dark black color. Do not be worried by this change.

Preventing anemia

Iron-deficiency anemia and other nutritional anemias can be prevented easily. Make sure your child is eating a well-balanced diet by following these suggestions:

- Do not give your baby cow's milk until he is over 12 months old.
- If your child is breast-fed, give him foods with added iron, such as cereal, when you begin feeding him solid foods. Before then, he will get enough iron from the breast milk. However, feeding him solid foods with too little iron will decrease the amount of iron he gets from the milk.

- If you formula-feed your baby, give him formula with added iron.
- Make sure your older child eats a well-balanced diet with foods that contain iron. Many grains and cereals have added iron (check labels to be sure). Other good sources of iron include egg yolks, red meat, potatoes, tomatoes, molasses, and raisins. Also, to increase the iron in your family's diet, use the fruit pulp in juices, and cook potatoes with the skins on.

With proper treatment, your child's anemia should improve quickly. Be sure to contact your pediatrician if you think your child might be anemic.

The information contained in this publication should not be used as a substitute for the medical care and advice of your pediatrician. There may be variations in treatment that your pediatrician may recommend based on individual facts and circumstances.

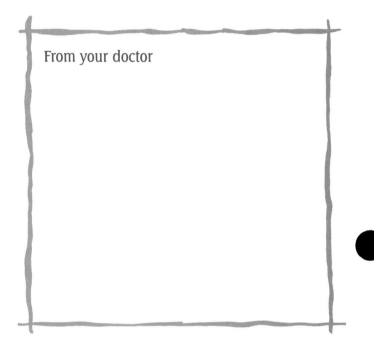

From your doctor

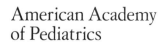

American Academy of Pediatrics

DEDICATED TO THE HEALTH OF ALL CHILDREN™

The American Academy of Pediatrics is an organization of 55,000 primary care pediatricians, pediatric medical subspecialists, and pediatric surgical specialists dedicated to the health, safety, and well-being of infants, children, adolescents, and young adults.

American Academy of Pediatrics
PO Box 747
Elk Grove Village, IL 60009-0747
Web site — http://www.aap.org

Bronchiolitis and Your Young Child
Guidelines for Parents
Adapted from *Caring for Your Baby and Young Child: Birth to Age 5*

Respiratory illnesses caused by viruses are some of the most common health problems in infancy. The common cold is the one we see most often. Bronchiolitis is another. Because of its symptoms, bronchiolitis can be scary for parents as well as children. This brochure explains what bronchiolitis is, as well as its causes, symptoms, and treatments.

What is bronchiolitis?

Bronchiolitis is an infection of the small breathing tubes (bronchioles) of the lungs. It occurs most often in infants. *Bronchiolitis* is sometimes confused with *bronchitis*, which is an infection of the larger, more central airways.

Bronchiolitis is almost always caused by a virus. The infection causes the small airways in the lungs to swell. This blocks the flow of air through the lungs and makes it hard for your baby to breathe. From October through March, bronchiolitis is often caused by *respiratory syncytial virus* (RSV) infection. During the other months, the illness is usually caused by other viruses.

Most adults and many children with RSV infections get only a cold. In infants the infection is more likely to lead to bronchiolitis. This is because their airways are smaller and are more easily blocked. Infants who develop bronchiolitis may develop asthma later in life. It is possible that RSV infection is the first trigger for the asthma. RSV is spread by contact with an infected person's mucus or saliva. It often spreads through families, child-care centers, and hospital wards. Careful hand washing can help prevent the spread of this infection.

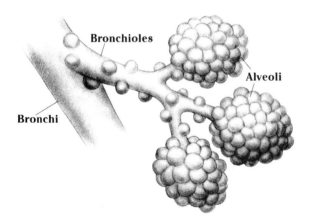

Signs and symptoms

A baby who develops bronchiolitis often starts off with signs of a cold, such as a runny nose, a mild cough, and a fever. After a day or two his cough may get worse. He will begin to breathe faster. The following signs may mean that he is having trouble breathing:

- He may widen his nostrils and squeeze the muscles under his rib cage to try to get more air in and out of his lungs.
- When he breathes he may grunt and tighten his stomach muscles.
- He will make a high-pitched whistling sound, called a wheeze, each time he breathes out.
- He may not take fluids well because he is working so hard to breathe that he has trouble sucking and swallowing.
- If it gets very hard for him to breathe, you may notice a bluish tint around his lips and fingertips. This tells you that his airways are so blocked that there is not enough oxygen getting into the blood.

If your baby shows any of these signs of trouble breathing, or if his fever lasts more than 24 hours (or is present at all in an infant under 3 months of age), call your pediatrician.

Also call your pediatrician if your baby develops any of the following signs or symptoms of dehydration:

- Taking less than her normal amount of fluids
- Dry mouth
- Crying without tears
- Urinating less often than normal

If you think your child has bronchiolitis and your child has any of the following conditions, call your pediatrician.

- Cystic fibrosis
- Congenital heart disease
- Bronchopulmonary dysplasia (seen in some infants who have been on a respirator as newborns)
- Immune deficiency disease (like AIDS)
- Organ transplant
- A cancer for which she is receiving chemotherapy

Home Treatment

There are no medications you can use to treat RSV infections at home. Antibiotics, which treat bacteria, are not helpful for bronchiolitis because it is almost always caused by a virus. However, you can ease your child's cold symptoms. Try the following suggestions:

To relieve stuffy nose and fever:

- Thin the mucus using mild salt-solution (saline) nose drops recommended by your pediatrician. *Never use nonprescription nose drops that contain any medication. Only use salt-solution nose drops.*

- Clear your baby's nose with a suction bulb. Squeeze the bulb part of the device first. Gently put the rubber tip into one nostril, and slowly release the bulb. This slight amount of suction will draw the clogged mucus out of the nose. This works best when your baby is under 6 months old.

- Place a cool-mist humidifier (vaporizer) in your baby's room. Set it close to her. Be sure to clean and dry the humidifier each day to keep bacteria or mold from growing. *Do not use hot water vaporizers since they can cause serious scalds or burns.*

- If your baby has a fever, give her acetaminophen. (Be sure to follow the recommended dosage for your child's age.) Do not give aspirin to your child. Aspirin has been associated with Reye syndrome, a disease that affects the liver and the brain. Never give her any other kind of cold medicine without first checking with your pediatrician.

To prevent dehydration:

- Make sure your baby drinks lots of fluid so he does not become dehydrated. He may prefer clear liquids rather than milk or formula. He may feed more slowly and may not tolerate solid foods very well because he is having trouble breathing.

Professional Treatment

If your baby is having mild to moderate trouble breathing, your pediatrician may try using a drug that opens up the breathing tubes, which seems to help some infants.

Some children with bronchiolitis need to be hospitalized, either for breathing problems or dehydration. Your pediatrician will treat your baby's breathing problems with oxygen and medication. The dehydration will be treated with a special liquid diet or with fluids given intravenously (directly into the blood stream).

Sometimes, pediatricians use a medication called *Ribavirin or Respigam* to treat RSV infection in an infants who has serious lung disease. This medicine is rarely needed if the baby is otherwise normal and healthy.

Very rarely an infant will not respond to any of these treatments. She might have to be put on a breathing machine (respirator). This usually is only a temporary measure to help her until her body is able to overcome the infection.

Prevention

The best way to protect your baby from bronchiolitis is to keep him away from the viruses that cause it. When possible, avoid close contact with children or adults who have colds. If your baby is in a child-care center where other children might have RSV, make sure that those who care for him wash their hands well and often.

When your baby has a cold, he needs a bit more attention to detect early signs of bronchiolitis or another serious infection. Be sure to call your pediatrician if you think your baby might have such a problem.

The information contained in this publication should not be used as a substitute for the medical care and advice of your pediatrician. There may be variations in treatment that your pediatrician may recommend based on individual facts and circumstances.

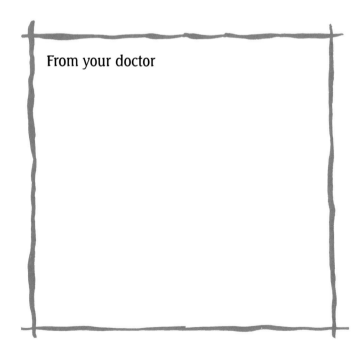

From your doctor

American Academy of Pediatrics

DEDICATED TO THE HEALTH OF ALL CHILDREN™

The American Academy of Pediatrics is an organization of 55,000 primary care pediatricians, pediatric medical subspecialists, and pediatric surgical specialists dedicated to the health, safety, and well-being of infants, children, adolescents, and young adults.

American Academy of Pediatrics
PO Box 747
Elk Grove Village, IL 60009-0747
Web site — http://www.aap.org

Common Childhood Infections

Part I Respiratory and Ear, Nose, and Throat Infections

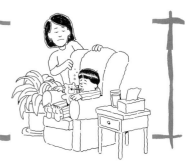

There was a time when childhood infections killed thousands of children. Today, vaccines protect against many of those infections, but you cannot immunize your child against every infectious disease. If you know the signs and symptoms of the most common childhood infections, you can at least help your sick child get better.

It is also important to know when to contact your pediatrician. Do so if you see signs of any of the following illnesses and are concerned (especially if your child is under 2 months of age). Use this brochure as a guide to common childhood infections.

Causes of infections

Most infections in children are caused by viruses, but they can also be caused by bacteria. Bacteria can live in certain parts of the body without causing any harm. They cause infections when they move to parts of the body where they do not belong. They can also come into the body from the outside; in the body they can cause an infection that requires treatment with an antibiotic.

Most viral diseases are not treated with an antibiotic because antibiotics do not work on viruses. Instead, the body gets rid of viruses on its own. When your child has a virus, your pediatrician will tell you how to make your child more comfortable. You should also make sure your child gets plenty of rest and eats a balanced diet.

Colds

We all know the symptoms of the common cold—sneezing, watery eyes, a cough, and a stuffy, runny nose. A child with a cold will often be cranky and have a mild fever and a headache.

Since there are hundreds of viruses that cause colds, there is still no vaccine for the common cold. Symptoms can be relieved with:

- a cool-mist vaporizer
- acetaminophen to bring down a fever
- decongestants
- lots of fluids

A cold usually lasts about a week. Any fever should appear at the beginning of the cold and then go away. Contact your pediatrician if:

- a fever continues or goes up during the week,
- symptoms seem to get worse after a week, or
- your child has problems breathing or ear pain.

Ear infection

Occasionally, children with colds will develop an earache. Since younger infants cannot complain of ear pain, be on the lookout for other signs. Fussiness, fever, or fluid draining from your child's ear may mean your child has an ear infection.

If your child has any of those symptoms, your pediatrician will examine her to determine if an ear infection is present. If there is one, he or she may prescribe an antibiotic to kill the bacteria that cause the infection. Be sure to give your child the full dose of the antibiotic for the whole time it is prescribed. This is important even if symptoms go away within a few days. You can give acetaminophen (in a dose recommended by your pediatrician) to ease any ear pain, but do not give aspirin. Aspirin has been linked with Reye syndrome, a serious disease that affects the liver and brain. After your child finishes the antibiotic, the pediatrician should check her ears again. Even after the pain and fever have gone, fluid can still remain. This can lead to more infections or future hearing problems.

Sinusitis

When your child has a cold, the sinuses around his nose often get stuffy and swollen. Sometimes the mucus in the sinuses may get infected with bacteria. When this happens, your child has a sinus infection. Sinusitis usually develops after your child has had a cold for at least 10 days. Signs of sinusitis are:

- persistent nasal discharge
- fever
- a cough during the day and night, that often gets worse at night
- tenderness in the face
- headaches

An antibiotic will destroy the bacteria that cause sinusitis.

Strep throat

Strep throat is a bacterial infection. On rare occasions it can lead to serious problems if not treated. Strep usually develops in children over 3 years of age. Signs of strep include a sore throat, fever, and swollen glands in the neck. (If there is also a skin rash, the condition is called **scarlet fever**.) Since many viruses can cause the same symptoms as strep, your pediatrician will need to test for strep to be sure your child has it. To do this, he or she will obtain a throat culture or do a rapid strep test.

If your child does have strep throat, your pediatrician will prescribe an antibiotic that will destroy the strep germ. After 24 to 36 hours of antibiotic treatment, your child is no longer contagious and should start to feel better. Remember to have your child finish all the medicine. If you stop treatment too early, the infection may come back or cause other problems.

If not treated, strep throat can lead to rheumatic fever. This can cause damage to the heart and swelling of the joints. Untreated strep throat can also lead to kidney disease and a number of other health problems.

Croup

Croup is a scary illness for most parents because of its symptoms. Your child may go to bed with a runny nose and mild cough, but wake up during the night with a cough that sounds like a seal's bark.

Croup is usually caused by a viral infection in and around the voice box. Your child's breathing may become noisy and labored, a condition called **stridor.** Your child may or may not have a fever.

Most cases of croup can be handled at home with the advice of your pediatrician. A cool-mist vaporizer may help. If you do not have one, turn on the hot water in your shower or bathtub and let the bathroom fill up with steam. Stay with your child in the bathroom while he breathes in the steam for a few minutes. Keep a close eye on your child so that he does not burn himself with the hot water. (Try sitting with your child on your lap, and read a short story to pass the time.) Or you could take your child for a walk in the cool night air. This may help your child to breathe better.

If your child has a severe case of croup, your pediatrician may recommend a hospital stay. During the stay, your child may need to be inside a plastic tent called a croup tent. To reduce the swelling around the voice box, doctors may give your child a cortisone medication or a medication to inhale.

Bronchiolitis

Bronchiolitis is a common disease of the lower respiratory tract (the bronchioles). It occurs most often in the winter. Bronchiolitis causes coughing, wheezing, and breathing trouble. It is most commonly found in children under 2 years of age. It often develops in infants and toddlers after they come into contact with someone who has an upper respiratory tract illness.

Bronchiolitis starts like a normal cold, with a runny nose and sneezing. After a few days, a child with bronchiolitis will develop a wheezy cough and trouble breathing. She may be cranky too. The cough and breathing problems may make it hard for her to eat. In some infants with severe bronchiolitis, symptoms appear much more quickly.

Bronchiolitis is usually caused by a virus that leads to swelling of the small bronchial tubes. This traps air and mucus in the lungs. Children with mild cases, especially those with a thick nasal mucus, may get some relief with a cool-mist vaporizer. A child who has a lot of trouble breathing may need to go to the hospital for oxygen and fluids. Sometimes medication may be used to help open the bronchial tubes and improve breathing.

A specific virus called respiratory syncytial virus (RSV) can cause bronchiolitis. If infection with RSV is severe or occurs in infants who also have a chronic illness (especially heart disease or lung disease), an antiviral agent called ribavirin (Virazole) can be used in the treatment.

Pneumonia

Pneumonia is an inflammation of the lungs. The symptoms vary based on the cause and severity of the illness. Viruses cause most pneumonias in children. Luckily these illnesses are mild. A child may have a cough, mild fever, and decreased appetite and energy. Viral pneumonias are often treated with acetaminophen for fever and are sometimes treated with bronchodilators (if there is wheezing). Bacterial pneumonias tend to have more severe symptoms, and they respond best to therapy with antibiotics, fluids, and humid air.

Pneumonia often occurs a few days after the start of an upper respiratory tract infection. If one of the more severe types of pneumonia develops, your child may suddenly have shaking chills; a high fever; difficult, rapid breathing; and other breathing problems. A cough may not develop until later. In many cases your pediatrician may need an x-ray to make sure that pneumonia is the cause of the symptoms.

Most cases of pneumonia can be safely treated at home. If the symptoms are severe or your child is under 6 months of age, however, he may need to go to the hospital for treatment.

Signs of infection in an infant

These are the signs of infection in an infant under 2 months of age. Since infections can be especially dangerous in a child this young, call your pediatrician right away if your child develops any of these symptoms:

- poor feeding
- poor color
- listlessness
- weak cry
- rectal temperature of at least 100.4°F
- breathing problems
- unusual fussiness
- sleeping more than usual
- vomiting or diarrhea

The information contained in this publication should not be used as a substitute for the medical care and advice of your pediatrician. There may be variations in treatment that your pediatrician may recommend based on individual facts and circumstances.

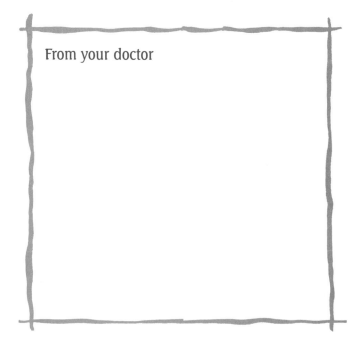

From your doctor

American Academy of Pediatrics

DEDICATED TO THE HEALTH OF ALL CHILDREN™

The American Academy of Pediatrics is an organization of 55,000 primary care pediatricians, pediatric medical subspecialists, and pediatric surgical specialists dedicated to the health, safety, and well-being of infants, children, adolescents, and young adults.

American Academy of Pediatrics
PO Box 747
Elk Grove Village, IL 60009-0747
Web site — http://www.aap.org

Common Childhood Infections

Part II Other Common Infections

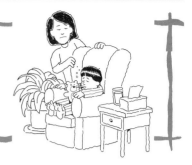

There was a time when childhood infections killed thousands of children. Today, vaccines protect against many of those infections, but you cannot immunize your child against every infectious disease. If you know the signs and symptoms of the most common childhood infections, you can at least help your sick child get better.

It is also important to know when to contact your pediatrician. Do so if you see signs of any of the following illnesses and are concerned (especially if your child is under 2 months of age). Use this brochure as a guide to common childhood infections.

Causes of infections

Most infections in children are caused by viruses, but they can also be caused by bacteria. Bacteria can live in certain parts of the body without causing any harm. They cause infections when they move to parts of the body where they do not belong. They can also come into the body from the outside; in the body they can cause an infection that requires treatment with an antibiotic.

Most viral diseases are not treated with an antibiotic because antibiotics do not work on viruses. Instead, the body gets rid of viruses on its own. When your child has a virus, your pediatrician will tell you how to make your child more comfortable. You should also make sure your child gets plenty of rest and eats a balanced diet.

Conjunctivitis (pinkeye)

Pinkeye is an infection that causes painful or itchy, red eyes. The undersides of your child's eyelids may also be irritated.

To treat pinkeye, your pediatrician may prescribe warm compresses and antibiotic drops or ointment. If the redness and swelling remain after a few days of treatment, it may mean a virus or allergy is causing the pinkeye.

Let your pediatrician know if your child has eye irritation with a high fever, sluggishness, or more severe swelling and redness around the eye. These could be signs of a more serious infection.

Not all pinkeye infections are contagious. Your pediatrician can let you know whether your child should stay out of school or the child care center until the infection clears.

Sty

A tender, local swelling and redness on your child's eyelid are usually signs of a sty. This is an infection in a gland of the eyelid. To treat a sty, apply warm compresses often. Let your pediatrician know if this does not work. He or she may then prescribe an antibiotic ointment or refer your child to an eye doctor who can drain the sty surgically. Sties are not very contagious.

Vomiting and diarrhea

Vomiting and diarrhea are the reasons many parents call the pediatrician. These illnesses are usually caused by viruses that infect the intestine. They usually last only about a day or two, but in some cases they can last up to a week.

If your child is throwing up, your pediatrician may tell you to not give food and fluid for a few hours. You can then give your child small sips of clear fluids, later followed by easy-to-digest foods. This will help prevent more vomiting, which can lead to dehydration.

Diarrhea is frequent, loose, watery stools. You may need to stop feeding your child solid foods and milk for 12 to 24 hours and instead give an oral electrolyte solution to prevent dehydration. You can buy this at your local drugstore.

Giardia is a parasite that infects the bowel and often causes prolonged diarrhea. It can be a problem, especially for those in child care centers and rural areas. If your child's diarrhea does not clear up, your pediatrician may test for *Giardia*. Disease caused by Giardia is treated with medication.

Mild vomiting and diarrhea rarely cause dehydration. However, if your child is dehydrated, she may:
- seem tired or have less energy
- produce less urine or tears
- have a dry mouth
- have sunken eyes

Some children may throw up many times over several days. If this occurs, and you notice any of the other symptoms listed previously, your pediatrician will want to examine your child. These symptoms may indicate dehydration or, less often, the first signs of a rare condition known as Reye syndrome. As Reye syndrome has been linked with taking aspirin during certain viral illnesses, you should never give aspirin to an infant or child.

If dehydration occurs, your child may need to have an intravenous (IV) tube inserted to receive fluids through her veins. To reduce the chance of dehydration, call your pediatrician early if your child has vomiting or diarrhea that will not go away.

Urinary tract infection (UTI)

Urinary tract infections (UTIs) are found in children from infancy through adolescence. A UTI occurs in the kidney or bladder and can cause the following symptoms:
- fever
- painful and frequent urination
- vomiting
- abdominal pain

Treatment of UTIs consists of taking an antibiotic for about 10 days. Even though your child shows signs of improvement within 1 to 2 days of starting to take an antibiotic, he must still finish the entire prescription.

X-rays and other tests are often needed to help determine the causes of the UTI.

Impetigo (skin infection)

Your child may have a skin infection called **impetigo** if a scratch turns into a yellow, oozing, crusty sore surrounded by redness. Impetigo can spread on the skin quickly. It can also spread to other people if they touch the infected skin lesions, by fingers, or from soiled clothing. This infection is most common in warm weather.

An antibiotic, taken by mouth or in ointment form, is used to treat impetigo.

If any of these illnesses or infections develop, remember that your pediatrician is your best source of help. Most important, if the illness or infection does not seem to go away, or appears to get worse, your pediatrician needs to know. Always call when you are concerned!

Signs of infection in an infant

These are the signs of infection in an infant under 2 months of age. Since infections can be especially dangerous in a child this young, call your pediatrician right away if your child develops any of these symptoms:

- poor feeding
- poor color
- listlessness
- weak cry
- rectal temperature of at least 100.4°F
- breathing problems
- unusual fussiness
- sleeping more than usual
- vomiting or diarrhea

The information contained in this publication should not be used as a substitute for the medical care and advice of your pediatrician. There may be variations in treatment that your pediatrician may recommend based on individual facts and circumstances.

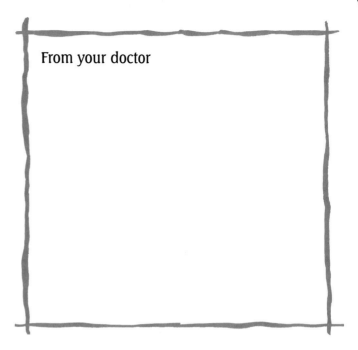

From your doctor

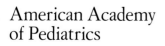

American Academy of Pediatrics

DEDICATED TO THE HEALTH OF ALL CHILDREN™

The American Academy of Pediatrics is an organization of 55,000 primary care pediatricians, pediatric medical subspecialists, and pediatric surgical specialists dedicated to the health, safety, and well-being of infants, children, adolescents, and young adults.

American Academy of Pediatrics
PO Box 747
Elk Grove Village, IL 60009-0747
Web site — http://www.aap.org

Croup and Your Young Child

Adapted from *Caring for Your Baby and Young Child: Birth to Age 5.*

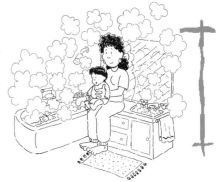

Croup is a common illness in young children. It can be scary for parents as well as children. This brochure explains the different types of croup and the causes, symptoms, and treatments.

What is croup?

Croup is an infection that causes a swelling of the voice box (larynx) and windpipe (trachea), making the airway just below the vocal cords become narrow. This makes breathing noisy and difficult.

Most children get infectious croup once or twice, and some children get croup whenever they have a respiratory illness. Children are most likely to get croup between 6 months and 3 years of age. After age 3, it is not as common because the windpipe is larger and swelling is less likely to get in the way of breathing. Croup can occur at any time of the year, but it is more common in the winter months.

Different types of croup

- *Viral croup* is the most common and is the result of a viral infection in the voice box and windpipe. This kind of croup often starts with a cold that slowly turns into a barking cough. Your child's voice will become hoarse and her breathing will get noisier. She may make a coarse musical sound each time she breathes in, called *stridor*. Most children with viral croup have a low fever, but some have temperatures up to 104°F.
- *Spasmodic croup* is usually caused by a mild upper respiratory infection or allergy. It can be scary because it comes on suddenly in the middle of the night. Your child may go to bed with a mild cold and wake up in a few hours, gasping for breath. He will be hoarse and have stridor when he breathes in. He also may have a cough that sounds like a seal barking. Most children with spasmodic croup do not have a fever. This type of croup can reoccur. It is probably similar to asthma and often responds to asthma medicines.

As your child's effort to breathe increases, he may stop eating and drinking. He also may become too tired to cough, although you will hear the stridor more with each breath. The danger with croup accompanied by stridor is that the airway will keep swelling. If this happens, it may reach a point where your child cannot breathe at all.

Stridor is common with mild croup, especially when a child is crying or moving actively. But if a child has stridor while resting, it can be a sign of severe croup.

Treatment

If your child wakes up in the middle of the night with croup, take her into the bathroom. Close the door and turn the shower on the hottest setting to let the bathroom steam up. Sit in the steamy bathroom with your child. Within 15 to 20 minutes, the warm, moist air should help her breathing. (She still will have the barking cough, though.)

For the rest of that night (and 2 to 3 nights after), try to use a cold-water vaporizer or humidifier in your child's room. Sometimes another attack of croup will occur the same night or the next. If it does, repeat the steam treatment in the bathroom. Steam almost always works. If it does not, take your child outdoors for a few minutes. Inhaling moist, cool night air may help open the air passages so that she can breathe more freely. If that does not help, call your pediatrician. If your child's breathing becomes a serious struggle or if your child looks blue, call for emergency medical services. (In most areas, dial 911.)

Never try to open your child's airway with your finger. Breathing is being blocked by swollen tissue out of your reach, so you cannot clear it away. Besides, putting your finger in your child's throat will only upset her. This can make her breathing even more difficult. For the same reasons, do not force your child to throw up. If she does vomit, hold her head down and then quickly sit her back up once she is finished.

Treating with medication

If your child has viral croup and is not breathing better after the steam treatment, your pediatrician may prescribe a steroid medication to reduce swelling. Steroids can be inhaled, taken by mouth, or given by injection. Treatment with a few doses of steroids should do no harm. For spasmodic croup, your pediatrician may recommend a bronchodilator to help your child's breathing.

Antibiotics, which treat bacteria, are not helpful because croup is almost always caused by a virus or allergy. Cough syrups are of little use too, because they do not affect the larynx or trachea, where the infection is located. These also may get in the way of your child coughing up the mucus from the infection.

If you are concerned that your child has croup, call your pediatrician even if it is the middle of the night. Also, listen closely to your child's breathing. Call for emergency medical services immediately if he

- Makes a whistling sound that gets louder with each breath
- Cannot speak or make verbal sounds for lack of breath
- Seems to be struggling to get a breath
- Has a bluish mouth or fingernails
- Has stridor when resting
- Drools or has extreme difficulty swallowing saliva

In the most serious cases, your child will not be getting enough oxygen into his blood. If this happens, he may need to go into the hospital. Luckily, these severe cases of croup do not occur very often.

Other infections

Another cause of stridor, barking cough, and serious breathing problems is acute epiglottitis (also known as supraglottitis). This is a dangerous infection with symptoms that can be a lot like those of croup. Luckily, the infection is less common now because there is a vaccine to protect against its cause, a bacterium called *Haemophilus influenzae* type b (Hib).

Acute epiglottitis usually affects children 1 to 5 years old and comes on suddenly with a high fever. Your child may seem very sick. She may have to sit up to be able to breathe. She also may drool because she cannot swallow the saliva in her mouth. If not treated, this disease could lead to complete blockage of your child's airway. If your pediatrician suspects acute epiglottitis, your child will go into the hospital for treatment with antibiotics. She will need a tube in her windpipe to help her breathe. Call your pediatrician immediately if you think your child has epiglottitis.

To protect against acute epiglottitis, your child should get the first dose of the Hib vaccine when she is 2 months old. This vaccine will also protect against meningitis (a swelling in the covering of the brain). Since the Hib vaccine has been available, the number of cases of acute epiglottitis and meningitis has decreased.

When croup persists or recurs frequently, your child may have some narrowing of the airway that is not related to an infection. This may be a problem that was present when your child was born, or one that developed later. If your child has persistent or recurrent croup, your pediatrician may refer you to a specialist for further evaluation.

Croup is a common illness during childhood. Although most cases are mild, croup can become serious and prevent your child from breathing. Contact your pediatrician if you suspect your child has croup. He or she will make sure your child is evaluated and treated properly.

The information contained in this publication should not be used as a substitute for the medical care and advice of your pediatrician. There may be variations in treatment that your pediatrician may recommend based on individual facts and circumstances.

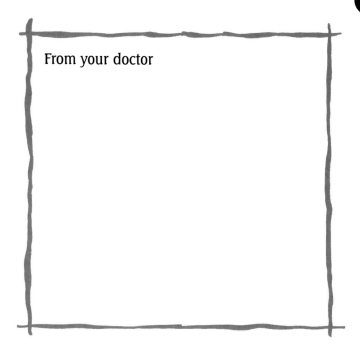

From your doctor

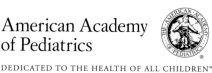

American Academy of Pediatrics

DEDICATED TO THE HEALTH OF ALL CHILDREN™

The American Academy of Pediatrics is an organization of 55,000 primary care pediatricians, pediatric medical subspecialists, and pediatric surgical specialists dedicated to the health, safety, and well-being of infants, children, adolescents, and young adults.

American Academy of Pediatrics
PO Box 747
Elk Grove Village, IL 60009-0747
Web site — http://www.aap.org

Diarrhea and Dehydration

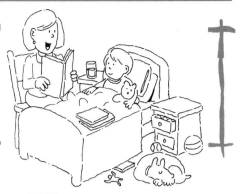

What is diarrhea?

Diarrhea is the passage of watery stools.

What causes diarrhea?

Most diarrhea in children is caused by one of several diarrhea-causing viruses and gets better by itself within a week. Although there can be many causes of diarrhea, the treatment suggested here is appropriate for acute illness (sudden onset, short lasting), which occurs most commonly.

A child with viral diarrhea has a fever and often starts the illness with some vomiting. Shortly after these symptoms appear, the child develops diarrhea. Often children with viral diarrhea "feel bad," but do not act ill.

You should call your pediatrician if your child is less than 6 months of age or has any of the following:

- blood in stool
- frequent vomiting
- abdominal pain
- urinates less frequently (wets fewer than 6 diapers per day)
- no tears when crying
- loss of appetite for liquids
- high fever
- frequent diarrhea
- dry, sticky mouth
- weight loss
- extreme thirst

It is not necessary to call your pediatrician if your child *continues* to look *well* even though there may be:

- frequent or large stools
- lots of intestinal gas
- green or yellow stools

How long will the diarrhea last?

Most of the time mild diarrhea lasts from 3 to 6 days. Occasionally a child will have loose stools for several days longer. As long as the child acts well and is taking adequate fluids and food, loose stools are not a great concern.

Mild illness and diet

Most children should continue to eat a normal diet including formula or milk while they have mild diarrhea. Breastfeeding should continue. If your baby seems bloated or gassy after drinking cow's milk or formula, call your pediatrician to discuss a temporary change in diet.

Special fluids for mild illness

These are not usually necessary for children with mild illness.

Moderate illness

Children with moderate diarrhea can be cared for easily at home with close supervision, special fluids, and your pediatrician's advice. Your pediatrician will recommend the amount and length of time that special fluids should be used. Later, a normal diet can be resumed. Some children are not able to tolerate cow's milk when they have diarrhea and it may be temporarily removed from the diet by your pediatrician. Breastfeeding should continue.

Special fluids for moderate illness

Special fluids have been designed to replace water and salts lost during diarrhea. These are extremely helpful for the home management of mild to moderately severe illness. Do not try to prepare these special fluids yourself. It is too easy to get confused by some of these complex recipes. You could accidentally make a bad fluid for your baby. Use a fluid that is made by one of the reputable manufacturers. The two most widely available products that you will find in nearly every pharmacy are:

- Pedialyte (Ross Laboratories)
- Infalyte (Mead Johnson Nutritionals)
- Other brands of special fluids are available and equally effective.
- Many drug stores have their own generic brands of special fluids. Ask the pharmacist for assistance.

If a child is not vomiting, these fluids can be used in very generous amounts until the child starts making normal amounts of urine again.

Severe illness

If your child develops the warning signs of illness listed in the previous column, he or she may require IV fluids in the emergency department for several hours to correct dehydration. Usually hospitalization is not necessary. Immediately seek your pediatrician's advice for the appropriate care if symptoms of severe illness occur.

Commonly asked questions:

Q. Should a child with diarrhea be fasted?

A. Absolutely not! Once she is rehydrated, let the child eat as much or as little of the usual diet as she wants. If she is vomiting, offer small amounts of liquids frequently.

Q. What about soft drinks, juices, or boiled skim milk?

A. A child with mild diarrhea can have regular fluids. But, if there is enough diarrhea to make your child thirsty, he must have special fluids (see Special fluids for moderate illness). Soft drinks, soda pop, soups, juices, sports drinks, and boiled skim milk have the wrong amounts of sugar and salt and may make your child sicker.

Q. What about anti-diarrhea medicines?

A. These medicines are not useful in most cases of diarrhea and can sometimes be harmful. Never use them unless they are recommended by your pediatrician.

Q. Which therapy is best?

A. Because diarrhea is so common, there are many different home remedies that have been tried through the years. Some of these old ideas may not be effective and some may actually make things worse. The recommendations in this brochure are based on the best information available at this time. If you have any questions about them, please check with your pediatrician.

Reminder–do's and don'ts

DO

- Watch for signs of dehydration which occur when a child loses too much fluid and becomes dried out. Symptoms of dehydration include a decrease in urination, no tears when baby cries, high fever, dry mouth, weight loss, extreme thirst, listlessness, and sunken eyes.
- Keep your pediatrician informed if there is any significant change in how your child is behaving.
- Report if your child has blood in his stool.
- Report if your child develops a high fever (more than 102°F or 39°C).
- Continue to feed your child if she is not vomiting. You may have to give your child smaller amounts of food than normal or give your child foods that do not further upset his or her stomach.
- Use diarrhea replacement fluids that are specifically made for diarrhea if your child is thirsty.

DON'T

- Try to make special salt and fluid combinations at home unless your pediatrician instructs you and you have the proper instruments.
- Prevent the child from eating if she is hungry.
- Use boiled milk or other salty broth and soups.
- Use "anti-diarrhea" medicines unless prescribed by your pediatrician.

From your doctor

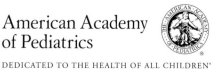
American Academy of Pediatrics

DEDICATED TO THE HEALTH OF ALL CHILDREN™

The American Academy of Pediatrics is an organization of 55,000 primary care pediatricians, pediatric medical subspecialists, and pediatric surgical specialists dedicated to the health, safety, and well-being of infants, children, adolescents, and young adults.

American Academy of Pediatrics
PO Box 747
Elk Grove Village, IL 60009-0747
Web site — http://www.aap.org

Copyright ©1996   American Academy of Pediatrics

Ear Infections and Children

Part I Symptoms, Treatment, and Complications

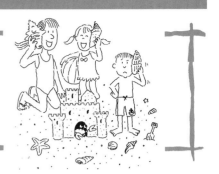

Next to the common cold, an ear infection is the most common childhood illness. In fact, most children have had at least one ear infection by the time they are 3 years old. Most of the time, ear infections clear up without causing any lasting problems. But, if they occur often or are not treated, they can lead to hearing loss or other damage. The American Academy of Pediatrics has developed this brochure to inform parents about the symptoms, treatments, and possible complications of *acute otitis media*, a common infection of the middle ear.

How do ear infections develop?

The ear has three main parts: the outer ear, middle ear, and inner ear (see illustration). A tiny tube, called the eustachian tube, connects the middle ear to the back of the throat and nose. When a child has a cold, nose or throat infection, or allergy, the eustachian tube can become blocked, causing a buildup of fluid in the middle ear. If this fluid becomes infected by bacteria or a virus, it can cause swelling of the eardrum and pain in the ear. This type of ear infection is called *acute otitis media.*

Often after the symptoms of acute otitis media clear up, fluid remains in the ear. Acute otitis media then develops into another kind of ear problem called *otitis media with effusion.* This condition is harder to detect than acute otitis media because, except for the fluid and some hearing loss that is usually mild, there are often no other noticeable symptoms. This fluid often lasts for up to 3 months and, in most cases, disappears on its own. The child's hearing then returns to normal.

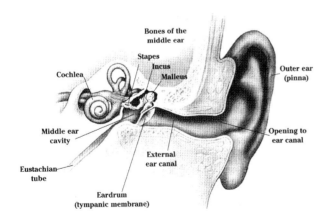

Cross-Section of the Ear

There are several risk factors for developing childhood ear infection, including:

Age. Infants and young children are more likely to get ear infections. The size and shape of their eustachian tubes make it easier for fluid to build up. Ear infections occur most often in children between 3 months and 3 years of age.

Also, the younger a child is at the time of the first ear infection, the greater the chance he or she will have repeated infections.

Sex. Although researchers are not sure why, boys have more ear infections than girls.

Heredity. Ear infections can run in families. Children are more likely to have repeated middle-ear infections if a parent or sibling also had repeated ear infections.

Colds/Allergies. Colds often lead to ear infections. Children in group child care settings have a higher chance of passing their colds to each other because they are exposed to more germs and viruses from the other children. Allergies that cause stuffy noses can also lead to ear infections.

Tobacco smoke. Children who breathe in someone else's tobacco smoke have a higher risk of developing health problems, including ear infections.

Bottle-feeding. Babies who are bottle-fed, especially while they are lying down, get more ear infections than breastfed babies. If you bottle-feed your child, hold his or her head above the stomach level during feedings. This keeps the eustachian tubes from getting blocked.

Parents can help reduce some of the risks of ear infections. For instance:

- Breastfeed instead of bottle-feed. Breastfeeding may decrease the risk of frequent colds and ear infections. If you do bottle-feed, do not give your child a bottle while he or she is lying down in the crib or playpen.
- Keep your child away from tobacco smoke, especially in your home or car.
- Try to keep your child's hands clean.

Symptoms of an ear infection

Your child may have a number of symptoms during an ear infection. Knowing what these symptoms are may help you treat some of them more quickly and get medical care, if needed.

Pain. The most common symptom of an ear infection is pain. While older children are able to tell you when their ears hurt, younger children may only appear irritable and cry. This may be more noticeable during feedings because sucking and swallowing may cause painful pressure changes in the middle ear. As a result of this discomfort, your child may have less of an appetite. A child with an ear infection may also have more trouble sleeping because lying down can increase ear pain.

There are other reasons besides an ear infection why your child's ears may hurt. In these cases, your child probably has an earache, not an ear infection. Ear pain can be caused by:

- an infection of the skin of the ear canal, often called "swimmer's ear"
- blocked or plugged eustachian tubes from colds or allergies
- a sore throat
- teething or sore gums

Fever. Another sign of an ear infection is a temperature ranging from 100°F to 104°F.

Ear drainage. You might also notice yellow or white fluid, possibly blood-tinged, draining from your child's ear. The fluid may have a foul odor and will look different from normal earwax (which is orange-yellow or reddish-brown). Pain and pressure often decrease after this drainage begins but this does not always mean that the infection is going away. If your child needs to travel in an airplane, or wants to swim, contact your pediatrician for specific instructions.

Difficulty hearing. During and after an ear infection, your child may have trouble hearing for several weeks. This occurs because the fluid behind the eardrum gets in the way of sound transmission. This is usually temporary and clears up after the fluid from the middle ear drains away. Because your child can have trouble hearing without other symptoms of an ear infection, watch for the following changes in behavior (especially during or after a cold) that may mean he or she cannot hear well:

- talking softly or in a muffled way
- saying "huh?" or "what?" more than usual
- not responding to sounds
- having more trouble understanding language in noisy rooms
- listening with the TV or radio turned up louder than usual

If you think your child may have difficulty hearing, contact your pediatrician. Being able to hear and listen to others talk helps a child learn speech and language. This is especially important during the first few years of life.

Treatment of ear infections

If your child has a fever, ear pain, or shows other symptoms of an ear infection, it is important to see your pediatrician. If your child's ears are infected, your pediatrician may prescribe an antibiotic. Be sure to follow your pediatrician's instructions closely. Make sure your child finishes the entire prescription. If you stop the medication too soon, some of the bacteria that caused the ear infection may still be present and cause an infection to start all over again. As the infection starts to clear up, your child might feel a "popping" in the ears. This is a normal sign of healing. Your child's ear pain and fever should go away within 2 days of starting the antibiotics. Children with ear infections do not need to stay home if they are feeling well, as long as a child care provider or someone at school can give them their medication properly.

Sometimes an ear infection does not go away even after your child takes an antibiotic. If your child still has fever or ear pain for more than 2 days, call your pediatrician. Your pediatrician may need to prescribe a different antibiotic.

To help with pain, your pediatrician may recommend an over-the-counter nonaspirin medicine, such as acetaminophen. Do not give aspirin to your child; it has been associated with Reye syndrome, a disease that affects the liver and brain. Your pediatrician might also suggest putting warm, not hot,

compresses against your child's ears to help relieve pain. (This is not recommended for young babies.) If your child is old enough to chew gum without swallowing it, give him or her sugarless gum to chew. Keep your child sitting up as much as possible; this may help lessen pressure on the middle ear and ease pain. An extra pillow at night may also help. (Never use pillows in a crib.) Avoid using over-the-counter cold medicines (decongestants and antihistamines) as they do not help clear up ear infections.

Complications from untreated ear infections

While your child is young and at higher risk for ear infections, it is important for you to know the symptoms and to get your child treatment if an infection develops. Although it is very rare, complications from untreated ear infections can develop, including:

- an infection of the inner ear that causes dizziness and imbalance (labyrinthitis)
- an infection of the skull behind the ear (mastoiditis)
- an infection of the membranes around the brain and spinal cord (meningitis)
- scarring or thickening of the eardrum
- facial paralysis
- permanent hearing loss

The information contained in this publication should not be used as a substitute for the medical care and advice of your pediatrician. There may be variations in treatment that your pediatrician may recommend based on individual facts and circumstances.

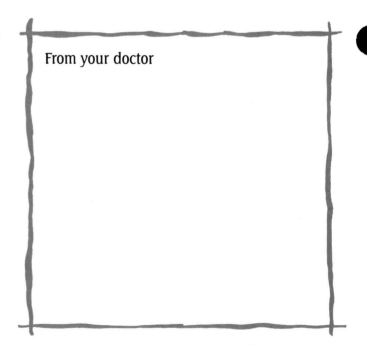

From your doctor

American Academy of Pediatrics

DEDICATED TO THE HEALTH OF ALL CHILDREN™

The American Academy of Pediatrics is an organization of 55,000 primary care pediatricians, pediatric medical subspecialists, and pediatric surgical specialists dedicated to the health, safety, and well-being of infants, children, adolescents, and young adults.

American Academy of Pediatrics
PO Box 747
Elk Grove Village, IL 60009-0747
Web site — http://www.aap.org

Ear Infections and Children

Part II Treatments for Repeated Ear Infections

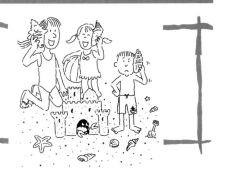

It is normal for children to have several ear infections when they are young—even as many as two separate infections within a few months. But, if your child has one ear infection after another, you may want to talk about other treatment options with your pediatrician.

Preventive treatment

With preventive antibiotic treatment, your child is given antibiotics for a long period of time to prevent ear infections from developing. These drugs are usually prescribed at a low dosage and taken once or twice a day. Although your child may still get ear infections while taking the antibiotics, they may occur less often. However, there is increasing concern that such antibiotic use may promote the spread of more dangerous antibiotic-resistant bacteria. Your pediatrician is the best judge of whether the benefits of this type of treatment outweigh the risks in your child's case.

Surgically inserted tubes

Another type of treatment for preventing repeated ear infections is an outpatient operation in which tubes are inserted through the eardrums. Tubes may also be used in cases of otitis media with effusion that last longer than 3 months and include some hearing loss. In this procedure, a small cut is made in the child's eardrum and fluid in the middle ear is drained out. Then a tiny plastic tube is fit into the slit. The tube acts as a ventilator, allowing air to get into the middle ear. This lessens the risk of harmful bacteria becoming trapped in the middle ear and causing another ear infection.

The tube is inserted using anesthesia in a surgeon's office or a hospital. Your pediatrician will decide whether to refer you to an ear, nose, and throat doctor (otolaryngologist) based on the following factors:

- how long your child has had fluid in his or her ears
- the number of recent ear infections your child has had
- failure of other treatments
- a significant hearing loss or other middle ear symptoms
- the age of your child

Most tubes come out of the eardrum on their own, between 6 to 18 months after they are put in. While the tubes are in, they do not require any special care. A child who has ear tubes, however, should not put his or her head under water when swimming.

Although repeated ear infections can be frustrating for you and your child, they are usually only a temporary problem and will likely improve as your child gets older. Most children stop getting ear infections by the time they are 4 years old.

Ear infections and hearing loss

Children who have had several ear infections may be more likely to suffer hearing loss. If your child is younger than 3 years of age and his or her hearing loss has lasted for more than 6 weeks, see your pediatrician. Long periods of hearing loss from an ear infection, although rare, may cause delays in speech and language development. This is especially critical in the first years of life when your child is learning to talk.

Hearing tests

In most cases of severe hearing loss, ear infections are not the cause. You should talk to your pediatrician about a hearing test if at any time you have doubts that your child may not be hearing normally. It is important to detect hearing loss as early as possible. Your child can have a hearing test at any age. Other health professionals may be involved in the testing. An audiologist will check to see how severe any hearing loss might be. A speech and language pathologist will test your child's speech and language skills and can recommend any special programs to help your child, if needed.

Your pediatrician may also suggest a hearing test if your child has had:

- repeated ear infections (more than 4 in a year)
- hearing loss for 6 weeks or longer
- middle ear fluid for more than 3 months

As a parent, you are the best person to recognize signs and symptoms in your child that suggest possible problems with hearing. Be sure to get treatment as soon as possible to help prevent any complications.

What if fluid remains in the middle ear?

If fluid stays in the middle ear for more than a few months, it may lead to repeated ear infections and can affect your child's hearing. If your child has had middle ear fluid in both ears for 3 months or longer, he or she should have a hearing test. Your pediatrician may refer your child to an ear, nose, and throat doctor (otolaryngologist) for further evaluation. He or she will let you know what treatment is needed.

Most ear infections that develop in children are minor. They are bothersome and uncomfortable, but they usually clear up without causing any lasting problems. It is important, however, that you contact your pediatrician at the first sign or symptom of an ear infection so that he or she can monitor the ear infection, decide when to check your child, and prescribe treatment, if necessary. If ear infections keep occurring or do not clear up on their own, they can cause other problems that may permanently affect your child's hearing and possibly speech. With proper care and treatment, ear infections can almost always be managed successfully.

The information contained in this publication should not be used as a substitute for the medical care and advice of your pediatrician. There may be variations in treatment that your pediatrician may recommend based on individual facts and circumstances.

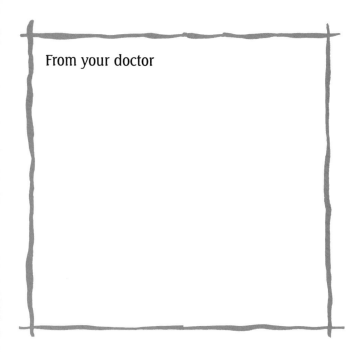

From your doctor

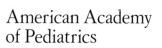

American Academy of Pediatrics

DEDICATED TO THE HEALTH OF ALL CHILDREN™

The American Academy of Pediatrics is an organization of 55,000 primary care pediatricians, pediatric medical subspecialists, and pediatric surgical specialists dedicated to the health, safety, and well-being of infants, children, adolescents, and young adults.

American Academy of Pediatrics
PO Box 747
Elk Grove Village, IL 60009-0747
Web site — http://www.aap.org

Febrile Seizures

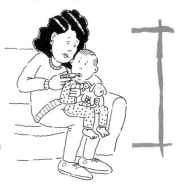

In some children, fevers can trigger seizures. Febrile seizures occur in 2% to 5% of all children between the ages of 6 months and 5 years. Seizures, sometimes called "fits" or "spells," are frightening, but they usually are harmless. The information in this brochure will help you understand febrile seizures and what happens if your child has one.

What is a febrile seizure?

A febrile seizure usually happens during the first few hours of a fever. The child may look strange for a few moments, then stiffen, twitch, and roll his eyes. He will be unresponsive for a short time, his breathing will be disturbed, and his skin may appear a little darker than usual. After the seizure, the child quickly returns to normal. Seizures usually last less than 1 minute but, although uncommon, can last for up to 15 minutes.

Febrile seizures rarely happen more than once within a 24-hour period. Other kinds of seizures (ones that are not caused by fever) last longer, can affect only one part of the body, and may occur repeatedly.

What do I do if my child has a febrile seizure?

If your child has a febrile seizure, act immediately to prevent injury.

- Place her on the floor or bed away from any hard or sharp objects.
- Turn her head to the side so that any saliva or vomit can drain from her mouth.
- Do not put anything into her mouth; she will not swallow her tongue.
- Call your pediatrician.

Will my child have more seizures?

Febrile seizures tend to run in families. The risk of having seizures with other episodes of fever depends on the age of your child. Children younger than 1 year of age at the time of their first seizure have about a 50% chance of having another febrile seizure. Children older than 1 year of age at the time of their first seizure have only a 30% chance of having a second febrile seizure.

Will my child get epilepsy?

Epilepsy is a term used for multiple and recurrent seizures. Epileptic seizures are not caused by fever. Children with a history of febrile seizures are at only a slightly higher risk of developing epilepsy by age 7 than children who have not had febrile seizures.

Are febrile seizures dangerous?

While febrile seizures may be very scary, they are harmless to the child. Febrile seizures do not cause brain damage, nervous system problems, paralysis, mental retardation, or death.

How are febrile seizures treated?

If your child has a febrile seizure, call your pediatrician right away. He or she will want to examine your child in order to determine the cause of your child's fever. It is more important to determine and treat the cause of the fever rather than the seizure. A spinal tap may be done to be sure your child does not have a serious infection like meningitis, especially if your child is younger than 1 year of age.

In general, physicians do not recommend treatment of a simple febrile seizure with preventive medications. However, this should be discussed with your pediatrician. In cases of prolonged or repeated seizures, the recommendation may be different.

Anti-fever drugs like acetaminophen and ibuprofen can help lower a fever, but they do not prevent febrile seizures. Your pediatrician will talk to you about the best ways to take care of your child's fever.

If your child has had a febrile seizure, do not fear the worst. These types of seizures are not dangerous to your child and do not cause long-term health problems. If you have concerns about this issue or anything related to your child's health, talk to your pediatrician.

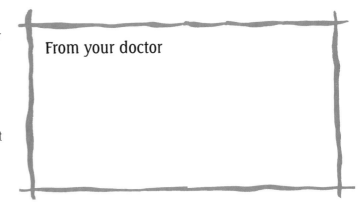

From your doctor

American Academy of Pediatrics

DEDICATED TO THE HEALTH OF ALL CHILDREN™

The American Academy of Pediatrics is an organization of 55,000 primary care pediatricians, pediatric medical subspecialists, and pediatric surgical specialists dedicated to the health, safety, and well-being of infants, children, adolescents, and young adults.

American Academy of Pediatrics
PO Box 747
Elk Grove Village, IL 60009-0747
Web site — http://www.aap.org

Fever and Your Child

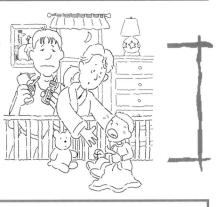

If your child has a fever, it is probably a sign that her body is fighting an infection. When your child becomes ill because of a virus or bacteria, her body may respond by increasing body temperature. It is important to remember that, except in the case of heat stroke, fever itself is not an illness—only a symptom of one. Fever itself also is not a sign that your child needs an antibiotic.

Many conditions, such as an ear infection, a common cold, the flu, a urinary tract infection, or pneumonia, may cause a child to develop a fever. In some cases, medication, injury, poison, or an extreme level of overactivity may produce a fever. An environment that is too hot may result in heat stroke, a potentially dangerous rise in body temperature. It is important to look for the cause of the fever.

Fevers are generally harmless and help your child fight infection. They can be considered a good sign that your child's immune system is working and the body is trying to rid itself of the infection.

The main purpose for treating fever is to help your child feel better. Reducing her temperature may make her more comfortable until the illness that has caused the fever has been treated or, more likely, run its course.

What is a fever?

A fever is a body temperature that is higher than normal. Your child's normal body temperature varies with his age, general health, activity level, the time of day, and how much clothing he is wearing. Everyone's temperature tends to be lower early in the morning and higher between late afternoon and early evening. Body temperature also will be slightly higher with strenuous exercise.

Most pediatricians consider any thermometer reading above **100.4°F (38°C)** a sign of a fever. This number may vary depending on the method used for taking your child's temperature. If you call your pediatrician, say which method you used.

Signs and symptoms of a fever

If your child has a fever, her heart and breathing rates naturally will speed up. You may notice that your child feels warm. She may appear flushed or perspire more than usual. Her body also will require more fluids.

Some children feel fine when they have a fever. However, most will have symptoms of the illness that is causing the fever. Your child may have an earache,

When to call your pediatrician right away

Call your pediatrician immediately if your child has a fever and
- Looks very ill, is unusually drowsy, or is very fussy
- Has been in an extremely hot place, such as an overheated car
- Has additional symptoms such as a stiff neck, severe headache, severe sore throat, severe ear pain, an unexplained rash, or repeated vomiting or diarrhea
- Has a condition that suppresses immune responses, such as sickle-cell disease or cancer, or is taking steroids
- Has had a seizure
- Is younger than 2 months of age and has a rectal temperature of

What if my child has a febrile seizure?

In some young children, fever can trigger seizures. These are usually harmless. However, they can be frightening. When this happens, your child may look strange for a few minutes, shake, then stiffen, twitch, and roll his eyes.
- Place him on the floor or bed, away from any hard or sharp objects.
- Turn his head to the side so that any saliva or vomit can drain from his mouth.
- Do not put anything into his mouth.
- Call your pediatrician.

Your pediatrician should always examine your child after a febrile seizure, especially if it is his first one. It is important to look for the cause of the febrile seizure.

More information about febrile seizures is available in *Febrile Seizures* on page 125.

a sore throat, a rash, or a stomachache. These signs can provide important clues as to the cause of your child's fever.

Managing a mild fever

A child older than 6 months of age who has a temperature below 101°F (38.3°C) probably does not need to be treated for fever, unless the child is uncomfortable. Observe her behavior. If she is eating and sleeping well and is able to play, you may wait to see if the fever improves by itself.

In the meantime,
- Keep her room comfortably cool.
- Make sure that she is dressed in light clothing.
- Encourage her to drink fluids such as water, diluted fruit juices, or a commercially prepared oral electrolyte solution.
- Be sure that she does not overexert herself.

Over-the-counter medications for fever

There are also medications you can give your child to reduce his temperature if he is uncomfortable. Both **acetaminophen** and **ibuprofen** are safe and effective in proper doses. Be sure to follow the correct dosage and medication schedule for your child. Remember, any medication can be dangerous if you give your child too much.

Ibuprofen should only be used for children older than 6 months of age. It should not be given to children who are vomiting constantly or are dehydrated. *Do not use aspirin to treat your child's fever. Aspirin has been linked with side effects such as an upset stomach, intestinal bleeding, and, most seriously, Reye syndrome.*

If your child is vomiting and unable to take medication by mouth, your pediatrician may recommend a rectal suppository for your child. Acetaminophen suppositories can be effective in reducing fever in a vomiting child.

Read the label on all medications to make sure that your child receives the right dose for his age and weight. To be safe, talk to your pediatrician before giving your child any medication to treat fever if he is younger than 2 years of age.

How to take your child's temperature

While you often can tell if your child is warmer than usual by feeling his forehead, only a thermometer can tell if he has a fever and how high the temperature is. There are several types of thermometers and methods for taking your child's temperature.

Mercury thermometers should not be used. The American Academy of Pediatrics (AAP) encourages parents to remove mercury thermometers from their homes to prevent accidental exposure to this toxin.

Rectal: If your child is younger than 3 years of age, taking his temperature with a rectal digital thermometer provides the best reading.

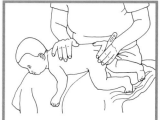

- Clean the end of the thermometer with rubbing alcohol or soap and water. Rinse it with cool water. Do not rinse with hot water.
- Put a small amount of lubricant, such as petroleum jelly, on the end.
- Place your child belly down across your lap or on a firm surface. Hold him by placing your palm against his lower back, just above his bottom.
- With the other hand, turn on the thermometer switch and insert the thermometer 0.5" to 1" into the anal opening. Hold the thermometer in place loosely with 2 fingers, keeping your hand cupped around your child's bottom. Do not insert the thermometer too far. Hold in place for about 1 minute, until you hear the "beep." Remove the thermometer to check the digital reading.

Oral: Once your child is 4 or 5 years of age, you may prefer taking his temperature by mouth with an oral digital thermometer.

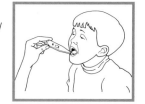

- Clean the thermometer with lukewarm soapy water or rubbing alcohol. Rinse with cool water.

- Turn on the switch and place the sensor under his tongue toward the back of his mouth. Hold in place for about 1 minute, until you hear the "beep." Check the digital reading.
- For a correct reading, wait at least 15 minutes after your child has had a hot
  or cold drink before putting the thermometer in his mouth.

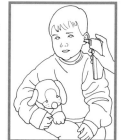

Ear: Tympanic thermometers, which measure temperature inside the ear, are another option for older babies and children.

- Gently put the end of the thermometer in the ear canal. Press the start button. You will get a digital reading of your child's temperature within seconds.
- While it provides quick results, this thermometer needs to be placed correctly in your child's ear to be accurate. Too much earwax may cause the reading to be incorrect.

Underarm (Axillary): Although not as accurate, if your child is older than 3 months of age, you can take his underarm temperature to see if he has a fever.

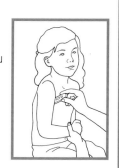

- Place the sensor end of either an oral or rectal digital thermometer in your child's armpit.
- Hold his arm tightly against his chest for about 1 minute, until you hear the "beep." Check the digital reading.

Other methods for taking your child's temperature are available. They are not recommended at this time. Ask your pediatrician for advice.

Sponging

Your pediatrician may recommend that you try sponging your child with lukewarm water in cases such as the following:

- Your child's temperature is above 104°F (40°C).
- She is vomiting and unable to take medication.
- She has had a febrile seizure in the past (see "What if my child has a febrile seizure?").

Sponging may reduce your child's temperature as water evaporates from her skin. Your pediatrician can advise you on this method.

Do not use cold water to sponge your child, as this could cause shivering. That could increase her temperature. Never add alcohol to the water. Alcohol can be absorbed into the skin or inhaled, causing serious problems such as a coma.

Usually 5 to 10 minutes in the tub is enough time for a child's temperature to start dropping. If your child becomes upset during the sponging, simply let her play in the water. If she is still bothered by the bath, it is better to remove her even if she has not been in long enough to reduce her temperature. Also remove her from the bath if she continues to shiver because shivering may increase body temperature.

Do not try to reduce your child's temperature to normal too quickly. This could cause the temperature to rebound higher.

Be sure to call your pediatrician if your child still "acts sick" once her temperature is brought down, or if you feel that your child is very sick. Also call if the fever persists for

- More than 24 hours in a child younger than 2 years of age
- More than 3 days in a child 2 years of age or older

The information contained in this publication should not be used as a substitute for the medical care and advice of your pediatrician. There may be variations in treatment that your pediatrician may recommend based on individual facts and circumstances.

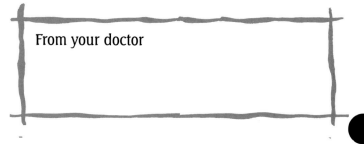

From your doctor

American Academy of Pediatrics

DEDICATED TO THE HEALTH OF ALL CHILDREN™

The American Academy of Pediatrics is an organization of 55,000 primary care pediatricians, pediatric medical subspecialists, and pediatric surgical specialists dedicated to the health, safety, and well-being of infants, children, adolescents, and young adults.

American Academy of Pediatrics
PO Box 747
Elk Grove Village, IL 60009-0747
Web site — http://www.aap.org

Copyright ©2001   American Academy of Pediatrics

A Guide to Children's Medications
Part I Prescription Medications

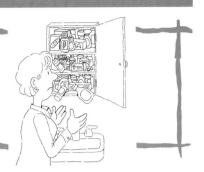

Cold medicines, allergy medications, antibiotics, and other prescriptions, syrups, creams, drops. Ever get confused over which medicines are made for children, when your child may need a prescription, or how much medicine to give your child? You are not alone. There are many medications that your child may need at one time or another. Some medications require a prescription from your pediatrician or other health care professional. Others, called over-the-counter medications, can be bought without a prescription. The following information will help you sort out the differences between prescription medications and over-the-counter medications, and when and how to use them.

Prescription medications

Prescription medications must be ordered by a doctor. If your child needs a prescription medication, it is very important that you understand the pediatrician's and pharmacist's instructions. The following list of questions will help you find out all you need to know:

- What is the name of the medication?
- How will this medication help my child?
- Do I need to do anything before giving this medication to my child?
- How much of the medication do I give my child?
- At what times of the day should I give the medication to my child?
- How long does my child have to take the medication?
- Should my child avoid certain foods or activities while using this medication?
- Should my child avoid other medications while using this medication?
- Are there any side effects that I should know about?
- Is there anything unusual about how my child is taking this medication (for example, is it a larger than usual dose)?
- Does this medication come in other forms that may be easier for my child to take, such as chewable tablets or liquid?
- Can this prescription be refilled? How many times?
- Is there any written information you can give me?
- What do I do if my child misses a dose?
- What do I do if I give my child too much?
- What if my child spits out the medication?
- Can you show me how to use this medication?

If your child goes to the hospital do the following:

- Bring your child's health records.
- If your child is taking any medications, bring them to the hospital in their original containers. Bring a record of when your child last took the medications.
- Ask about any medications your child is given while in the hospital.

Many medications come in less expensive forms. These are called generics. Often a generic can be used instead of a brand name. Other times it is more important to use the brand name. Talk to your pediatrician about the difference in using a generic instead of a brand name.

Ask as many questions as you need. If more questions come up after you leave your pediatrician's office, call the office or ask the pharmacist for clarification. If your child is old enough, make sure he understands what he must do as well.

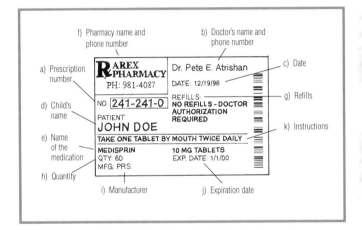

Read the label

Almost half of all parents do not correctly follow the directions on drug labels. However, labels have a lot of important information that you need to know. The illustration on this page shows the different parts of the label and what they mean.

a) Prescription number (you will need this number when calling the pharmacy for a refill or for insurance forms).

b) Doctor's name and phone number.

c) Today's date.

d) Your child's name—this medicine is only for the child whose name is on the label. Do not give medications to another child even if the other child has similar symptoms.

e) Name of the medication or the main ingredient—make sure this matches what your pediatrician told you. There may also be information on the strength of the medication (ie, 10 mg tablets).

f) Pharmacy name and phone number.

g) Refills—the label will show a number of how many refills are permitted. The label may also state "no refills—Dr authorization required," which means you have to talk to your pediatrician if you need more.

h) QTY—"quantity" or how much is in the package

i) MFG—"manufacturer" or who makes it

j) Expiration date—do not use the medication past this date. Do not save unused prescriptions. If your child gets sick again, talk to your pediatrician.

k) Instructions—this is information about how often and when your child needs to take the medicine. Instructions on labels can be confusing. Talk to your pediatrician for specific instructions and make sure they match what is on the label. The following are some common instructions you may find on a label:

- "Take full course"—means that your child should finish taking the entire contents of the prescription even if she is feeling better. This is especially true if your child is taking antibiotics. The infection can come back if you stop too soon.
- "Take with food"—means that you should give the medicine to your child after she has eaten a meal. Some medications work better when the stomach is full.
- "Take four times a day"—means to take the medicine four times throughout the day (for example, at breakfast, lunch, dinner, and before bed). This is different than "Take every four hours," which adds up to 6 times in a 24-hour period (for example, 6 AM, 10 AM, 2 PM, 6 PM, 10 PM, and 2 AM). If you are confused about when to give your child's medications, talk to your pediatrician or pharmacist. Most medicines do not have to be precisely timed in order to be effective, but some do.
- "Take as needed as symptoms persist"—means the medicine can be taken when symptoms are present.

The package may also have brightly colored warning labels with additional information. The following are examples:
- Safe storage instructions, such as "keep refrigerated"
- Instructions for use, such as "shake well before using"
- Possible side effects, such as "may cause drowsiness"

Common prescription medications for children

Antibiotics—used for bacterial infections like strep throat, some types of ear infections, sinus infections, urinary tract infections, and skin infections. Antibiotics are very safe but can have some side effects including skin rash, loose stools, stomach upset, staining of urine, or even mild to severe allergic reactions. Be sure to tell your pediatrician if your child has any side effects from antibiotics. Antibiotics (such as penicillin, amoxicillin, sulfas, and many others) can cure bacterial infections. Viral infections like colds and flu are not treated with antibiotics. New strains of bacteria have become resistant to some antibiotics because the antibiotics have been overused. When your child is sick, antibiotics are not always the answer. Your pediatrician will let you know if an antibiotic would help your child.

Ear preparations—commonly used for infections of the ear canal, like swimmer's ear. They may cause minor side effects.

Eye preparations—for conjunctivitis (pink eye) or allergies. Some children may get puffy eyes from using these medications.

Skin preparations—for skin infections, burns, lice, rashes, and acne. When used correctly, these medicines usually have no side effects. Certain lice medications can be toxic. Talk to your pediatrician if using a medication for lice.

Analgesics—used to relieve pain. Analgesics can have many side effects including stomach upset, ringing in the ears, dizziness, irritability, and nervousness. Since young children cannot always tell you if they are feeling these symptoms, talk to your pediatrician if your child acts unusual after taking these medications.

Inhalers—used to treat asthma. Include bronchodilators, inhaled steroids, and a drug called cromolyn sodium.

Liquid medicines

Many children's medicines come in liquid form because they are easier to swallow than pills. But they must be used correctly. Too often parents misread the directions, giving children several times the recommended dosage. This can be very dangerous, especially if given over a period of several days. Read the instructions carefully. Call your pediatrician if you are not sure how much, how often, or for how long to give medicines to your child.

When giving your child a liquid medication, do not use standard tableware tablespoons and teaspoons because they usually are not accurate. Instead, use one of the measuring devices listed below (many children's medications come with one). These can help you give the right amount of medicine to your child.

Syringes and oral droppers—These can be very helpful when giving medicine to an infant. Simply squirt the medicine between your child's tongue and the side of his mouth. This makes it easier for him to swallow. Avoid squirting the medicine into the back of your child's throat—he is more likely to gag and spit the medicine out. If you have a syringe that has a plastic cap, throw the cap into the trash so that it does not fall off in your child's mouth causing a choking hazard. You do not need to re-cap the syringe.

Dosing spoons—These can be useful for older children who will open their mouths and "drink" from the spoon.

Medication cups—These often come as caps on liquid cold and flu medicines.

Taking medicines safely

You can help prevent overdose or poisoning by following these tips:
- Always use good light. Giving medicine in the dark increases the risk that you will give the wrong medicine or the wrong dose.
- Read the label before you open the bottle, after you remove a dose, and again before you give it. This routine can ensure your child's safety.
- Always use child-resistant caps and lock all medications away from your child.
- Give the correct dose. Children are not just small adults. Never guess how much to give your child based on her size.
- Never play doctor. Do not increase the dose just because your child seems sicker than last time.
- Always follow the weight and age recommendations on the label. If it says not to give it to children younger than age 2, don't. Check with your pediatrician.
- Do not confuse the abbreviations for tablespoon (TBSP or T) and teaspoon (tsp or t).
- Avoid making conversions. If the label calls for 2 teaspoons and you have a dosing cup labeled only with ounces, do not use it. Use an appropriate measuring device.
- Be sure your pediatrician knows if your child is taking more than one medication at a time.
- Supervise your children if they are old enough to take medicine by themselves. Never let young children take medicine by themselves.
- Before using any medication, always check for signs of tampering. Do not use any medicine from a package that shows cuts, tears, or other imperfections.

It is not always easy to give medicine to a child. You may find your infant or toddler hates the taste and spits out the medicine or refuses to swallow it. Try adding a little sugar or juice to the dosing device to make it taste better. However, do not mix medications into a bottle of milk or a bowl of cereal. Your child may only eat part of it, or it may settle to the bottom and never get into his mouth. Older children may be more willing to take chewable tablets over liquid medicines. Although most children's medicines are flavored to make them taste better, avoid calling them candy. It might make your toddler decide to take them on his own.

Talk to your pediatrician if you have any questions or concerns about giving your child medications. Keep your pediatrician informed about any changes in how your child is feeling or if your child has any reactions to the medications.

The information contained in this publication should not be used as a substitute for the medical care and advice of your pediatrician. There may be variations in treatment that your pediatrician may recommend based on individual facts and circumstances.

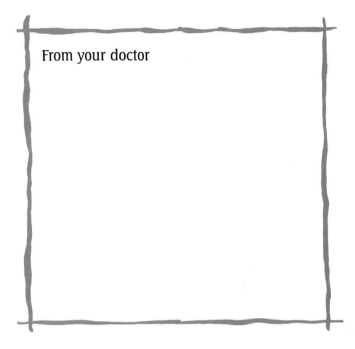

From your doctor

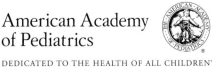

American Academy
of Pediatrics

DEDICATED TO THE HEALTH OF ALL CHILDREN™

The American Academy of Pediatrics is an organization of 55,000 primary care pediatricians, pediatric medical subspecialists, and pediatric surgical specialists dedicated to the health, safety, and well-being of infants, children, adolescents, and young adults.

American Academy of Pediatrics
PO Box 747
Elk Grove Village, IL 60009-0747
Web site — http://www.aap.org

A Guide to Children's Medications

Part II Over-the-counter Medications

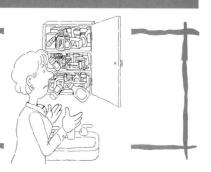

Over-the-counter medications

Over-the-counter medications (OTCs) can be bought at your local drug store or grocery store without a doctor's order. This does not mean that OTCs are harmless. Like prescription medications, OTCs can be very dangerous to a child if given incorrectly. You need to read and understand the instructions before giving OTCs to your child.

Common OTCs for children

The following list describes some common OTCs for children. Talk to your pediatrician before giving any medications to your child.

Fever reducer or pain reliever (acetaminophen, ibuprofen)

If your child has a mild fever but is playing, drinking fluids, and generally acting well, there is no reason to treat the fever. However, if your child complains of headaches, body aches, or seems irritable, there are fever reducers such as acetaminophen and ibuprofen that may help him feel better. They can also help relieve minor pain from bangs and bumps, or tenderness from an immunization.

Given in the correct dosage, acetaminophen and ibuprofen have few side effects and are quite safe. They come in drops for infants, liquid ("elixir") for toddlers, and chewable tablets for older children. Acetaminophen also comes in suppositories for the child who is vomiting and cannot keep down medicine taken by mouth. Remember, the infant drops are stronger than the liquid elixir for toddlers. Too many parents make the mistake of giving higher doses of the infant drops to a toddler thinking the drops are not as strong. Be sure the type you give your child is appropriate for her weight and age.

Ibuprofen tends to be more effective than acetaminophen in treating high fevers (103°F or higher). However, never give it to a child who is dehydrated or vomiting continuously. Also, children who are sensitive to aspirin, have a kidney disease, asthma, or an ulcer should not take ibuprofen.

A warning about aspirin

Never give aspirin to your child unless your pediatrician specifically instructs you to use it. Aspirin has been linked to Reye's syndrome, a serious and sometimes fatal liver disorder, especially when given to children with the flu or chicken pox. For more information on Reye's syndrome, or for a list of medications that contain aspirin, contact the National Reye's Syndrome Foundation at 800/233-7393.

Ibuprofen should not be used with any other pain reliever or fever reducer, unless directed by a doctor. Read the instructions and talk to your pediatrician about dosage to avoid giving your child too much for too long.

Antihistamines

Antihistamines can relieve runny noses, itchy eyes, and sneezing due to allergies (but not colds). They also relieve itching from chickenpox or insect bites and may even control hives or other allergic reactions. They can make some children sleepy. In other children they may cause irritability and nervousness. For that reason, avoid giving an antihistamine for the first time at bedtime. If you do, your child may have difficulty sleeping. If your child has asthma, check with your pediatrician before using antihistamines.

Mild cortisone cream

Insect bites, mild skin rashes, poison ivy, or small patches of eczema usually respond to cortisone cream. Never use it for chickenpox, burns, infections, open wounds, or broken skin. Check with your pediatrician before using it repeatedly or using it on your child's face.

Cough syrups

Coughing helps the lungs clear out germs. A cough is "productive" if it sounds like mucus is being brought up. You can best relieve it by humidifying the air in your child's bedroom to loosen mucus. Be sure to clean the humidifier frequently to prevent mold and bacteria buildup. Some cough medicines, called expectorants, may also help loosen mucus. Sometimes, a cough may be dry and annoying, and may keep your child awake. However, avoid using cough suppressants, as coughing is necessary to clear the lungs. Check with your pediatrician before giving your child cough medicines or expectorants, especially for use in infants. Cough syrups may not relieve cough caused by asthma.

Cold remedies

Combinations of antihistamines and decongestants can have side effects such as hyperactivity, sleeplessness, and irritability. Giving your child more than one cold medicine to treat different symptoms can be dangerous. Some of the same ingredients may be in each product. Also, many cold medicines contain acetaminophen. If you are already giving your child acetaminophen in addition to the cold medicine, this can lead to overdose. Read labels carefully. Check with your pediatrician before giving your child any cold medicines.

Nose drops (saltwater/saline)

Infants and toddlers cannot sniffle or blow their nose. If your child is sleeping well and eating happily, there is no need to treat her stuffy nose. But if your child is unable to sleep or eat because of thick mucus, saltwater nose drops can help clear the nose. Put a drop or two into a nostril at a time. Using a bulb syringe, squeeze the bulb, put the tip gently into your child's nostril, then let go. This will suction out the drops, along with the mucus. Be careful, overuse of a bulb syringe can be irritating to a child's nose.

Nose drops (decongestant)

Decongestant nose drops can shrink the membranes in the nose and make breathing easier. However, they should never be given to an infant because too much of the medication can be absorbed through the membranes of the nose.

Also, the more they are used, the less effective they become and symptoms can return. If your older child can't eat or sleep because of nasal stuffiness, use decongestant nose drops only for a brief time. Talk to your pediatrician if your child's symptoms do not improve.

Medications used for common GI problems

There are many OTC medications for heartburn, gas, constipation, and diarrhea. Most of these conditions usually go away by themselves or by a temporary change in diet. Before using any medicine for constipation or diarrhea, talk to your pediatrician. Repeated bouts of diarrhea or chronic constipation can be due to serious underlying problems.

Liquid medicines

Many children's medicines come in liquid form because they are easier to swallow than pills. But they must be used correctly. Too often parents misread the directions, giving children several times the recommended dosage. This can be very dangerous, especially if given over a period of several days. Read the instructions carefully. Call your pediatrician if you are not sure how much, how often, or for how long to give medicines to your child.

When giving your child a liquid medication, do not use standard tableware tablespoons and teaspoons because they usually are not accurate. Instead, use one of the measuring devices listed below (many children's medications come with one). These can help you give the right amount of medicine to your child.

Syringes and oral droppers—These can be very helpful when giving medicine to an infant. Simply squirt the medicine between your child's tongue and the side of his mouth. This makes it easier for him to swallow. Avoid squirting the medicine into the back of your child's throat—he is more likely to gag and spit the medicine out. If you have a syringe that has a plastic cap, throw the cap into the trash so that it does not fall off in your child's mouth causing a choking hazard. You do not need to re-cap the syringe.

Dosing spoons—These can be useful for older children who will open their mouths and "drink" from the spoon.

Medication cups—These often come as caps on liquid cold and flu medicines.

Taking medicines safely

You can help prevent overdose or poisoning by following these tips:

- Always use good light. Giving medicine in the dark increases the risk that you will give the wrong medicine or the wrong dose.
- Read the label before you open the bottle, after you remove a dose, and again before you give it. This routine can ensure your child's safety.
- Always use child-resistant caps and lock all medications away from your child.
- Give the correct dose. Children are not just small adults. Never guess how much to give your child based on her size.
- Never play doctor. Do not increase the dose just because your child seems sicker than last time.
- Always follow the weight and age recommendations on the label. If it says not to give it to children younger than age 2, don't. Check with your pediatrician.

- Do not confuse the abbreviations for tablespoon (TBSP or T) and teaspoon (tsp or t).
- Avoid making conversions. If the label calls for 2 teaspoons and you have a dosing cup labeled only with ounces, do not use it. Use an appropriate measuring device.
- Be sure your pediatrician knows if your child is taking more than one medication at a time.
- Supervise your children if they are old enough to take medicine by themselves. Never let young children take medicine by themselves.
- Before using any medication, always check for signs of tampering. Do not use any medicine from a package that shows cuts, tears, or other imperfections.

It is not always easy to give medicine to a child. You may find your infant or toddler hates the taste and spits out the medicine or refuses to swallow it. Try adding a little sugar or juice to the dosing device to make it taste better. However, do not mix medications into a bottle of milk or a bowl of cereal. Your child may only eat part of it, or it may settle to the bottom and never get into his mouth. Older children may be more willing to take chewable tablets over liquid medicines. Although most children's medicines are flavored to make them taste better, avoid calling them candy. It might make your toddler decide to take them on his own.

Talk to your pediatrician if you have any questions or concerns about giving your child medications. Keep your pediatrician informed about any changes in how your child is feeling or if your child has any reactions to the medications.

The information contained in this publication should not be used as a substitute for the medical care and advice of your pediatrician. There may be variations in treatment that your pediatrician may recommend based on individual facts and circumstances.

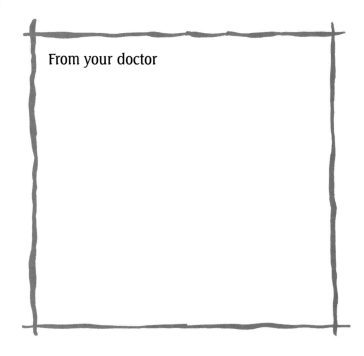

From your doctor

American Academy of Pediatrics

DEDICATED TO THE HEALTH OF ALL CHILDREN™

The American Academy of Pediatrics is an organization of 55,000 primary care pediatricians, pediatric medical subspecialists, and pediatric surgical specialists dedicated to the health, safety, and well-being of infants, children, adolescents, and young adults.

American Academy of Pediatrics
PO Box 747
Elk Grove Village, IL 60009-0747
Web site — http://www.aap.org

Copyright ©1999 American Academy of Pediatrics

How to Help Your Child With Asthma

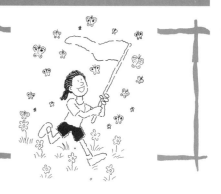

One out of 10 children in the United States has asthma. In fact, asthma is one of the main reasons children are admitted to the hospital and miss school. The number of children with asthma has increased in the last 20 years. There also has been a rise in the number of children who have died of asthma. As a parent, you need to know about asthma symptoms and how to tell if your child's asthma is getting worse. Your child's pediatrician can help you and your child learn what asthma is and how to prevent and treat asthma symptoms. Prevention and early treatment of asthma may help reduce the number of days your child is absent from school or in the hospital.

What is asthma?

Asthma is a chronic disease of the tubes that carry air to the lungs. These "airways" become narrow and their linings become swollen, irritated, and inflamed. Children with asthma can be sensitive to irritants including colds and other viral infections, cigarette smoke, cold air, and particles or chemicals in the air. Allergies to dust, animals, pollens, and molds can also be irritants.

Recognizing asthma

It is important to know the first signs that your child's airways are narrowing. For younger children, *first signs* of airway narrowing may include the following:

- Coughing at night
- Fast breathing or trouble breathing that causes your child to use extra muscles in the neck, abdomen, and chest to help "push" air out
- Noisy breathing or difficulty exhaling (wheezing)
- Refusing to participate in physical activities with peers

A cough may be the first and sometimes the only asthma symptom. Symptoms of asthma can be different for each person. They can appear quickly or develop slowly. Some children have symptoms of asthma often enough that they have to take medication every day. Other children may just need medication once in a while.

For children over 5 or 6 years of age, you can measure the amount of air they can breathe with the use of a simple device called a *peak flow meter*.

The peak flow meter will help you measure the flow of air from your child's lungs so that you can tell if the airways are narrowed. Your pediatrician can show you and your child how to use a peak flow meter and how to find out your child's "personal best" peak flow rate. You can use the peak flow meter on a regular basis to see when your child's asthma is getting worse and how well treatment is working. For additional information, see the section on peak flow rate meters in this brochure.

What to do if your child has symptoms of asthma

If your child has symptoms of asthma, talk to your pediatrician about how to control them. Controlling asthma symptoms will help your child feel better, be able to run and play normally, and take part in sports and other physical activi-

ties. Your pediatrician will help you learn what triggers your child's asthma so that you and your child can reduce or eliminate asthma attacks at home, child care, or school.

Be sure to ask your pediatrician for a written asthma action plan that includes advice about the following:

- How to prevent or reduce asthma symptoms
- How to recognize asthma symptoms and look for worsening of asthma symptoms
- What treatment should be given first
- What to do if the symptoms get worse
- What to do in an emergency

Asthma and children under 5 years of age

Studies show that as many as 80% of children with asthma develop symptoms before age 5. However, it can be difficult to diagnose a child of this age with asthma. In many young children, what may seem to be asthma symptoms are often respiratory infections caused by viruses.

Any sign or symptoms of asthma in an infant or child should be closely monitored by you and your child's pediatrician. The type of treatment will vary depending on your child's age, size, and symptoms. Whatever treatment you and your pediatrician decide is best, make sure any adult who cares for your child is informed and instructed about how and when to give your child his medicine.

Asthma triggers

Certain things cause, or trigger, asthma "attacks" or make asthma worse. Some of the asthma triggers are

1. Infections of the airways
   - Viral infections of the nose and throat
   - Other infections, such as pneumonia or sinus infections
2. Irritants in the environment (outside or indoor air you breathe)
   - Cigarette and other smoke
   - Air pollution
   - Cold air, dry air
   - Sudden changes in the weather
3. Things your child may be allergic to (allergens)
   - Animal dander
   - Pollens
   - Mold
   - House dust mites
   - Cockroaches
4. Exercise
5. Emotional stress

What medications are used to treat asthma?

There are different kinds of asthma medications. Your pediatrician will choose the best medications for your child and talk to you about when to use them. Some of these medications are used daily. Others are used only during asthma attacks. There are two groups of asthma medications—long-term control and quick relief.

1. **Long-term Control** (Prevention): When the airway becomes inflamed, it can cause swelling and pain. Use of long-term control or prevention drugs is one way to help reduce or prevent these symptoms.
2. **Quick Relief** (Rescue): Bronchodilators relax muscles so they can open up narrowed airways. These drugs help relieve the feeling of tightness in the chest, wheezing, and breathlessness.

These drugs are usually inhaled in an aerosol (mist) form, but also can be given by injection. Aerosol or dry powder forms can be delivered by an inhaler directly into the mouth.

The dry powder form cannot be used by younger children. The aerosol form can be used by younger children, but they may need to use a tube called a spacer to increase the efficiency of the aerosol. Younger children may also use a mask or might find a nebulizer or compressor easier to use.

If you have difficulty paying for the costs of medications, supplies, and services that your child needs, ask your pediatrician about programs that may be able to help you.

How can I tell if my child's asthma is not being controlled?

The following are signs that current treatment may not be effective. Talk to your pediatrician if any of the following occur:

- Symptoms such as coughing, wheezing, chest tightness, and shortness of breath occur more frequently (especially at night, even waking the child from sleep).
- Large changes in peak flow rate measurements occur (more than 20% change between morning and evening measurements).
- Medications do not seem to help your child's cough or breathing problems.
- Your child's asthma attacks last longer and do not easily improve with treatment.
- Your child's asthma attacks quickly become severe.
- You frequently have to take your child to your pediatrician or the hospital emergency room for treatment of acute asthma.

Mild, moderate, and severe asthma symptoms

It is important to learn to recognize when your child's asthma symptoms are getting worse or becoming severe. At times your child's airways may become more irritated and narrowed. If this happens, your child may suddenly start to cough, have difficulty breathing, or sense a gradual worsening of asthma symptoms. This is usually called an asthma "attack." During asthma attacks, the airways are more obstructed and the air flow is decreased. Your child's treatment is based on the severity of asthma symptoms and the degree of airway obstruction.

Signs of mild, moderate, or severe asthma attacks are described below. Discuss your child's specific symptoms with your pediatrician to decide which category best describes your child's symptoms. Knowing how severe your child's symptoms are will help you and your pediatrician decide on the best possible treatment plan for your child.

Signs indicating that your child may be having a MILD asthma attack are

- Breathing is mildly difficult.
- Breathing is slightly faster than usual.
- Speaking in complete sentences is still easily done.
- Mild complaints of wheezing, coughing, shortness of breath, or tightness in the chest.
- Peak flow rate is 80% to 100% of the child's personal best.
- No "drawing in" of muscles between the ribs is noticeable.
- Awareness of surroundings is normal and the child is alert.

Signs indicating that your child may be having a MODERATE asthma attack are

- Breathing is moderately difficult.
- Breathing is faster than usual.
- Speaking is affected because of difficulty breathing (phrases or partial sentences are spoken).
- Moderate complaints of wheezing, coughing, shortness of breath, or tightness in the chest.
- Peak flow rate is 60% to 80% of the child's personal best.
- Slight to moderate "drawing in" of muscles between the ribs is necessary to breathe.
- Awareness of surroundings is normal, and the child is alert.

Signs indicating that your child may be having a SEVERE asthma attack are

- Breathing is extremely difficult.
- Breathing is very fast or very slow with a lot of distress (labored breathing).
- Speaking is affected because of difficulty breathing (single words or short sentences are spoken).
- Severe complaints of wheezing, coughing, shortness of breath, or tightness in the chest.
- Peak flow rate is less than 60% of the child's personal best.
- "Drawing in" of the neck, abdomen, and chest muscles is needed in order to breathe. Level of awareness has decreased (child may be drowsy, anxious, or irritable).

Where can I learn more about asthma?

For more information, contact the following organizations:

American Lung Association
800/LUNG USA (800/586-4872)
Call for the office nearest you.
Web site: www.lungusa.org

Asthma and Allergy Foundation of America
1125 15th St NW, Suite 502
Washington, DC 20005
800/7-ASTHMA (800/727-8462)

National Heart, Lung, and Blood Institute (NHLBI)
9000 Rockville Pike
Bethesda, MD 20892
301/951-3260
Web site: www.nhlbi.nih.gov/

Peak flow rate meters

The peak flow meter measures the amount of air flow in the airways (breathing tubes). The peak flow rate is the rate of air flowing through the breathing tubes when a person blows air out as quickly and forcefully as possible into the peak flow meter. There are many kinds of peak flow meters. The same peak flow meter should be used every time to make sure the changes in air flow are measured correctly. Peak flow rate measurements help determine if the airway is closing or opening up.

Peak flow rates *decrease* (the numbers on the scale go down) when your child's asthma is getting worse or is out of control. Peak flow rates *increase* (the numbers on the scale go up) when the asthma treatment is working and the airways are opening up. The use of peak flow rate measurements will help you recognize when your child's airway is narrowing, so asthma treatment can be started early. Peak flow rates can also help you identify some of the "triggers" for your child's asthma so they can be avoided.

There are differences in peak flow rate measurements at different times of the day. Measuring your child's peak flow rate twice a day or more shows you how much your child's peak flow rate changes throughout the day. Children of different sizes and ages have different peak flow rate measurements.

How to measure peak flow rate

1. Have your child stand, take a deep breath, and fill her lungs with air.
2. Have your child blow into the peak flow meter as fast and as hard as possible.
3. Read the number on the peak flow meter scale, and write down the number on a piece of paper.
4. Measure the peak flow rate again, and write down the numbers. (Measure the peak flow rate a total of three times.)
5. At a time when your child is able to do her best, draw a circle around the best (highest) of the three measurements. This is your child's "personal best" peak flow rate. This value may need to be changed periodically as your child grows or improves or both.

Your child's peak flow rate

Fill in the following information, and keep it for future reference.

Your pediatrician suggests you measure your child's peak flow rate
_____ twice daily, morning and evening
_____ or
_____ at the time of asthma symptoms

Your child's **personal best** peak flow rate is _____

Your child's GREEN (safety) asthma zone is _____
(90% or more of personal best peak flow rate)

Your child's YELLOW (caution) asthma zone is _____
(70% to 90% of personal best peak flow rate)

Your child's RED (danger) asthma zone is _____
(less than 70% of personal best peak flow rate)

The information contained in this publication should not be used as a substitute for the medical care and advice of your pediatrician. There may be variations in treatment that your pediatrician may recommend based on individual facts and circumstances.

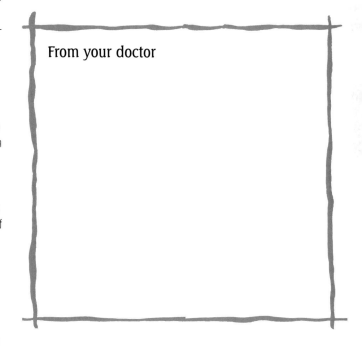

From your doctor

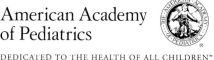

Influenza
Guidelines for Parents

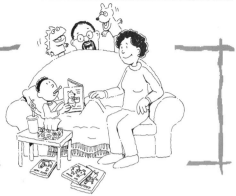

The flu — every child seems to get it at some time or another. But what is the flu? Can it be prevented? Should my child get a flu shot? These are just a few of the most common questions parents have about influenza (the flu). The following information will help you understand what influenza is, how to prevent it, and treatments that are now available.

What is the flu?

The flu is an illness caused by a virus. There are three different flu viruses, types A, B, and C. Types A (the most common) and B (usually milder) cause the usual epidemics of the flu. Flu viruses usually strike between December and early April. Because each of the types of flu virus has different strains, every year the flu is slightly different. It can infect people several times during their lifetime.

The flu can last a week or even longer. Your child usually will feel the worst during the first 2 or 3 days and may have any of the following symptoms:

- A sudden fever (usually above 101°F)
- Chills and shakes with the fever
- Extreme tiredness
- Headache and body aches
- Dry, hacking cough
- Sore throat
- Vomiting and belly pain
- Stuffy, runny nose

There are usually no serious complications from the flu. However, sometimes an ear infection, a sinus infection, or pneumonia may develop. Talk to your pediatrician if your child says that his ear hurts, he feels congested in his face and head, his cough persists, or his fever lasts beyond 3 to 4 days.

How the flu is spread

The flu is spread from person to person in the following ways:

- Direct hand-to-hand contact
- Indirect contact (for example, if your child touches an infected surface like a toy or a doorknob and then puts her hand to her own eyes, nose, or mouth)
- Virus droplets being passed through the air from coughing or sneezing

The flu spreads very easily, especially in preschool and school-age children. Adults who spend time with children are exposed easily and can get the disease. The virus usually is transmitted just as symptoms begin or in the first several days of the illness.

Treatment

In children older than 1 year of age, type A influenza can be treated with antiviral agents if given in the first day or two of the illness. This can speed recovery. Under some circumstances, antiviral agents can be taken before exposure to the flu and can prevent illness. This is particularly important for children with other health problems who have not had the flu shot. Antibiotics can be used to fight bacterial infections but have *no* effect on viruses, including the influenza viruses. Extra bed rest, extra fluids, and light, easy-to-digest meals can also help your child feel better.

If your child is uncomfortable because of fever, acetaminophen in proper doses for age and weight will help him feel better.

Do not give aspirin to your child for the flu. An increased risk of developing Reye syndrome (an illness that can seriously affect the liver and the brain) is associated with aspirin use during bouts of the flu and many other diseases caused by viruses.

Do not give your child over-the-counter cough or cold medicines without checking with your pediatrician.

Prevention

Good hygiene is the best way to prevent the flu from spreading to other family members. If your child has the flu, the following will help prevent its spread:

- Teach your child to cover her mouth and nose with a tissue or her sleeve, but not with her hands, when coughing or sneezing. If your child is old enough, teach her how to blow her nose properly.
- Use facial tissues for runny noses and to catch sneezes. Throw them in the trash after each use.
- Avoid kissing your child on or around the mouth or face, though she will need plenty of hugs while she is sick.
- Make sure everyone washes her hands before and after coming in close contact with someone with the flu.
- Wash dishes and utensils in hot, soapy water or in the dishwasher.
- Do not let children share pacifiers, cups, utensils, washcloths, or towels. Never share toothbrushes.
- Use disposable paper cups in the bathroom and kitchen.
- Disinfect. Viruses can live for more than 30 minutes on doorknobs, toilet handles, countertops, even on toys. Use a disinfectant or soap and hot water to keep these areas clean.
- Do not smoke around your child. Children who are exposed to tobacco smoke cough and wheeze more and have a harder time getting over the flu.

Influenza vaccine

There are safe and effective vaccines to protect against the flu. However, they are mainly recommended for children with health problems that make it risky for them to get the flu. This includes children with the following:

- Heart disease
- Lung disease, including asthma
- Immune problems, such as human immunodeficiency virus (HIV) infection
- Blood diseases
- Cancer
- Chronic kidney disease
- Metabolic diseases, such as diabetes
- Long-term aspirin therapy, such as with rheumatoid arthritis

©2002 American Academy of Pediatrics

Children 6 months or older with these health problems should get a flu shot each fall, as should everyone in the household. All young children may benefit from a flu shot. Your pediatrician can recommend what is best for your child.

For children younger than 9 years of age, the vaccine requires two injections, given 1 month apart the first year it is given. After that, only one dose is needed. The best time to get the flu vaccine is in late October to early December before the flu season starts. Vaccination should begin earlier for those needing two shots.

Because the strains of flu are different every year, a new flu vaccine is developed each year as well. The vaccine is made from killed flu viruses and helps the immune system fight the flu. Most children are immune within 2 weeks of getting the vaccine. Side effects are almost always minor and include soreness at the site of the injection and a low-grade fever. The flu shot cannot cause influenza.

> **Important note:** Even though there are few side effects to the vaccine, production of the vaccine involves the use of eggs. If your child has had a serious allergic reaction to eggs or egg products, he should be skin tested before getting the vaccine. If skin testing confirms hypersensitivity, the vaccine usually should not be given.

Scientists are working on the development of a nasal spray flu vaccine. This will be a painless and effective way to protect children from the flu.

Influenza or cold?

Both the flu and colds are caused by viruses and share many symptoms, but there are differences. A child with a common cold usually has a lower fever, a runny nose, and only a small amount of coughing. Children with the flu usually feel much sicker, achy, and miserable. Also, the flu tends to strike more quickly than a cold. Stomach upsets and vomiting are more common with the flu than with a cold. Children who have colds usually have enough energy to play and keep up with their usual day-to-day routines. The flu, on the other hand, keeps most children in bed for several days.

When to call the pediatrician

An older child with the flu usually does not need to see the pediatrician unless the condition becomes more serious. If your child is 3 months of age or younger, however, call your pediatrician if she has a fever. For a child older than 3 months of age who has been exposed to the flu, call your pediatrician if your child experiences any of the following:

- Difficulty breathing
- Blue lips or nails
- A cough that just will not go away (for more than 1 week)
- Pain in the ear
- Continued or new onset of fever after 3 to 4 days of illness

If your child seems extremely sick or his condition does not improve, call your pediatrician.

The information contained in this publication should not be used as a substitute for the medical care and advice of your pediatrician. There may be variations in treatment that your pediatrician may recommend based on individual facts and circumstances.

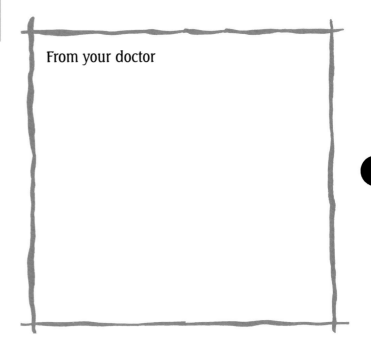

From your doctor

The American Academy of Pediatrics is an organization of 55,000 primary care pediatricians, pediatric medical subspecialists, and pediatric surgical specialists dedicated to the health, safety, and well-being of infants, children, adolescents, and young adults.

American Academy of Pediatrics
PO Box 747
Elk Grove Village, IL 60009-0747
Web site — http://www.aap.org

American Academy of Pediatrics

DEDICATED TO THE HEALTH OF ALL CHILDREN™

Lyme Disease

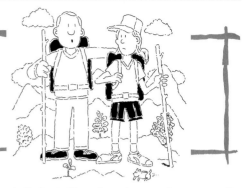

In the past 20 years, Lyme disease has quickly become an important public health problem in some areas of the United States. Since its discovery in Lyme, Connecticut, in 1975, thousands of cases of the disease have been reported across the United States and around the world. By knowing more about the disease and how to prevent it, you can help keep your family safe from the effects of Lyme disease.

What is Lyme disease?

Lyme disease is an infection caused by a bacteria called a *spirochete*. The disease is spread to humans by the bites of deer ticks infected with this bacteria. Deer ticks are tiny black-brown creatures no bigger than a poppy seed. They live in forests or grassy, wooded, marshy areas near rivers, lakes, or oceans. Many people who have been infected with Lyme disease were bitten by deer ticks while hiking or camping, or during other outdoor activities in the summer or fall months.

Where is Lyme disease most common?

The deer ticks that are infected with Lyme disease are commonly found in areas that have very low and high seasonal temperatures and high humidity. In the United States, Lyme disease is more common in the following regions:

- **Northeast** (Massachusetts, Rhode Island, Connecticut, New York, New Jersey, Delaware, Pennsylvania, and Maryland)
- **North central states** (Wisconsin, Minnesota, Illinois, Indiana, and Michigan)
- **West Coast** (California)

Lyme Disease Risk

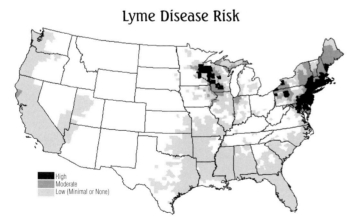

High
Moderate
Low (Minimal or None)

How will I know if my child has Lyme disease?

The first and most obvious symptom of Lyme disease is a rash surrounded by a light ring or halo, resembling a target. This is where your child was bitten and it may appear from 3 to 30 days *after* the bite occurred. Some people may have many rashes, and others may not notice a rash at all. Most people who develop the rash will not feel anything, but for others the rash may hurt,

itch, burn, or feel warm to the touch. The rash most commonly appears on the groin, thighs, trunk, and armpits.

Other symptoms that often accompany the rash include
- Headache
- Chills
- Fever
- Fatigue
- Swollen glands
- Aches and pains in the muscles or joints
  If your child develops the rash along with any of the symptoms listed above, call your pediatrician.

How serious is Lyme disease?

For most people, Lyme disease can be easily recognized and treated. If left untreated, Lyme disease can progress and become worse. In very rare cases, it can cause problems with vision, facial muscles, and can cause permanent damage to joints or the nervous system.

How is Lyme disease treated?

Lyme disease is most often treated with antibiotics (usually penicillin or tetracycline) prescribed by your pediatrician. The antibiotics are usually taken by mouth (pills), but also can be given intravenously (directly into the bloodstream through a vein) in more severe cases. Both early and late stages of the disease can be treated with antibiotics; however, late stages of the disease may be more difficult to treat.

How can I prevent Lyme disease?

If you live or work in a region where Lyme disease is a problem, or if you visit such an area, you will need to know how to protect your child from the ticks that carry the infection. Use the following suggestions when your child is in or around a grassy, wooded area while camping, hiking, or participating in any other outdoor activity, especially in the months between April and October.

- **Cover arms and legs.** Have your child wear a long-sleeved shirt, and tuck his pants into his socks.
- **Wear a hat** to help keep ticks away from the scalp. Keep long hair pulled back.
- **Wear light-colored clothing** to make it easier to spot ticks.
- **Wear enclosed shoes or boots.** Avoid wearing sandals in an area where ticks may live.
- **Use insect repellent.** Products with *DEET* are effective against ticks and can be used on the skin. However, large amounts of DEET can be harmful to your child if it is absorbed through the skin. Look for products that contain no more than 10% DEET. Wash the DEET off with soap and water when your child returns indoors. Products with *permethrin* can be used on clothing, but *cannot* be applied to the skin.

Ticks and how to remove them

Ticks do not fly, jump, or drop from trees. They hide in long grass and small trees, bushes, or shrubs waiting for an animal or person to brush by. Then, they attach themselves to the animal or person's skin. When a tick is found on a person (or a household pet), it should be removed as completely as possible using the following steps:

1. **Grasp the tick as close to the skin as possible** with a tweezers. Be careful not to squeeze the tick's body.
2. **Slowly pull the tick away from the skin.**
3. **After the tick is out, clean the bitten area** with rubbing alcohol or other first aid ointment.

- **Stay on cleared trails whenever possible.** Avoid wandering from a trail or brushing against overhanging branches or shrubs.
- **After coming indoors, check for ticks.** This will only take a couple minutes. Ticks often hide behind the ears or along the hairline. It may take up to 48 hours for a person to become infected, so removing any ticks soon after they have attached themselves can help reduce the chances of becoming infected.

Keep in mind, ticks can be found right in your own backyard, depending on where you live. Removing leaves and keeping your yard clear of brush and tall grass may reduce the number of ticks. Talk to a licensed professional pest control expert about other steps you can take to reduce ticks in your yard.

Is there a vaccine for Lyme disease?

In 1998, the Food and Drug Administration (FDA) approved the first vaccine for Lyme disease. The vaccine should be considered by people between the ages of 15 and 70 who live or work in an area that may be a high risk for Lyme disease. *The vaccine is not available for children under 15 years of age, and it is not recommended for pregnant women.*

The vaccine consists of three injections over a 12-month period. The vaccine cannot be used to treat Lyme disease, and it is not effective against any other diseases carried by ticks. Some people may have a temporary reaction to the vaccine that includes the following:

- Redness or swelling at the injection site
- Headache
- Fever
- Chills
- Fatigue
- Joint or muscle pain

Lyme disease is a health concern in some areas of the United States and not much of a problem in others. Be aware of whether there is a risk of Lyme disease wherever you and your family spend time outdoors. If you live in an area where Lyme disease has become a problem, take the steps listed in this brochure to protect your family members. Consider the vaccine for members of your family between the ages of 15 and 70. If you have any questions about the disease or the vaccine, talk to your child's pediatrician or your doctor.

The information contained in this publication should not be used as a substitute for the medical care and advice of your pediatrician. There may be variations in treatment that your pediatrician may recommend based on individual facts and circumstances.

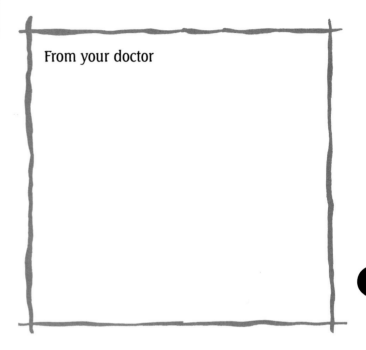

From your doctor

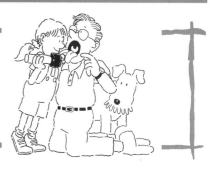

Tonsils and the Adenoid

In years past, it was very common for children to have their tonsils and the adenoid taken out. Today, doctors know much more about tonsils and the adenoid and are more careful about recommending removal.

Tonsils and the adenoid: what are they?

The **tonsils** are oval-shaped, pink masses of tissue on both sides of the throat. Tonsils can be different sizes for different children. They can be large or small. There is no "normal" size. You can usually see the tonsils by looking at the back of the mouth with a flashlight. Pressing on the tongue may help, but this makes many children gag. The **uvula**, a fleshy lobe that hangs down in the back of the mouth, should not be mistaken for the tonsils.

The **adenoid** is often referred to as "adenoids." This is incorrect because the adenoid is actually a single mass of tissue. The adenoid is similar to the tonsils and is located in the very upper part of the throat, above the uvula and behind the nose. This area is called the *nasopharynx*. The adenoid can be seen only with special mirrors or instruments passed through the nose.

Both the tonsils and the adenoid are part of your body's defense against infections. Since similar tissues in other parts of the body do the same job, removal of the tonsils or the adenoid does not harm the body's ability to fight infection.

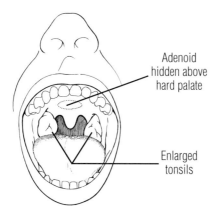

Adenoid hidden above hard palate

Enlarged tonsils

What is tonsillitis?

Tonsillitis is an inflammation of the tonsils usually due to infection. There are several signs of tonsillitis, including:
- Red and swollen tonsils
- White or yellow coating over the tonsils
- A "throaty" voice
- Sore throat
- Uncomfortable or painful swallowing
- Swollen lymph nodes ("glands") in the neck
- Fever

What are the symptoms of an enlarged adenoid?

It is not always easy to tell when your child's adenoid is enlarged. Some children are born with a larger adenoid. Others may have temporary enlargement of their adenoid due to colds or other infections. This is especially common among young children. Constant swelling or enlargement can cause other health problems such as ear and sinus infections. Some signs of adenoid enlargement are:
- Breathing through the mouth instead of the nose most of the time
- Nose sounds "blocked" when the child talks
- Noisy breathing during the day
- Snoring at night

Both the tonsils *and* the adenoid may be enlarged if your child has the symptoms mentioned above, along with any of the following:
- Breathing stops for a short period of time at night during snoring or loud breathing (this is called "sleep apnea").
- Choking or gasping during sleep.
- Difficulty swallowing, especially solid foods.
- A constant "throaty voice," even when there is no tonsillitis.

Treatment

If your child shows any of these signs or symptoms of enlargement of the tonsils or the adenoid, and doesn't seem to be getting better over a period of weeks, talk to your pediatrician. In many children, the tonsils and adenoid become enlarged without obvious infection. They often shrink without treatment.

According to the guidelines of the American Academy of Pediatrics, your pediatrician may recommend surgery for the following conditions:
- Tonsil or adenoid swelling that makes normal breathing difficult (this may or may not include sleep apnea).
- Tonsils that are so swollen that your child has a problem swallowing.
- An enlarged adenoid that makes breathing uncomfortable, severely alters speech and possibly affects normal growth of the face. In this case, surgery to remove only the adenoid may be recommended.
- Your child has repeated ear or sinus infections despite treatment. In this case, surgery to remove only the adenoid may be recommended.
- Your child has an excessive number of severe sore throats each year.
- Your child's lymph nodes beneath the lower jaw are swollen or tender for at least six months, even with antibiotic treatment.

How do I prepare my child for surgery?

Though it is not as common as it once was, some children need to have their tonsils and/or adenoid taken out. If your child needs surgery, make sure he or she knows what will happen before, during, and after surgery. Don't keep the surgery a secret from your child. Surgery can be scary, but it's better to be honest than to leave your child with fears and unanswered questions.

The hospital may have a special program to help you and your child get familiar with the hospital and the surgery. If the hospital allows, try to stay with your child during the entire hospital visit. Let your child know you'll be nearby during the entire operation. Your pediatrician can also help you and your child understand the operation and make it less frightening in the process. A little ice cream afterwards won't hurt either.

The information contained in this publication should not be used as a substitute for the medical care and advice of your pediatrician. There may be variations in treatment that your pediatrician may recommend based on individual facts and circumstances.

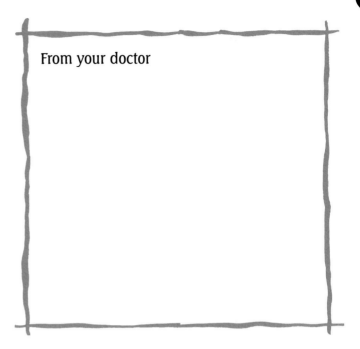

From your doctor

American Academy of Pediatrics

DEDICATED TO THE HEALTH OF ALL CHILDREN™

The American Academy of Pediatrics is an organization of 55,000 primary care pediatricians, pediatric medical subspecialists, and pediatric surgical specialists dedicated to the health, safety, and well-being of infants, children, adolescents, and young adults.

American Academy of Pediatrics
PO Box 747
Elk Grove Village, IL 60009-0747
Web site — http://www.aap.org

Copyright ©1997, Updated 3/99
American Academy of Pediatrics

©2002 American Academy of Pediatrics

Treating Jaundice in Healthy Newborns

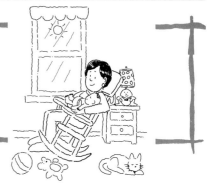

You may have been told that your child has "jaundice" and you probably have many questions about this condition. Jaundice is a common condition in newborn infants that usually shows up shortly after birth. In most cases, it goes away on its own. If not, it can be treated easily. This information has been developed by the American Academy of Pediatrics to help you understand this common condition and how it is treated.

What is jaundice?

A baby has jaundice when bilirubin, which is produced naturally by the body, builds up faster than a newborn's liver can break it down and get rid of it in the baby's stool. This happens because of one or more of the following reasons:

- The baby's developing liver is not yet able to remove the bilirubin from the blood
- More bilirubin is being made than the liver can handle
- Too much of the bilirubin is reabsorbed from the intestines before the baby gets rid of it in the stool

Too much bilirubin makes a jaundiced baby's skin look yellow. This yellow color will appear first on the face, then on the chest and stomach, and, finally, on the legs.

What is bilirubin?

Everyone's blood contains hemoglobin found in red blood cells. Red blood cells live only a short time and, as they die, the oxygen-carrying substance (hemoglobin) is changed to yellow bilirubin. Normal newborns have more bilirubin because their liver is not efficient at removing it. Older babies, children, and adults get rid of this yellow blood product quickly, usually through bowel movements.

Can jaundice hurt my baby?

Jaundice can be dangerous if the bilirubin reaches too high a level in the blood. The level at which it becomes dangerous will vary based on a child's age and if there are other medical conditions. A small sample of your baby's blood can be tested to measure the bilirubin level. Other tests may be needed to see if your baby has a special reason to make extra bilirubin that is causing the jaundice.

How do I know if my baby has jaundice?

Parents should be aware of any changes in their newborn's skin color or the coloring in the whites of their child's eyes. Look at the baby under natural daylight or in a room that has fluorescent lights. A quick and easy way to test for jaundice is to press gently with your fingertip on the tip of your child's nose or forehead. If the skin looks white (this is true for babies of all races), there is no jaundice. If you see a yellowish color, contact your pediatrician to check your baby to see if significant jaundice is present.

How is jaundice treated?

Mild to moderate levels of jaundice do not require any treatment. If high levels of jaundice do not clear up on their own, your baby may be treated with special lights or other treatments. These special lights help get rid of the bilirubin by altering it to make it easier for your baby's liver to get rid of it. This treatment may require that your baby stay in the hospital for a few days. Some pediatricians treat babies with these lights at home. If your baby needs light therapy, talk to your pediatrician about how long the treatment lasts and where it will be done.

Another treatment is more frequent feedings of breastmilk or formula to help pass the bilirubin out in the stools. Increasing the amount of water given to a child is not sufficient to pass the bilirubin because it must be passed in the stools. Rarely, babies may require treatment of their blood to remove bilirubin. For example, in a few cases of very high bilirubin levels, a blood exchange is done to give a baby fresh blood and remove the bilirubin. Your pediatrician will give you more details if other treatments are necessary. Once your child's bilirubin level goes down, it is unlikely that it will increase again. However, if your child continues to look yellow after 3 weeks of life, talk to your pediatrician as other tests may need to be done.

What effect does breastfeeding have on jaundice?

Most breastfed babies do not have a problem with jaundice that requires interruption of breastfeeding. However, if your baby develops jaundice that lasts a week or more, your pediatrician may ask you to temporarily stop breastfeeding for a day or two. If you must temporarily stop breastfeeding, talk to your pediatrician about pumping your breasts so you can keep producing breast milk and can restart nursing easily.

If your baby has jaundice, do not be alarmed. Remember that jaundice in a *healthy* newborn is not serious and usually clears up easily. If your baby has a very serious case of jaundice and other medical problems, your pediatrician will talk to you about other treatments.

The information contained in this publication should not be used as a substitute for the medical care and advice of your pediatrician. There may be variations in treatment that your pediatrician may recommend based on individual facts and circumstances.

American Academy of Pediatrics

DEDICATED TO THE HEALTH OF ALL CHILDREN™

The American Academy of Pediatrics is an organization of 55,000 primary care pediatricians, pediatric medical subspecialists, and pediatric surgical specialists dedicated to the health, safety, and well-being of infants, children, adolescents, and young adults.

American Academy of Pediatrics
PO Box 747
Elk Grove Village, IL 60009-0747
Web site — http://www.aap.org

Copyright ©1995   American Academy of Pediatrics

Urinary Tract Infections in Young Children

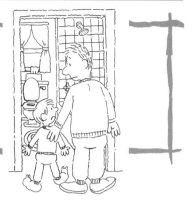

Urinary tract infections (UTIs) are common in young children. UTIs may go untreated because the symptoms may not be obvious to the child or to parents. These infections can lead to serious health problems. From this brochure, parents can learn more about urinary tract infections—what they are, how children get them, and how they are treated.

The urinary tract

The urinary tract makes and stores urine. It is made up of the kidneys, ureters, bladder, and the urethra. The kidneys produce urine. Urine travels from the kidneys down two narrow tubes called the ureters to the bladder. The bladder is a thin muscular bag that stores urine until it is time to empty urine out of the body. When it is time to empty the bladder, a muscle at the the bottom of the bladder relaxes. Urine then flows out of the body through a tube, called the urethra. The opening of the urethra is at the end of the penis in boys and above the vaginal opening in girls.

Urinary tract infections

Normal urine has no germs (bacteria). However, bacteria can get into the urinary tract from two sources: the skin around the rectum and genitals and the bloodstream from other parts of the body. Bacteria may cause infections in any or all parts of the urinary tract, including the following:

- the urethra (called "urethritis")
- the bladder (called "cystitis")
- the kidneys (called "pyelonephritis")

UTIs are common in infants and young children. About 3 percent of girls and 1 percent of boys will have a UTI by 11 years of age. A young child with a high fever and no other symptoms, has a 1 in 20 chance of having a UTI. The frequency of UTIs in girls is much greater than in boys. Uncircumcised boys have slightly more UTIs than those who have been circumcised.

Symptoms

Symptoms of UTIs may include the following:

- fever
- pain or burning during urination
- need to urinate more often, or difficulty getting urine out
- urgent need to urinate, or wetting of underwear or bedding by a child who knows how to use the toilet
- vomiting, refusal to eat
- abdominal pain
- side or back pain
- foul-smelling urine
- cloudy or bloody urine
- unexplained and persistent irritability in an infant
- poor growth in an infant

Diagnosis

If your child has symptoms of a UTI, your pediatrician will do the following:

- ask about your child's symptoms
- ask about any family history of urinary tract problems
- ask about what your child has been eating and drinking (certain foods can irritate the urinary tract and cause similar symptoms)
- examine your child
- get a urine sample from your child

Your pediatrician will need to test your child's urine to see if there are bacteria or other abnormalities. There are several ways to collect urine from a child.

- The preferred method to diagnose a UTI is to place a small tube, called a catheter, through the urethra into the bladder. Urine flows through the tube into a special urine container.
- Another method is to insert a needle through the skin of the lower abdomen to draw urine from the bladder. This is called needle aspiration.
- If your child is very young or not yet toilet trained, the pediatrician may place a plastic bag over the genitals to collect the urine. Since bacteria can contaminate the urine and give a false test result, this method is used only to screen for infection.
- An older child may be asked to urinate into a container.

Your pediatrician will discuss with you the best way to collect your child's urine.

Treatment

UTIs are treated with antibiotics. The way your child receives the antibiotic depends on the severity and type of infection. If your child has a fever or is vomiting and unable to keep fluids down, the antibiotics may be put directly into the bloodstream or muscle using a needle. This is usually done in the hospital. Otherwise, the antibiotics can be given by mouth, as liquid or pills.

UTIs need to be treated right away for the following reasons:

- to get rid of the infection
- to prevent the spread of the infection
- to reduce the chances of kidney damage

Infants and young children with UTIs usually need to take antibiotics for 7 to 14 days, sometimes longer. Make sure your child takes all the medicine your pediatrician prescribes. Do not stop giving your child the medicine until the pediatrician says the treatment is finished, even if your child feels better. UTIs can return if not fully treated.

Follow-up

After your child finishes the antibiotics, your pediatrician may want to test another urine sample to make sure the bacteria are gone. In addition, your pediatrician will want to make sure the urinary tract is normal and that the infection did not cause any damage. Several tests are available to do this, including the following:

Kidney and bladder ultrasound: Uses sound waves to examine the bladder and kidneys.

Voiding cystourethrogram (VCUG): A catheter is placed into the urethra and the bladder is filled with a liquid that can be seen on X-rays.

Intravenous pyelogram: A liquid that can be seen on X-rays is injected into a vein and then travels into the kidneys and bladder.

Nuclear scans: Radioactive materials are injected into a vein to see if the kidneys are normal. There are many kinds of nuclear scans, each giving different information about the kidneys and bladder. The radioactive materials give no more radiation than other kinds of X-rays.

Keep in mind, UTIs are common and most are easy to treat. Early diagnosis and prompt treatment are important because untreated or repeated infections can cause long-term medical problems. Talk to your pediatrician if you suspect that your child might have a UTI.

The information contained in this publication should not be used as a substitute for the medical care and advice of your pediatrician. There may be variations in treatment that your pediatrician may recommend based on individual facts and circumstances.

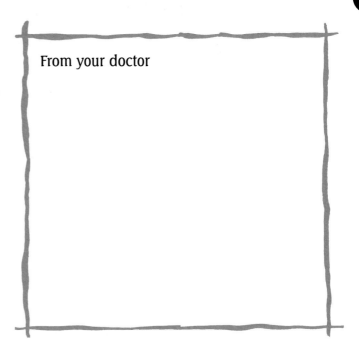

From your doctor

American Academy
of Pediatrics

DEDICATED TO THE HEALTH OF ALL CHILDREN™

The American Academy of Pediatrics is an organization of 55,000 primary care pediatricians, pediatric medical subspecialists, and pediatric surgical specialists dedicated to the health, safety, and well-being of infants, children, adolescents, and young adults.

American Academy of Pediatrics
PO Box 747
Elk Grove Village, IL 60009-0747
Web site — http://www.aap.org

Your Child and Antibiotics
Unnecessary Antibiotics CAN Be Harmful

About antibiotics

Antibiotics are among the most powerful and important medicines known. When used properly they can save lives, but used improperly, they can actually harm your child. Antibiotics should not be used to treat viral infections.

Bacteria and viruses

Two main types of germs—bacteria and viruses—cause most infections. In fact, viruses cause most coughs and sore throats and all colds. Bacterial infections can be cured by antibiotics, but common viral infections never are. Your child recovers from these common viral infections when the illness has run its course.

Resistant bacteria

New strains of bacteria have become resistant to antibiotics. These bacteria are not killed by the antibiotic. Some of these resistant bacteria can be treated with more powerful medicines, which may need to be given by vein (IV) in the hospital, and a few are already untreatable. The more antibiotics prescribed, the higher the chance that your child will be infected with resistant bacteria.

How bacteria become resistant

Each time we take antibiotics, sensitive bacteria are killed, but resistant ones may be left to grow and multiply. Repeated use and improper use of antibiotics are some of the main causes of the increase in resistant bacteria. These resistant bacteria can also be spread to others in the family and community.

When are antibiotics needed, and when are they not needed?

This complicated question is best answered by your doctor, and the answer depends on the specific diagnosis. Here are a few examples:

Ear infections. There are several types; most need antibiotics, but some do not.

Sinus infections. Most children with thick or green mucus do not have sinus infections. Antibiotics are needed for some long-lasting or severe cases.

Cough or bronchitis. Children rarely need antibiotics for bronchitis.

Sore throat. Most cases are caused by viruses. Only one main kind, strep throat, requires antibiotics. This kind must be diagnosed by a laboratory test.

Colds. Colds are caused by viruses and may sometimes last for 2 weeks or more. Antibiotics have no effect on colds, but your doctor may have suggestions for comfort measures while the illness runs its course.

The infection may change

Viral infections may sometimes lead to bacterial infections. But treating viral infections with antibiotics to prevent bacterial infections does not work, and may lead to infection with resistant bacteria. Keep your doctor informed if the illness gets worse or lasts a long time, so that proper treatment can be given, as needed.

Commonly asked questions

What can I do to protect my child from antibiotic-resistant bacteria?

Use antibiotics only when your doctor has determined that they might be effective. Antibiotics will not cure most colds, coughs, sore throats, or runny noses—children fight off colds on their own.

If mucus from the nose changes from clear to yellow or green, does this mean that my child needs an antibiotic?

Yellow or green mucus does not mean that your child has a bacterial infection. It is normal for the mucus to get thick and change color during a viral cold.

Does this mean I should never give my child antibiotics?

Antibiotics are very powerful medicines, and should be used to treat bacterial infections. If an antibiotic is prescribed, make sure you take the entire course and never save antibiotics for later use.

How do I know if my child has a viral or bacterial infection?

Ask your doctor. If you think that your child might need treatment, you should contact your doctor. But remember, colds are caused by viruses, and should not be treated with antibiotics.

You can protect your child from resistant bacteria
A prescription for parents:

Learn about the differences between bacterial and viral infections, and talk to your child's doctor about them. Understand that antibiotics should not be used for viral infections.

The information contained in this publication should not be used as a substitute for the medical care and advice of your pediatrician. There may be variations in treatment that your pediatrician may recommend based on individual facts and circumstances.

American Academy of Pediatrics

DEDICATED TO THE HEALTH OF ALL CHILDREN™

The American Academy of Pediatrics is an organization of 55,000 primary care pediatricians, pediatric medical subspecialists, and pediatric surgical specialists dedicated to the health, safety, and well-being of infants, children, adolescents, and young adults.

American Academy of Pediatrics
PO Box 747
Elk Grove Village, IL 60009-0747
Web site — http://www.aap.org

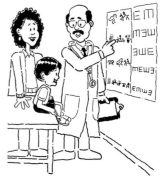

Your Child's Eyes

Part I Visual Development and Warning Signs

The American Academy of Pediatrics has developed this information to emphasize the importance of regular eye examinations in infancy and childhood. The information below describes the normal function and development of an infant's eye and vision. It gives an overview of warning signs and other problems that should be evaluated by your pediatrician or ophthalmologist. Regular eye exams at proper age intervals are the key to maintaining your child's healthy vision. The earlier the visual problems are detected, the better the outcome.

Visual development

At birth, babies have not yet attained normal adult vision—but they can see. Newborns can make out large shapes and faces but are unable to distinguish fine details. Faces have strong visual appeal. Because the visual system is immature, your baby probably cannot distinguish between pastel colors or subtle variations in shading, but can see bright, strong colors in contrasting patterns of light and dark.

Your baby's visual development is very dramatic during the first year of life. Vision usually develops rapidly so that by the age of 3 to 4 months, most infants can see small objects. Some babies can distinguish between various colors (especially red and green) by this time.

They can focus clearly on close and distant objects and can distinguish a real human face from one that is drawn.

By 4 months, the baby's eyes should be well aligned (work together) to give the perception of depth or binocular vision. By 12 months, a child's vision reaches normal adult levels. Vision does not develop exactly on the same schedule in all infants, but the overall pattern of development is the same. Because visual development is so rapid during the first year, early detection of visual problems is critical so that permanent visual impairment does not occur.

Warning signs that may indicate a problem
(Infants up to 1 year of age)

If your baby can't make steady eye contact by 2 or 3 months of age, or seems unable to see, you should consult your pediatrician. A constant crossing of the eyes or one eye that turns out is usually abnormal; however, most babies do occasionally cross their eyes during their first 6 months of life. Babies older than 3 months of age can usually follow or "track" an object with their eyes as it moves across their field of vision. You can test this by holding a colored object, like a toy or a ball, in front of your baby until he or she can see it. Then, slowly move the object and watch as your baby's eyes follow. Be careful to avoid clues aided by voices or other sounds.

Warning signs for your preschool child

The presence of any of the following requires immediate consultation with your pediatrician or ophthalmologist. If the eyes become misaligned (strabismus), the child should be evaluated immediately. This may be a situation that is easily corrected with glasses or it may represent a more serious eye disorder. The presence of a white pupil suggests a number of eye disorders ranging from a cataract to a tumor of the eye. Immediate evaluation is indicated. The sudden development of pain and redness in one eye or both eyes can represent a number of different conditions ranging from simple pink eye to blinding eye problems. If this occurs, a simple visit to your pediatrician will generally result in the correct diagnosis and proper treatment.

Warning signs at any age

No matter how old your child is, if you spot any one of the following, consult your pediatrician:

- Your child's eyes flutter quickly from side-to-side or up-and-down (nystagmus).
- The eyes are always watery.
- The eyes are always sensitive to light.
- Any change in the eyes from their usual appearance.
- You see white, grayish-white, or yellow-colored material in the pupil.
- There is redness in either eye that doesn't go away in several days.
- There is continued pus or crust in either eye.
- The eyes look crossed, turn out, or don't focus together (strabismus).
- Your child often rubs the eye(s).
- Your child often squints.
- Your child often tilts (or turns) his or her head.
- The eyelid(s) appears to droop.
- The eye(s) appears to bulge.

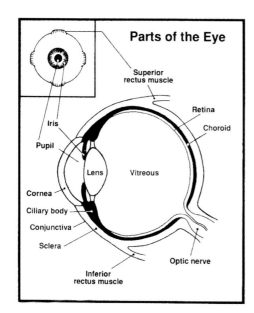

Parts of the Eye

Superior rectus muscle

Retina

Choroid

Iris

Pupil

Lens

Vitreous

Cornea

Ciliary body

Conjunctiva

Sclera

Optic nerve

Inferior rectus muscle

Vision screening information

Vision screening is a very important factor in identifying vision-threatening conditions. The American Academy of Ophthalmology and the American Academy of Pediatrics recommend that children be screened in four stages:

1. **In the newborn nursery:** Pediatricians and ophthalmic practitioners should examine all infants prior to their discharge from the nursery to check for infections and structural defects, cataracts, or glaucoma. All children with multiple medical problems or with a history of prematurity and/or oxygen exposure should be examined by an ophthalmologist.

2. **By the age of 6 months:** Pediatricians should screen infants at the time of their well-baby visits to check for alignment (eyes working together).

3. **At the age of 3 to 4 years:** All children should be examined by a pediatrician. At this age, the visual acuity is checked and the eyes are examined for any other abnormality that may cause a problem with the child's educational development. Any abnormality requires referral to an ophthalmologist.

4. **At the age of 5 years and older:** Pediatricians should screen children annually if this is not provided by school personnel or volunteer organizations. Visual acuity is tested as well as evaluation of other ocular functions.

Learning disabilities

Learning disabilities are quite common in childhood years and have many causes. The eyes are often suspected but are almost never the cause of learning problems. Your pediatrician may refer you for an evaluation by an educational specialist to pinpoint the exact cause.

When should your child's eyes be checked?

Pediatricians check the eyes shortly after birth as part of the newborn examination. Your baby's eyes also will be examined later during health supervision visits. The doctor looks for eye disease and checks to see if the eyes are functioning properly. Children with a family history of serious vision problems are more likely to have eye problems.

Fortunately, most babies have normal, healthy eyes. When problems occur, early detection and treatment make it more likely that the child's vision will develop normally. If your pediatrician detects problems, he or she may refer your child to an ophthalmologist for further evaluation and care.

Vision care is an important part of preventive health care for children. The American Academy of Pediatrics is dedicated to working for a better future for your children. Join us by making sure your children receive regular eye examinations.

The information contained in this publication should not be used as a substitute for the medical care and advice of your pediatrician. There may be variations in treatment that your pediatrician may recommend based on individual facts and circumstances.

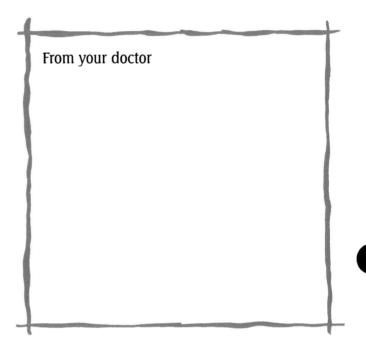

From your doctor

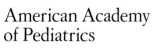 American Academy of Pediatrics

DEDICATED TO THE HEALTH OF ALL CHILDREN™

The American Academy of Pediatrics is an organization of 55,000 primary care pediatricians, pediatric medical subspecialists, and pediatric surgical specialists dedicated to the health, safety, and well-being of infants, children, adolescents, and young adults.

American Academy of Pediatrics
PO Box 747
Elk Grove Village, IL 60009-0747
Web site — http://www.aap.org

Your Child's Eyes

Part II Specific Problems That Require Further Evaluation

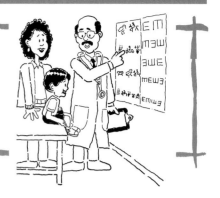

Falsely misaligned eyes (pseudostrabismus)

Sometimes infants appear to have crossed eyes, yet the eyes are truly straight. The cause for pseudostrabismus is presence of a wide nasal bridge or extra folds of skin between the nose and the inside of the eye that make the child have a cross-eyed appearance. Most children outgrow this problem, but you should contact your doctor for an examination. Your pediatrician can tell whether a child has misaligned eyes or just pseudostrabismus, but in some instances, a visit to an ophthalmologist is necessary for further tests.

Misaligned eyes (strabismus)

With strabismus, the eyes are not aligned. Strabismus is quite common and occurs in about 4% of children. One eye may gaze straight ahead while the other eye turns inward, upward, downward, or outward. When an eye turns inward, the child has "crossed" eyes (esotropia). There are two common causes for esotropia. Some children are born with crossed eyes (or develop it shortly after birth), and in this situation the muscles are too tight. Treatment for this most commonly involves surgery on the eye muscles, generally performed prior to the age of 2.

The second most common cause for esotropia is excessive farsightedness. This problem can be present at birth, but most commonly occurs between the age of 2 and 6 years. This type of esotropia is corrected with glasses.

When an eye turns outward, the child has exotropia. Exotropia may be present from birth, but most commonly is seen in children 2 to 7 years of age. Generally the eyes turn out on rare occasions at first but with time more frequent outward turning of the eyes is noted. Children with exotropia occasionally squint one eye when exposed to bright sunlight. The treatment for large amounts of exotropia is usually eye muscle surgery.

Children with misaligned eyes will generally turn off the vision in the turned eye so that they are not plagued with double vision. Children with strabismus should have a careful examination by an ophthalmologist because untreated strabismus may lead to a lazy eye (amblyopia) or loss of depth perception. Rarely, strabismus may indicate a more serious condition, such as cataract or eye tumor (retinoblastoma).

Lazy eye (amblyopia)

Lazy eye is reduced vision from lack of use in an otherwise normal eye. It usually happens only in one eye. Any condition that prevents a clear image can interfere with the development of vision and result in amblyopia.

Amblyopia is common, affecting about 2% of children. Some causes of amblyopia include strabismus, droopy eyelids (ptosis), cataracts, or refractive errors. Because early treatment offers the best results, your pediatrician will refer you to an ophthalmologist.

Cataract (cloudy lens)

A cataract is a clouding of the eye's normally clear lens. The lens is located behind the pupil and helps focus images on to the back of the eye (retina). Cataracts may be present at birth or may appear later in life. Injury may also cause this condition. Early detection and treatment are crucial in infants and children so that normal visual development can occur. For this reason, most cataracts should be surgically removed soon after they are discovered. It should be noted that cataracts in infants and children are uncommon and not related to cataracts that occur in adults.

Glaucoma (elevated eye pressure)

Glaucoma is a condition in which the pressure inside the eye is too high. If left untreated, glaucoma will eventually lead to total blindness. Warning symptoms are extreme sensitivity to light, tearing, and persistent pain. Signs include an enlarged eye, cloudy cornea, and lid spasm. If any of these are present, your pediatrician will refer you to an ophthalmologist immediately. Glaucoma in childhood usually requires surgery to prevent blindness.

Tearing

The tear duct system, which allows the tears to drain from the eyes into the nose, usually opens in the first few months of life. In some infants, however, the system remains blocked, resulting in the eyes overflowing with tears and collecting mucus. Tearing may result from other ocular conditions, the most serious of which is glaucoma (see above). If your child suffers from continued tearing or watering from the eyes, please consult your pediatrician. Gentle massage of the tear duct can occasionally assist in relieving the blockage. If massage and observation are unsuccessful, a tear duct probe or more involved surgery is occasionally required.

Ptosis (droopy eyelids)

Ptosis refers to a situation in which the eyelids are not as open as they should be. This situation is caused by a weakness of a muscle that opens the upper eyelid. When ptosis is mild, it is just a cosmetic problem. However, ptosis can interfere with vision if it is severe enough to block the vision in the eye. In infancy, it is important that ptosis be eliminated so that vision will develop normally. Correction of ptosis usually requires surgery on the eyelid(s).

Blepharitis (swollen eyelids)

Blepharitis refers to an inflammation in the oily glands of the eyelid. This usually results in swollen eyelids and excessive crusting of the eyelashes, most evident in the morning. Tenderness of the eyelids and a foreign body sensation in the eye may occur as well. Blepharitis can be treated with warm compresses and eyelid scrubs using baby shampoo. If an infection is present, antibiotics may be necessary. If any of these findings are present, please consult your pediatrician.

"Pink eye" (conjunctivitis)

Pink eye appears as a reddening of the white part of the eye. It is usually associated with excessive tearing, a discharge, and a foreign body sensation in the eyes. Conjunctivitis has many causes and can occur at any age. In infants and children, pink eye is usually caused by a viral or bacterial infection. In older children, it may also be caused by allergy. Depending on the cause of conjunctivitis, eye drops or ointment may be indicated. If your child has conjunctivitis, regular hand washing will help prevent the spread of the infection to other family members. If conjunctivitis occurs, call your pediatrician's office.

Corneal abrasion (scratched cornea)

A corneal abrasion refers to a scratch of the front clear surface of the eye (cornea). These abrasions are very painful and usually associated with light sensitivity and tearing. Treatment consists of antibiotics to prevent infection and a patch to allow for the healing of the scrape. This may be monitored by your pediatrician although more serious injuries often need follow up by an ophthalmologist.

Nearsightedness (myopia)

Children who are "nearsighted" see objects that are close to them clearly, but objects that are far away are unclear. Nearsightedness is very rare in infants and toddlers, but becomes more common in school-age children. Eyeglasses will help clear the vision but will not "cure" the problem. Despite using glasses, near-sightedness will generally increase in amount until the mid-teenage years so that periodic follow-up examinations by an ophthalmologist are indicated.

Farsightedness (hyperopia)

A small degree of farsightedness is normal in infants and children. It does not interfere with vision and requires no correction. It is only when the farsightedness becomes excessive, or causes the eyes to cross, that glasses are required.

Astigmatism

Astigmatism is the result of an eye that has an irregular corneal shape. Astigmatism may result in blurred vision. Children with astigmatism may need glasses if the amount of astigmatism is large.

The information contained in this publication should not be used as a substitute for the medical care and advice of your pediatrician. There may be variations in treatment that your pediatrician may recommend based on individual facts and circumstances.

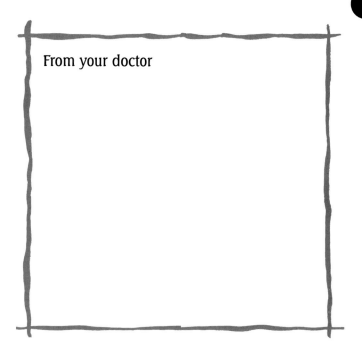

From your doctor

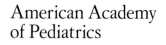
American Academy
of Pediatrics

DEDICATED TO THE HEALTH OF ALL CHILDREN™

The American Academy of Pediatrics is an organization of 55,000 primary care pediatricians, pediatric medical subspecialists, and pediatric surgical specialists dedicated to the health, safety, and well-being of infants, children, adolescents, and young adults.

American Academy of Pediatrics
PO Box 747
Elk Grove Village, IL 60009-0747
Web site — http://www.aap.org

SECTION FOUR

Feeding and Nutrition

Calcium and You

Facts for Teens

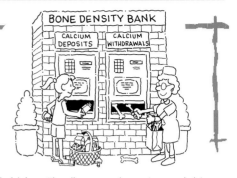

As you grow, you need calcium to build a healthy body. It keeps you strong so you can do well at things like sports, dancing, and school activities.

Getting plenty of calcium while you are young also makes you strong and keeps you looking good for your entire lifetime.

In fact, your body's need for calcium is very high between the ages of 9 and 18 years. However, most young people in the United States do not get enough calcium in their diets.

What is calcium?

Calcium is a mineral that many parts of your body require. Its main job is **to build strong bones and teeth.** About 99% of your body's calcium is in your bones and teeth. A very small amount of calcium is in body fluids such as blood. But this small amount performs vital functions, including the following:

- Keeping a strong heart beat
- Controlling blood pressure
- Making muscles move
- Helping blood clot
- Sending nerve messages

If you make the right choices, the food you eat will provide the calcium you need. If you do not get enough calcium, your body will take calcium from your bones to support other vital functions, weakening the bones.

Why do my bones need calcium?

Bones provide the basic support structure (skeleton) for your body and protect vital organs such as your heart and lungs.

Although bones may appear lifeless, they are alive and growing. Existing bone constantly is being renewed through a process called remodeling. Your body needs a good supply of calcium to fuel this process.

The "bone bank"

Bones serve as a "bank" for calcium. When you are young, your body can deposit calcium in your "bone bank" by increasing your **bone density.** Density means how closely packed together the materials in your bones are. Dense bones are strong bones.

As you get older, you lose the ability to bank calcium. By the time you reach about 30 years of age, your bones reach their **peak bone density.** That means your bones are as dense (or packed with calcium) as they will get — for life.

After that time, **you can no longer deposit extra calcium in your bone bank.** Instead your body withdraws calcium from your bone bank.

Why should I bank calcium?

Having a good supply of calcium stored in your bones means that there will be plenty for growing, rebuilding bones, and performing the many body functions that require it. You are much less likely to break bones that are packed with calcium.

In addition, you are saving calcium that you will need to withdraw from the bone bank when you are older. People who do not store enough calcium when

they are young are at high risk for getting diseases such as osteoporosis later in life.

Osteoporosis is a disease of older people that can make bones so fragile that they can break from the stress of merely bending over. It can result in a hunched-over appearance. People with osteoporosis may not realize they have the disease until 1 or more bones fracture. By this time, it is usually too late to undo the bone damage.

Is calcium all I need for strong bones?

Calcium does not work alone. After you eat or drink foods that contain calcium, your body must absorb the calcium through your intestines. You need a small amount of **vitamin D** for this to happen. Rickets, a disease that softens bones, can develop if your body does not absorb enough calcium.

Sources of vitamin D include the following:

- Sunlight. (Your body makes vitamin D when your skin is exposed to sunlight.)
- Milk fortified with vitamin D.

In addition, some juices or other products may be fortified with vitamin D. Check nutrition labels to learn which foods are fortified with vitamin D.

Exercise is important as well. Studies show that regular, weight-bearing exercise helps you build strong bones. Combined with a balanced diet, exercise does the following:

- Helps your body make hormones that protect bones
- Generates electrical activity that promotes bone growth and repair
- Boosts the flow of blood and nutrients to your bones

How much calcium do I need?

The amount of calcium that your body needs varies according to age. The greatest need is during late childhood and the teenage years.

The American Academy of Pediatrics recommends the following daily intake of calcium:

Age	Calcium need (mg per day)	Servings of milk to meet need
4–8 years	800	3 servings
9–18 years	1,300	4 servings
19–50 years	1,000	3–4 servings

How can I get calcium?

The best way to get the calcium that you need is by **eating and drinking foods that naturally contain calcium.** Many foods contain calcium.

Milk and other dairy products are good sources of calcium. They naturally offer the most calcium per serving. For example, 1 cup of milk has about the same amount of calcium as 4 cups of broccoli.

Most teenagers can get the calcium they need with 4 daily servings of dairy products, plus some green vegetables. Keep the following tips in mind:

- Low-fat and nonfat dairy products are super sources of calcium.
- Chocolate (or any flavor) milk has as much calcium as plain milk.
- Dark green, leafy vegetables such as kale and turnip greens are low in calories and are high in calcium.
- Tofu, broccoli, chickpeas, lentils, canned sardines, salmon, and other fish with bones also are good sources of calcium.
- Calcium-fortified foods such as juices and cereals can help boost the calcium in your diet. However, remember to limit the amount of juice that you drink each day to 8 to 12 ounces (1½ cups).

The tables at the end of this brochure show the amount of calcium in a variety of foods.

Calcium supplements

Certain medical conditions, diets, or lifestyle choices can make it hard for you to get enough calcium by eating the right foods. In some cases, your pediatrician may recommend a calcium supplement, such as a daily dose of a calcium-containing antacid tablet or liquid.

Lactose intolerance

A few young people have lactose intolerance, which means they have trouble digesting lactose (the sugar in milk). Milk with reduced lactose is available to help these teens. Nondairy foods that are rich in calcium, as well as calcium-fortified foods, also can be good choices for people who have lactose intolerance. In some cases, your pediatrician may recommend a calcium supplement.

However, most of the people who have lactose intolerance have only partial lactose intolerance. They can digest dairy products in small amounts with a meal. Aged cheeses and yogurts in which the lactose is broken down can provide good sources of calcium for them. Lactase preparations that make the lactose easier to digest also are available.

Can I get too much calcium?

It is unlikely that you would get too much calcium through your diet. However, it is important to watch how much calcium you get if you take supplements and eat many calcium-fortified foods.

Calcium boosters

On the go

- Order milk or milk shakes instead of soda at restaurants or school cafeterias.
- Choose foods with cheese, such as pizza, tacos, cheeseburgers, or grilled cheese sandwiches.
- Top salads, chips, or soups with cheese.
- Select yogurt or ice cream.

At home

- Choose easy, calcium-rich snacks such as cheese sticks, chocolate milk, yogurt, and pudding.
- Create special drinks with milk. Add flavorings. Make shakes.
- Use low-fat yogurt — on its own or with fresh fruit — as a topping for pancakes or waffles, and in shakes, salad dressings, dips, and sauces.
- Add milk to soups and hot cereals.
- Eat calcium-rich vegetables with cheese or yogurt-based dips.
- Sprinkle cheese on pastas, chili, and popcorn.
- Top sandwiches with a slice of cheese.
- Rely on favorites such as macaroni and cheese, pizza, and tacos.

Calcium blockers

The amount of calcium that your body gets can be thrown out of balance by the following:

- **Drinking a lot of soda (pop or soft drinks)** — Studies show that this may make you more prone to bone fractures. That may be because of the high phosphorus content of sodas. (Phosphorus may make it difficult for your body to absorb calcium, even if you eat or drink enough.) It also may be because sodas are taking the place of calcium-rich drinks and foods in many teenagers' diets.
- **Fad diets** — Some diets do not provide enough calories or offer a variety of foods. This may keep your body from getting enough calcium as well as many other nutrients it needs.
- **Vegetarian diets** — Teens who choose vegetarian diets that exclude dairy products must be very careful to include enough calcium.
- **Excess alcohol** — This can reduce the absorption of calcium in your intestines. It also can damage your liver, decreasing your body's ability to use vitamin D.
- **Diseases of the pancreas, small intestine, or liver** — Diabetes is an example.
- **Certain medications** — Medications such as steroids, anticonvulsants, and antacids that contain aluminum can interfere with calcium absorption.
- **Excess protein, salt, or phosphorus in your diet** — These may block calcium absorption.

- Experiment with calcium-rich foods that may be new to you and your family. Try sardines, tofu, slivered almonds, and salmon with bones.
- Try calcium-fortified juice and calcium-fortified waffles or cereal for breakfast.

Making low-fat calcium choices

Watching how much fat you eat and drink is also important. While you need to include some fat in your diet, no more than 30% of your daily calorie intake should come from fat.

However, you can easily increase the calcium and lower the fat in your diet at the same time.

There are many good sources of calcium that are either low in fat or have no fat at all. The following are examples:

- Nonfat dairy products such as milk, yogurt, and cheese
- Low-fat dairy products such as milk, yogurt, and cheese

How to read food labels

Nutrition labels can help you choose foods that are high in calcium. These labels are on food packages.

The labels list the amount of calcium in a serving as **"% Daily Value,"** not as **milligrams (mg).**

100% of the Daily Value = 1,000 mg of calcium per day

The Daily Value is an amount that applies mainly to adults. Remember, if you are between the ages of 9 and 18 years, you need 1,300 mg of calcium per day.

To find out how many milligrams (mg) of calcium are in a serving, place a "0" at the end of the number listed for the Daily Value. For example, a serving of calcium-fortified orange juice might list the amount of calcium as 30% of the Daily Value.

30% Daily Value = 300 mg calcium

In general, a food that lists a Daily Value of 20% or more for calcium is high in calcium. Any food that contains less than 5% of the Daily Value is low in calcium.

- Calcium-rich vegetables
- Calcium-fortified foods such as orange juice

Removing fat from a food does not take away calcium.

Making trade-offs in your food choices is another option to keep in mind. For example, if you go for a thick, chocolate milk shake, skip the fatty French fries.

Counting calcium

If you are between the ages of 9 years and 18 years, you need about **1,300 mg of calcium each day.** Keep track of what you eat for a few days to see if you are getting enough calcium.

If a medical condition or restricted diet may be keeping you from getting the calcium you need, talk to your pediatrician.

The following tables show the amount of calcium in a variety of foods from several food groups. Calcium amounts may vary. Check nutrition labels on products for exact amounts.

Milk Group	Calcium (mg)
* Milk, regular or low fat, 1 cup	300
Chocolate milk, 1 cup	300
Yogurt, 1 cup	300–415
American cheese, 2 oz	348
Cheddar cheese, 1½ oz	300
Cottage cheese, ½ cup	77
Mozzarella cheese, 1½ oz	275
Parmesan cheese, ¼ cup	338
Ricotta cheese, part skim, ½ cup	337
Swiss cheese, 1½ oz	408
Milk shake, 10 fl oz	319–344
Ice cream, ½ cup	88
Ice cream, soft-serve, ½ cup	113
Frozen yogurt, ½ cup	103
Pudding, instant, ½ cup	151
Soy milk, calcium-fortified, 1 cup	300
Rice milk, calcium-fortified, 1 cup	300

Prepared Foods	Calcium (mg) (Verify on label.)
Bean burrito	57
Cheese enchilada	324
Cheeseburger	182
Lasagna with meat, 2½" by 2½"	460
Macaroni & cheese, ½ cup	180
Pizza, cheese, 1 slice	220
Taco, 1 small	221

*Low-fat milk has as much or more calcium than whole milk.

Protein Group	Calcium (mg)
Almonds, chopped, 1 oz	66
White beans, ½ cup	113
Salmon, canned with bones, 2 oz	110
Sardines, 2 oz	248
Tofu, calcium-fortified, 1 cup	260

Fruits	Calcium (mg)
Orange juice, calcium-fortified	300
Orange, 1 medium	50
Prunes, dried, ¼ cup	22
Raisins, ¼ cup	22

Vegetables	Calcium (mg)
Bok choy (Chinese cabbage) ½ cup	79
Broccoli, cooked, ½ cup	35
Broccoli, raw, 1 cup	35
Carrots, raw, 1 medium	27
Kale, cooked, ½ cup	45
Mustard greens, cooked, ½ cup	64
Sweet potatoes, mashed, ½ cup	44
Turnip greens, cooked, ½ cup	98

Grains	Calcium (mg) (Verify on label.)
Bread, whole wheat, 1 slice	25
Cereal, ready-to-eat, 1 oz	48
Farina, enriched, ½ cup	95
Tortilla, corn, 1 medium	60
Waffle, enriched, 4-inch	77

The information contained in this publication should not be used as a substitute for the medical care and advice of your pediatrician. There may be variations in treatment that your pediatrician may recommend based on individual facts and circumstances.

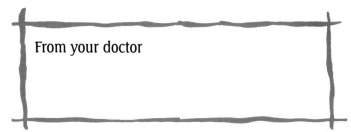

From your doctor

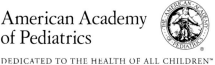

American Academy of Pediatrics

DEDICATED TO THE HEALTH OF ALL CHILDREN™

The American Academy of Pediatrics is an organization of 55,000 primary care pediatricians, pediatric medical subspecialists, and pediatric surgical specialists dedicated to the health, safety, and well-being of infants, children, adolescents, and young adults.

American Academy of Pediatrics
PO Box 747
Elk Grove Village, IL 60009-0747
Web site — http://www.aap.org

Copyright ©2001   American Academy of Pediatrics

Feeding Kids Right Isn't Always Easy
Tips for Preventing Food Hassles

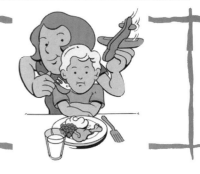

Feeding Kids—What's Your Role?

While parents are the best judges of **what** children should eat and **when**, children are the best judges of **how much** they should eat.

Here are **five** important feeding jobs for parents and caregivers:

1. Offer a variety of healthful and tasty foods. Be adventurous!
2. Serve meals and snacks on a regular schedule.
3. Make mealtime pleasant.
4. Teach good manners at the table.
5. Set a good example.

Happy encounters with food at any age help set the stage for sensible eating habits throughout life. Handling food and eating situations positively encourages healthful food choices.

This brochure gives helping hints for food and nutrition for young children. For specific advice, talk to your child's pediatrician or a registered dietitian.

Mealtime: Not a Battleground

"Clean your plate."
"No dessert until you eat your vegetables."
"If you behave, you can have a piece of candy."

To parents and caregivers, these phrases probably sound familiar. However, food should be used as nourishment, not as a reward or punishment. In the long run, food bribery usually creates more problems than it solves.

Did You Know That…

…encouraging your child to wash his or her hands thoroughly before meals may help prevent foodborne illness?

Here are six common childhood eating situations. Try these simple tips to make mealtime a more pleasant experience.

Feeding Challenges…	Feeding Strategies…
Food Jags: Eats one and only one food, meal after meal	Allow the child to eat what he or she wants if the "jag" food is wholesome. Offer other foods at each meal. After a few days, the child likely will try other foods. Don't remove the "jag" food, but offer it as long as the child wants it. Food jags rarely last long enough to cause any harm.
Food Strikes: Refuses to eat what's served, which can lead to "short-order cook syndrome"	Have bread, rolls or fruit available at each meal, so there are usually choices that the child likes. Be supportive, set limits and don't be afraid to let the child go hungry if he or she won't eat what is served. Which is worse, an occasional missed meal or a parent who is a perpetual short-order cook?
"The TV Habit": Wants to watch TV at mealtime	Turn off the television. Mealtime TV is a distraction that prevents family interaction and interferes with a child's eating. Value the time spent together while eating. Often it is the only time during the day that families can be together. An occasional meal with TV that the whole family can enjoy is fine.
The Complainer: Whines or complains about the food served	First ask the child to eat other foods offered at the meal. If the child cannot behave properly, have the child go to his or her room or sit quietly away from the table until the meal is finished. Don't let him or her take food along, return for dessert or eat until the next planned meal or snack time.
"The Great American White Food Diet": Eats only bread, potatoes, macaroni, and milk	Avoid pressuring the child to eat other foods. Giving more attention to finicky eating habits only reinforces a child's demands to limit foods. Continue to offer a variety of food-group foods. Encourage a taste of red, orange or green foods. Eventually the child will move on to other foods.
Fear of New Foods: Refuses to try new foods	Continue to introduce and reinforce new foods over time. It may take many tries before a child is ready to taste a new food… and a lot of tastes before a child likes it. Don't force children to try new foods.

Mealtime Is More Than Food

Youngsters are too smart to heed the old saying "Do as I say, not as I do." Children learn by imitating what they see. Adults who eat poorly can't expect their children to eat well. Set a good example by eating meals at regular times and by making healthful and tasty food choices.

Parents and caregivers are "gatekeepers," who control what foods come into the house. Having lots of healthful foods around helps children understand that these food choices are a way of life.

Mealtime is family time. Children learn many things as you eat together. And pleasant social encounters with food help develop good food habits.

Three, Two, One ... Let's Eat!

Prepare children for meals. A five-minute warning before mealtime lets them calm down, wash their hands and get ready to eat. A child who is anxious, excited or tired may have trouble settling down to eat.

Consistent food messages encourage children to eat and help prevent arguments over food. Try these simple steps:

- Be a smart gatekeeper. Buy a variety of foods you want the child to eat. Be adventurous with food!
- Be flexible. Don't worry if the child skips a meal.
- Be sensible. Set an example by eating a variety of healthful foods yourself.
- Let children make their own food choices from the healthful choices you provide.

Occasional Meal Skipping and Finicky Food Habits Are Okay

Well-meaning adults often view a child's odd food and eating behaviors as a problem. However, childhood food jags, a fear of new foods and other feeding challenges are usually part of normal development.

There's no need to worry if a child skips a meal or won't eat the vegetables on his or her plate. Keep the big picture in mind. Offer a variety of healthful, tasty and nourishing foods. Over time, a child will get everything needed to grow and develop normally. Plenty of food variety and a relaxed, happy atmosphere at mealtime are the "ingredients" for a well-fed child.

Children often use the table as a stage for showing their independence. Sometimes, food is not the issue at all. The eating process is just one more way children learn about the world.

Work Up an Appetite!

Active play, along with eating right, promotes good health ... and a healthy appetite! And it is the best exercise for toddlers and young children.

Making a snowman, playing tag, throwing balls, riding a bike and taking a nature walk are healthful and fun for the whole family. Don't just watch. Join in and be active, too. When you're physically active, you set a good example.

This brochure was developed as part of the **HEALTHY START...Food to Grow On** program, an information and education campaign that promotes healthful food choices and eating habits for healthy children ages two years and over. The **HEALTHY START** program was produced as a cooperative effort by the American Academy of Pediatrics (AAP), The American Dietetic Association (ADA), and the Food Marketing Institute (FMI).

For a referral to a registered dietitian and food and nutrition information, call the ADA's National Center for Nutrition and Dietetics Consumer Nutrition Hot Line at (800) 366-1655. For answers to your food and nutrition questions from a registered dietitian, please dial (900) CALL-AN-RD or (900) 225-5267.

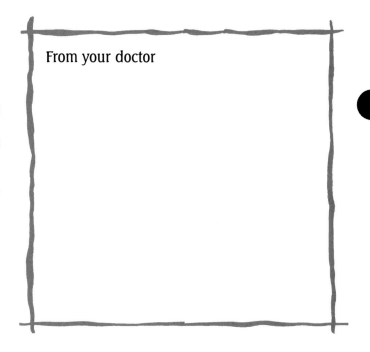

From your doctor

American Academy of Pediatrics

DEDICATED TO THE HEALTH OF ALL CHILDREN™

The American Academy of Pediatrics is an organization of 55,000 primary care pediatricians, pediatric medical subspecialists, and pediatric surgical specialists dedicated to the health, safety, and well-being of infants, children, adolescents, and young adults.

American Academy of Pediatrics
PO Box 747
Elk Grove Village, IL 60009-0747
Web site — http://www.aap.org

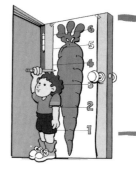

Growing Up Healthy
Fat, Cholesterol and More

Children and Heart Disease: A Generation at Risk

Many Americans consume too many calories and too much fat, especially saturated fat, and cholesterol. These eating patterns are one cause of America's high rates of obesity and heart disease. As a parent or caregiver, you can help your child develop eating and physical activity habits to stay healthy now—and throughout life.

What's a Parent to Do?

Food and physical activity habits begin at home. Although many things influence children, adults are still the most important role models for developing healthful eating and lifestyle habits.

The information in this brochure provides eating and physical activity guidelines for healthy children ages two years and over. For specific food and nutrition advice, talk to your child's pediatrician or a registered dietitian.

Food Guide Pyramid for Young Children
A Daily Guide for 2- to 6-Year-Olds

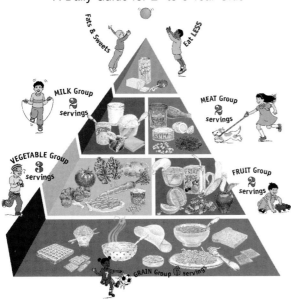

Fat in Food: How Much for Children?

If heart disease runs in your family, your child is at greater risk for heart disease in adulthood. To help protect your child from heart disease later in life, help him or her learn healthful eating and lifestyle habits during childhood.

Most nutrition experts agree that childhood is the best time to *start* cutting back on total fat, saturated fat and cholesterol. But adult goals aren't meant for young children under the age of two years. Fat is an essential nutrient that supplies energy, or calories, they need for growth and active play.

Between the ages of two and five, as children eat with their family, encourage them to gradually choose foods with less fat and saturated fat. By age five, their overall food choices, like yours, should be low in fat.

You might wonder: how is saturated fat different than other fat? It's more solid at room temperature. Saturated fats come mostly from animal sources, such as butter, cheese, bacon and meat, as well as stick margarine.

Caution: A low-fat eating plan is not advised for children under two years of age because of special needs for rapid growth and development during these years.

Pyramid Way to Healthful Eating

For healthful eating, offer foods from the five major food groups of the Food Guide Pyramid. Encourage nutrient-rich foods with less fat: grain products; fruits; vegetables; low-fat dairy foods; and lean meats, poultry, fish, and cooked dry beans.

Most young children—age two and over—need the minimum number of servings from each food group. Although children will decide how much they can eat, a child-size serving is one-fourth to one-third the size of an adult portion. That's about one measuring tablespoon per year of the young child's age.

Good Nutrition: It's a Juggling Act

Chances are that some of your child's favorite foods are higher in fat and energy (or calories) compared to the amount of nutrients they provide. Any food that supplies energy and nutrients can fit into a nutritious eating plan for your child.

Follow this nutrition advice: Offer your child many different food-group foods. Be flexible; what children eat over several days, not one day or one meal, is what counts. Help your child eat sensibly. Here are ways to be sensible about fat, saturated fat and cholesterol in food choices:

Food Group...	Most Days...	Some Days...
Bread, Cereal, Rice and Pasta	bagel or English muffin	doughnut or danish
	pretzels, baked chips	regular corn chips
	graham crackers, crackers, fig bars, vanilla wafers	chocolate chip cookies, cupcakes
Vegetable	baked potato	french fries
	raw vegetables	creamy cole slaw
Fruit	fresh fruit and juice —	
Milk, Yogurt and Cheese	reduced-fat cheese	cheese
	low-fat frozen yogurt or ice cream	ice cream
Meat, Poultry, Fish, Dry Beans, Eggs and Nuts	baked and grilled chicken	fried chicken
	baked fish	fried fish sticks

Smart Ideas for the Whole Family

Try these simple tips to limit extra fat, saturated fat and cholesterol:

- Have plenty of fresh fruits and vegetables available and ready to eat.
- Offer skim or I% milk* and low-fat yogurt. Choose cheeses that are lower in fat.
- Include starchy foods, such as potatoes, rice, pasta, and whole-grain breads and cereals often.
- Choose lower fat or fat-free toppings like grated parmesan cheese, herbed cottage cheese and nonfat/low-fat gravy, sour cream, or yogurt.
- Select lean meats, such as skinless chicken and turkey, fish, lean beef cuts (round, loin, lean ground beef) and lean pork cuts (tenderloin, chops, ham). Trim off all visible fat, and remove skin from poultry before eating.
- Choose margarine and vegetable oils made from canola, corn, sunflower, soybean and olive oils. Choose tub and liquid margarine, rather than regular margarine in sticks, too.
- Try angel food cake, frozen fruit bars, and low-fat/fat-free frozen desserts such as fudge bars, yogurt or ice cream.
- Use nonstick vegetable sprays when cooking.
- Use fat-free cooking methods, such as baking, broiling, grilling, poaching or steaming, when preparing meat, poultry or fish.
- Serve vegetable- and broth-based soups. Or use skim or 1% milk* or evaporated skim milk when making cream soups.
- Use the Nutrition Facts label on food packages to find foods with less fat per serving. Be sure to check serving size as you make choices. Remember that the % Daily Values on food labels are based on calorie levels for adults.

Parent Tip: Forget "Forbidden" Foods

Forcing children to eat food doesn't work. Neither does forbidding foods. Foods that are "forbidden" just may become more desirable for children.

It's important for both children and adults to be sensible and enjoy all foods, but not to overdo on any one type of food. Sweets and higher-fat snack foods in appropriate portions are okay. Just make sure your child is offered wise food choices from all the food groups.

Caution:

- Restricting a child's eating pattern too much may harm growth and development, or encourage undesirable eating behaviors.
- Before making any drastic changes in a child's eating plan or physical activity habits, talk to your child's pediatrician or a registered dietitian.
- Don't restrict fat or calories for children under two years of age, except on the advice of your child's pediatrician.

* Children *under* two years old should only drink whole milk.

Teach Good Habits by Example

Children learn more from ACTIONS than from WORDS. Practice what you preach. Your actions will make you healthier, too!

Get Up and Move...Turn Off That Tube!

Too much television usually results in not enough physical activity or creative play. Pediatricians recommend limiting TV time to no more than one or two hours each day.

Be active. Join your children in doing other activities. These activities will please almost any young child:

- Playing tag
- Jumping rope
- Throwing balls
- Riding a tricycle or bicycle
- Pulling a wagon
- Flying a kite
- Digging in the sand
- Making a snowman

- Ice skating or sledding
- Jumping in leaves
- Playing on swings
- "Driving" a toy truck
- Swimming
- Walking with the family
- Dancing
- Pushing a toy shopping cart

This brochure was developed as part of the **HEALTHY START...Food to Grow On** program, an information and education campaign that promotes healthful food choices and eating habits for healthy children ages two years and over. The **HEALTHY START** program was produced as a cooperative effort by the American Academy of Pediatrics (AAP), The American Dietetic Association (ADA), and the Food Marketing Institute (FMI).

For a referral to a registered dietitian and food and nutrition information, call the ADA's National Center for Nutrition and Dietetics Consumer Nutrition Hot Line at (800) 366-1655. For answers to your food and nutrition questions from a registered dietitian, please dial (900) CALL-AN-RD or (900) 225-5267.

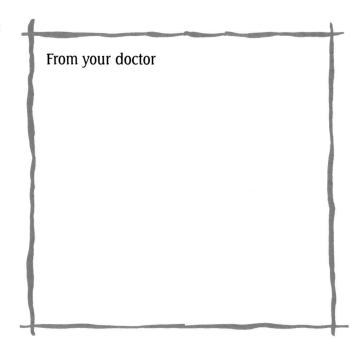

From your doctor

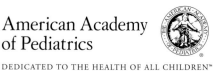

American Academy of Pediatrics

DEDICATED TO THE HEALTH OF ALL CHILDREN™

The American Academy of Pediatrics is an organization of 55,000 primary care pediatricians, pediatric medical subspecialists, and pediatric surgical specialists dedicated to the health, safety, and well-being of infants, children, adolescents, and young adults.

American Academy of Pediatrics
PO Box 747
Elk Grove Village, IL 60009-0747
Web site — http://www.aap.org

Right from the Start
ABC's of Good Nutrition for Young Children

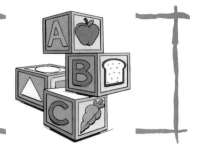

Good Nutrition: The Results Are Worth It

Proper nutrition begins at the supermarket with the foods you buy and continues at home as you prepare and serve meals. Giving your child a healthy start with good eating habits promotes his or her lifelong health.

This brochure focuses on feeding young children. It is meant to help you set the stage for healthful eating habits and food choices. The ABCs of good family nutrition start with love and common sense.

For specific advice about food and nutrition for young children, talk to your child's pediatrician or a registered dietitian.

Active Play Is Important to Health

Along with proper nutrition, your child needs physical activity for lifelong health. In the form of active play, physical activity not only promotes your child's appetite. It also helps develop a sense of well-being and confidence in his or her physical activities. From the early childhood years, encourage your child to live an active life.

Actions Speak Louder Than Words

As children grow and develop, they watch for clues about food choices. Youngsters often copy food habits, likes and dislikes. When you make wise food choices, your actions speak louder than words.

The ABCs of Good Nutrition

A variety of foods provides the nutrients that young children need to build strong bodies and stay healthy. Food also supplies the energy that children need to grow normally, play, learn and explore the world around them.

Offering a variety of tasty foods is the best way to supply the nutrition that a growing child needs.

A wide variety of foods are part of the five different food groups. Each food group makes special nutrient contributions. And each nutrient has certain jobs in the body.

Foods from all the groups work together to supply energy and nutrients necessary for health and growth. No one food group is more important than another. For good health, you and your child need them all.

Eating Right: The Pyramid Way

The Food Guide Pyramid is a practical eating guide that emphasizes food from five major food groups. It's flexible and realistic. And it's meant for all healthy people, ages two and over.

By following the advice of the Pyramid, children get the nutrients and energy from food that they need for growth and good health.

The Food Guide Pyramid shows the variety of foods within each food group and the number of servings that are right for your child. Most children—over two years—need the *minimum number of servings from each food group.*

Food Guide Pyramid for Young Children

A Daily Guide for 2- to 6-Year-Olds

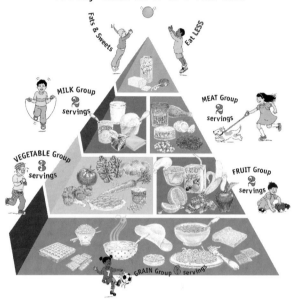

Some Pyramid Foods to Choose

- *From the Bread, Cereal, Rice and Pasta Group:* a whole-grain bread, crackers, cereal, grits, pasta, rice, bagel, tortilla, cornbread, pita bread, muffin, English muffin, matzo crackers, rice cake, pancakes, breadsticks, pretzels
- *From the Vegetable Group:* asparagus, beets, bok choy, broccoli, carrots, cauliflower, collard greens, corn, cucumber, green and red peppers, green beans, jicama, kale, okra, peas, potato, pumpkin, snow peas, squash, spinach, sweet potato, tomato, vegetable juices, zucchini
- *From the Fruit Group:* apple, applesauce, apricot, banana, berries, cantaloupe, fruit cocktail, figs, fruit juices, grapefruit, kiwifruit, mango, nectarine, orange, papaya, peach, pear, plum, pineapple, raisins*, prunes, starfruit, strawberries, tangerine, watermelon
- *From the Milk, Yogurt and Cheese Group:* skim, 1%, 2% and whole** milk, yogurt, cheese, string cheese, cottage cheese, pudding, custard, frozen yogurt, ice milk, calcium-fortified soybean milk
- *From the Meat, Poultry, Fish, Dry Beans, Eggs and Nuts* Group:* lean cuts of beef, veal, pork, ham and lamb; skinless chicken and turkey; fish; shellfish; cooked beans (kidney beans, black-eyed peas, pinto beans, lentils, black beans); refried beans (made without lard); peanut butter; eggs; reduced-fat deli meats; tofu; nuts*; peanuts*

---

* Raisins, nuts, peanuts and seeds are not recommended for children under four years of age because they are a choking hazard. Small pieces of hard, uncooked fruits and vegetables also pose a choking hazard to children under age four.

** Children under two years of age should *only* drink whole milk.

How Do I Know If My Child Is Eating Enough?

Children eat when they are hungry and usually stop when they are full. Some parents worry because young children appear to eat very small amounts of food, especially when compared to adult portions. A child who is growing well is getting enough to eat.

To check your child's eating pattern, pay attention to his or her food choices.

- Make sure no one food group is completely left out. If this happens for a few days, don't worry. But prolonged neglect of a food group could keep your child from getting enough nutrients.
- Encourage your child to be adventurous and eat a variety of foods within the food groups, too. Even within a food group, different foods provide different nutrients.

Child-Size Servings: Be Realistic

For youngsters, adult-size servings can be overwhelming. Offering child-size servings encourages food acceptance.

Here's an easy guide to child-size servings:

- Serve one-fourth to one-third of the adult portion size, or one measuring tablespoon for each year of the young child's age.
- Give less than you think the child will eat. Let the child ask for more if he or she is still hungry.

Snacks Count, Too

Snacks make up an important part of childhood nutrition. Children must eat frequently. With their small stomachs, they cannot eat enough at meals alone for their high energy needs. Three meals and two or three healthful snacks a day help youngsters meet their daily nutrition needs.

To make the most of snacks, parents and caregivers should control the type of snack and time it is served.

Type. Offer a variety of food-group snacks. Choose mostly snack foods that supply enough nutrients to justify their energy, or calories. Picking snack foods from the five food groups of the Food Guide Pyramid is the best way to do this.

Timing. Plan snacks. Schedule snacks around normal daily events, and space them at least two hours before meals. Children should learn to get and feel hungry, instead of feeling full all the time.

Quick and Smart Snack Food Ideas

For more nutrition, mix and match snacks from more than one food group:

- Fresh, frozen or canned fruit (banana, strawberries, cantaloupe pieces, orange sections, apple slices) or fruit juice
- Raw vegetables (baby carrots, cucumber slices, zucchini sticks, broccoli florets*)
- Vegetable soup
- Graham, animal crackers or fig bars
- Soft pretzels or breadsticks
- English muffin or bagel
- Low-fat yogurt or string cheese
- Skim or 1% milk** (flavored or unflavored)
- Turkey or meat cubes
- Hard-cooked egg

* Raisins, nuts, peanuts and seeds are not recommended for children under four years of age because they are a choking hazard. Small pieces of hard, uncooked fruits and vegetables also pose a choking hazard to children under age four.

** Children under two years of age should *only* drink whole milk.

This brochure was developed as part of the **HEALTHY START...Food to Grow On** program, an information and education campaign that promotes healthful food choices and eating habits for healthy children ages two years and over. The **HEALTHY START** program was produced as a cooperative effort by the American Academy of Pediatrics (AAP), The American Dietetic Association (ADA), and the Food Marketing Institute (FMI).

For a referral to a registered dietitian and food and nutrition information, call the ADA's National Center for Nutrition and Dietetics Consumer Nutrition Hot Line at (800) 366-1655. For answers to your food and nutrition questions from a registered dietitian, please dial (900) CALL-AN-RD or (900) 225-5267.

The information contained in this publication should not be used as a substitute for the medical care and advice of your pediatrician. There may be variations in treatment that your pediatrician may recommend based on individual facts and circumstances.

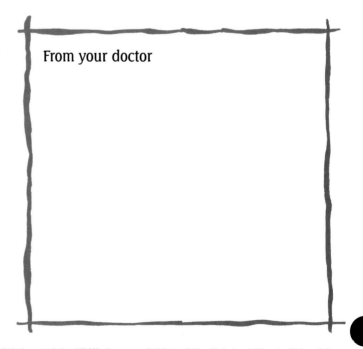

From your doctor

American Academy of Pediatrics

DEDICATED TO THE HEALTH OF ALL CHILDREN™

The American Academy of Pediatrics is an organization of 55,000 primary care pediatricians, pediatric medical subspecialists, and pediatric surgical specialists dedicated to the health, safety, and well-being of infants, children, adolescents, and young adults.

American Academy of Pediatrics
PO Box 747
Elk Grove Village, IL 60009-0747
Web site — http://www.aap.org

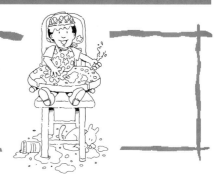

Starting Solid Foods

Adapted from *Caring for Your Baby and Young Child: Birth to Age 5*

Until now, your baby's diet has been made up of breast milk and/or formula. But once your child reaches 4 to 6 months of age, you can begin adding solid foods. This brochure has been developed by the American Academy of Pediatrics to give parents information on how to introduce solid foods to their infants. The information in this brochure is based on the Academy's parenting manual *Caring for Your Baby and Young Child: Birth to Age 5.*

When can my baby eat solid foods?

Most babies are ready to eat solid foods at 4 to 6 months of age. Before this age, most babies do not have enough control over their tongues and mouth muscles. Instead of swallowing the food, they push their tongues against the spoon or the food. This tongue-pushing reflex helps babies when they are nursing or drinking from a bottle. Most babies lose this reflex at about 4 months of age. Energy needs of babies increase around this age as well, making this an ideal time to introduce solids.

You may start solid foods at any feeding. At first you may want to pick a time when you do not have many distractions. However, keep in mind that as your child gets older, she will want to eat with the rest of the family.

Feeding your baby solid foods

To prevent choking, make sure your baby is sitting up when you introduce solid foods. If your baby cries or turns away when you give him the food, do not force the issue. It is more important that you both enjoy mealtimes than for your baby to start solids by a specific date. Go back to nursing or bottle-feeding exclusively for a week or two, then try again.

It is important for your baby to get used to the process of eating — sitting up, taking bites from a spoon, resting between bites, and stopping when full. Always use a spoon to feed your baby solid foods. Some parents try putting solid foods in a bottle or infant feeder with a nipple. This is not a good idea. Feeding your baby this way can cause choking. It also greatly increases the amount of food your baby eats and can cause your baby to gain too much weight. These early experiences will help your child learn good eating habits throughout life.

How to start

Start with half a spoonful or less and talk to your baby through the process ("Mmm, see how good this is!"). Your baby may not know what to do at first. She may look confused or insulted, wrinkle her nose, roll the food around her mouth, or reject it altogether. This is a normal reaction, because her feedings have been so different up to this point.

One way to make eating solids for the first time easier is to give your baby a little milk first, then switch to very small half-spoonfuls of food, and finish with more milk. This will prevent your baby from getting frustrated when she is very hungry.

Do not be surprised if most of the first few solid-food feedings wind up on your baby's face, hands, and bib. Increase the amount of food gradually, with just a teaspoonful or two to start. This allows your baby time to learn how to swallow solids.

What kinds of foods should my baby eat?

For most babies it does not matter what the first solid foods are. Many pediatricians recommend cereals first. The first cereals usually are offered in this order:
- Rice cereal
- Oatmeal cereal
- Barley cereal

It is a good idea to give your baby wheat and mixed cereals last, because they may cause allergic reactions in very young babies.

You can use premixed baby cereals in a jar or dry cereals to which you add breast milk, formula, or water. The premixed foods may be easier to use, but the dry ones are richer in iron and allow you to control the thickness of the cereal. Whichever type of cereal you choose, make sure that it is made for babies. Only baby foods contain the extra nutrients your child needs at this age.

Once your baby learns to eat one food, gradually give him other foods such as
- Infant cereals
- Fruit
- Strained vegetables
- Meat

Give your baby eggs last, because they occasionally cause allergic reactions. Babies are born with a preference for sweets. The order of introducing foods does not change this.

Give your baby one new food at a time, and wait at least 2 to 3 days before starting another. After each new food, watch for any allergic reactions such as diarrhea, rash, or vomiting. If any of these occur, stop using the new food and talk with your pediatrician.

Within 2 or 3 months of starting solid foods, your baby's daily diet should include the following foods each day:
- Breast milk or formula
- Cereal
- Vegetables
- Meats
- Fruits

Finger foods

Once your baby can sit up and bring her hands or other objects to her mouth, you can give her finger foods to help her learn to feed herself. To avoid choking, make sure anything you give your child is soft, easy to swallow, and cut into small pieces. Some examples include small pieces of banana, wafer-type cookies, or crackers; and well-cooked and cut-up yellow squash, peas, and potatoes. Do not give your baby any food that requires chewing at this age.

At each of your child's daily meals, she should be eating about 4 ounces, or the amount in one small jar of strained baby food. (Do not give your child foods that are made for adults. These foods often have added salt and preservatives.)

If you want to give your baby fresh food, use a blender or food processor, or just mash softer foods with a fork. All fresh foods should be cooked with no added salt or seasoning. Though you can feed your baby raw bananas (mashed), most other fruits and vegetables should be cooked until they are soft. Refrigerate any

Warning: do not home-prepare beets, turnips, carrots, spinach, or collard greens

In some parts of the country, these vegetables have large amounts of nitrates, chemicals that can cause an unusual type of anemia (low blood count) in young infants. Baby food companies are aware of this problem and screen the produce they buy for nitrates. They also avoid buying these vegetables in parts of the country where nitrates have been found. Because you cannot test for this chemical yourself, it is safer to use commercially prepared forms of these foods, especially while your child is an infant. If you choose to prepare them at home anyway, serve them fresh and do not store them. Storage of these foods may actually increase the amount of nitrates in them.

food you do not use and look for any signs of spoilage before giving it to your baby. Fresh foods are not bacteria-free, so they will spoil more quickly than food from a can or jar.

What can I expect after my baby starts solids?

When your child starts eating solid foods, his stools will become more solid and variable in color. Due to the added sugars and fats, they will have a much stronger odor too. Peas and other green vegetables may turn the stool a deep-green color; beets may make it red. (Beets sometimes make urine red as well.) If your baby's meals are not strained, his stools may contain undigested pieces of food, especially hulls of peas or corn, and the skin of tomatoes or other vegetables. All of this is normal. Your child's digestive system is still immature and needs time before it can fully process these new foods. If the stools are extremely loose, watery, or full of mucus, however, it may mean the digestive tract is irritated. In this case, reduce the amount of solids and let him build a tolerance for them a little more slowly. If the stools continue to be loose, watery, or full of mucus, consult your pediatrician to see if your child has a digestive problem.

Should I give my baby juice?

Babies do not need juice. Babies less than 6 months of age should not be given juice. However, if you choose to give your baby juice, do so only after she is 6 months of age and offer it only in a cup, not in a bottle. Limit juice intake to no more than 4 ounces a day and offer it only with a meal or snack. Any more than this can fill up your baby, giving her less of an appetite for other, more nutritious foods, including breast milk or formula. Too much juice also can cause diaper rash, diarrhea, or excessive weight gain. To help prevent tooth decay, avoid putting your child to bed with a bottle.

Give your child extra water if she seems to be thirsty between feedings. During the hot months when your child is losing fluid through sweat, offer water two or more times a day. If you live in an area where the water is fluoridated, these feedings also will help prevent future tooth decay.

Junior foods

When your child reaches about 8 months of age, you may want to introduce "junior" foods. These are slightly coarser than strained foods and are packaged in larger jars — usually 6 to 8 ounces. They require more chewing than baby foods. You also can expand your baby's diet to include soft foods such as puddings, mashed potatoes, yogurt, and gelatin. As always, introduce one food at a time, then wait 2 or 3 days before trying something else to be sure your child does not develop an allergic reaction.

As your baby's ability to use his hands improves, give him his own spoon and let him play with it at mealtimes. Once he has figured out how to hold the spoon, dip it in his food and let him try to feed himself. But do not expect much in the

beginning, when more food is bound to go on the floor and high chair than into his mouth. A plastic cloth under his chair will help minimize some of the cleanup.

Be patient, and resist the temptation to take the spoon away from him. For a while you may want to alternate bites from his spoon with bites from a spoon that you hold. Your child may not be able to use a spoon on his own until after his first birthday. Until then, you may want to fill the spoon for your child but leave the actual feeding to him. This can help decrease the mess and waste.

Good finger foods for babies include the following:

- Crunchy toast
- Well-cooked pasta
- Small pieces of chicken
- Scrambled egg
- Ready-to-eat cereals
- Small pieces of banana

Offer a variety of flavors, shapes, colors, and textures, but always watch your child for choking in case he bites off a piece that is too big to swallow.

Because children often swallow without chewing, do not offer children younger than 4 years of age the following foods:

- Chunks of peanut butter
- Nuts and seeds
- Popcorn
- Raw vegetables
- Hard, gooey, or sticky candy
- Raisins
- Chewing Gum

Other firm, round foods like grapes, cooked carrots, hot dogs, meat sticks (baby food "hot dogs"), or chunks of cheese or meat always should be cut into **very small** pieces. Before cutting a hot dog, remove the slippery peel.

Choosing a high chair

Select a chair with a wide base, so it cannot be tipped over if someone bumps against it.

If the chair folds, be sure it is locked each time you set it up.

Whenever your child sits in the chair, use the safety straps. This will prevent your child from slipping down and causing serious injury or even death. Never allow your child to stand in the high chair.

Do not place the high chair near a counter or table. Your child may be able to push hard enough against these surfaces to tip the chair over.

Never leave a young child alone in a high chair and do not allow older children to climb or play on it, as this could tip it over.

A high chair that hooks on to a table is not a good substitute for a more solid one. If you plan to use this type of chair when you eat out or when you travel, look for one that locks on to the table. Be sure the table is heavy enough to support your child's weight without tipping. Also, check to see whether your child's feet can touch a table support. If your child pushes against the table, it may dislodge the seat.

Good eating habits start early

Babies and small children do not know what foods they need to eat. Your job as a parent is to offer a good variety of healthy foods. Watch your child for cues that she has had enough to eat. Do not overfeed!

Begin to build good eating habits. Usually eating five to six times a day (three meals and two to three snacks) is a good way to meet toddlers' energy needs. Children who "graze," or eat constantly, may never really feel hungry. They can have problems from eating too much or too little.

If you are concerned that your baby is *already* overweight, talk with your pediatrician before making any changes to her diet. During these months of rapid growth, your baby needs a balanced diet that includes fat, carbohydrates, and protein. It is not wise to switch a baby under 2 years of age to skim milk, for example, or to other low-fat substitutes for breast milk or formula. A better solution might be to slightly reduce the amount of food your child eats at each meal. This way, your child will continue to get the balanced diet she needs.

Your pediatrician will help you determine if your child is overfed, not eating enough, or eating too many of the wrong kinds of foods. Because prepared baby foods have no added salt, you do not have to worry about salt at this age. However, be aware of the eating habits of others in your family. As your baby eats more and more "table foods," she will imitate the way you eat, including using salt and nibbling on snacks. For your child's sake as well as your own, cut your salt use and watch how much fat you consume. Provide a good role model by eating a variety of healthy foods.

The information contained in this publication should not be used as a substitute for the medical care and advice of your pediatrician. There may be variations in treatment that your pediatrician may recommend based on individual facts and circumstances.

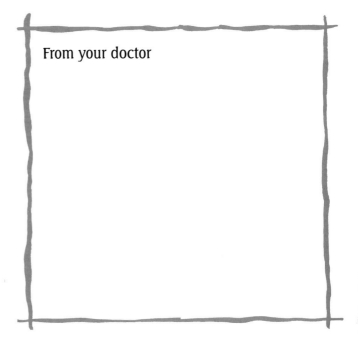

From your doctor

American Academy of Pediatrics

DEDICATED TO THE HEALTH OF ALL CHILDREN™

The American Academy of Pediatrics is an organization of 55,000 primary care pediatricians, pediatric medical subspecialists, and pediatric surgical specialists dedicated to the health, safety, and well-being of infants, children, adolescents, and young adults.

American Academy of Pediatrics
PO Box 747
Elk Grove Village, IL 60009-0747
Web site — http://www.aap.org

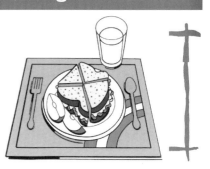

What's to Eat?

Healthy Foods for Hungry Children

The Food Guide Pyramid—A Menu for Good Health

Ask anyone who cares for children—feeding kids can be challenging! The Food Guide Pyramid is a tool for helping you plan meals and snacks for your family. The advice is given for one day*. This brochure gives meal suggestions that are tasty, convenient and nutritious. From breakfast through dinner, these ideas will please even the fussiest eater. For specific food and nutrition advice, talk to your child's pediatrician or a registered dietitian.

*The amount of food and number of servings children need daily from each food group depends on their age and how active they are.

Active Play is Important, Too!

Physical activity, along with proper nutrition, promotes lifelong health. Active play is the best exercise for kids! Parents can join their children and have fun while being active, too. Some fun activities for parents and kids to do together include playing on swings, riding tricycles or bicycles, jumping rope, flying a kite, making a snowman, swimming or dancing.

Food Guide Pyramid for Young Children

A Daily Guide for 2- to 6-Year-Olds

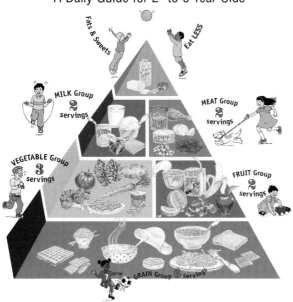

Off to a Good Start...The Breakfast Bonus

Breakfast provides energy to carry a child through an active morning. Children who skip breakfast may not concentrate well at school or may lack energy to play. Not everyone enjoys traditional breakfast foods, such as cereal and toast. These breakfast ideas are a little different:

- Breakfast shake: combine skim or 1% milk*, fruit and ice in a blender.
- Frozen banana: dip a banana in yogurt, then roll it in crushed cereal. Freeze.
- Peanut butter spread on crackers, a tortilla, apple slices or jicama slices.
- Leftover spaghetti, chicken or pizza: serve hot or cold!

* Skim and 1% milk are recommended for children over two years old. Children under two years of age should only drink whole milk.

Cereal Choices

Cereal with milk is the number-one breakfast favorite. Check the Nutrition Facts label—found on most packaged foods—for the amount of iron, other nutrients and fiber. Look at the % Daily Values to find how much.

If your child prefers a sweet taste, you might jazz up unsweetened cereal with sliced peaches or bananas, strawberries, or blueberries.

Lunches Worth Munchin'

Children who help make their own lunches are more likely to eat them. Include these brown bag perks to make lunches fun!

- Use cookie cutters to cut sandwiches in fun, interesting shapes.
- Decorate lunch bags with colorful stickers.
- Put a new twist on a sandwich favorite. Top peanut butter with raisins, bananas or apple slices.
- For color and crunch, use a variety of veggies as "sandwich toppers": cucumber slices, sprouts, grated carrots or zucchini.

Brown Bag Food Safety

Remember the golden rule for food safety:

Keep Hot Foods Hot and Cold Foods Cold.

When there's no refrigerator to store a bag lunch, keep food safe by:

- Tucking an ice- or freezer-pack into the lunch bag. Or use an insulated container to keep hot foods hot.
- Adding a box of frozen fruit juice.
- Freezing the sandwich bread and filling—or other freezable foods—the night before.

You may also help prevent food-borne illness by:

- Encouraging your child to wash his or her hands thoroughly before meals.

Did You Know That...

Most regular deli meats, such as salami and bologna, are very high in fat. Try reduced-fat deli meats. Turkey breast, ham and roast beef are usually lower-fat choices. Check the Nutrition Facts label on packaged meats to learn the fat content.

Pretzels, baked tortilla chips and baked potato chips are virtually fat-free and make a good alternative for potato chips and other high-fat snacks.

The Meal Dilemma... Dealing with Picky Eaters

Even the most nutritious meal won't do any good if a child refuses to eat it. Some youngsters are naturally finicky eaters. Others eat only certain foods—or refuse food—as a way to assert themselves. If your child refuses one food from a group, try offering a substitute from the same food group of the Food Guide Pyramid. Try these ideas to make your family meals happy ones:

If Your Child Refuses...	Instead Try...
Green vegetables	Deep-yellow or orange vegetables
Milk	Chocolate milk, cheese, yogurt
Beef	Chicken, turkey, fish, pork

- Boost the nutritional value of prepared dishes with extra ingredients. Perhaps add nonfat dry milk to cream soups, milkshakes and puddings. Or mix grated zucchini and carrots into quick breads, muffins, meatloaf, lasagna and soups.
- Serve a food your child enjoys along with a food that he or she has refused to eat in the past.
- Try serving a food again if it was refused before. It may take many tries before a child likes it.
- Let children help with food preparation. It can make eating a food more fun.
- Add eye appeal. Cut foods into interesting shapes. Or create a smiling face on top of a casserole with cheese, vegetables or fruit strips.
- Set a good example by eating well yourself. Whenever possible, eat meals as a family.

How Much Food Is Enough?

Some parents worry because young children seem to eat small amounts of food, especially when compared with adult portions. Don't worry about how little a child eats. A child who is growing well is getting enough to eat.

Hungry And In a Hurry? Food for Fast Times

When it comes to food, families want convenience. It's no surprise that fast-food restaurants are so popular. However, some fast foods supply a lot of fat and calories. These tips help you get the most from foods that are fast:

- Most fast foods can fit within a healthful eating plan. Children and adults can afford to eat these foods every once in a while if other food choices are sensible. Try these ways to enjoy them:
  Share: split an order of fries with other family members.
  Choose food-group foods: in combination meals, substitute fruit juice or skim or l% milk* for soft drinks.

Balance high-fat choices with low-fat choices: order a small hamburger and the salad bar for your child. Kids like the fresh fruit, carrot sticks and broccoli florets.
- Most fast-food spots offer lower-fat choices: salad bar (low-fat dressing), plain baked potatoes (topped with salad bar veggies), chili, skim or 1% milk*, low-fat frozen yogurt, English muffins, fruit juice and grilled (non-fried) chicken sandwiches.
- Supermarkets offer a variety of nutritious foods that are fast. Ready-made deli sandwiches (made with reduced-fat deli meats), fresh fruits and the salad bar are some "fast foods" from the grocery store.

* Children under two years of age should *only* drink whole milk.

Microwave Magic—Safely!

A microwave oven can help you cook in a healthful way. Vegetables cooked in a microwave oven stay nutrient-rich. For one reason, nutrients don't dissolve in any cooking water; short cooking time is another factor. Meat, fish and poultry dishes can be cooked or reheated with little or no added fat.

Microwaving also can help you cook faster and easier. But it can pose potential hazards—especially when children cook with the microwave oven. BURNS are the most common microwave injury. Children can be burned by:

- Removing dishes from the microwave oven—*make sure they use a pot holder.*
- Spilling hot foods—*keep the oven out of a young child's reach.*
- Opening microwave popcorn packages and other containers—*show older children how to open the container so steam escapes away from their hands and face.*
- Eating food that is cooked unevenly or has "hot spots"—*show older children how to stir food well before tasting it, or let food "rest" so that heat distributes evenly.*

Here's a common sense rule for microwave ovens: *If children are too young to read or follow written directions, they are too young to use a microwave oven without supervision.*

This brochure was developed as part of the **HEALTHY START...Food to Grow On** program, an information and education campaign that promotes healthful food choices and eating habits for healthy children ages two years and over. The **HEALTHY START** program was produced as a cooperative effort by the American Academy of Pediatrics (AAP), The American Dietetic Association (ADA), and the Food Marketing Institute (FMI).

For a referral to a registered dietitian and food and nutrition information, call the ADA's National Center for Nutrition and Dietetics Consumer Nutrition Hot Line at (800) 366-1655. For answers to your food and nutrition questions from a registered dietitian, please dial (900) CALL-AN-RD or (900) 225-5267.

American Academy of Pediatrics

DEDICATED TO THE HEALTH OF ALL CHILDREN™

The American Academy of Pediatrics is an organization of 55,000 primary care pediatricians, pediatric medical subspecialists, and pediatric surgical specialists dedicated to the health, safety, and well-being of infants, children, adolescents, and young adults.

American Academy of Pediatrics
PO Box 747
Elk Grove Village, IL 60009-0747
Web site — http://www.aap.org

Copyright ©1991, Updated 1996
American Academy of Pediatrics

SECTION FIVE

Behavior and Psychosocial Issues

Adoption:

Guidelines for Parents   Part I   Adopting a Young Child

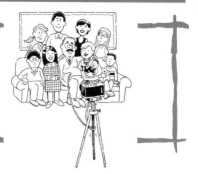

If you have recently adopted or soon will be adopting a child, you are probably experiencing many different emotions. The excitement and delight of a new addition to the family is often mixed with concern or even fear of what lies ahead.

There are many different types of adoption. Children often are adopted by a relative or a stepparent. More and more families are adopting children of another race, country, or culture. Many families adopt older children from foster homes, but most children who are adopted come into their new families as infants or very young children. The fact is, children of any age or background who are adopted will bring special issues and challenges to your family that biological parents never face.

By better understanding the role adoption plays in your child's growth and development, you can help your child accept his own uniqueness and learn to be proud of who he is and how he helped form your family.

Better early than never

Talk to your child about her adoption as soon as she is able to understand—usually between ages 2 and 4. The word adopted should become a part of your child's vocabulary early on. These early discussions give you practice in talking about adoption and show your child that it is OK to bring up the topic. If you are uneasy that your child is not biologically yours, she will feel it.

Just as any child delights in the story of the day she was born, a child who is adopted will treasure details of how she came into the family. While going through the adoption process, keep a scrapbook or journal the same way an excited mother does during pregnancy. Keep track of important dates and steps in the process. Take pictures of the people and places involved in your child's earlier life. Details about your child's earlier life and the adoption process will help make both easier to understand.

Share with your child the joy you felt at bringing her home that very first day. Many families even celebrate the arrival or adoption date every year, in addition to a birthday. It shows that the child came to the family in a different way, but is just as valued and loved.

The longer you wait to discuss adoption with your child, the harder it will be. Any level of openness you can build when your child is very young will help as your child grows and begins to ask more difficult questions about her adoption.

If talking with your child about adoption is difficult, talk to your pediatrician. He or she can be a valuable source of support and understanding.

Is anything different?

As he grows into adulthood, your child may be asked questions by other people that he will not be able to answer. They may be simple, innocent questions such as, "Where did you get those big, blue eyes?" or "Do you look more like your mom or your dad?"

They could be questions on a form to be filled out at the doctor's office or when joining an athletic team at school, such as, "Has any blood relative ever had cancer? Diabetes?" or "What is your ethnic background?"

The most painful questions may be the ones the child asks himself. "Who am I?" "Where did I come from?" "Why did my parents give me away?"

Sooner or later, these questions or others like them will come up. Many children who are adopted simply don't have the answers.

Being adopted can play a vital role in the development of your child's self-image. It becomes a basic part of who he is. Some children who are adopted grow up feeling different from other children. Those differences are real. Many adopted children have two sets of parents. Some may have been denied affection or even basic nutrition or medical care. Whatever the circumstances, it is important to recognize that your child's life experience has been quite different from that of other children.

Keep no secrets

As the years pass, your child will become more concerned about his place in your family. This may be especially true around ages 9 through 12, when most children become very worried about appearance and fitting in. Your child may begin to ask questions about his own appearance, his background, and the adoption and its circumstances. The following are some common questions your child may ask:

- "Did I grow in your body, Mommy?"
- "Why did my birth mother give me away?"
- "Did she and my birth father love each other?"
- "What was my name before I was adopted?"
- "What nationality am I?"
- "Do I have brothers or sisters?"
- "How much did it cost to adopt me?"

- **Do your best to answer questions honestly and in a way that will be easy for your child to understand at her age.** They may be painful questions for you to think about, but it is normal for children who are adopted to ask them. It is important to develop trust between you and your child. The more your child trusts you, the easier it will be for her to come to you with questions. If your child feels that talking about these questions makes you uncomfortable, she may keep them inside. She may then wonder, imagine, and perhaps fear the worst. Your child may also seek the answers elsewhere, perhaps from a relative or friend who may not give accurate information. Dealing with these issues openly is very important for your child. Be honest and as informative as you can. You may not know the answers for some questions. Be honest about that too.
- **Avoid responding with your own worries** like "Why do you want to know?" or "Are you unhappy with our family?" Your child's curiosity is healthy and natural. It should not be discouraged or seen as a threat to you—it's normal. Questioning your child's loyalties may only confuse him further. If your child believes talking about his adoption will hurt you, he will avoid it.

- **Don't force the issue on your child**. Some children are curious from the very beginning. Others may be afraid to bring it up. The best you can do is create an atmosphere in the family that lets your child know it is OK to talk about adoption. In a loving, supportive environment, when your child is ready to know more, she will ask.

Relatives, friends, and strangers

Even when adoption is handled well at home, there may be relatives who are not quite as understanding. This is particularly important when the child is from a different race or country. Some friends or relatives may disapprove of or even resist accepting your child into the family.

Explain to your relatives that your child is as much a part of the family as anyone else. You may not change their minds or correct old thinking, but it is important to show loyalty to your child. For a child to feel loved and welcomed, he needs to be treated like a full member of the family. Do not settle for anything less.

Questions from strangers can also be tricky. When a stranger innocently asks, "Where did he get those big blue eyes?," and everyone in the family has small brown eyes, tell the truth. Say simply, "From his mother." It may not be necessary to share personal information with a stranger, but don't lie. If your child hears you lying to a stranger, he may assume there is something about being adopted that he should be ashamed of, something that needs to be covered up.

You do not have to introduce your child as "my adopted son." He is simply your son. However, if a question comes up about differences in appearance or ethnicity, offer a simple, but honest explanation. When you are proud of your child's identity, he too, will learn to appreciate his own value.

Facing the past

It can be very difficult to talk with your child about the past. It may be painful to think about or acknowledge your child's other identity. Children who are adopted need to belong and to feel connected to their roots. Having kind and loving adoptive parents does not erase the past. Sooner or later, many adopted children want to know where they came from and why they were placed for adoption.

As your child gets older, make sure she knows where to look for information about the adoption. It is a good idea to keep copies of your child's important papers accessible to her at any time. She may want to look them over in private and in her own time. Someday, she may want to read through them with you. In some cases, she may never have the desire to see the papers at all. But it is important that the choice be hers and that the option be available to her.

Preparing for the future

As your child grows into adulthood, he may begin thinking about searching for his birth family. He may begin to feel less dependent on you, and more able to search for information on his own. Some states have programs available to help adults who were adopted get information about their adoption. Only a few states have open records. Check with your state government to find out about the laws concerning adoption records.

Birth mothers and fathers also may conduct searches. The pain or guilt of giving up a child may become too much to bear over the years. Many have gone on to raise other children and may feel a need for information about the child they placed for adoption.

It is important for you to consider the possibility that the birth parents may one day play a role in your child's life. By establishing an open, loving, and supportive relationship with your child, the issues that may emerge in the teen and adult years will often be much easier to manage. Search and reunion can bring pain and joy for everyone involved. The child, no matter what age, needs the continuing love and support of his adoptive family.

Your family, your child

Raising a family today is difficult. Raising a child who is adopted can present unique challenges. If the child misbehaves, gets into trouble, or has problems at school, it is tempting to blame adoption. The fact is, all children sometimes misbehave or get into trouble. It is possible your child's problems have nothing to do with adoption at all. They may simply be a normal part of growth.

As your child grows, he is influenced by family, the community, friends, school, and society in general. He is also influenced by the genes passed to him from his birth mother and father. There is no research that can tell us which is more important, but we know that both are powerful. Adoption is an important part of who your child is, but keep in mind that many other factors will affect who he becomes.

Helping your child accept the fact that he is different, yet just like everyone else, may not sound easy, but it is important to try. Talking openly and truthfully with your child about his adoption, his birth parents, and his feelings is the key. Adoption gives both you and your child a tremendous gift—the gift of each other. With love, honesty, and patience, you and your child will form a relationship that is as deep and meaningful as any bond between a parent and child.

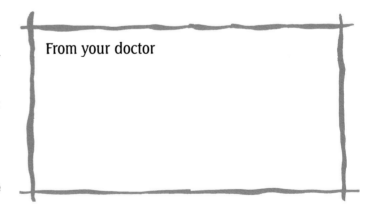

From your doctor

American Academy of Pediatrics

DEDICATED TO THE HEALTH OF ALL CHILDREN™

The American Academy of Pediatrics is an organization of 55,000 primary care pediatricians, pediatric medical subspecialists, and pediatric surgical specialists dedicated to the health, safety, and well-being of infants, children, adolescents, and young adults.

American Academy of Pediatrics
PO Box 747
Elk Grove Village, IL 60009-0747
Web site — http://www.aap.org

Copyright ©1999   American Academy of Pediatrics

Adoption:
Guidelines for Parents Part II Adopting an Older Child

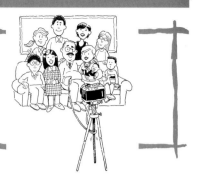

If you have recently adopted or soon will be adopting a child, you are probably experiencing many different emotions. The excitement and delight of a new addition to the family is often mixed with concern or even fear of what lies ahead.

There are many different types of adoption. Children often are adopted by a relative or a stepparent. More and more families are adopting children of another race, country, or culture. Many families adopt older children from foster homes, but most children who are adopted come into their new families as infants or very young children. The fact is, children of any age or background who are adopted will bring special issues and challenges to your family that biological parents never face.

By better understanding the role adoption plays in your child's growth and development, you can help your child accept his own uniqueness and learn to be proud of who he is and how he helped form your family.

Adopting the older child

Becoming a new parent is tough, but becoming a new parent of a school-age child or adolescent can be tougher.

An older child may bring problems from the past into his new family. He may have lived in a number of foster homes, each affecting him in some way. He may have lived with one or both birth parents for a time. There may be a history of drug, alcohol, physical, or sexual abuse. He may have been separated from siblings. Many factors could have affected your child's life before he came to your home. Following are some suggestions that will help you deal with them:

- **Learn as much as you can about your child's background** and that of his birth parents. The adoption agency can help you gather as much information as possible. By learning everything you can about your child and his past, you may become more aware of problems that may lie ahead. Keep in mind, it is impossible for you or the adoption agency to know everything your child may have gone through.

- **Keep a connection to your child's past.** It is important that your child feel connected in a positive way to the life she had before coming to your home. Keep in touch with someone she knew; a grandparent, relative, friend, or neighbor. If possible, put together a "life book" by collecting mementos and photos of your child's previous home, school, and people she was close to. These things will be important as your child adjusts to her new life.

- **Don't be afraid to seek help.** Adoptive parents should understand that an older child with serious problems may need professional help to resolve these issues. Constant and persistent love can work wonders for most children, however, in some cases, love may not be enough.

- **Don't blame yourself.** An older child may rebel against his new family. This anger is usually because of the child's past losses. These problems are not your fault. Remind yourself that you are part of the solution as you help your child work out his issues. Most of all, be patient.

- **Talk to your pediatrician.** He or she may be able to help or suggest counselors or support groups.

Relatives, friends, and strangers

Even when adoption is handled well at home, there may be relatives who are not quite as understanding. This is particularly important when the child is from a different race or country. Some friends or relatives may disapprove of or even resist accepting your child into the family.

Explain to your relatives that your child is as much a part of the family as anyone else. You may not change their minds or correct old thinking, but it is important to show loyalty to your child. For a child to feel loved and welcomed, he needs to be treated like a full member of the family. Do not settle for anything less.

Questions from strangers can also be tricky. When a stranger innocently asks, "Where did he get those big blue eyes?," and everyone in the family has small brown eyes, tell the truth. Say simply, "From his mother." It may not be necessary to share personal information with a stranger, but don't lie. If your child hears you lying to a stranger, he may assume there is something about being adopted that he should be ashamed of, something that needs to be covered up.

You do not have to introduce your child as "my adopted son." He is simply your son. However, if a question comes up about differences in appearance or ethnicity, offer a simple, but honest explanation. When you are proud of your child's identity, he too, will learn to appreciate his own value.

Facing the past

It can be very difficult to talk with your child about the past. It may be painful to think about or acknowledge your child's other identity. Children who are adopted need to belong and to feel connected to their roots. Having kind and loving adoptive parents does not erase the past. Sooner or later, many adopted children want to know where they came from and why they were placed for adoption.

As your child gets older, make sure she knows where to look for information about the adoption. It is a good idea to keep copies of your child's important papers accessible to her at any time. She may want to look them over in private and in her own time. Someday, she may want to read through them with you. In some cases, she may never have the desire to see the papers at all. But it is important that the choice be hers and that the option be available to her.

Preparing for the future

As your child grows into adulthood, he may begin thinking about searching for his birth family. He may begin to feel less dependent on you, and more able to search for information on his own. Some states have programs available to help adults who were adopted get information about their adoption. Only a few states have open records. Check with your state government to find out about the laws concerning adoption records.

Birth mothers and fathers also may conduct searches. The pain or guilt of giving up a child may become too much to bear over the years. Many have gone on to raise other children and may feel a need for information about the child they placed for adoption.

It is important for you to consider the possibility that the birth parents may one day play a role in your child's life. By establishing an open, loving, and supportive relationship with your child, the issues that may emerge in the teen and adult years will often be much easier to manage. Search and reunion can bring pain and joy for everyone involved. The child, no matter what age, needs the continuing love and support of his adoptive family.

Your family, your child

Raising a family today is difficult. Raising a child who is adopted can present unique challenges. If the child misbehaves, gets into trouble, or has problems at school, it is tempting to blame adoption. The fact is, all children sometimes misbehave or get into trouble. It is possible your child's problems have nothing to do with adoption at all. They may simply be a normal part of growth.

As your child grows, he is influenced by family, the community, friends, school, and society in general. He is also influenced by the genes passed to him from his birth mother and father. There is no research that can tell us which is more important, but we know that both are powerful. Adoption is an important part of who your child is, but keep in mind that many other factors will affect who he becomes.

Helping your child accept the fact that he is different, yet just like everyone else, may not sound easy, but it is important to try. Talking openly and truthfully with your child about his adoption, his birth parents, and his feelings is the key. Adoption gives both you and your child a tremendous gift—the gift of each other. With love, honesty, and patience, you and your child will form a relationship that is as deep and meaningful as any bond between a parent and child.

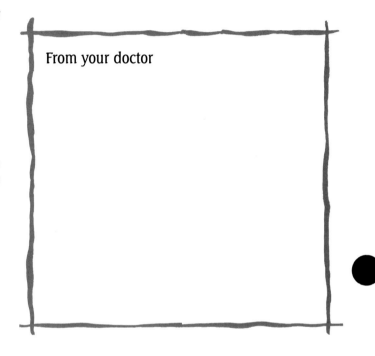

From your doctor

American Academy of Pediatrics

DEDICATED TO THE HEALTH OF ALL CHILDREN™

The American Academy of Pediatrics is an organization of 55,000 primary care pediatricians, pediatric medical subspecialists, and pediatric surgical specialists dedicated to the health, safety, and well-being of infants, children, adolescents, and young adults.

American Academy of Pediatrics
PO Box 747
Elk Grove Village, IL 60009-0747
Web site — http://www.aap.org

Adoption:

Guidelines for Parents Part III Additional Resources

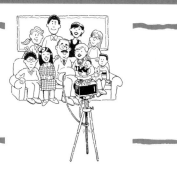

"Who are my real parents?"

Early on, many parents find themselves dealing with the question of who the child's "real" or "natural" parents are. Relatives or friends may ask if you have met the child's "real" parents. Your child herself may even ask about her "real" mother or father. Let your child know that the words mother and father have more than one meaning.

A mother is someone who gives birth to a child, but a mother is also someone who loves, nurtures, and guides a child to adulthood. She takes care of the child's needs every day, changes the diapers, and dries the tears. Being a father also can have different meanings.

Find other words that everyone in your family is comfortable with. The terms birth mother and father are very common. Biological parents is also used frequently. Remember, both sets of parents are "real" and deserve to be recognized for who they are and the roles they have played in the child's life.

A note from your pediatrician... international adoptions

Parents who adopt children from other countries need to be aware of the special medical needs their child may have. Your pediatrician recommends the following:

- Immunizations should meet US standards.
- Test for infectious diseases (such as HIV, hepatitis B and C, syphilis, tuberculosis, and parasites) and nutritional disorders (such as lead poisoning, anemia, rickets, and iodine deficiency), even if testing was done in another country before the adoption.
- Have your child's vision, hearing, and developmental abilities (such as language) assessed as soon as possible.

"You are special because..."

Adoptive parents often tell their child she is special because she was "chosen" or that she was "given up out of love." Though the parents mean well, these statements may be confusing to the child.

For most parents, adoption is not the first choice. Most adoptions in the United States are by parents who first tried to conceive and were unable to do so. Sooner or later, children learn this. Telling the child she is even more special because she is "chosen" may be recognized by the child as bending the truth. Some children may feel that being chosen means they must always be the best at everything.

Being told she was given up out of love may raise questions about what love is and whether others who love her will leave too.

The most important thing for your child to know is that she is wanted — not any more than a biological child would be and not any less. Any attempt to make the adopted child feel more special than a biological child may have quite a different, unintended effect.

Every child in the family should be treated the same by you, your spouse, the siblings, and your relatives. Children who are adopted may feel different from other members of the family. Her appearance, her performance in school, or her athletic ability may be quite different. But she is, first and foremost, your child. What makes her special is not that she was adopted, but that she is yours.

A word about...open adoptions

When there is contact between birth parents and adoptive parents during the adoption process, it is considered an "open adoption." This can mean simply exchanging names and addresses or, in fully open adoptions, the birth parents may have ongoing communication with or even visit the child.

In an open adoption, your young child may not understand the relationships between the two sets of parents. There are fewer secrets in an open adoption, but just as many difficult questions. It is important to address the issues mentioned in this brochure and provide your child with the guidance and support she needs.

For more information

There are many quality resources available to find out more about adoption. The following are just a few:

Books

Adopting the Hurt Child: Hope for Families with Special-Needs Kids; by Gregory C. Keck, Regina M. Kupecky (Pinon Press, 1998)

The Adoption Triangle; by Arthur D. Sorosky, Annette Baran, and Reuben Pannor (Corona, 1989)

Being Adopted; The Lifelong Search for Self; by David M. Brodzinsky, Marshall Schechter, and Robin Marantz Henig (Anchor, 1993)

Birthmothers: Women Who Have Relinquished Babies for Adoption Tell Their Stories; by Merry Bloch Jones (Chicago Review, 1993)

How It Feels to Be Adopted; by Jill Krementz (Knopf, 1988)

Journey of the Adopted Self; by Betty Jean Lifton (BasicBooks, HarperCollins, 1995)

Let's Talk About It: Adoption; by Fred Rogers (Paper Star, 1998)

Raising Adopted Children; by Lois R. Melina (HarperCollins, 1998)

Real Parents, Real Children; by Holly van Gulden and Lisa M. Bartels-Rabb (Crossroad, 1995)

Talking With Young Children About Adoption; by Mary Watkins, Susan Fisher (Yale University Press, 1995)

Organizations

Adoptive Families of America (AFA)
2309 Como St
St Paul, MN 55108
800/372-3300
http://www.AdoptiveFam.org

American Adoption Congress (AAC)
1000 Connecticut Ave, NW
Suite 9
Washington, DC 20036
202/483-3399
http://www.american-adoption-cong.org

Child Welfare League of America (CWLA)
440 First Street, NW
Third Floor
Washington, DC 20001
202/638-2952
http://www.cwla.org

North American Council on Adoptable Children (NACAC)
970 Raymond Ave, Suite 106
St Paul, MN 55114-1149
651/644-3036
E-mail: NACAC@aol.com

These resources were chosen to represent a broad range of viewpoints. Inclusion on this list does not imply an endorsement by the American Academy of Pediatrics. The Academy is not responsible for the content of the resources mentioned above. Addresses and phone numbers are as current as possible, but may change at any time.

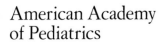

American Academy of Pediatrics

DEDICATED TO THE HEALTH OF ALL CHILDREN™

The American Academy of Pediatrics is an organization of 55,000 primary care pediatricians, pediatric medical subspecialists, and pediatric surgical specialists dedicated to the health, safety, and well-being of infants, children, adolescents, and young adults.

American Academy of Pediatrics
PO Box 747
Elk Grove Village, IL 60009-0747
Web site — http://www.aap.org

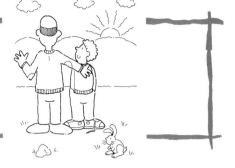

Alcohol:
Your Child and Drugs

Children are challenged at younger ages than ever before to try drugs. Use of tobacco, marijuana, and cocaine are serious problems. However, one of the most abused drugs in our society is alcohol. Alcohol is a drug because it acts as a depressant on the nervous system and is very addictive. Though it's illegal for people under age 21 to drink, we all know that most teenagers are no strangers to alcohol. Many of them are introduced to alcohol during childhood.

Why parents should worry

- About 1 out of 5 fifth graders have been drunk.
- Four out of 10 sixth graders say there is pressure from other students to drink.
- Nearly 80% of high school seniors report having used alcohol.

Alcohol is often the first drug that young people try. Some parents may breathe a sigh of relief when they find out their teen is "only" drinking alcohol. Since alcohol is legal and found in most American homes, parents may think it isn't dangerous. Not true. Alcohol can be very harmful.

Childhood drinking begins early, often between 11 and 13 years of age, and sometimes even younger. Alcohol is often called a "gateway drug." When young people like the feeling they get from alcohol, they may be interested in trying other drugs later. This can lead to multiple drug use, which is very dangerous. The use of alcohol, by itself or with other drugs, can harm your child's normal growth and development.

Even if a teenager only drinks occasionally, intoxicated behavior can be lethal. Just one drink can impair decision making and slow down reaction time in any situation. Alcohol is linked with a variety of risky behaviors, such as:

- **Crime and serious violence.**
- **Early sexual activity, multiple partners, sexually transmitted diseases including AIDS, and unintended teenage pregnancy.**
- **Fetal Alcohol Syndrome.** Drinking during pregnancy can cause a baby to be born with major birth defects. No one knows exactly how much alcohol is too much during pregnancy, but the more a mother drinks, the greater the risk to her baby.
- **Drunk driving.** It is the leading cause of death for young adults, aged 15 to 24 years. In one study, an estimated 6% to 14% of drivers under 21 years of age who were stopped at roadside checkpoints had been drinking. This age-group makes up only one fifth of the licensed drivers in the United States, yet they are involved in almost half of all fatal car crashes.

Why young people drink

Young people drink alcohol for a variety of reasons.
1. Curiosity. They have heard that getting drunk is fun and they want to find out for themselves.
2. They see drinking as a "rite of passage"—something to be experienced on the way to adulthood.
3. To get drunk. This explains why they often drink until they are out of control. Binge drinking (consuming five or more drinks in a row for males, four for females) is alarmingly common. Sixteen percent of 8th graders, 25% of 10th graders, and 30% of seniors have reported binge drinking.
4. To fit in with friends who are already using alcohol.
5. To feel relaxed and to boost self-confidence.
6. To escape problems, such as depression, family conflict, trouble in school or with a boyfriend or girlfriend.

Stages of alcohol use

The same pattern of use and abuse exists for alcohol as with other drugs such as marijuana or cocaine. Experts have noted the following stages of alcohol use:

Stage 1:

Experimenting with alcohol. There may be strong peer pressure to use alcohol "just for fun" and to be part of the group. Most use happens on weekends. There often is no change in behavior between uses.

Stage 2:

Actively seeking alcohol. Alcohol is used to produce good feelings during times of stress. Usage occurs during the week. Schoolwork may suffer. Changes in behavior may include:

- an increase in time spent alone
- a decline in communication with family members, frequent arguing, and a high level of secretiveness
- changes in dress and grooming
- changes in choice of friends
- repeated or unexplained injuries or fights
- poor sleeping habits and a lack of energy
- irregular eating habits
- bloodshot eyes
- mood changes, including irritability and depression
- running away from home
- attempting suicide

Keep in mind that some of these symptoms occur from time to time in normal, nonalcohol-using teens, and none alone is proof of alcohol or drug use. However, a combination of any of the above symptoms may signal a problem.

 ©2002 American Academy of Pediatrics

Stage 3:

Preoccupation with alcohol. There is an almost total loss of control over the use of alcohol. Attempts to limit alcohol use at this stage can cause withdrawal symptoms of depression, moodiness, and irritability. Alcoholic beverages may disappear from the home. There is a danger of turning to other drugs or stronger forms of liquor. Family possessions may also disappear as the alcohol user seeks money to support his habit. There may be trouble with the law for these same reasons.

The good news

Most adolescents never move beyond the first stage of alcohol use. Whether they do or not depends for the most part on their personality, their family, and their community. For those who do move to the advanced stages, the entire process can take months or years. Many young people and adults receive help too late. This is why early detection is so important.

How to prevent alcohol use and abuse

As with any disease, prevention is the best treatment. Parents must learn the facts about teen alcohol use and abuse to help their children remain alcohol free.

Parents who drink

Parents who choose to use alcohol must be careful how it is used in the home. Having a drink should never be shown as a way to cope with problems. Don't drink in unsafe conditions—driving the car, mowing the lawn, using the stove, etc. Don't encourage your child to drink or to join you in having a drink. Never make jokes about getting drunk; make sure that your children understand that it is neither funny nor acceptable. Show your children that there are many ways to have fun without alcohol. Happy occasions and special events don't have to include drinking.

Parents should set a good example at home by limiting their own use of alcohol and other drugs. Parents who don't drink should be aware that this alone will not guarantee their children and teenagers won't use alcohol. Parents who are alcoholics or problem drinkers place their children at increased risk of alcohol dependence. Studies suggest that alcoholism may run in the family. One out of 5 young adults with an alcoholic parent is likely to become an alcoholic too.

Education about alcohol should begin early. Parents can help their children resist alcohol use in these ways:

- **Give your child a sense of confidence.** This is the best defense against peer pressure. Build your child's self-esteem with praise and avoid frequent criticism.
- **Listen** to what your child says. Pay attention, and be helpful during periods of loneliness or doubt.
- **Know who your child's friends are** and make a point to get to know them.

- **Provide parental supervision.** Don't allow your teen to attend parties where alcohol is being served. Insist that a parent be present at parties to supervise. Contact other parents to arrange alcohol-free social events.
- **Offer a "free call home."** Drinking and driving may lead to death. Make sure your child knows not to ride with a driver who has been drinking. Let him know that he can call home without fear of consequences that night. Discuss the incident the next day.
- **Help your child learn to handle strong emotions and feelings.** Model ways to control stress, pain, or tension.
- **Talk about things that are important issues for your child,** including alcohol, drugs, and the need for peer-group acceptance.
- **Encourage enjoyable and worthwhile outside things to do;** avoid turning leisure time into chores.
- **Join your child in learning all you can about preventing alcohol abuse.** Programs offered in schools, churches, and youth groups can help you both learn more about alcohol abuse.

Your pediatrician understands that good communication between parents and children is one of the best ways to prevent alcohol use. If talking with your teenager about alcohol is difficult, your pediatrician may be able to help open the lines of communication. If you suspect your child is using alcohol or any other drug, ask your pediatrician for advice and help.

The information contained in this publication should not be used as a substitute for the medical care and advice of your pediatrician. There may be variations in treatment that your pediatrician may recommend based on individual facts and circumstances.

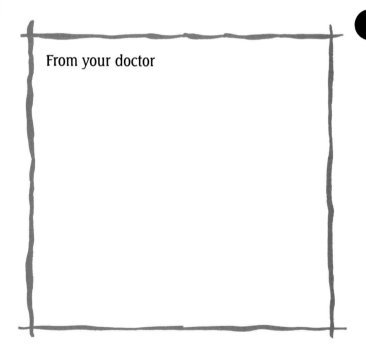

From your doctor

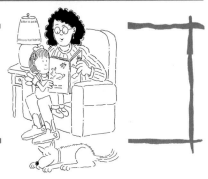

Child Sexual Abuse:
What It Is and How To Prevent It

Sexual abuse of children is more common than most people realize. At least 1 out of 5 adult women and 1 out of 10 adult men report having been sexually abused in childhood. By educating yourself and your children about sexual abuse, you can help prevent it from happening to your children and better cope with it if it does.

What is child sexual abuse?

Sexual abuse is when an adult or an older child forces sexual contact on a younger child. The abuser may use physical abuse, bribery, threats, tricks, or take advantage of a younger child's lack of knowledge. Any of the following acts by an adult or older child are sexual abuse:

- Fondling a child's genitals
- Getting a child to fondle their genitals
- Mouth to genital contact with a child
- Rubbing their genitals on a child
- Penetrating a child's vagina or anus
- Showing their genitals to a child
- Showing pornographic or "dirty" pictures or videotapes to a child
- Using a child as a model to make pornographic materials

Could my child be sexually abused? By whom?

Children are abused most often by adults or older children whom they know and who can influence their behavior by exerting power over them. In 8 out of 10 reported cases, the abuser is someone the child knows. The abuser is often an authority figure whom the child trusts or loves.

How would I know if my child is being sexually abused?

Many parents expect their son or daughter to tell them or another trusted adult about being sexually abused. Abusers often threaten or convince the child not to tell anyone about it. The child may believe that the abuse is his fault and that he will be punished if someone finds out. A child's first statements about abuse may be vague and incomplete. He may just hint about the problem to see if he would get in trouble. Abused children may tell a friend about it. The friend may then tell an adult. Children may tell about abuse after a personal safety program at their school. Parents may suspect abuse because of the child's behavior. You should be aware of the following behavioral changes in your child that may be symptoms of sexual abuse:

- Noticeable, new fear of a person (even a parent) or certain places
- Unusual or unexpected response from the child when asked if she was touched by someone
- Drawings that show sexual acts
- Abrupt changes in behavior, such as bed-wetting or loss of bowel control
- Sudden awareness of genitals
- Sexual acts and words shared with other children or animals

- Questions about sexual activity that are beyond the child's development
- Changes in sleep habits, such as nightmares in young children
- Constipation, or refusal to have bowel movements

Physical signs of abuse may include the following:

- Anal or genital redness, pain, or bleeding
- Unusual discharge from the anus or vagina
- Sexually transmitted diseases such as gonorrhea, chlamydia, or genital warts
- Repeated urinary tract infections in females
- Pregnancy, in older females

What should I do if my child reveals sexual abuse to me?

Children tend to ignore things that make them feel uncomfortable, rather than recognize them as warning signs. If your child talks about abuse, listen carefully and take it very seriously. When a child's plea for help is ignored, not believed, or punished, she may not risk telling again. As a result, the child could remain a victim of abuse for months or years. Teach your child that it is OK to talk about uncomfortable feelings.

If your child reveals abuse, you should take the following steps:

1) **Face the issue.** Listen to your child's reasons for revealing the abuse. Tell your child the abuse is not her fault. Give her extra love, comfort, and reassurance. If you are angry, make sure she knows you are not angry with her, and you will help her. Let your child know how brave she is to tell you and that you understand how scared she feels. This is even more important if the child has been abused by a close and trusted relative or family friend.

2) **Take charge of the situation.** Protect the child from further abuse.

3) **Discuss the problem** with a pediatrician and a counselor who can provide support.

4) **Report abuse to the police or local child protection service agency.** Ask about crisis support help.

Can I deal with sexual abuse in my family without contacting the authorities?

Parents should not try to stop or treat sexual abuse themselves. If abuse is suspected, parents should follow the steps above and get help.

What will happen to the child and to the abuser if sexual abuse is reported?

Sexual abuse is against the law. It is a crime, no matter who the abuser is. Cases are investigated by the police, a social service agency, or both. With the help of a doctor, they will decide whether sexual abuse took place. Depending on the circumstances, the police may let social services manage the case, especially if the child is very young, shows no signs of physical injury, or the abuser is young or a family member. When a child is abused by a nonfamily member, the matter must be handled by the police.

After sexual abuse is reported, what happens next depends on the circumstances of the case. Preventing further abuse of the child is the first concern of the authorities. The abuser may be referred for treatment. The child and the entire family may also be referred to a treatment program. If the suspected abuser lives in the home and faces criminal charges, authorities will recommend that the suspected abuser leave the home. In any case, the child can usually stay in the home as long as her family will take the necessary steps to protect her from further abuse by asking the abuser to leave the home while the problem is investigated. Whatever the circumstances, the child and family will need a lot of support from relatives and friends.

What parents can do to prevent sexual abuse

The American Academy of Pediatrics encourages you to take the following steps:

- **Talk** to your child about sexual abuse. If your child's school sponsors a sexual abuse program, discuss what he learned.

- **Teach** your child which body parts are private (parts covered by a bathing suit) and the proper names of those parts. Let him know that his body belongs to him. Tell him to yell "no" or "stop" to anyone who may threaten him sexually.

- **Listen** when your child tries to tell you something, especially when it seems hard for him to talk about it. Make sure your child knows it's OK to tell you about any attempt to molest him or touch him in a way that made him feel uncomfortable, no matter who the abuser may be. Let him know he can trust you and that you will not be angry with him if he tells you.

- **Give** your child enough time and attention. Weekly family meetings can be used to talk about all good and bad experiences.

- **Know** the adults and children with whom your child is spending time. Be careful about allowing your child to spend time alone or in out-of-the-way places with other adults or older children. Make visits to your child's caregiver without notice. Ask your child about his visits to the caregiver or with child sitters.

- **Never** let your child enter a stranger's home without a parent or trusted adult. Door-to-door fund-raising is particularly risky for unsupervised children.

- **Check** to see if your child's school has an abuse prevention program for the teachers and children. If it doesn't, start one.

- **Tell** someone in authority if you suspect that your child or someone else's child is being abused.

Your child's teacher or school counselor can help you teach your child to avoid or report sexual abuse. They know how this can be done without upsetting or scaring your child. Your pediatrician also understands the importance of communication between parents and children. He or she is trained to detect the signs of child sexual abuse and is familiar with resources in the community. Ask your pediatrician for advice on how to protect your children.

For further information on child sexual abuse or other forms of abuse, please contact:

Prevent Child Abuse America
PO Box 2866
Chicago, IL 60690-9950
800/556-2722
Web site: http://www.childabuse.org

Talking with your child

Measures to protect your children from sexual abuse should begin early, since many child abuse cases involve preschoolers. The guidelines below offer topics to discuss with your children depending on their ages.

Age	Prevention Plan
18 months–3 years	Teach your child the proper names for body parts.
3–5 years	Teach your child about private parts of the body (parts covered by a bathing suit) and how to yell "no" to sexual advances. Use coloring books or reading books with examples. Give simple, easy-to-understand answers to questions about sex. Play the "What if…?" game. Ask your child what she would do in certain situations.
5–8 years	Discuss safety away from home and the difference between being touched in private parts of the body and other touching. Encourage your child to talk about scary experiences, including requests to touch someone else's private parts or look at pornography. Play the "What if…?" game. Ask your child what she would do in certain situations.
8–12 years	Stress personal safety and give examples of possible problem areas, such as video arcades, malls, locker rooms, and out-of-the-way places outdoors. Start to discuss rules of sexual conduct that are accepted by the family. Discuss basic facts about human reproduction.
12–18 years	Continue to stress personal safety and potential problem areas. Discuss the prevention of rape, date rape, sexually transmitted diseases, and unintended pregnancy. Talk about the effects of drugs and alcohol on sexual behavior.

The information contained in this publication should not be used as a substitute for the medical care and advice of your pediatrician. There may be variations in treatment that your pediatrician may recommend based on individual facts and circumstances.

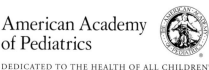

American Academy of Pediatrics

DEDICATED TO THE HEALTH OF ALL CHILDREN™

The American Academy of Pediatrics is an organization of 55,000 primary care pediatricians, pediatric medical subspecialists, and pediatric surgical specialists dedicated to the health, safety, and well-being of infants, children, adolescents, and young adults.

American Academy of Pediatrics
PO Box 747
Elk Grove Village, IL 60009-0747
Web site — http://www.aap.org

Choosing Child Care: What's Best for Your Family?

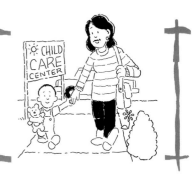

With increasing demands on the family, parents look to quality child care to help them manage family and work. About 70% of parents have their children in some form of child care. These families may be headed by two parents with two incomes available, or they may be headed by single parents who must provide income as well as take care of their children.

The American Academy of Pediatrics offers the following advice to help you find the care best suited for your child and family.

Finding quality child care is important. Standards for child care settings may vary depending on the type of child care. Use the following list of questions when visiting child care settings to help you decide the child care option that is best for you and your child.

What to look for

1. Do the child:staff ratios and the size of groups meet or exceed recommended levels? (See chart.)
2. Does the staff appear to enjoy caring for the children?
3. Is the center or home bright, cheerful, and well ventilated? Is all equipment clean, safe, and well maintained?
4. Do the children in the program appear to be happy?
5. Is the noise level in the child care areas comfortable?
6. Do the adults and the children often talk with each other? Are children encouraged to talk with each other?
7. Is the indoor space large enough? Look for 50 square feet, measured wall-to-wall, per child.
8. Is there a sleeping or quiet area large enough for all the children to rest during nap time? (There should be at least 3 feet of space between children sleeping in a head-to-toe manner.)
9. Does each child have a place for his or her own belongings?
10. Are infants always fed in an upright position and, until they can sit by themselves for feeding, held by an adult? (No bottles are allowed in bed or propped.)
11. Is all the food nutritious, well prepared, well served, and age-appropriate? Are you able to check the menus and meal plans in advance?
12. Are there many toys present that are accessible, safe, and appropriate for your child's age group?
13. Is there protective surfacing under indoor climbing equipment? Indoor climbers require the same types of impact-absorbing materials and fall zones as those installed outdoors.
14. Is there an outside play area that is free of sharp edges, pinch points, sharp rocks, and ditches?
15. Is the outside area free of hazards such as hard surfaces, sharp rocks, high climbers, tall slides, unprotected seesaws and merry-go-rounds, and unsafe swings?
    a. Is equipment age-appropriate, properly installed, and well maintained?
    b. Is there impact-absorbing material such as soft sand, wood chips, smooth gravel, or specially manufactured rubber mats under and at least 6 feet out from equipment?
16. Are there individual cribs, beds, cots, or mats to sleep on? Do sleeping children stay within view of caregivers?
17. Is there a clean diaper-changing area for infants and toddlers? Is a sink within the caregiver's reach near the diaper-changing surface?
18. Are the toilets and sinks clean and easy to reach? Can children reach clean towels, liquid soap, and toilet paper?
19. Do caregivers wash hands after changing diapers, wiping a runny nose, or helping a child with toileting?
20. Do caregivers make sure that children wash their hands after toileting, playing outside, and before meals?
21. Does each child have his or her own separate wash cloth and towel?
22. Are there sinks in each room, with a separate sink for food preparation and hand washing?
23. Does the center or home appear to be clean and safe for your child?

Age	Child:Staff ratio	Maximum group size
Birth–24 months	3:1	6
25–30 months	4:1	8
31–35 months	5:1	10
3 year olds	7:1	14
4 year olds	8:1	16
5 year olds	8:1	16
6–8 year olds	10:1	20
9–12 year olds	12:1	24

What to ask

1. Is the child care center or home licensed or registered with local government? Has the program achieved accreditation by a nationally recognized independent group of early childhood professionals? (Ask to see a current document and find out what type of inspection or review was done.)
2. Are you welcome to visit the facility during normal operating hours before and after registering your child in the program?
3. Can you see all areas your child will use?
4. Is there a written plan for play and learning activities that includes active play, quiet play, nap or rest time, and snacks and meals? (Ask to see it.)
5. Are there daily opportunities for inside and outside play, and are children supervised at all times?
6. Is television viewing limited to short times and age-appropriate programs?
7. Does the center offer parenting education classes or other family support?
8. Is each child assigned to one caregiver who is primarily responsible for his or her care and whereabouts, even if other caregivers are sometimes involved?
9. Does the caregiver regularly meet with parents? (Ask how often.)
10. Is there a written policy about discipline? (Ask to read it.)
11. Is smoking banned from the child care center or home?
12. Are there written policies and plans for the care of ill children that include the responsibilities of parents? (Ask to see the policies.)
13. Is there a quiet, well-supervised arrangement for the care of ill children until parents pick them up?
14. Will the caregivers give prescribed medications to your child? (If yes, under what conditions?)
15. Is there a health specialist, such as a pediatrician, who serves as a consultant for the child care program?
16. Are staff members and volunteers trained in child development?
17. Are you comfortable with the experience and qualifications of the staff?
18. Are the staff members and volunteers trained in first aid, injury prevention, emergency response to choking, and prevention of infections?
19. Does the caregiver perform monthly evacuation and emergency drills and monthly playground checks?
20. What are the arrangements if a caregiver gets sick or has to be away?
21. Can you get recommendations and advice from parents whose children are currently in the program?
22. Did the center explain to you all the costs and fees involved with your child's care?

Different children, different care

The key to good child care is whether the caregiver can adapt to the needs of children and families. Not all children of the same age are at the same level of development; each child has unique character traits. A good caregiver understands these personal and developmental differences and creates a program to meet each child's needs.

Infants (birth to 12 months)

When your child is an infant, the number of caregivers should be limited. Your child can only form a trusting relationship with a few people. Most young infants thrive when they have steady, positive relationships with their caregivers. Close contact aids your child's social and emotional growth. Your infant becomes used to a certain tone of voice, way of being held, etc. The caregiver also learns to recognize your infant's cues for distress, hunger, and playfulness. Even if more than one adult works with the group, one adult should have primary responsibility for your child.

Toddlers (12 months to 3 years)

Toddlers need a safe and supervised child care area to explore. They need many ways to express their growing independence under the watchful eye of a caregiver.

Toddlers learn language by listening to adults and repeating what they say. Television and other sources of steady background noise should be limited to no more than 1 to 2 hours of exposure. More may interfere with the interactions required to learn to talk. The caregiver should be positive, avoiding shouting and rude comments.

Since toddlers are just starting to learn about sharing, many clean, sturdy, and safe toys should be out at all times. There should be no toys or pieces smaller than 1 1/4 inches in diameter that can break off and cause a child to choke.

Preschool children (3 to 5 years)

Preschool children can take care of many of their basic needs. Most can wash their hands, brush their teeth, undress, and feed themselves. Many also can use the bathroom alone, although some still need adult help. Preschoolers are starting friendships. They are using language skills to express their needs and relate to other children. They need a balance between quiet play, active play, group play, and individual time.

Children learn by doing. A child care setting should have lots of objects for children to use in a variety of ways so they learn more about the world. Preschoolers show interest in colors, shapes, and numbers. Caregivers should encourage interest in these areas. Learning should be fun, not forced.

If your child gets sick

Children sometimes get sick while in child care. Make sure that you can always be reached by your child care provider. Many times children are allowed to stay with their child care provider as long as they can participate in most of the activities. If the child needs extra rest, there must be a place to lie down and still be observed.

Sometimes children need medications while they are at child care. Both prescription and over-the-counter medications should have a pharmacy label with the child's name, dosage, and expiration date. The child care provider should know when and how to safely give the medication and properly record each dose.

School-age children (5 to 12 years)

School-age children in child care before school need quiet play at that time. Ideally, your child should eat a balanced breakfast at home; this is good family time and enables you and your child to talk about the day ahead.

After school, children have just come from a structured school environment. After a nutritious snack, these children need active, imaginative play as well as the chance to socialize. Activities should be age-appropriate on safe playgrounds. While many of these children enjoy competition, programs should be geared toward self-improvement. Programs should also allow children to make friends, help them learn to get along with others, and work to better their self-esteem. Look for after-school programs that offer some separate activities for older and younger children every day. Vans used to pick up children should be safe and require the use of seat belts.

Children with physical, developmental, or emotional problems may need special care. Discuss your child's needs with your pediatrician and caregiver to help your child function well in a positive environment.

Ask your pediatrician for advice about the best child care setting. Your pediatrician can help you and your child's caregiver plan for your child's special needs, development, age-appropriate activities, toilet training, and safety.

Types of child care

Caregivers can be family members, close friends, or trusted employees. You can choose from three types of care:

- **In-home care** services bring the caregiver into your home.
- **Family child care** is offered in the home of the caregiver.
- **Center-based care** usually takes place outside the home in a facility designed for young children. You should consider the pros and cons of each type of care.

In-home care can be very convenient. Many home care providers can arrange their schedules to match your needs. Since the caregiver comes to your home, your child does not have to adjust to a new setting. This gives you greater control over your child's environment. Also, your child can receive more individual attention, especially if the caregiver is not expected to do housekeeping. Home care may lessen your child's exposure to seasonal illnesses, because of exposure to fewer children.

Skilled in-home providers are difficult to find. You will need a backup plan for the times when the caregiver is sick or goes on vacation. You alone are the judge of the caregiver's character, health, and skill. It is hard to know for sure what the caregiver does when you are not there. In some urban areas, agencies may provide training, placement, and supervision for in-home providers.

The training of home care providers should include emergency response to choking and first aid. The caregiver should provide you with a daily schedule and a daily report. Plan frequent opportunities for someone to observe the caregiver's interactions with your child.

Family child care takes place in the caregiver's home. Many family child care providers who offer child care have young children of their own. Caregivers may care for children who are the same age or for children of all ages.

Check to see that the home is clean and safe. Also, make sure that the caregiver and the caregiver's children are healthy. Television watching should be limited to 1 or 2 hours per day. Carefully review how the caregiver handles meals and discipline.

Including the caregiver's own children, a child care home should not have more than six children per adult caregiver. (In some states, group homes allow more children when at least two adults are available at all times.) The total number of children should be less when infants and toddlers are included. Unlike child care center recommendations, a single caregiver within the family care setting should care for no more than two children younger than 2 years of age. Since there is only one adult, backup care in an emergency situation must be close by. In some areas, caregivers belong to a network of family child care providers who may provide backup help.

Family child care providers usually work alone. This makes it hard to judge their work. Look for caregivers who are licensed or registered with the state and have their home visited by an inspector. Family caregivers can be accredited through the National Association for Family Child Care (NAFCC).

Center-based care has many names—child care center, preschool, nursery school, or learning center. Center-based care also may have different sponsors, including churches, schools, colleges, universities, social service agencies, Head Start, independent owners and chains, and employers.

Regardless of what type of child care center you choose, there are some basic things to consider:

- All centers should be licensed and inspected regularly for health, safety, cleanliness, staffing, and program content. Just because a center is licensed, do not assume it is regularly inspected. Check to see how often the center you are considering had announced and unannounced inspections in the past year and what was checked. To find out about the regulations in your area, contact your city, county, or state department of social services.
- Caregivers and center directors should have basic training and experience in early childhood development. Check to see if the center is accredited by state or national organizations. Several independent groups of early childhood care and education professionals offer accreditation. For centers, these are the National Association for the Education of Young Children (NAEYC) or the National Child Care Association (NCCA). (Although it is reassuring to know that a caregiver is accredited, some very good caregivers may not be accredited by either of these organizations. You might suggest that they apply for accreditation.)
- Look for age-appropriate toys, a daily schedule that is used, and joyful interactions between children and staff. Parents should be able to make unannounced visits to the center to see their child, and receive quick notification if their child gets sick or is injured.
- Be sure to check the center's special programs and published policies, including its policies on sick children. Centers have the advantage of covering a caregiver's illness or vacation.
- Look for centers that have two caregivers per room, a window or glass door for supervisors to view activities, and ongoing staff training.

Paying for child care can be quite an investment, so families must budget ahead. Although the cost seems high, consider how much the caregiver should earn for professionally meeting your family's child care needs and helping your child develop normally. Ask your company for assistance from:

- direct payment through cafeteria plans
- dependent-care spending accounts (tax savings)
- voucher programs
- company discounts

Whatever type of child care you choose—in-home, family, or center-based be sure to consider these factors:

- **Quality of adult/child relationships**—Are staff members specially trained in child development and early education? Are children cared for in small groups and given activities according to their level of development? Are there enough trained adults available to children on a regular basis?
- **Location**—How far will the care be from home? From work? Is this convenient for both parents? Can both parents easily get there in an emergency?
- **Hours**—What hours of care are needed? What happens if you are late in picking up your child?
- **Alternative arrangements**—What happens if your child is sick? When the caregiver cannot come? What if the child care program is closed? What pediatric medical care is available to the program?
- **Consistency**—Are the program's policies on meals, discipline, and toilet training the same as your views at home? Will your child be able to have a stable relationship with one caring adult?
- **Parent responsibility**—It is ultimately your responsibility to ensure that your child receives the best care. Talk with the caregiver on a regular basis. Plan to spend time with your child and the caregiver every day, both before you leave and when you return. When problems occur, your home caregiver or staff at the child care center should be able and willing to help you work through the situation. If problems persist and you suspect your child's health or safety is in question, find another child care arrangement for your child right away.

Preparing your child

Most young infants, up to 7 months, adapt to caring adults and seldom have problems adjusting to good child care. Older infants may be upset when left with strangers. They will need extra time and your support to "get to know" the caregiver.

Some children show changes in behavior when they start child care. Toddlers may cry, pout, refuse to go to child care, or act angry in other ways. Preschoolers may regress and behave like a younger child. They may be more wakeful at night. This behavior usually goes away after a few days or weeks in high-quality child care.

You can reduce your child's fears about starting child care. Visit the program or family child care home with your child before beginning care. Show your child that you like and trust the caregiver. Arrange a visit with in-home providers while you are at home or when you need child care for a short time. Some children like to carry a reminder of home when they go to child care. A family photograph or small toy can be helpful. Talking to your child about child care and the caregiver is helpful. Preparation and familiarity make any new experience easier for children. There also are storybooks about child care that you and your child can read together. (Check with your local library.)

After a child has been in child care, a sudden change in caregivers may be upsetting. This can happen even if the new caregiver is kind and competent. If you are concerned about your child's feelings, you may want to arrange a meeting with the caregiver or ask your pediatrician for advice. Parents need to help the caregivers and the child deal with any changes in the child's routine at home or child care.

Good child care helps children grow in every way and promotes their physical, social, and mental development. It offers support to working parents. Your pediatrician wants your child to grow and develop with enjoyment in a setting that supports you as a parent.

For further information on child care and early education, contact:
- National Association for the Education of Young Children, 1509 16th Street, NW, Washington, DC 20036-1426.
- National Association of Child Care Resource and Referral Agencies, 1319 F Street, NW, Suite 810, Washington, DC 20004
- Child Care Aware: 800/424-2246

The information contained in this publication should not be used as a substitute for the medical care and advice of your pediatrician. There may be variations in treatment that your pediatrician may recommend based on individual facts and circumstances.

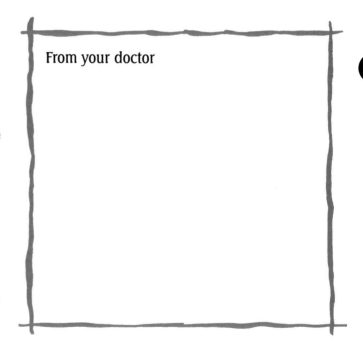

From your doctor

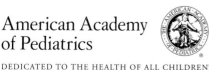

American Academy of Pediatrics

DEDICATED TO THE HEALTH OF ALL CHILDREN™

The American Academy of Pediatrics is an organization of 55,000 primary care pediatricians, pediatric medical subspecialists, and pediatric surgical specialists dedicated to the health, safety, and well-being of infants, children, adolescents, and young adults.

American Academy of Pediatrics
PO Box 747
Elk Grove Village, IL 60009-0747
Web site — http://www.aap.org

Copyright ©1997   American Academy of Pediatrics

Cocaine: Your Child and Drugs

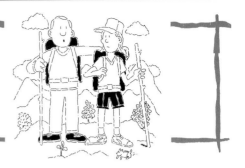

Cocaine use in the United States

Cocaine use by teens is a major problem and concern in America today. Many young people think that drugs are not all that harmful and that using cocaine is a symbol of status and success. They also think that trying cocaine is a step toward becoming an adult. The American Academy of Pediatrics has developed this information to help you learn about the dangers of cocaine use.

What is cocaine?

Cocaine is made from the leaves of the South American cocoa bush. The leaves are soaked in chemicals until they break down into cocaine crystals. These crystals are dried and crushed into a bitter, white powder.

How is cocaine used?

As a powder, cocaine is usually inhaled, or "snorted," through the nose. A less common method is to inject it directly into a vein. Cocaine can also be smoked in a pipe after it is hardened into a paste. This is called "free-basing."

Cocaine is also sold in a nugget form for as little as $5 to $15. This type of cocaine, called "crack," is also smoked. Users can make their own crack from a mixture of cocaine powder, baking soda, and water. Crack cocaine is much more powerful than cocaine in powder form.

The "high" from smoking crack cocaine is more intense and habit-forming than from snorting cocaine powder.

What are the effects of cocaine?

While most people know the effects of alcohol and marijuana, very few know the facts about cocaine. Cocaine is a powerful stimulant. It affects the nervous system and causes a user's heart rate and blood pressure to increase very quickly. Cocaine triggers pleasure centers in the brain and makes the user feel instantly alert. It also creates a false sense of joy (a "high"). But this "high" is short-lived—from 5 to 30 minutes, depending on how the drug is taken. As the drug's effects wear off, users may feel anxious, depressed, and tired. Marijuana, alcohol, sleeping pills, or "uppers" are sometimes used to ease cocaine's effects.

Is cocaine addictive?

The cocaine "high" tempts users to want more of the drug once its effects start to wear off. The more a person uses cocaine, the greater the desire to keep using it. The amount of cocaine needed to get high depends on how it is used, how long the person has been using it, and the strength (potency) of the drug. Cocaine is highly addictive. In laboratory tests, monkeys have starved or died because they chose cocaine instead of food and water. Smoking cocaine or crack increases the risk of addiction. When a person smokes cocaine, the lungs transfer the drug quickly into the bloodstream and it goes straight to the brain.

What are the dangers of cocaine?

Cocaine causes the user's heart rate and blood pressure to increase. The more cocaine used, the more intense this becomes. For some people, even small amounts of cocaine can cause dangerous increases in heart rate and abnormal heart rhythms. When this happens, the heart may not be able to pump enough blood to the brain, and a cocaine user can die.

In young people, cocaine can cause:
- Emotional problems
- School problems
- Low motivation
- Isolation from friends or family
- Family conflicts

Some cocaine users even turn to stealing or prostitution to support this costly drug habit. Pregnant women who use cocaine may have miscarriages, or their babies may be born with severe birth defects.

Stages of drug use

There are several stages of drug use. Be aware of any changes in your child's behavior that may indicate a problem with drugs.

Experimenting with drugs. In this stage, a person tries a drug such as cocaine in search of "fun." There is often strong peer pressure to enter this stage. Assuming there are no initial physical problems, there is usually no change in behavior, except for secret activities meant to hide the cocaine use.

Actively seeking drugs. In this stage, a person needs more cocaine to get the same feelings. This is called tolerance and is a sign of addiction. A person may use cocaine daily to get "high" and escape reality. Behavior begins to change and schoolwork may slip. Problems at home and school may lead the person to use more cocaine. Because cocaine is highly addictive, occasional users can quickly become frequent users.

Preoccupation with drugs. In this stage, there is a significant loss of control over drug use, and the user may become angry or isolated without cocaine. Heavy drug use is costly, and a user may lie and steal from family or friends to pay for cocaine. This may lead to trouble with the law.

Whether or not someone becomes a heavy user often depends on the reasons for trying cocaine in the first place. Recognizing the signs of abuse and getting help from family members, pediatricians, teachers, youth groups, or clergy are the first steps in helping your child recover from drug abuse or addiction.

How to help your child resist drugs

Sooner or later most youngsters will find themselves in a situation in which they must decide whether or not to take drugs. Follow these guidelines to help your child learn to resist this pressure:

- Build your child's self-esteem with plenty of praise and love.
- Avoid being overly critical when your child makes mistakes.
- Talk openly with your child about important topics like drugs and drug use.
- Help your child deal with peer pressure, strong emotions, and feelings.
- Encourage your child to get involved in hobbies, school clubs, and other activities.
- Spend leisure time with your child.

Remember, parents who use and abuse drugs place their children at higher risk for drug abuse. Make sure you set a good example at home by:

- Limiting your use of alcohol
- Not smoking cigarettes
- Using over-the-counter drugs sparingly and only according to directions on the label or from your physician

Despite your best efforts, your teen may still use or abuse drugs. Some warning signs of drug abuse include:

- Changes in choice of friends
- Changes in dress and appearance
- Frequent arguments and unexplained violent actions
- Changes in sleeping or eating habits
- Skipping school
- Falling grades
- Runaway and delinquent behavior
- Legal problems
- Suicide attempts

Positive, honest communication between you and your child is one of the best ways to help prevent drug use. If talking to your teen becomes a problem, your pediatrician may be able to help open the lines of communication. If you suspect your child is using cocaine or any other drug, talk to your pediatrician about how you can help.

The information contained in this publication should not be used as a substitute for the medical care and advice of your pediatrician. There may be variations in treatment that your pediatrician may recommend based on individual facts and circumstances.

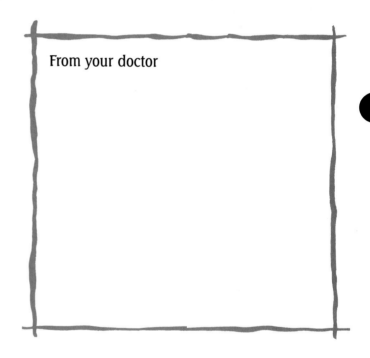

From your doctor

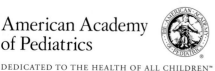

American Academy of Pediatrics

DEDICATED TO THE HEALTH OF ALL CHILDREN™

The American Academy of Pediatrics is an organization of 55,000 primary care pediatricians, pediatric medical subspecialists, and pediatric surgical specialists dedicated to the health, safety, and well-being of infants, children, adolescents, and young adults.

American Academy of Pediatrics
PO Box 747
Elk Grove Village, IL 60009-0747
Web site — http://www.aap.org

Discipline and Your Child

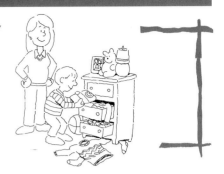

As a parent, it is your job to teach your child the difference between acceptable and unacceptable behavior. But getting your child to behave the way you want is not as hard as you think. This brochure will help you learn effective ways to discipline your child.

Because learning takes time, especially for a young child, you may find that it takes several weeks of working on a behavior before you see a change. Try not to get frustrated when you do not see the results of your efforts right away.

Discipline vs punishment

Many parents think discipline and punishment are the same thing. However, they are really quite different. Discipline is a whole system of teaching based on a good relationship, praise, and instruction for the child on how to control his behavior. Punishment is negative; an unpleasant consequence for doing or not doing something. Punishment should be only a very small part of discipline.

Effective discipline should take place all the time, not just when children misbehave. Children are more likely to change their behavior when they feel encouraged and valued, not shamed and humiliated. When children feel good about themselves and cherish their relationship with their parents, they are more likely to listen and learn.

Encourage good behavior from infancy

You can begin laying the groundwork for good behavior from the time your child is born. When you respond to your infant's cries, you are teaching her that you are there, you can be counted on when she needs you, and that she can trust you. When your child is about 2 months of age, start to modify your responses and encourage your baby to establish good sleeping patterns by letting her fall asleep on her own. By keeping a reasonably steady schedule, you can guide her toward eating, sleeping, and playing at times that are appropriate for your family. This lays the groundwork for acceptable behavior later on.

Once your baby starts to crawl (between 6 and 9 months of age) and as she learns to walk (between 9 and 16 months of age), safety is the most critical discipline issue. The best thing you can do for your child at this age is to give her the freedom to explore certain things and make other things off-limits. For example, put childproof locks on some cabinets, such as those that contain heavy dishes or pots, or poisonous substances like cleaning products. Leave other cabinets open. Fill the open cabinets with plastic containers or soft materials that your child can play with. This feeds your baby's need to explore and practice, but in safe ways that are acceptable to you.

You will need to provide extra supervision during this period. If your child moves toward a dangerous object, such as a hot stove, simply pick her up, firmly say, "no, hot" and offer her a toy to play with instead. She may laugh at first as she tries to understand you but, after a few weeks, she will learn.

Discipline issues become more complex at about 18 months of age. At this time, a child wants to know how much power she has and will test the limit of that power over and over again. It is important for parents to decide—together—what those limits will be and stick to them. Parents need to be very

clear about what is acceptable behavior. This will reduce the child's confusion and her need to test. Setting consistent guidelines for children when they are young also will help establish important rules for the future.

If you and your partner disagree, discuss it with each other when you are not with your child. Do not interfere with each other when your child is present. This upsets the child or teaches her to set the adults up against each other which can cause more problems.

Tips to avoid trouble

One of the keys to effective discipline is avoiding power struggles. This can be a challenge with young children. It is best to address only those issues that truly are important to you. The following tips may help:

- **Offer choices whenever possible.** By giving acceptable choices, you can set limits and still allow your child some independence. For example, try saying, "Would you like to wear the red shirt or the blue one?"
- **Make a game out of good behavior.** Your child is more likely to do what you want if you make it fun. For example, you might say, "Let's have a race and see who can put his coat on first."
- **Plan ahead.** If you know that certain circumstances always cause trouble, such as a trip to the store, discuss with your child ahead of time what behavior is acceptable and what the consequences will be if he does not obey. Try to plan the shopping trip for a time when your child is well rested and well fed, and take along a book or small toy to amuse him if he gets bored.
- **Praise good behavior.** Whenever your child remembers to follow the rules, offer encouragement and praise about how well he did. You do not need any elaborate system of rewards. You can simply say, "Thank you for coming right away," and hug your child. Praise for acceptable behavior should be frequent, especially for young children.

Strategies that work

Of course you cannot avoid trouble all of the time. Sooner or later your child will test you. It is your child's way of finding out whether you can be trusted and really will do what you say you will do if she does not listen to you.

When your child does not listen, try the following techniques. Not only will they encourage your child to cooperate now, but they will teach her how to behave in the future as well.

Natural consequences. When a child sees the natural consequences of her actions, she experiences the direct results of her choices. (But be sure the consequences do not place her in any danger.) For example, if your child drops her cookies on purpose, she will not have cookies to eat. If she throws and breaks her toy, she will not be able to play with it. It will not be long before your child learns not to drop her cookies and to play carefully with her toys.

When you use this method, resist the urge to lecture your child or to rescue her (by getting more cookies, for example). Your child will learn best when she learns for herself and will not blame you for the consequences she receives.

 191

Logical consequences. Natural consequences work best, but they are not always appropriate. For example, if your child does not pick up her toys, they may be in the way. But chances are she will not care as much as you do. For older children, you will need to step in and create a consequence that is closely connected to her actions. You might tell her that if she does not pick up her toys, then you will put them away where she will not be allowed to play with them again for a whole day. Children less than 6 years of age need adult help picking up yet can be asked to assist with the task. If your child refuses your request for help, take her by the hand as you silently finish the job. This insistence that your child participate, along with your silence, becomes a clear consequence for your child.

When you use this method, it is important that you mean what you say and that you are prepared to follow through *immediately*. Let your child know that you are serious. You do not have to yell and scream to do this. You can say it in a calm, matter-of-fact way.

Withholding privileges. In the heat of the moment, you will not always be able to think of a logical consequence. That is when you may want to tell your child that, if she does not cooperate, she will have to give something up she likes. The following are a few things to keep in mind when you use this technique:

- Never take away something your child truly needs, such as a meal.
- Choose something that your child values that is related to the misbehavior.
- For children younger than 6 or 7 years of age, withholding privileges works best if done immediately following the problem behavior. For instance, if your young child misbehaves in the morning and you withhold television viewing for that evening, your child probably will not connect the behavior with the consequence.
- Be sure you can follow through on your promise.

Time-out. Time-out should be your last resort and you should use it only when other responses do not work. Time-outs work well when the behavior you are trying to punish is clearly defined and you know when it occurred. Time-outs also can be helpful if you need a break to stay calm. You can use a time-out with a child as young as 1 year old. Follow these steps to make a time-out work:

1. Choose a time-out spot. This should be a boring place with no distractions, such as a chair. Remember the main goal is to separate the child from the activity and people connected with the misbehavior. It should allow the child to pause and cool off. (Keep in mind that bathrooms can be dangerous and bedrooms may become playgrounds.) Decide which 2 or 3 behaviors will be punished with time-out and explain this to your child.

2. When your child does something she knows will result in a time-out, you may warn her once (unless it is aggression). If it happens again, send her to the time-out spot *immediately*. Tell her what she did wrong in as few words as possible. A rule of thumb is 1 minute of time out for every year of your child's age. (For example, a 4-year-old would get a 4-minute time-out.) But even 15 seconds will work. If your child will not go to the spot on her own, pick her up and carry her there. If she will not stay, stand behind her and hold her gently but firmly by the shoulders or restrain her in your lap and say, "I am holding you here because you have to have a time-out." Do not discuss it any further. It should only take a couple of weeks before she learns to cooperate and will choose to sit quietly rather than be held down for time-out.

3. Once your child is capable of sitting quietly, set a timer so that she will know when the time-out is over. If fussing starts again, restart the timer. Wait until your child stops protesting before you set the timer.

4. When the time is up, help your child return to a positive activity. Your child has "served her time." Do not lecture or ask for apologies. If you need to discuss her behavior, wait until later to do so.

Tips to make discipline more effective

You will have days when it seems impossible to get your child to behave. But there are ways to ease frustration and avoid unnecessary conflict with your child.

- **Be aware of your child's abilities and limitations.** Children develop at different rates and have different strengths and weaknesses. When your child misbehaves, it may be that he simply cannot do what you are asking of him or he does not understand what you are asking.
- **Think before you speak.** Once you make a rule or promise, you will need to stick to it. Be sure you are being realistic. Think if it is really necessary before saying "no."
- **Remember that children do what "works."** If your child throws a temper tantrum in the grocery store and you bribe him to stop by giving him candy, he will probably throw another tantrum the next time you go. Make an effort to avoid reinforcing the wrong kinds of behavior, even with just your attention.
- **Work toward consistency.** No one is consistent all of the time. But try to make sure that your goals, rules, and approaches to discipline stay the same from day to day. Children find frequent changes confusing and often resort to testing limits just to find out what the limits are.
- **Pay attention to your child's feelings.** If you can figure out why your child is misbehaving, you are one step closer to solving the problem. It is kinder and helps with cooperation when you let your child know that you understand. For example, "I know you are feeling sad that your friend is leaving, but you still have to pick up your toys." Watch for patterns that tell you misbehavior has a special meaning, such as your child is feeling jealous. Talk to your child about this rather than just giving consequences.
- **Learn to see mistakes—including your own—as opportunities to learn.** If you do not handle a situation well the first time, don't despair. Think about what you could have done differently, and try to do it the next time. If you feel you have made a real mistake in the heat of the moment, wait to cool down, apologize to your child, and explain how you will handle the situation in the future. Be sure to keep your promise. This gives your child a good model of how to recover from mistakes.

Set an example

Telling your child how to behave is an important part of discipline, but *showing* her how to behave is even more significant. Children learn a lot about temper and self-control from watching their parents and other adults interact. If they see adults relating in a positive way toward one another, they will learn that this is how others should be treated. This is how children learn to act respectfully.

Even though your children's behavior and values seem to be on the right track, your children will still challenge you because it is in their nature and is a part of growing up. Children are constantly learning what their limits are, and they need their parents to help them understand those limits. By doing so, parents can help their children feel capable and loved, learn right from wrong, develop good behavior, have a positive approach toward life, and become productive, good citizens.

Why spanking is not the best choice

The American Academy of Pediatrics recommends that if punishment is needed, alternatives to spanking should be used.

Although most Americans were spanked as children, we now know that it has several important side effects.

- It may seem to work at the moment, but it is no more effective in changing behavior than a time-out.
- Spanking increases children's aggression and anger instead of teaching responsibility.
- Parents may intend to stay calm but often do not, and regret their actions later.
- Because most parents do not want to spank, they are less likely to be consistent.
- Spanking makes other consequences less effective, such as those used at child care or school. Gradually, even spanking loses its impact.
- Spanking can lead to physical struggles and even escalate to the point of harming the child.
- Children who continue to be spanked are more likely to be depressed, use alcohol, have more anger, hit their own children, approve of and hit their spouses, and engage in crime and violence as adults.
- These results make sense since spanking teaches the child that causing others pain is justified to control them—even with those they love.

If you are having trouble disciplining your child or need more information on alternatives to spanking, talk to your pediatrician.

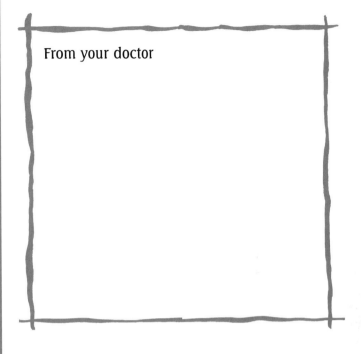

From your doctor

American Academy of Pediatrics

DEDICATED TO THE HEALTH OF ALL CHILDREN™

The American Academy of Pediatrics is an organization of 55,000 primary care pediatricians, pediatric medical subspecialists, and pediatric surgical specialists dedicated to the health, safety, and well-being of infants, children, adolescents, and young adults.

American Academy of Pediatrics
PO Box 747
Elk Grove Village, IL 60009-0747
Web site — http://www.aap.org

Copyright ©1998, Updated 1/02   American Academy of Pediatrics

Divorce and Children

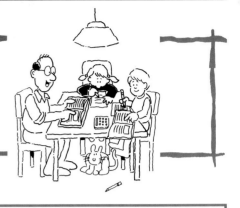

Every year, more than one million children in the United States experience the divorce of their parents. The average divorce takes place within the first 7 years of marriage, so many of these children are under the age of 6. For many children, divorce can be as difficult as the death of a parent. The entire family is faced with the challenge of adjusting to a new way of life. When this happens, children need the guidance, patience, and love of both parents to help them through.

Put your child first

The most important factor in how divorce affects a child's life is how parents treat each other and their children during and after the divorce. Keep in mind, divorce is a major event in your child's life, one that she has no control over. Parents must work together to make the changes as easy as possible for everyone. Even as the marriage ends, your role as a parent continues. In fact, it becomes more important than ever. Set aside your differences with your child's other parent and *put your child first*, by following these suggestions:

- **Never force your child to take sides.** Every child will have loyalties to both parents.
- **Do not involve your child in arguments** between the two of you.
- **Do not criticize each other in front of your child** or when your child might be listening to a conversation you are having with someone else. Even if you find out the other parent is saying bad things about you, explain to your child that when people get angry they sometimes say things that are hurtful.
- **Discuss your concerns and feelings with your child's other parent** when and where your child cannot hear.
- **Avoid fighting in front of your child.**

Making it easier

As a parent, there are many things you can do to help your child adjust to the changes in your family, including the following:

Talk with your child early and often

This is a very important way for you to help your child through difficult times. Being able to share his fears, worries, and feelings with you can make your child feel safe and special. The earlier you tell him what is happening and the more often you talk, the more comfortable he will feel. When talking with your child about the divorce, follow these guidelines:

- **Be completely honest and open** about the circumstances. Talk about the divorce in simple terms. For example, "Your dad and I are having some trouble getting along" or "Your mother and I are thinking we may need to separate."

How children react to divorce

Reactions to a divorce can vary depending on your child's age, sex, temperament, past experiences, and family support. The following are normal ways that your child may react to a separation or divorce. If any of these behaviors become excessive, talk to your pediatrician.

Children under 3 years of age may:
- Be sad
- Be afraid of others
- Not want to be separated from one parent
- Have problems eating or sleeping
- Have trouble with toilet training
- Have outbursts or tantrums
- Blame themselves for the divorce—especially children between 3 and 5 years of age.

School-age children may:
- Be moody or angry
- Have problems eating or sleeping
- Seem distracted and faraway
- Not do as well in school
- Have tantrums
- Be more aggressive or angry
- Express their sadness and wish for parents to get back together
- Worry about divided loyalty to their parents

Adolescents may:
- Withdraw emotionally from family and/or friends
- Become aggressive or angry
- Engage in risky behaviors such as sexual experimentation or use of drugs
- Worry about the financial effects of divorce on the family
- Have problems eating or sleeping
- Feel depressed

- **Make sure your child knows he is not responsible.** Children will often think it is their fault that one parent has left. They may blame themselves or feel alone, unwanted, or unloved. Let your child know the changes are not his fault, that you love him and will not leave him.
- **Try not to blame your ex-spouse** or show your anger. Explain that parents sometimes make adult decisions to live separately.

- **Be patient with questions.** You do not have to have all the answers. Sometimes just carefully listening to your child's concerns is more helpful than talking. Following are questions you might expect from your child:
  –Why are you getting divorced?
  –Will you ever get back together again?
  –Where am I going to live?
  –Will we move?
  –Will I have to change schools?
  –Was the divorce my fault?
  –How often will I see Daddy/Mommy?
  –Are we going to be poor?

Give your child the reassurance he needs to feel safe and loved. If needed, don't hesitate to get help from your pediatrician or a family counselor.

A word about....custody

Custody arrangements can be one of the most difficult issues in a divorce. Today, parents are able to work out a wide variety of custody and visitation arrangements. *Physical custody* defines where the child lives and can be split between both parents. Even if physical custody remains with one parent, the other parent can share *legal custody*. Legal custody allows a parent to share in key decisions such as a child's schooling, medical treatment, and religion.

Although mothers are still more likely to maintain custody of the child, more and more fathers are now taking on this role. While there is no evidence that one form of custody is better than another, all children need a stable place where they feel secure.

Even more important than custody is that both parents remain as involved as possible. Ideally, both parents should play a role in the child's life by helping with homework, attending athletic or other after-school events, and contributing emotional and financial support. The parents should work together to arrange a flexible schedule for visits. Neither parent should be prevented from taking part in raising the child. Make sure your child knows that it is OK to love both parents.

If you are having custody disagreements, consider calling a mediator to help settle disagreements. Mediators can be found by contacting a lawyer or family court.

Allow your child to be a child

Resist using your child as a replacement for your ex-spouse. Avoid pressuring children with statements like, "You are the man in the family now" or "Now I have to depend on you." Children have a right to enjoy childhood and grow up at a normal pace. As they grow older, they will be able to take on more responsibility and help around the house. Don't expect too much too soon.

Child support

According to the US Department of Health and Human Services, millions of female-headed households do not receive child support. In some cases, one parent does not want money from the other parent. In others, the parent may not be able or willing to pay or perhaps cannot even be found. Many times, the parent with custody simply does not enforce the child support agreement.

The financial burden of raising a child should not fall on one parent alone. Both parents have a financial obligation to their child. However, even when child support is paid, money issues may still be a problem between parents. Remember, if either parent uses money as a weapon, it is the child who is caught in the cross fire.

Contact your state's child support enforcement agency for guidelines on what parents *must* pay for child support. If your child's other parent will not cooperate, your state or local government may take action to force payment. State agencies can also help if your child's other parent has suddenly moved and you do not know where he or she is living. In most cases, it is often helpful to talk with an attorney.

For more information, contact:
Department of Health and Human Services
Office of Child Support Enforcement
370 L'Enfant Promenade, SW
Washington, DC 20447
202/401-9373

Web site: http://www.acf.dhhs.gov/
programs/cse/index.ht

Respect the relationship between your child and the other parent

Allow your children to spend time with their other parent without making them feel guilty or disloyal to you. When a parent leaves, many children are afraid the other one may leave too. Reassure your children that you both still love them even though they may only be living with one parent at a time. It is important to let your children show their love to both parents. Unless your ex-spouse is unfit to parent, try not to let your differences keep your children away from him or her. Remember, one of the most important ways to help your children cope with a separation or divorce is to help them maintain a strong, loving relationship with both parents.

Keep your child's daily routine simple and predictable

Many divorced parents feel guilty that the divorce has upset their children. They find it hard to discipline the children when they need it. Making rules, setting a good example, and providing emotional support can be difficult. Giving in to your child's demands will not help. Anger or difficult behavior may be part of your child's attempts to cope with the divorce. Set sensible limits. Schedule meals, chores, and bedtime at regular times so that your child knows what to expect each day. Parents living separately should agree on a set of consistent rules for both households. It is also very important to live up to your promises to visit or spend time with your child. A routine weekly or monthly schedule may be comforting to your child.

Use help from the outside

Children often turn to neighbors, grandparents, and peers for comfort and attention. These relationships can offer support and stability to children as well as needed relief to a parent. Teachers or school social workers who are aware of the divorce and understand the child's problems may also be able to give a helping hand.

For parents too, the changes are not easy. Many adults going through a divorce experience depression. If you are suffering from anxiety or depression as a result of a divorce or separation, don't be afraid to see a counselor. It is important for parents to be healthy so they can be available to their children during this difficult time. Social agencies, mental health centers, women's centers, and support groups for divorced or single parents are helpful. There are also many informative books and articles about divorce for both parents and children (see "For More Information"). Your pediatrician is very aware of the effects that separation and divorce may have on emotions and behavior. He or she can help you find ways to cope with the stress you and your children are feeling.

Adjusting to a new life

Children have great strength and the ability to bounce back from rough times. After a divorce, children may even develop much closer relationships with each parent. In time, most children learn to accept the changes brought on by divorce. The challenge becomes much easier though, when both parents provide the understanding, support, and love that all children need from their mothers and fathers, even after they separate.

For more information

There are many excellent books available on coping with divorce for both you and your children. Here are just a few to look for at your local library or bookstore. Please note: Not all of these materials have been reviewed by the American Academy of Pediatrics.

Preschoolers:

The Dinosaurs Divorce: A Guide for Changing Families
by Laurene Krasny Brown and Marc Brown (Little Brown & Co, 1988)

It's Not Your Fault, Koko Bear
by Vicki Lansky (Book Peddlers, 1998)

School-age kids:

The Boys and Girls Book About Divorce
by Richard Gardner (Bantam, 1970)

How It Feels When Parents Divorce
by Jill Krementz (Knopf, 1988)

Why Are We Getting a Divorce?
by Peter Mayle (Crown Publishers, 1988)

Parents:

Caring for Your Baby and Young Child: Birth to Age 5
from the American Academy of Pediatrics (Bantam, 1998)

Caring for Your School-Age Child: Ages 5–12
from the American Academy of Pediatrics (Bantam, 1995)

Caring for Your Adolescent: Ages 12–21
from the American Academy of Pediatrics (Bantam, 1991)

Vicki Lansky's Divorce Book for Parents
by Vicki Lansky (Book Peddlers, 1996)

The American Academy of Pediatrics also offers a brochure called *Single Parenting: What You Need to Know* that you might find helpful. Please ask your pediatrician.

From your doctor

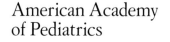

American Academy of Pediatrics

DEDICATED TO THE HEALTH OF ALL CHILDREN™

The American Academy of Pediatrics is an organization of 55,000 primary care pediatricians, pediatric medical subspecialists, and pediatric surgical specialists dedicated to the health, safety, and well-being of infants, children, adolescents, and young adults.

American Academy of Pediatrics
PO Box 747
Elk Grove Village, IL 60009-0747
Web site — http://www.aap.org

Eating Disorders

Part I Anorexia Nervosa

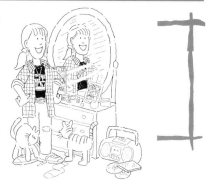

Guidelines for Teens

Eating is something that most people look forward to. It can mean experiencing good food, doing something healthy for your body, and spending time with family or friends. Many social events such as parties and holidays also involve food. But, for a person who has an eating disorder, eating brings about very different feelings. Constant thoughts about eating and an intense fear of gaining weight become an obsession for a person who has an eating disorder.

Living with an eating disorder is very hard. The road to recovery is not easy but, with treatment, a person can recover and go on to lead a healthy life. Without help, a person with an eating disorder can have a number of medical problems, become very sick, and even die. The American Academy of Pediatrics has developed this brochure to help you learn about some common eating disorders, their causes, symptoms, and possible courses of treatment.

What is an eating disorder?

The two most common eating disorders are *anorexia nervosa* and *bulimia nervosa*. Anorexia is self-starvation. Bulimia is a disorder in which a person eats large amounts of food ("bingeing") and then rids the body of that food before it can be absorbed ("purging"). A person who is bulimic purges either by vomiting or using laxatives or diuretics (water pills). Some people have symptoms of both anorexia and bulimia.

There is no single cause of an eating disorder. Many factors may be involved and are different for each person. Some factors include:

- Feeling insecure
- An excessive desire to be in control
- A distorted body image (feeling fat) and striving for the perfect body
- A family history of depression or an eating disorder
- Severe family problems
- A history of sexual abuse
- Extreme social pressures
- Pressure from activities such as running, gymnastics, wrestling, or ballet

Most anorexics and bulimics are girls; however, boys can suffer from these disorders as well. Adolescents experience many social pressures, especially from the media, to be thin. This pressure to be thin or to diet can be especially strong for teens if their friends are dieting or trying to lose weight. It is easy for teens to get over-the-counter diet pills to reduce their appetite so that they do not eat as much—a practice that can become habit-forming. Diet pills can raise blood pressure, cause kidney damage, make a person dizzy or hallucinate, or even lead to fatal stroke.

It is important, however, for both girls and boys to understand that not everyone has the type of body that is superthin. In fact, only a small number do. If a person is not meant to be naturally thin, that person needs to accept that fact and learn to like his or her body the way it is. It is important to have a healthy attitude toward weight and to feel good about oneself.

Anorexia nervosa

Anorexia is an eating disorder that mainly affects females between 14 and 18 years of age. A person with this disorder has such an intense fear of becoming fat that she hardly eats anything and becomes dangerously thin. Anorexics often weigh as little as 80 to 100 pounds. Many anorexics also over-exercise and may abuse diet pills to keep from gaining weight. If the condition gets worse, anorexics can die from suicide, heart attack, or starvation.

How does an anorexic behave?

When a person develops anorexia nervosa, her behavior changes, especially in regard to eating. A person with anorexia may:

- Eat only "safe" foods, usually those low in calories and fat.
- Cut up food into very small pieces.
- Spend more time playing with food than eating it, such as rearranging it on the plate throughout a meal.
- Buy, prepare, and cook food only for others.

As the anorexic becomes more obsessed with food, her personality changes as well. She may become more self-centered, as all her energy and focus is on herself and staying thin. In addition, a person with anorexia may:

- Exercise compulsively.
- Wear baggy clothing to hide extreme thinness, or complain that normal clothing is too tight.
- Spend less time with friends and family, becoming more isolated, withdrawn, and secretive.
- Develop rituals to keep her mind off her hunger, such as chewing each bite of food 30 times before swallowing.
- Get angry if she is not able to exercise or if her daily routine is disturbed.

How does anorexia affect the body?

When the body is being starved of food, many physical changes occur that can lead to kidney and liver damage, very low blood pressure, and heart failure. Other physical changes that can happen include:

- The constant feeling of being cold because the body has lost the fat and muscle it needs to keep warm. This may make the anorexic exercise even more in an attempt to get warm. Eyes become vacant and hollow.
- Bones stick out and the skin shrinks around the bones, often making the stomach seem like it is sticking out (leading the anorexic to still think that she is fat or overweight).
- Hair on the head falls out, while fine hair appears on other parts of the body for warmth.
- Hair and fingernails become brittle and skin becomes dry and rough due to a lack of protein and vitamins in the diet.

- Menstrual periods stop (or do not start at all if a girl developed anorexia before her first period). This puts the anorexic at higher risk of developing osteoporosis, a disease that causes bones to become brittle and break more easily.
- Pain in the abdomen, constipation, and bloating. Stunted growth, resulting in permanent short stature.
- Anemia.

Who can be affected by anorexia nervosa?

Teens who develop anorexia are usually good students, even overachievers. They try to get along with others, tend to be perfectionists, and do not like to admit they need help with anything. To others they appear to be in control. However, they are actually unsure of themselves, are self-critical, and have low self-esteem. They are very concerned about whether other people like them and about pleasing others. Some of these negative feelings may come from having a poor body image (the way a person feels about how his or her body looks).

Many young people think that losing weight will make them feel better about how they look. This is why most people who develop anorexia start by dieting. The message they get from our culture, including the media, is that a slim body is attractive and desirable. They may also start dieting in response to some kind of major life change, like puberty or going away to college. Because anorexics have low self-esteem, they do not feel confident that they can handle these changes. They do not feel like they have control. Dieting makes them feel better about themselves and becomes something they are able to do well on their own. Over time, the dieting is really no longer about food, but becomes a way for the anorexic to feel like she has control over her life.

Recognize signs of anorexia

Recognizing the early signs of anorexia is important for successful treatment. Otherwise, it may be too late. If someone answers yes to any of the following statements, that person should get help right away.

- I cannot stop dieting, even though my family and friends warn me that I have lost too much weight.
- Even though I have lost a lot of weight, when I look in the mirror I still think that certain parts of my body are fat.
- I cannot stop exercising.
- I do not get my menstrual period monthly.

Treatment for eating disorders

The chance of successfully treating someone who has an eating disorder is much higher if the disorder is detected early and the person begins to get help. Treatment depends on many things, including the person's willingness to cooperate, family and support structure, and the stage of the disorder.

Successful treatment of eating disorders involves many health professionals who work together by treating a certain aspect of the disorder. Treatment begins with a visit to a pediatrician, who will examine the person's medical condition to see how the eating disorder has affected the body. If the effects are severe, the person may need to be hospitalized for treatment.

In treating anorexia, increasing the person's weight is crucial. If the anorexic needs to be hospitalized, her treatment will focus on getting her weight back up to a normal level. If she refuses to eat, she may need a feeding tube to get the proper nutrients into her body. Hospitalization often helps the anorexic slowly change her behavior so that when she returns home, she can gain weight slowly with outpatient pediatric and psychiatric treatment. A person with bulimia may need hospitalization to control the cycles of bingeing and purging and to replace needed nutrients in the body.

Counseling is necessary to help a person with an eating disorder understand how she uses food as a way of handling problems and feelings. It will help her improve her self-image (including body image) and develop independence so that she can take control of her life in positive ways. A mix of individual therapy and family therapy is usually most effective in treating eating disorders. Since an eating disorder usually affects a person's entire family, a therapist can try to help family members understand the disorder. The therapist can also help families create a supportive home environment for the person with an eating disorder. Occasionally, people who have eating disorders also have problems with alcohol abuse or other substance abuse, and may need to be treated for those as well.

Anorexia and bulimia are both very serious eating disorders that do not go away by themselves. However, eating disorders are treatable with help. A person with an eating disorder needs professional help to recover and become healthy again.

For other resources and help with eating disorders, contact the following organizations:

National Association of Anorexia Nervosa
  and Associated Disorders
Box 7
Highland Park, IL 60035
847/831-3438

American Anorexia/Bulimia Association
418 E 76th St
New York, NY 10021
212/734-1114

Anorexia Nervosa and Related Eating Disorders
Box 5102
Eugene, OR 97405
503/344-1144

Some people who struggle with eating disorders alternate between anorexic and bulimic behaviors. About half of all people who have anorexia at one time or another develop some symptoms of bulimia (mainly the bingeing and purging). The following information shows some of the ways in which the disorders are alike and different.

Similarities of people with eating disorders:

- Distorted body image
- Strong-willed, determined nature
- Obsessive thoughts about food, eating, and body shape
- Depression
- Excessive exercise
- Overachiever, perfectionist
- Difficulty concentrating
- Poor self-esteem
- Self-destructive behavior
- Irritability
- Vomiting and use of laxatives and/or diuretics to keep weight off

Differences between people with eating disorders:

Anorexia

- Age range: persons 14 to 18 years old
- Severe weight loss
- Shockingly thin body
- Withdrawn personality
- Denial of hunger
- Sexual inactivity
- No menstrual periods
- Denial of eating disorder
- Strong resistance to treatment
- Death from starvation or suicide

Bulimia

- Age range: persons 15 to 24 years old
- Slight weight changes
- Normal weight appearance
- Outgoing personality
- Pronounced hunger
- Sexual activity
- Irregular menstrual periods
- Awareness of eating disorder
- Accepting to treatment
- Death from low potassium or suicide

The information contained in this publication should not be used as a substitute for the medical care and advice of your pediatrician. There may be variations in treatment that your pediatrician may recommend based on individual facts and circumstances.

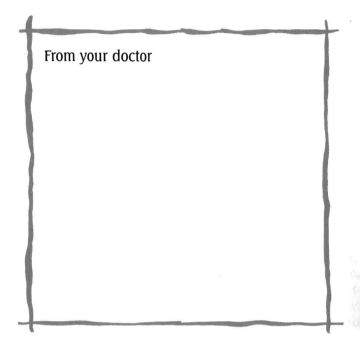

From your doctor

American Academy of Pediatrics

DEDICATED TO THE HEALTH OF ALL CHILDREN™

The American Academy of Pediatrics is an organization of 55,000 primary care pediatricians, pediatric medical subspecialists, and pediatric surgical specialists dedicated to the health, safety, and well-being of infants, children, adolescents, and young adults.

American Academy of Pediatrics
PO Box 747
Elk Grove Village, IL 60009-0747
Web site — http://www.aap.org

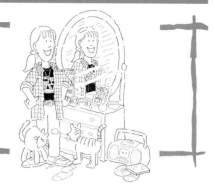

Eating Disorders

Part II Bulimia Nervosa

Guidelines for Teens

Eating is something that most people look forward to. It can mean experiencing good food, doing something healthy for your body, and spending time with family or friends. Many social events such as parties and holidays also involve food. But, for a person who has an eating disorder, eating brings about very different feelings. Constant thoughts about eating and an intense fear of gaining weight become an obsession for a person who has an eating disorder.

Living with an eating disorder is very hard. The road to recovery is not easy but, with treatment, a person can recover and go on to lead a healthy life. Without help, a person with an eating disorder can have a number of medical problems, become very sick, and even die. The American Academy of Pediatrics has developed this brochure to help you learn about some common eating disorders, their causes, symptoms, and possible courses of treatment.

What is an eating disorder?

The two most common eating disorders are *anorexia nervosa* and *bulimia nervosa*. Anorexia is self-starvation. Bulimia is a disorder in which a person eats large amounts of food ("bingeing") and then rids the body of that food before it can be absorbed ("purging"). A person who is bulimic purges either by vomiting or using laxatives or diuretics (water pills). Some people have symptoms of both anorexia and bulimia.

There is no single cause of an eating disorder. Many factors may be involved and are different for each person. Some factors include:

- Feeling insecure
- An excessive desire to be in control
- A distorted body image (feeling fat) and striving for the perfect body
- A family history of depression or an eating disorder
- Severe family problems
- A history of sexual abuse
- Extreme social pressures
- Pressure from activities such as running, gymnastics, wrestling, or ballet

Most anorexics and bulimics are girls; however, boys can suffer from these disorders as well. Adolescents experience many social pressures, especially from the media, to be thin. This pressure to be thin or to diet can be especially strong for teens if their friends are dieting or trying to lose weight. It is easy for teens to get over-the-counter diet pills to reduce their appetite so that they do not eat as much—a practice that can become habit-forming. Diet pills can raise blood pressure, cause kidney damage, make a person dizzy or hallucinate, or even lead to fatal stroke.

It is important, however, for both girls and boys to understand that not everyone has the type of body that is superthin. In fact, only a small number do. If a person is not meant to be naturally thin, that person needs to accept that fact and learn to like his or her body the way it is. It is important to have a healthy attitude toward weight and to feel good about oneself.

Bulimia nervosa

Bulimia nervosa is another eating disorder that is harmful to a person's physical and mental health. Bulimia and anorexia share some of the same symptoms. As with anorexia, food and staying thin become an obsession, but the bulimic does not starve herself. Instead, the bulimic gets an uncontrollable urge to binge (eat a large amount of food in a short period of time) and then purge this food from her body.

Bulimia usually develops between the ages of 15 and 24. Like anorexia, it affects mostly females. A bulimic's weight is usually within the range of what is normal for her size and height, but it tends to go up and down a lot because of all the bingeing and purging.

How does a person with bulimia behave?

A bulimic no longer has full control over eating. She may be afraid to eat in restaurants or with other people because she cannot control the urges to binge or the urges to purge after eating normal amounts of food. This fear may cause her to avoid social situations and isolate herself from other people. Bulimics may also change in other ways by:

- Becoming very secretive about food, spending a lot of time thinking about and planning the next binge, and setting aside certain times to binge.
- Stealing food or hoarding it in strange places, such as under the bed or in closets.
- Bingeing on foods with distinct colors in order to know when they are later thrown up.
- Spending a lot of time, energy, and money, because bulimia is a time-consuming and expensive addiction.

How does bulimia affect the body?

The following changes may be signs that a person has bulimia:

- Teeth start to decay from contact with stomach acids during vomiting.
- Weight goes up and down.
- Menstrual periods become irregular.
- The face and throat look puffy and swollen.
- Periods of dizziness and blackouts occur.
- Dehydration due to loss of body fluids occurs. The bulimic may need to be hospitalized if this happens.
- Constant upset stomach, constipation, and sore throat may be present.
- Damage to vital organs, such as the liver and kidneys, heart failure, and death can occur.

Who can be affected by bulimia?

People who develop bulimia often have a hard time dealing with and controlling impulses, stress, and anxieties. Like anorexics, they are not happy with their body image and think they are overweight or fat. This leads them to start dieting, but then, in response to anxiety and other emotions, they give in to their impulses and cravings for food by bingeing.

During a binge, a person with bulimia may eat between 3,000 and 7,000 calories, often in less than a few hours. Depression, boredom, or anger often trigger a binge. Eating during a binge is almost robot-like. The bulimic chews and swallows without paying attention to what the food tastes like or whether she is hungry or full. Binges usually end when there is no more food to eat, when the stomach hurts so much from eating, or when something such as a phone call breaks the bulimic's concentration on bingeing.

After eating large amounts of food, the bulimic feels guilty and is afraid of gaining weight. To ease her guilt and fear, she purges the food from her body by vomiting or taking pills that cause diarrhea. After bingeing she may turn to extreme exercise or strict dieting. This period of "control" lasts until the next binge, and then the cycle starts all over again. Bulimia becomes an attempt to control two very strong impulses - the desire to be thin and the desire to eat. Other factors that may lead to bulimia include:

- Depression
- Substance abuse
- Childhood physical abuse or sexual abuse

Treatment for eating disorders

The chance of successfully treating someone who has an eating disorder is much higher if the disorder is detected early and the person begins to get help. Treatment depends on many things, including the person's willingness to cooperate, family and support structure, and the stage of the disorder.

Successful treatment of eating disorders involves many health professionals who work together by treating a certain aspect of the disorder. Treatment begins with a visit to a pediatrician, who will examine the person's medical condition to see how the eating disorder has affected the body. If the effects are severe, the person may need to be hospitalized for treatment.

In treating anorexia, increasing the person's weight is crucial. If the anorexic needs to be hospitalized, her treatment will focus on getting her weight back up to a normal level. If she refuses to eat, she may need a feeding tube to get the proper nutrients into her body. Hospitalization often helps the anorexic slowly change her behavior so that when she returns home, she can gain weight slowly with outpatient pediatric and psychiatric treatment. A person with bulimia may need hospitalization to control the cycles of bingeing and purging and to replace needed nutrients in the body.

Counseling is necessary to help a person with an eating disorder understand how she uses food as a way of handling problems and feelings. It will help her improve her self-image (including body image) and develop independence so that she can take control of her life in positive ways. A mix of individual therapy and family therapy is usually most effective in treating eating disorders. Since an eating disorder usually affects a person's entire family, a therapist can try to help family members understand the disorder. The therapist can also help families create a supportive home environment for the person with an eating disorder. Occasionally, people who have eating disorders also have problems with alcohol abuse or other substance abuse, and may need to be treated for those as well.

Anorexia and bulimia are both very serious eating disorders that do not go away by themselves. However, eating disorders are treatable with help. A person with an eating disorder needs professional help to recover and become healthy again.

For other resources and help with eating disorders, contact the following organizations:

National Association of Anorexia Nervosa
  and Associated Disorders
Box 7
Highland Park, IL 60035
847/831-3438

American Anorexia/Bulimia Association
418 E 76th St
New York, NY 10021
212/734-1114

Anorexia Nervosa and Related Eating Disorders
Box 5102
Eugene, OR 97405
503/344-1144

Some people who struggle with eating disorders alternate between anorexic and bulimic behaviors. About half of all people who have anorexia at one time or another develop some symptoms of bulimia (mainly the bingeing and purging). The following information shows some of the ways in which the disorders are alike and different.

Similarities of people with eating disorders:

- Distorted body image
- Strong-willed, determined nature
- Obsessive thoughts about food, eating, and body shape
- Depression
- Excessive exercise
- Overachiever, perfectionist
- Difficulty concentrating
- Poor self-esteem
- Self-destructive behavior
- Irritability
- Vomiting and use of laxatives and/or diuretics to keep weight off

Differences between people with eating disorders:

Anorexia
- Age range: persons 14 to 18 years old
- Severe weight loss
- Shockingly thin body
- Withdrawn personality
- Denial of hunger
- Sexual inactivity
- No menstrual periods
- Denial of eating disorder
- Strong resistance to treatment
- Death from starvation or suicide

Bulimia
- Age range: persons 15 to 24 years old
- Slight weight changes
- Normal weight appearance
- Outgoing personality
- Pronounced hunger
- Sexual activity
- Irregular menstrual periods
- Awareness of eating disorder
- Accepting to treatment
- Death from low potassium or suicide

The information contained in this publication should not be used as a substitute for the medical care and advice of your pediatrician. There may be variations in treatment that your pediatrician may recommend based on individual facts and circumstances.

From your doctor

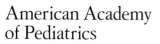
American Academy of Pediatrics

DEDICATED TO THE HEALTH OF ALL CHILDREN™

The American Academy of Pediatrics is an organization of 55,000 primary care pediatricians, pediatric medical subspecialists, and pediatric surgical specialists dedicated to the health, safety, and well-being of infants, children, adolescents, and young adults.

American Academy of Pediatrics
PO Box 747
Elk Grove Village, IL 60009-0747
Web site — http://www.aap.org

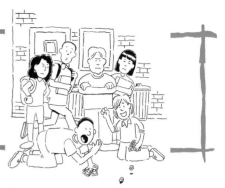

Gambling:
Not a Safe Thrill

A generation ago, most people felt gambling was not a wholesome activity. Today, many Americans have embraced gambling as a fun and relaxing form of entertainment. Most people who gamble do not end up as problem gamblers. Responsible, casual gambling for adults is not harmful. However, for young people, gambling can become a serious addiction.

Gambling is now legal in 48 out of 50 states. Compulsive gambling is considered by many experts to be the "addiction of the 90s." Consider these statistics

- About 90% of high school seniors have gambled at least once.
- Two-thirds of all students from ages 12 to 18 gamble regularly.
- There are nearly 8 million compulsive gamblers in the United States today. More than 1 million of them are teens.

Gambling should not be seen as a "safe thrill." Parents need to be aware of the danger gambling poses to young people and the warning signs of problem gambling.

How do teens gamble?

Any game of chance or skill that is played for money is gambling. Most forms of gambling are illegal for anyone under the age of 18. However, teens find their own ways to gamble, including the following:

- Playing cards or dice games for money
- Playing games of skill for money (pool, basketball, pogs)
- Buying lottery tickets and scratch cards
- Playing casino- and arcade-type games (like pull tabs and slot machines)
- Placing bets on sports events
- Gambling on the Internet

Why do teens gamble?

Gambling is promoted as fun and exciting; an easy way to "strike it rich." Many young people hope that if they can win big money, all their problems will be solved. As legalized gambling spreads to almost every community, it is easy for young people to get caught up in the promises of wealth and power. Adults do, too. In the United States, 80% of adults participate in some form of gambling.

Who is the typical teen gambler?

Today, many communities rely on gambling casinos as a major source of income. Teens in these communities may be at greater risk for developing problems with gambling than other teens. However, teen gambling can be found anywhere—in cities and small towns, among the wealthy and the poor.

It's not easy to "spot" a teen gambler. They look no different than their friends. They often are very outgoing and social. In addition, teen gamblers tend to be

- Highly motivated, energetic
- Smart
- Competitive, risk-takers
- Good students, hard working
- Perfectionists
- Confident

Teens who develop problems with gambling may often have other issues, such as difficulties with their family life, problems with other addictions like alcohol or drugs, or engage in other high-risk behaviors.

What is compulsive gambling?

When gambling moves beyond fun and games and starts becoming the focus of a person's life, it is considered compulsive gambling. There are three phases of compulsive gambling.

The winning phase

- Gambling is fun and exciting.
- Winning makes the gambler feel like a "big shot."
- Losses are thought of as "bad luck."
- All the gambler thinks about is gambling.
- The gambler thinks gambling is the most exciting thing in life.
- Free time, lunch breaks, or recess are often spent gambling.

The losing phase

- The gambler starts to lose, often borrowing money to cover losses.
- Self-esteem decreases.
- The gambler may lie to friends and family about gambling.
- The gambler may begin to sell possessions to cover bets.
- The gambler begins to miss school, work, or other important events to gamble.

The desperation phase

- The gambler becomes obsessed with gambling.
- Severe mood swings, lying, cheating, and stealing may occur.
- School failure is common.
- Nothing or nobody comes before a bet.
- Suicide may be attempted as a way out.

How can I tell if my son or daughter is having a problem with gambling?

Look for the following warning signs:

- Finding gambling "stuff" like lottery tickets, betting sheets, casino chips
- Excessive TV sports watching and an overly intensive interest in the outcome of sports events
- Visits to a casino, despite being underage
- Excessive "checking in" or spending time on the Internet
- Unexplained debts

- Flaunts large amounts of money or buys expensive items
- Absences from school or work
- Anxiety and nervousness
- Stealing for gambling money

What parents can do

You are the best role model for your children. Take a close look at your own attitudes and habits. Do you spend your last dollar on lottery tickets? Do you make frequent visits to the casino with hopes of striking it rich? While gambling may be okay for you, you may be sending a message to your teen that gambling is a safe and healthy activity.

Talk to your children about gambling. Remind them that gambling is illegal for teens. Be clear about how you feel about gambling, and let them know what you expect of them. Help your children develop ways to resist gambling and develop interests in other activities.

Identifying a gambling problem early is the key to successful treatment. If you feel your teen may have a problem, there are people in your community who can help, including the following:

- Pediatricians
- Counselors
- Teachers
- Elders or Clergy

Compulsive gambling is like other addictions. Outside help may be the only way a person can stop. Talk to your pediatrician for information about treatment options, like individual counseling or family therapy, that can give compulsive gamblers the strength they need to quit.

Resources

For more information on treatment options, support groups, or other educational materials, contact

North American Training Institute
314 W Superior St, Suite 702
Duluth, MN 55802
218/722-1503
www.nati.org
www.wannabet.org (a Web site for kids on gambling)

Gambler's Anonymous
International Service Office
PO Box 17173
Los Angeles, CA 90017
213/386-8789
www.gamblersanonymous.org

The National Council on Problem Gambling, Inc
Nationwide Helpline
800/522-4700
10025 Governor Warfield Pkwy, Suite 311
Columbia, MD 21044
www.ncpgambling.org/

Trimeridian, Inc
A national organization dedicated to providing comprehensive research, diagnostic, treatment, prevention, and education resources for individuals, families, and employers affected by problem gambling.
655 W Carmel Dr, Suite 120
Carmel, IN 46032
800/777-NOGAMBLE
www.trimeridian.com/

Please note: Inclusion on this list does not imply an endorsement by the American Academy of Pediatrics. The Academy is not responsible for the content of the resources mentioned above. Addresses, phone numbers, and Web site addresses are as current as possible, but may change at any time.

The information contained in this publication should not be used as a substitute for the medical care and advice of your pediatrician. There may be variations in treatment that your pediatrician may recommend based on individual facts and circumstances.

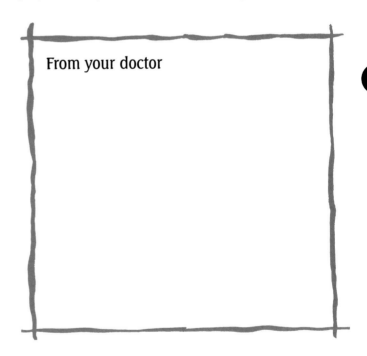

From your doctor

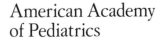

American Academy of Pediatrics

DEDICATED TO THE HEALTH OF ALL CHILDREN™

The American Academy of Pediatrics is an organization of 55,000 primary care pediatricians, pediatric medical subspecialists, and pediatric surgical specialists dedicated to the health, safety, and well-being of infants, children, adolescents, and young adults.

American Academy of Pediatrics
PO Box 747
Elk Grove Village, IL 60009-0747
Web site — http://www.aap.org

Healthy Communication With Your Child

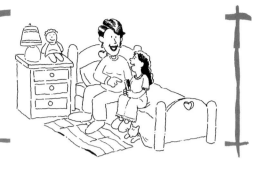

Many parents think that the main purpose of communication is to get information to their children. Telling children to eat their vegetables and reminding them to look both ways before crossing the street are expressions of love and caring. That is sending *information* about diet and safety. But communication has another important function. Communication is a two-way bridge that connects you and your child's feelings. Healthy communication—the kind that builds a strong two-way bridge—is crucial in helping your child develop a healthy personality and good relationships with you and others. It gives your child a chance to become a happy, safe, healthy person, no matter what happens. The American Academy of Pediatrics has developed this brochure to help you understand what healthy communication is and how to practice it.

Why is healthy communication important?

Healthy communication is important because it helps your child:
- Feel cared for and loved
- Believe she matters and is important to you
- Feel safe and not all alone with his worries
- Learn to tell you what she feels and needs directly in words
- Learn how to manage his feelings safely so that he does not act on feelings without thinking (or overreact)
- Talk to you openly in the future

Healthy communication also helps you:
- Feel close to your child
- Know your child's needs
- Know you have powerful tools to help your child grow
- Manage your own stress and frustrations with your child

What are the building blocks of healthy communication?

Building the two-way bridge of communication requires:
- **Being available**—Children need to feel that their parents are available to them. This means being able to spend time with your child. Even spending 10 minutes a day communicating with each of your children alone makes the bridge of communication stronger. Being available also means quickly getting yourself into a quiet and "tuned-in" mood before you start listening to your child or talking about something important. Being able to understand and talk about *your* feelings as well as your child's is another important part of being available.
- **Being a good listener**—Being a good listener helps your child feel loved, even when he is upset and you can't do anything to fix the problem. Ask your child for his ideas and feelings before beginning to talk about yours. Also, try to understand exactly what he is saying to you. What your child is trying to tell you is important to him, even when it may not be to you. You do not have to agree with what your child is saying to be a good listener. It helps your child calm down, so later he can listen to you.

- **Showing empathy**—This means tuning in to your child and letting her know you appreciate her feelings. You can show empathy even if you disagree with your child. Empathy is about appreciating feelings for their own sake. It is not about who is right or wrong. Showing empathy means checking out whether you understand what your child is feeling. Ask whether your understanding of how she is feeling is right.
- **Being a good sender**—Be a good *listener* first. If your child already feels heard and cared for, he will be in a better mood to listen to you.

  Make sure that what you say, your tone of voice, and what you do all send the same message. For example, if you laugh when you say "NO!", your child will be confused and will not know what you really want.

  Use *words* to communicate what you want your child to do. Even when setting limits with a toddler you can use words while holding him back.

  Use feeling words when you praise your child's behavior. For example, you can say "I am so happy!" when your child puts away her toys. It is also helpful to use "you" and point out the good behavior (as in "You have done a great job with your homework!"). Encourage your child to praise herself as well. Praise helps children get through the bad times.

  Use "I" statements to tell your child what displeases you about her behavior. For example, saying "When I couldn't find you, I felt worried and angry" is better than saying in an angry tone "You disappeared! Where were you?" Tell your child what you feel and think. Don't tell your child what she should think or feel.
- **Being a good role model**—Young children learn better by copying what their parents do than by being told. Children will copy your way of communicating. If you yourself use a lot of feeling words, it will help your child to learn to do the same. When parents use feeling words instead of screaming, doing something hurtful, or calling someone a name, children learn that using feeling words is a better way to deal with strong feelings. Saying feelings rather than acting on them helps children control themselves. You can help your child learn to label his feelings by deciding what feeling words are OK to say at home or in school.

The flip side of healthy communication: verbal abuse

Children usually bounce back quickly when they are hurt. For example, your child may cry when she falls and scrapes a knee, but ten minutes later she has forgotten all about the fall and is running outside again. The same thing might happen when someone at school calls your child a name. If it only happens once, your child will probably forget it. However, children who suffer the same type of hurts over and over again do not bounce back quickly. Children who are verbally abused are deeply hurt by what their parents say and by how they say it.

What is verbal abuse?

There are three kinds of verbal abuse:

- **Name-calling, frequent criticism, and blaming:** Criticism is making "you" statements and calling your child names. For example, saying "You are stupid" is name-calling and criticism; saying "I am upset with you and I wish you would stop doing that" is not. Criticizing, name-calling, and blaming only make things worse in the long run.

- **Violating children's boundaries, yelling, threatening to hurt or abandon them, and lying:** Sometimes, a parent's strong emotions are too much for a young child to handle. Children build walls between themselves and their parents when this happens. Children who back up, hide, or put their hands over their ears are often trying to protect themselves from too much strong emotion. They are usually not trying to show disrespect.

  Children are not little adults. They cannot block out screaming and loudness the way adults can. Loud talking or yelling while standing over children makes them feel very scared and unsafe. It hurts their emotions, just as physical abuse hurts their bodies and emotions. Yelling and loudness are even more hurtful when children are tired, sick, hungry, or scared about something. The younger the child is, the more this is true.

  Children believe threats of harm or threats that you will leave them. Threats scare children more than you can imagine. They do not help your child behave better.

  Lying also violates your child's boundaries. Children will believe lies because they do not usually have enough information to be able to tell lies from the truth.

- **Silence**—Children feel long silences (hours or days) very strongly. They do not know what these silences mean. Children read horrible things into their parents' silences. Silence sends a strong message of anger or dislike. It makes your child feel confused and helpless. It you are silent because you are depressed, it is better to tell your child that you are sad or ill and that it is not about him. When you are silent, you are not being a good sender.

Parents may get silent because:
- They are afraid that they will say something that will make things worse.
- They do not know what to say or do.
- They have such strong feelings of anger or sadness that they can't talk.
- They are ill.
- Their own parents used silence to control them.

Parents verbally abuse children because they:
- Never learned healthy communication.
- Do not know other ways to control their children's behavior.
- Do not know that children are hurt by verbal abuse and that it makes things worse.
- Have not learned how to manage their own strong feelings.
- Are under a lot of stress.
- Think their children need to develop a "thick skin" to survive.
- Were treated the same way by their parents, teachers, and other adults.

Preventing verbal abuse: handling parental stress and anger

Parenting is a very hard job. There are times when you will feel so stressed that you think you can't handle one more thing. At those times, a crying baby, a toddler throwing a temper tantrum, or a fifth-grader refusing to do her homework might push you over the edge. It is important to find ways to help your child to behave that do not involve hurting her feelings. It is also important to find ways to prevent stress, and to calm yourself down when you are stressed, so that you do not say or do something harmful to your child.

Here are some things you might do to calm yourself:
- Take a few deep breaths very slowly.
- Wait 5 minutes before starting to talk to your child.
- Try to find a word to label your feeling.
- Say it to yourself or write it down.
- Share your feelings with your spouse or another adult. Call a friend.
- Keep your attention on the present. Don't add up past problems.

Parents who are under a lot of stress may find it hard to control strong feelings like anger, fear, frustration, or helplessness. They may not realize that their anger is a reaction to feeling worried, confused, hurt, or overwhelmed with stress. For example, you would probably feel worried if your child got lost in the supermarket. If you were in a rush, you might be angry when you find her. You might yell at your child for having wandered away instead of saying "I was worried that I might not find you!" When you can learn to calm down and figure out what is really making you angry, you can avoid hurting your child out of anger.

Some people find that using the RETHINK© method helps them control their anger before they say or do something they might regret.

RETHINK© stands for:

Recognize your feelings.

Empathize with the other person.

Think of the situation differently. Use humor.

Hear what the other person is saying.

Integrate your love with your angry thoughts.

Notice your body's reaction to feeling anger and to calming down.

Keep your attention on the present problem.

Using RETHINK© can help you get control over your anger before you lash out at your child. If using the RETHINK© method or trying other ways to calm yourself does not work, try talking to your spouse, your pediatrician, or a counselor, minister, parent, or close friend. There is nothing to be ashamed of in admitting you need help in controlling your anger. All parents get frustrated and angry with their children. Asking for help with the difficult job of parenting is *always* better than losing control.

American Academy of Pediatrics

DEDICATED TO THE HEALTH OF ALL CHILDREN™

The American Academy of Pediatrics is an organization of 55,000 primary care pediatricians, pediatric medical subspecialists, and pediatric surgical specialists dedicated to the health, safety, and well-being of infants, children, adolescents, and young adults.

American Academy of Pediatrics
PO Box 747
Elk Grove Village, IL 60009-0747
Web site — http://www.aap.org

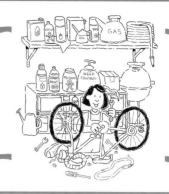

Inhalant Abuse: Your Child and Drugs
Guidelines for Parents

When you think of young people using drugs, alcohol and marijuana probably come to mind first. Some young people do use those drugs, but each year more are abusing another group of substances that you may know little about. These are called inhalants. The abuse of inhalants is also called solvent abuse, huffing, sniffing, glue sniffing, or volatile substance abuse.

There are over 1,000 inhalants—common products most often found in the home, office, and classroom. These products are legal because they have a useful purpose. They are also safe when used for that purpose. But when young people misuse them by breathing them into their lungs, inhalants are poison. Over time, the abuse of inhalants can cause severe permanent damage to the body, especially the brain. **The scariest thing about inhalants is that your child could die from using them only once.**

Read this brochure to learn more about inhalants so that you can talk with your child about them. Educating young people about their dangers is an important step in preventing inhalant abuse. This brochure also describes the signs and symptoms of inhalant abuse. If you suspect your child is abusing inhalants, it is important to get help and, if necessary, treatment right away.

Common inhalants and how they are used

Hair spray. Gasoline. Spray paint. Glue. Typewriter correction fluid. You probably have at least one of these products in your home. These are just a few of the inhalants that are poisonous when children:

- Sniff or inhale them directly from the cans, bottles, or other containers they are in.
- Spray them into a bag, empty soft drink can, or other container and breathe them in. (Gases like nitrous oxide are often inhaled from balloons.)
- Spray or pour them onto a cloth or piece of clothing and inhale deeply from the fabric.

There are three general types of inhalants: solvents, gases, and nitrites.

- **Solvents** are usually liquid. They are found in household and industrial products, such as glues, paints, and polishes.
- **Gases** are found in many household and commercial products. Aerosol sprays like hair spray and spray paint, as well as medical gases like nitrous oxide, fall into this category. Almost all pressurized aerosol sprays can be abused.
- **Nitrites** are found in room deodorizers.

Inhalant abuse is on the rise

Inhalant abuse is a growing problem—one that deserves parents' attention. While the use of some drugs is declining, inhalant abuse is on the rise among children and teens. In the past decade it has nearly doubled. Adolescents 12 to 14 years of age are most likely to abuse inhalants, and almost 20% of eighth-graders have tried some form of them. Most young people who ever try inhalants do so before their second year of high school.

A household guide to inhalants

Here is a list of only a few of the common household products that are dangerous when inhaled:

Kitchen
Cooking spray
Typewriter correction fluid
Disinfectants
Fabric protectors
Felt-tip markers
Furniture polish and wax
Oven cleaners

Bathroom
Air fresheners
Spray deodorants
Hair sprays
Nail polish removers

Garage/Workshop
Pressurized aerosol sprays
Butane
Gasoline
Glues and adhesives
Paints and paint thinners
Refrigerants (freon)
Rust removers
Spray paints

Why do children abuse inhalants?

There are many reasons why inhalants appeal to children. They are cheap, easy to get, and easy to hide. For a few dollars, a can of butane offers a quick high. Or a child can sit in class and secretly sniff correction fluid. Because inhalants are legal, kids can easily make excuses if they are caught with them.

Another appeal of inhalants is the social part of using them. Kids enjoy abusing inhalants with other kids, and most inhalant abuse is thought to be done with friends.

Reasons why children use inhalants

- Low cost
- Way to rebel against parents
- Easy to get and hide

- Peer pressure or influence
- Not illegal to possess, so kids can make excuses if they are caught with inhalants
- Public is not aware of the dangers

Signs and symptoms of inhalant abuse

- Breath and clothing that smells like chemicals
- Spots or sores around the mouth
- Paint or stains on body or clothing
- Drunk, dazed, or glassy-eyed look
- Nausea, loss of appetite
- Anxiety, excitability, irritability

Prevention of inhalant abuse

Although some states have laws to try and deal with inhalant abuse, such laws are not always easy to enforce. Since inhalants are legal and kids can get them from so many different ways, it is not possible to make inhalants entirely off-limits. The best way to fight inhalant abuse is to educate your child about how harmful these products are. Explain how they can cause both short- and long-term health problems, further drug abuse, and death. It is important to start talking with children at a young age, because inhalant abuse often starts as young as 8 or 9 years old. Parents and teachers should also be able to recognize the warning signs of inhalant abuse.

Help prevent your child from turning to inhalants and other drugs by taking these steps:

Set a good example at home. As a parent, you are the best role model for your child. Parents who use drugs also place their children at higher risk for drug use.

Build self-esteem and confidence. Praise your child often. Encourage your son or daughter to set goals and make decisions to achieve them. With each success and your constant support, your child will become more confident in what he or she can do. Children with self-confidence feel good about themselves without needing drugs.

Help your child develop different interests. Encourage your child to read, have hobbies, play sports, or join clubs. These activities can keep your son or daughter from using drugs out of boredom or from having too much free time. Young people will find that they can have a lot of fun and feel good without drugs. Take an active interest in your child's interests and in his or her friends.

Help your child resist peer pressure. Being independent and self-confident can help your child resist pressure from friends to abuse inhalants. To foster independence, show confidence in your child's ability to make his or her own decisions. Encourage your child to make his or her own judgments, no matter what friends or others say or do.

Talk openly and often. Talk about things that are important to and relevant in your child's life. This includes discussing drugs and how some kids might use them to be accepted by their peers. Educating your pre-teen or teen about the dangers of drugs, including inhalant abuse, works best through talking rather than lecturing.

Treatment of inhalant abuse

When children are abusing inhalants, many times their parents do not find out until the abuse has already become a habit. Chronic inhalant abusers are hardest to treat because they often have many serious personal and social problems. They also have difficulty staying off inhalants and have very high rates of relapse. All of these reasons can keep chronic inhalant abusers from benefiting from many drug abuse treatment programs.

Toxic chemicals from inhalants stay in the body for weeks. Because of this, when chronic abusers stop using inhalants they may feel the effects of withdrawal for weeks. Withdrawal is the body's way of getting over its physical addiction to inhalants. During withdrawal from inhalants, a person may have:

- Hand tremors
- Excess sweating
- Constant headaches
- Nervousness

Treatment for inhalant abusers is usually long-term, sometimes as long as 2 years. It must address the many social problems most inhalant abusers have and involves:

- Support of the child's family
- Moving the child away from unhealthy friendships with other abusers
- Teaching and fostering better coping skills
- Building self-esteem and self-confidence
- Helping the child adjust to school or another learning setting

Inhalant abuse is a difficult form of substance abuse to treat. It is best to recognize and start treatment before the problem becomes a habit. Parents and educators need to be able to recognize the signs of inhalant abuse, especially because most abusers do not seek treatment on their own.

Parents also play the most important role in helping their children to resist abusing inhalants in the first place. The most effective prevention of inhalant abuse is through the education of parents, teachers, and school-aged children.

Information for you and your child

What are the effects of inhalants?

One thing that all inhalants have in common is that they contain chemicals that were never meant for people to consume. So why would anyone breathe toxic chemicals on purpose? Just like the users of other drugs, inhalant abusers try to get "high" from the chemicals.

The effects of inhalants usually last only a few minutes, unless users inhale repeatedly. At first, inhalants have a stimulating effect. Then if the users keep inhaling, they may feel dazed, dizzy, and have trouble walking. Sometimes users get aggressive or think they see things that are not there. Stronger chemicals or repeated inhaling can cause people to pass out. A user can also die suddenly from using inhalants.

When someone uses an inhalant, large amounts of toxic chemicals enter the lungs and pass from the bloodstream into the brain. There they damage and kill brain cells. The amount of fumes a young person inhales greatly exceeds what is considered safe even in a workplace setting. It takes at least 2 weeks for the body to get rid of some of the chemicals in inhalants. Inhalants exit the body mainly through exhaling, which is why an inhalant abuser's breath often smells like chemicals. Inhalants also pass out of the body through urine.

Short-term effects of inhalants are:

- Headaches, nausea, vomiting
- Loss of balance
- Dizziness
- Slurred and slow speech
- Mood changes
- Hallucinations

Over time, inhalants can cause more serious damage, such as:

- Loss of concentration
- Short-term memory loss
- Hearing loss
- Muscle spasms
- Permanent brain damage
- Death

How do inhalants kill?

No one can predict how much of an inhalant will kill. A young person can use a certain amount one time and seem fine, but his or her next use could be fatal.

The Texas Commission on Drugs and Alcohol Abuse reports the following ways that inhalants can kill:

- Asphyxia—Solvent gases can cause a person to stop breathing from a lack of oxygen.
- Choking—Users can choke on their own vomit.
- Suffocation—This is more common among users who inhale from plastic bags.
- Injuries—Inhalants can cause people to become careless or aggressive. This often leads to behaviors that can injure or kill, such as operating a motor vehicle dangerously or jumping from great heights. Teens also can get burned or even be killed if someone lights a cigarette while they are huffing butane, gasoline, or some other flammable substance.
- Suicides—Coming down from an inhalant high causes some people to feel depressed, which may lead them to take their own lives.
- Cardiac arrest—Chemicals from inhalants can make the heart beat very fast and irregularly, then suddenly stop beating. This is called cardiac arrest. One reason why this might happen is that inhalants somehow make the heart extra-sensitive to adrenaline. (Adrenaline is a hormone that the body produces, usually in response to fear, excitement, or surprise.) A sudden rush of adrenaline combined with inhalants can make the heart stop instantly. This "Sudden Sniffing Death," as it is called, is responsible for more than half of all deaths due to inhalant abuse.

Another very real danger of inhalants is that they often lead young people to try other drugs whose effects are even more intense and last longer.

The information contained in this publication should not be used as a substitute for the medical care and advice of your pediatrician. There may be variations in treatment that your pediatrician may recommend based on individual facts and circumstances.

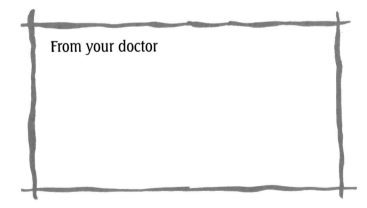

From your doctor

American Academy of Pediatrics

DEDICATED TO THE HEALTH OF ALL CHILDREN™

The American Academy of Pediatrics is an organization of 55,000 primary care pediatricians, pediatric medical subspecialists, and pediatric surgical specialists dedicated to the health, safety, and well-being of infants, children, adolescents, and young adults.

American Academy of Pediatrics
PO Box 747
Elk Grove Village, IL 60009-0747
Web site — http://www.aap.org

The Internet and Your Family

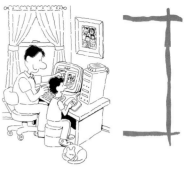

Not long ago, computers were huge machines that occupied entire rooms. Today's desktop and laptop computers give us our own personal windows to the world. The stunning growth of the Internet has placed knowledge and information at our fingertips. The possibilities for learning and exploring on the Internet are endless. Being able to use technology is fast becoming a requirement for success in today's society. Teaching your child the basic skills of working with computers will provide tools she will need in our changing world.

It is critical that your child have your guidance when learning to use the Internet. Even if your child is an experienced computer user, he needs your involvement, your experience, and your judgment. Although children can use the Internet to tap into the Library of Congress or view pictures of the surface of Mars, not all material on the Internet is appropriate for children. As a parent, you can guide and teach your child in a way that no one else can. Regardless of your technological know-how, you can make sure your child's experience on the Internet is safe, educational, and fun.

What is the information superhighway?

The Internet, sometimes called the information superhighway, is a giant network of computers that connects people and information all over the world. The term *on-line* means being connected to the Internet. The World Wide Web (often shortened to WWW or the Web) is the most popular part of the Internet because it includes pictures and sound as well as text.

What can my child and I find on the Internet?

A computer that is connected to the Internet allows you to turn your home, community center, local library, or school into a place of unlimited information. The Internet can help you and your child do the following:
- **Find educational resources**, including up-to-the-minute news, important documents, photos, and research.
- **Get help with homework** through on-line encyclopedias, reference materials, and access to experts.
- **Improve computer skills** necessary to find information, solve problems, and communicate with others.
- **Connect with places around the world** to exchange e-mail with on-line pen pals and learn about other countries and cultures.
- **Locate parenting information** and swap ideas with other families.
- **Learn and have fun together** by sharing interesting and enjoyable experiences.

Surfing the Net

When you go to the Internet, you may have a specific address in mind or you may browse through the Web, just as you would a library or a catalog. This is often called "surfing the Net." Following are several ways to get around on the Web:

- **Using Web addresses**. Every Web site has its own unique address. By typing the address in the space provided, your Web browser will take you there. Make sure you type the address exactly as specified.
- **Following links.** Many sites include *hyperlinks* to other related sites. By clicking on the highlighted area, you can connect to another Web site without having to type its address.
- **Using search engines.** Search engines are programs that can enable you to search the Internet using keywords or topics. For example, if you or your child are interested in finding information about Abraham Lincoln, simply click on a search engine and enter his name. A list of several Web sites will come up for you to explore.

Other Internet uses

E-mail—Electronic mail is by far the most popular activity on-line. You and your child can exchange notes with friends and family. Most Internet service providers offer e-mail accounts and allow you to choose your own e-mail address.

Listservs—By using e-mail, you can participate in a *listserv* (a discussion group focusing on a topic that interests you). Subscribing to a listserv allows you to read all messages sent by other members of the group. You can also send your own responses that will be read by everyone else. Most listservs are run by an administrator or moderator. A list of listservs and how to subscribe to them can be found at http://www.liszt.com.

Usenet newsgroups—Usenet is a system of thousands of special interest groups that allow people to post messages for anyone else to read. Readers can respond by posting a general message or sending e-mail to the author of an earlier message. Unlike listservs, Usenet groups do not require you to subscribe. Your Internet service provider will let you search for newsgroups that interest you by using keywords (for example, try "parenting").

A caution about newsgroups: Most newsgroups are not moderated. No one keeps the discussion focused on the topic or has control over inappropriate behavior. Some topics may not be suitable for children.

Setting rules of the road

Just like you have rules for how your children should deal with strangers and which TV shows, movies, and videos they are allowed to watch, it is important to have a set of rules when they use the Internet. Be wary of people on the Net who can be mean, rude, or even criminal. To keep your child's time on the Internet safe, productive, and fun, follow these guidelines:
- Set limits on the amount of time your child can spend on-line each day or week. Consider using an alarm clock or timer in case you or your child loses track of time.
- Do not let surfing the Net take the place of homework, playing outside or with friends, and pursuing other interests.

Visit us at www.aap.org

The award-winning Web site of the American Academy of Pediatrics pro-vides a wide range of helpful information for parents. The site is updated daily with the latest on children's health and safety. A search engine allows parents to search the site's thousands of pages of information for specific topics. The site includes:

- You and Your Family—a special section dedicated to the needs of par-ents and children of all ages
- The latest information on immunizations, car seat safety, Sudden Infant Death Syndrome, breastfeeding, and dozens of other topics
- Where We Stand—Presenting the Academy's positions on children's health and safety issues
- Excerpts from AAP child care books and brochures
- The latest research and reports on children's health issues
- Information on new state and federal legislation
- A catalog of AAP publications with on-line ordering
  Check out **http://www.aap.org** often for the latest in children's health and safety.

- Make sure your child knows that people on-line are not always who they say they are and that on-line information is not necessarily private.
- Teach your child the following:
  NEVER give out personal information (including name, address, phone number, age, race, school name or location, or friends' names) without your permission.
  NEVER use a credit card on-line without your permission.
  NEVER share passwords, even with friends.
  NEVER arrange a face-to-face meeting with someone she meets on-line, unless you approve of the meeting and go with your child to a public place. Teenagers in particular need to be aware of the risks.
  NEVER respond to messages that make her feel confused or uncomfortable. Your child should ignore the sender, end the commun-ication, and tell you or another trusted adult right away.
  NEVER use bad language or send mean messages on-line.

Caring about content

Even without trying, your child may come across material on the Internet that is obscene, violent, hate-filled, racist, or offensive in other ways. One type of material, child pornography, is even illegal. If you or your child encounter child pornography, you should report it to the National Center for Missing and Exploited Children at 1-800-THE LOST (843-5678) or visit its Web site at http://www.missingkids.org.

Though other material is not illegal, you should take the following steps to keep it away from your child:

- Make sure your child understands what you consider appropriate for him and what areas are off limits. Set clear rules and enforce them.
- Look into software or services that can filter or block offensive Web sites and material. Also, many Internet service providers offer site blocking, restrictions on e-mail, and other controls for parents. Be aware, however, that many children are smart enough to find ways around these restrictions. Nothing can replace supervision.
- Make a point to participate in your child's on-line time. Put the computer in the living room or family room. Stay involved and monitor what your child is doing.
- Find out what the Internet use policies are at your child's school or at your local library

Information: the good and the bad

Anyone can put information on the Internet and not all of it is reliable. Some people and organizations are very careful about the accuracy of the information they post, others are not. Some give false information on purpose. Remind your children not to copy on-line information and claim it is their own.

As the Internet grows, so does the trend of on-line advertising. Steer your child to non-commercial sites and other places that do not sell products to children. Teach your child to recognize the advertising and marketing of prod-ucts and services. Encourage your child to think about who created the ads and why they are there. Discuss questions like the following:

- What is the product being advertised?
- How are they trying to get you to buy the product?
- Is there something about the product they are not telling you?

There is an almost unlimited amount of information, products, and services available on the Internet, and it continues to grow. It is important to be aware of the potential risks involved in going on-line. By setting clear rules and using common sense, you can help your child take advantage of the vast resources the Internet offers, while at the same time having fun and staying safe.

Other great places to visit

Following is just a sampling of interesting, informative sites available to you and your family. This is not a complete list and the American Academy of Pediatrics is not responsible for the content of the sites mentioned here. The addresses are as current as possible, but may change at any time. If an address does not work, use a search engine to find the updated link.

Children with special needs

Computers should be accessible to everyone and special equipment is available to help children with special needs. A joystick, for example, can make operating a computer easier for a child with limited mobility. Special keyboards, screens, and computerized-voice products can allow a child with special needs to enjoy the benefits of using a computer. For more information, contact:

The ERIC Clearinghouse on Disabilities and Gifted Education 800/328-0272 (TTY 703/264-9449) or http://www.cec.sped.org/ericec.htm

The Starbright Foundation 310/442-1560 or http://www.starbright.org

For parents

Family Education Network
http://www.familyeducation.com
Focusing on helping children succeed in school

FedWorld
http://www.fedworld.gov
Reference for federal government information on the Web

I Am Your Child
http://www.iamyourchild.org
The I Am Your Child campaign stresses the importance of a child's first years, and is sponsored by Rob Reiner's Families and Work Institute

Media Literacy from NCADI
http://www.health.org
National Clearinghouse for Alcohol and Drug Information site providing tools to use media literacy to help youth think for themselves and resist powerful media messages about alcohol and drugs

NetParents
http://www.netparents.org
Information on Internet security and blocking software

YouthInfo
http://youth.os.dhhs.gov
Focuses mainly on adolescents. Sponsored by the US Department of Health and Human Services

For children

50+ Great Sites for Kids and Parents
http://www.ala.org/parentspage/greatsites/50.html
Sponsored by the American Library Association. Directory of many sites for children of all ages.

Exploratorium
http://www.exploratorium.edu
Puzzles, games, and experiments

The Internet Public Library: Reference Center
http://www.ipl.org/ref
Includes an "Ask a Question" feature and a teen collection

Jean Armour Polly's 100 Extraordinary Experiences for Internet Kids
http://www.well.com/user/polly/ikyp.exp.html
Fun, interesting, and educational adventures on the Internet

The Library of Congress
http://www.loc.gov
Includes historical collections, databases, and access to other government information systems

My Virtual Reference Desk
http://www.refdesk.com
Dozens of links to dictionaries, encyclopedias, and other reference materials.

Public Broadcasting System
http://www.pbs.org
Information and activities related to PBS children's programming

Steve Savitsky's Interesting Places for Kids
http://www.starport.com/places/forKids/
Unusual links for kids

Health and medical sites

Note: On-line advice should never replace your pediatrician.

Centers for Disease Control
http://www.cdc.gov
Information on preventing and controlling disease, injury, and disability

Healthfinder
http://www.healthfinder.gov
US Government sponsored site that can help you search for health information, resources, and services

Mayo Clinic
http://www.mayohealth.org
Health information and advice from one of the world's most renowned medical research institutions

Medsite
http://www.medsite.com
A medical search engine that reviews medical Web sites and helps make medical information more accessible

National Institutes of Health
http://www.nih.gov
Extensive information on preventing, detecting, diagnosing, and treating disease and disability

National Organization for Rare Disorders (NORD)
http://www.rarediseases.org
Dedicated to helping people with rare "orphan" diseases and assisting the organizations that serve them

US Department of Health and Human Services
http://www.dhhs.gov
Information on more than 250 programs protecting the health of Americans

Adapted from the US Department of Education booklet "Parents Guide to the Internet." For the complete publication, see http://www.ed.gov/pubs/parents/internet/.

The information contained in this publication should not be used as a substitute for the medical care and advice of your pediatrician. There may be variations in treatment that your pediatrician may recommend based on individual facts and circumstances.

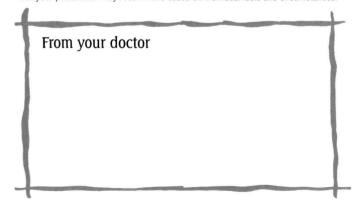

From your doctor

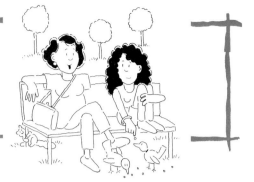

Marijuana:
Your Child and Drugs

Young people today can face strong peer pressure to try drugs. As a parent, you are your child's first and best protection against drug use. The first step is to become informed yourself. The American Academy of Pediatrics has developed this brochure to help you learn about marijuana and how you can help your child withstand pressure to use it.

Marijuana comes from the cannabis plant and looks like dried leaves. It is smoked either in a pipe or a hand-rolled cigarette, called a "joint." Other common names for marijuana are pot, weed, grass, herb, and reefer.

Marijuana is fairly easy for young people to get. It also tends to be the first illegal drug they try. After smoking marijuana, teens may go on to try "harder" drugs, such as cocaine and LSD.

Teens' use of marijuana has gone up in recent years. Among high school students, marijuana is one of the most widely abused drugs. A 1995 national survey of American high school seniors showed that:

- 41% have used marijuana at some time in their lives
- 21% used it in the past 30 days
- 4.6% use marijuana every day
- 88% said the drug is fairly easy or very easy to get

About one third of marijuana smokers start using the drug by sixth grade.

These statistics are cause for concern. Another concern is that marijuana today is about 25 times stronger than it was in the 1960s. THC, the main ingredient in marijuana, builds up in the body over time. The more a person smokes, the more THC builds up. It can take several weeks for the body to get rid of chemicals from just one marijuana cigarette. Besides THC, marijuana contains more than 400 other chemicals that can be health hazards.

Some short-term effects of smoking marijuana include:

- Calm, relaxed, sleepy feeling
- Increased appetite
- Dry, bloodshot eyes; dry throat and mouth
- Increased heart rate
- Slowed reaction time
- Poor short-term memory
- Anxiety, panic attacks, or paranoia

Why young people are at risk

Over time, marijuana may cause serious physical effects in teens who are still growing and maturing. These include:

- Lower sperm count and testosterone levels in males (Testosterone is a hormone that controls hair and penis growth, muscle mass, and voice changes during puberty.)
- Irregular menstrual periods and ovulation in females, which can lead to infertility
- Heart and lung damage
- Cancer

- Memory problems
- Psychological dependence on the drug

Marijuana can make it difficult for a person to think, listen, speak, remember things, solve problems, and form concepts. It can also affect how well your teen does in school. Heavy, chronic marijuana smokers often have less drive and ambition.

The effects of marijuana can make driving or playing sports risky. This is because marijuana impairs complex motor skills and the ability to judge speed and time. Using drugs like marijuana increases the risk of injury, such as from vehicle crashes.

In adolescence, sexual feelings are evolving and changing. Smoking marijuana can confuse these feelings and cause your teen to take sexual chances. This could lead to an unplanned pregnancy or a sexually transmitted disease (including HIV, the virus that causes AIDS).

Why do young people try marijuana?

There are many reasons why young people use drugs. Some of the most common reasons are:

- To fit in with their friends
- To avoid dealing with strong emotions or problems
- Because they are curious
- To rebel and be different
- For a quick way to feel good and have fun
- Because some media show drug use as "cool" or normal and not having any bad effects

Some teens may think using marijuana will make them "cool" or seem more adult-like. They need to know that marijuana use is not a normal step in growing up, despite what their peers may say.

Stages of marijuana use

There are three stages of drug use that can occur:

- **Casual use.** There is strong peer pressure to enter this stage, where a teen usually smokes marijuana to feel good and have fun. He or she still limits drug use in this stage.
- **Heavier use.** The user enters this stage when he or she starts to build a tolerance to marijuana. This is when a person needs more and more of a drug to get the same effects as before. You may notice behavior changes in this stage (see the box on the next page). Your teen's schoolwork also may slip. Problems that develop at home and at school because of drug use may cause a teen to use even more drugs.
- **Dependency.** In this stage there is a real loss of control over drug use. The user now feels that he or she needs marijuana to get through the day. Without it, he or she may become angry or withdrawn. Because heavy use is costly, a teen may lie and steal from family and friends to be able to buy marijuana. This could lead to trouble with the law.

Whether or not someone becomes a heavy user will depend on his or her reasons for smoking marijuana in the first place. Being able to recognize the signs of abuse is the first step in getting help for your teen.

Signs your child may be using marijuana

Your child:

- Has red eyes; uses eye drops a lot
- Is hungry often and even gains weight
- Is less motivated and has an "I don't care" attitude
- Withdraws from the family; spends more time in his or her room or away from home
- Forgets things; has trouble paying attention or communicating
- Buys things like CDs and T-shirts with pro-marijuana messages or symbols
- Starts missing school or shows a drop in school grades
- Has new friends and interests; gives up old hobbies, sports, or other activities

How to help your child say "no" to marijuana

Talk with your teen about drugs: Young people who do not know the facts about drugs may try them just to see what they are like. After you become informed, talk with your teen about marijuana and its harmful effects. Try to get your teen to share any questions and concerns he or she has. Be sure to really listen to your teen; do not lecture or do all the talking.

Help your teen handle peer pressure: Peers and friends can strongly influence your teen to try marijuana. As a parent, your influence can be just as strong to help your teen be independent and resist peer pressure. Tell him or her that it is okay to say "no" to marijuana and mean it. Your teen might respond to friends by saying, "I tried marijuana and didn't like it," or "I would get in a lot of trouble if my parents ever found out." Practice these and other responses with your son or daughter. If a friend is offering the marijuana, it may be harder to say "no." Your teen can suggest other things to do with that friend. This shows that your teen is rejecting the drug, not the friend.

Help your teen deal with emotions: During the teen years, many young people face strong emotions for the first time. These new feelings can be hard to cope with, and your teen may sometimes get depressed or anxious. He or she may turn to marijuana to escape such feelings and forget problems. It is important to talk with your teen about any concerns and problems he or she is facing. Assure your teen that everything has an upside, and things do not stay "bad" for very long. Point out that even after using marijuana or other drugs, the same problems and hassles are still there.

Enhance your teen's self-confidence: Praise the positive qualities in your teen often. Encourage your son or daughter to set goals and make personal decisions to achieve them. With each success, your teen will gain more confidence. Applaud effort as well as success. As your teen becomes more responsible, you can still provide guidance, emotional support, and security when needed. Becoming responsible also means facing the results of one's actions—good or bad. Making mistakes is a normal part of growing up; so try not to be too critical when your son or daughter makes a mistake.

Instill strong values in your teen. Teach your son or daughter the values that are important to your family. Also teach him or her to think of these values when deciding what is right and wrong. Explain that these are the standards your family lives by, despite what other people are doing.

Be a good role model: As a parent, you should avoid use of marijuana and other drugs. You are the best role model for your teen. Make a stand against drug issues—your teen will listen.

Encourage healthy ways to have fun: Young people are always looking for ways to have fun. They can also get bored easily. Drugs offer what seems to be a carefree "high" with little or no effort. Help your teen develop an interest in different hobbies, clubs, and activities. Look for healthy ways to reduce boredom and too much free time. Take an active interest in what is important to your teen.

Realize that not all young people will resist the lure of drugs. If your teen is using marijuana, he or she needs your help. Know the signs of marijuana use. Being able to recognize these signs is the first step in getting help for your teen. Pediatricians, family members, teachers, youth groups, mental health professionals, and clergy can provide support for your teen to stop smoking marijuana. If the problem is too much for you to handle on your own, get professional help. Your teen may need counseling, a support group, and/or a treatment program.

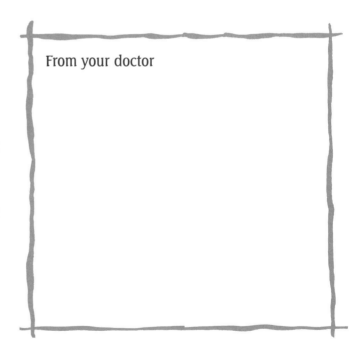

From your doctor

American Academy of Pediatrics

DEDICATED TO THE HEALTH OF ALL CHILDREN™

The American Academy of Pediatrics is an organization of 55,000 primary care pediatricians, pediatric medical subspecialists, and pediatric surgical specialists dedicated to the health, safety, and well-being of infants, children, adolescents, and young adults.

American Academy of Pediatrics
PO Box 747
Elk Grove Village, IL 60009-0747
Web site — http://www.aap.org

Copyright ©1992, Updated 3/96
American Academy of Pediatrics

Media History

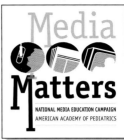
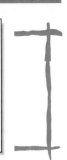

Please check one answer for each question. If the question does not apply to your family (ie, you do not own a VCR, video game player, or computer), leave that section blank.

Child's Name _____

Date _____

Television

Does your child watch more than 1 to 2 hours of TV per day?   ☐ Frequently   ☐ Sometimes   ☐ Never

Do you watch TV with your child or know what your child is watching?   ☐ Frequently   ☐ Sometimes   ☐ Never

Do you discuss TV shows with your child?   ☐ Frequently   ☐ Sometimes   ☐ Never

Does your child have a TV in his or her room?   ☐ Yes   ☐ No

Do you limit your child's watching of TV shows that often contain violence, sex, foul or explicit language, or images of tobacco or alcohol use?   ☐ Frequently   ☐ Sometimes   ☐ Never

Do you have rules about when TV can be watched?   ☐ Yes   ☐ No

Do you allow your child to eat meals or snacks while watching TV?   ☐ Yes   ☐ No

Does your child ask you to buy products he or she sees advertised on TV?   ☐ Frequently   ☐ Sometimes   ☐ Never

Movies and Videos

Do you allow your child to watch movies or videos that are R-rated?   ☐ Frequently   ☐ Sometimes   ☐ Never

Do you read movie reviews to know the content of PG-13 movies?   ☐ Frequently   ☐ Sometimes   ☐ Never

Does your child have nightmares or trouble sleeping after watching movies?   ☐ Frequently   ☐ Sometimes   ☐ Never

How often does your child watch music videos on TV?   ☐ Frequently   ☐ Sometimes   ☐ Never

Radio, CDs, Cassette Tapes

Are you familiar with the type of music your child listens to?   ☐ Yes   ☐ No

Have you talked to your child about lyrics that you object to?   ☐ Yes   ☐ No

Do you set limits on the types of music your child listens to?   ☐ Yes   ☐ No

Video and Computer Games

Are you familiar with the types of games your child plays?   ☐ Yes   ☐ No

Do you check a game's rating before you rent or buy it?   ☐ Yes   ☐ No

Do you allow your child to own or rent games with violent content?   ☐ Frequently   ☐ Sometimes   ☐ Never

Do you limit the number of hours your child plays these games?   ☐ Frequently   ☐ Sometimes   ☐ Never

Internet and Computer On-line Services

Do you monitor Internet and on-line computer use?   ☐ Frequently   ☐ Sometimes   ☐ Never

Does your child have a computer in his or her room?   ☐ Yes   ☐ No

Are you familiar with the types of chat rooms and Web sites your child visits?   ☐ Yes   ☐ No

Do you talk to your child about the best use of the Internet?   ☐ Frequently   ☐ Sometimes   ☐ Never

Have you purchased blocking software that prevents your child from visiting inappropriate/ pornographic Web sites?   ☐ Yes   ☐ No

Books

Do you read to your child or does your child read at least once a day?   ☐ Yes   ☐ No

Do you provide your child with a variety of reading materials?   ☐ Yes   ☐ No

Do you talk to your child about the books that you read together or that your child is reading on his or her own?   ☐ Frequently   ☐ Sometimes   ☐ Never

Do you have any specific concerns about:

Your child's use of tobacco,
alcohol, or illicit drugs?   ☐ Yes   ☐ No

Your child's own sense
of body image or sexuality?   ☐ Yes   ☐ No

Displays of aggressive
behavior or use of foul
language?   ☐ Yes   ☐ No

The information contained in this publication should not be used as a substitute for the medical care and advice of your pediatrician. There may be variations in treatment that your pediatrician may recommend based on individual facts and circumstances.

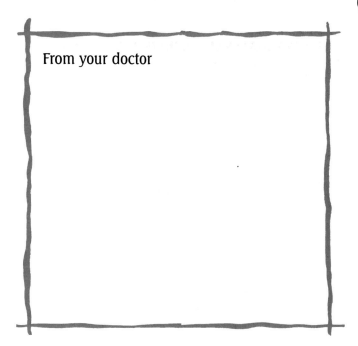

From your doctor

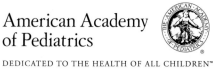

American Academy
of Pediatrics

DEDICATED TO THE HEALTH OF ALL CHILDREN™

The American Academy of Pediatrics is an organization of 55,000 primary care pediatricians, pediatric medical subspecialists, and pediatric surgical specialists dedicated to the health, safety, and well-being of infants, children, adolescents, and young adults.

American Academy of Pediatrics
PO Box 747
Elk Grove Village, IL 60009-0747
Web site — http://www.aap.org

Copyright ©2000   American Academy of Pediatrics

©2002 American Academy of Pediatrics

The Ratings Game:
CHOOSING YOUR CHILD'S ENTERTAINMENT

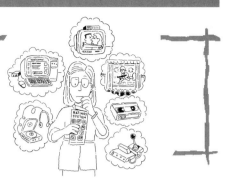

Even before reaching middle school age, your child will spend tens of thousands of hours watching television, movies, and videos; listening to the radio, CDs, and cassettes; playing video and computer games; and surfing the Internet. But TV, movies, music, games, and the Internet are much more than entertainment. They are a source of information, and they help teach our children about the world in which we live. As children have more and more entertainment options to choose from, it becomes even more important for parents to become involved in making choices.

To help parents make informed choices, many entertainment companies are now using *ratings systems*. Movies have used ratings for years, but ratings are now being given to TV programs, video and computer games, and music. Ratings are designed to give parents more information about the content of the program, movie, music, or game. The ratings are usually based on the amount of violence, sex, nudity, strong language, or drug use your child will see or hear.

Why do we need ratings?

Ratings have become more common because research has shown how much children are influenced by what they see and hear, especially at very young ages. The effects don't seem to go away as the child gets older. One study of 8-year-old boys found that those who watched violent TV programs growing up were most likely to be involved in aggressive, violent behavior by age 18 and serious criminal behavior by age 30.

Young children who see violent acts in movies, shows, and games may not be able to tell the difference between "make-believe" and real life. They may not understand that *real* violence hurts and kills people. When the "good guys" or heroes use violence, children may learn that it is okay to use force to solve problems. Younger children may even become more afraid of the world around them.

Most entertainment companies are now providing ratings for their products. However, it is up to you to protect your child from the effects of exposure to violence, as well as sex, drug use, and even strong language. Look for ratings and warning labels. Use them to make smart decisions about what your child sees and hears. Ratings can be useful tools, but watch and listen *with* your child to discuss the content and meaning of the shows they watch, music they hear, or games they play.

Movies

When you think of ratings systems, the one used by the Motion Picture Association of America (MPAA) probably comes to mind. Though movie producers are not required to use the rating system, most movies that make it to the big screen have one of the following MPAA ratings:

G | GENERAL AUDIENCES — All Ages Admitted — Contains very little violence; no nudity, sex, or drug use. May contain some tobacco or alcohol use.

PG | PARENTAL GUIDANCE SUGGESTED — SOME MATERIAL MAY NOT BE SUITABLE FOR CHILDREN — May contain adult themes, alcohol and tobacco use, some profanity, violence, or brief nudity.

PG-13 | PARENTS STRONGLY CAUTIONED — Some Material May Be Inappropriate for Children Under 13 — Contains more intense themes, violence, nudity, sex, or language than a PG film, but not as much as an R. May contain drug use scenes.

R | RESTRICTED — UNDER 17 REQUIRES ACCOMPANYING PARENT OR ADULT GUARDIAN — Contains adult material. May include graphic language, violence, sex, nudity, and drug use.

NC-17 — NO ONE 17 AND UNDER ADMITTED — Children should not be admitted. Contains violence, sex, drug abuse, and other behavior that most parents would consider off-limits to children.

This is the oldest, most well-known, and widely used rating system for any form of media, but it is not perfect. For example, the ratings divide children into three age groups (under 13, 13 to 17, and over 17). However, a PG movie that contains some violence or nudity will have a much different effect on a 5-year-old child than it would a 12-year-old. Find out as much as you can about a movie before letting your child watch. Read reviews, check the Internet, talk to friends who have seen it. Choose carefully when considering movies with PG-13, PG, and sometimes even G ratings. If you aren't sure, see the movie first, and decide if it is appropriate for your child.

Videos

Along with cable television, the use of VCRs and videotaped movies in the home has made it much more difficult to control your child's viewing. Children have easier access to R-rated movies than ever before. Most video stores have no way to prevent a child from renting or buying inappropriate material. Younger children are also more likely to watch the same movies many times. Just as a young child will sit and watch her favorite television show every day, she is just as likely to watch the same videotape over and over.

Movies from the video store are rated with the same system used for movies in the theater. Read the package and pay attention to the rating. Decide what movies are appropriate for your child depending on her age and maturity. Set rules and apply them at home, as well as at the theater. Talk to the manager of your local video store about setting stricter rules for renting videos rated anything more than G. For suggestions of quality children's videos, contact the Coalition for Quality Children's Media at 505/989-8076 or on the Web at http://www.cqcm.org.

Keep in mind, *children under 17 years of age should not be allowed to view R-rated movies.* The rating states that children under 17 should not view these films without a parent or guardian; however, these films often contain graphic violence, drug use, sex, nudity, and inappropriate language. Even though the rating system seems to suggest a younger child may watch an R-rated movie when a parent is present, it is *not* recommended they watch at all. *No child 17 years of age or under should be allowed to watch a movie rated NC-17.*

Television

The television industry has adopted a set of ratings called the TV Parental Guidelines to help parents select programs for their children. Channels that have agreed to use the ratings show them for 15 seconds at the start of a program. They may also be found in your local TV listings. The ratings apply to all TV programs, *except news and sports.* (Keep in mind that news programs often contain violence that may be inappropriate for viewing by young children.) Instead of flipping through channels, use the following ratings to help you and your child choose TV shows:

 The program is suitable for all children. Whether animated or live-action, it is designed for a young audience, including ages 2 to 6. The program is not expected to frighten younger children.

 The program is suitable for children aged 7 and older who can tell the difference between make-believe and reality. The program may contain mild fantasy or comedic violence that could frighten children under 7.

 The program is suitable for children aged 7 and older who can tell the difference between make-believe and reality. The program contains fantasy violence more intense or combative than TV-Y7. Violence is the central theme of the program and the fighting is presented in an exciting way. Violent acts are glorified, and violence is used as an acceptable, effective way to solve a problem. Programs can be cartoons, live-action, or a combination of both.

 General Audience. Most parents would find this program suitable for all ages. There is little or no violence, no strong language, and little or no sexual content.

    Parental guidance is suggested. The program contains material that parents may find unsuitable for younger children. It may have an inappropriate theme, and it may contain moderate violence (V), some sexual content (S), and strong language (L) or suggestive dialogue between characters (D).

    Parents are strongly cautioned. The program contains some material that many parents would find unsuitable for children under 14. It contains intense violence (V), sexual content (S), and strong language (L) or intensely suggestive dialogue (D).

 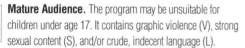   **Mature Audience.** The program may be unsuitable for children under age 17. It contains graphic violence (V), strong sexual content (S), and/or crude, indecent language (L).

Starting in 2000, all new television sets with screens **13 inches or larger** will have a computer device called the *v-chip*. The v-chip allows parents to block programs from their televisions. TVs with screens smaller than 13 inches will not have the v-chip. If your child is allowed to watch TV alone, choose a set that is at least 13 inches so you can use the v-chip to block programs.

TV for toddlers

The first two years of your child's life are especially important in the growth and development of your child's brain. During this time, children need good, positive interaction with other children and adults. Too much television can negatively affect early brain development. This is especially true at younger ages, when learning to talk and play with others is so important.

Until more research is done about the effects of TV on very young children, the American Academy of Pediatrics does not recommend television for children aged 2 or younger. For older children, the Academy recommends no more than 1 to 2 hours per day of educational, nonviolent programs.

Computer games

The Entertainment Software Rating Board (ESRB) assigns ratings* to games for personal computers and home video systems. The ratings are as follows:

 Early Childhood. Suitable for ages 3 and older. Does not contain inappropriate material.

 Everyone. Suitable for ages 6 and older. May contain minimal violence, some comic mischief (such as slapstick comedy), or some crude language. (E is a new rating. Older games may still carry the rating K-A, Kids to Adults, which is also suitable for ages 6 and older.)

 Teen. Suitable for ages 13 and older. May contain violence, mild or strong language, or suggestive themes.

 Mature. Suitable for ages 17 and older. May contain more intense violence, language, or sexual themes.

 Adults Only. Suitable only for adults. May contain graphic sex or violence. Not intended to be rented or sold to anyone under the age of 18.

 Rating Pending. Game has not yet been rated.

On the back of the game package, the ESRB also includes a brief description of the content to give parents more information about the game. For example, an EC rating might come with the description "Edutainment," which means educational entertainment. Other content descriptors include the following:

- Informational
- Suggestive themes
- Comic mischief
- Mature sexual themes
- Mild violence
- Strong sexual content
- Violence
- Mild language
- Realistic violence
- Strong language
- Nudity
- Hate speech
- Use of tobacco and alcohol
- Strong hate speech

* Please be advised that the ESRB rating icons, "EC," "K–A," "E," "T," "M," "AO," "RP" are copyrighted works and certification marks owned by the Interactive Digital Software Association and the Entertainment Software Rating Board and may only be used with their permission and authority. Under no circumstances may the rating icons be self-applied to any product that has not been rated by the ESRB. For information regarding whether a product has been rated by the ESRB, please call the ESRB at (212) 759-0700 or 1-800-771-3772.

A word about...the Internet

The rapid growth of the Internet has placed knowledge and information at your child's fingertips. However, not all information on the Internet is appropriate for children. Anyone can set up a Web site and post information on any topic. You might be surprised how easy it is for your child to locate information that contains graphic sex, violence, or drug use.

Internet companies are still in the process of creating a universal ratings system for material posted on the Net. Until a system is created, there are many options available to parents. The Recreational Software Advisory Council on the Internet (RSAC*i*) offers a system to Web site developers on a voluntary basis. Most Internet browsers are already set up to use RSAC*i*. For more information, visit the Web site at http://www.rsac.org. The Entertainment Software Rating Board offers a rating system as well. Visit http://www.esrb.org to find out more.

There also are many services and software products available that allow parents to block or filter inappropriate Web sites and material. Ask your Internet service provider about site blocking, restrictions on e-mail, and other controls for parents.

It is very important that your child have your help and supervision when using the Internet. Even if your child is an experienced computer user, he needs your involvement and your supervision.

Computer game companies rate their games voluntarily, but most now use the ESRB system. Some games may also carry a rating by the Recreational Software Advisory Council (RSAC). Their system assigns a score based on a scale of 0 to 4 in the categories of Violence, Sex, Nudity, and Language. The rating score appears on the front of the game package.

Coin-operated video games

All new coin-operated video games are labeled with a Parental Advisory Disclosure Message that appears in the artwork of the game or on a color sticker on the machine. The labels come in the following colors:

Green — Suitable for all ages
Yellow — Mild
Red — Strong

Yellow and red stickers indicate content in one of the following four categories:
- Animated violence
- Life Like violence
- Sexual content
- Language

For example, a yellow sticker with the description "Sexual Content Mild" means the game contains sexually suggestive references or material. A red sticker that reads "Life Like Violence Strong" means the game contains scenes involving human-like characters in combat situations that may result in pain, injury, or death to one or many characters.

SEXUAL CONTENT MILD	LIFE LIKE VIOLENCE STRONG

Music

The Recording Industry Association of America has a Parental Advisory Program that is also voluntary. Each record company uses its own guidelines to determine which recordings will be labeled with a parental advisory.

If a record company decides to use the advisory, it is required to use a standard black and white logo reading

 The logo is smaller than 1-inch square and should be located on the front of the CD, cassette, album, or videocassette.

If you have any doubt about the content of lyrics in the music your child chooses, listen to the music before allowing your child to buy it. Many music stores will allow you to listen to CDs before buying. Check out the Internet too. Most record companies and recording artists have their own Web sites where you may be able to read song lyrics or even hear samples of recent recordings.

Protect your child

Your child will be exposed to all forms of entertainment and media at a very young age. By helping your child develop the skills to question what they see and hear in the media, you can protect your child from the many negative messages in movies, television, music, and games. Follow these guidelines:

1. **Use the ratings.** Help children and teens choose movies, shows, videos, music, Web sites, and computer and video games that are appropriate for their ages and interests. Get into the habit of checking the content ratings and parental advisories for all media. Use the ratings as a guide, but watching and listening yourself are the best ways to decide which movies, shows, games, or CDs are suitable for your child. *Keep in mind that companies do not have to use ratings. Beware of products that have no ratings, and find out more about them before letting your child watch, play, or listen.*

2. **Set time limits.** Limit your child's total screen time to no more than 1 or 2 hours per day. This includes TV, movies, video and computer games, and surfing the Internet. Consider using a timer to enforce the rule.

3. **Watch *with* your child.** Whenever possible, participate in your child's TV, video game, music, or computer time, and discuss what she sees and hears. When you share your child's experiences, you can talk to her about the messages she is receiving. Discuss how the messages compare with the values you are teaching your child.

4. **Keep TV sets, VCRs, video games, and computers out of your child's bedroom.** Instead, put them where you can be involved and monitor the activity. Do not let your child watch TV while doing homework or eating meals.

5. **Know how much is too much.** It is easy to overlook the messages children are getting from media. There are signs that TV, movies, or games may be having too much of an impact on your child's behavior. If your child has a problem with any of the following behaviors, talk to your pediatrician, and take a look at how much TV, movies, or computer games may be affecting him:
   - Poor school performance
   - Hitting or pushing other kids often
   - Aggressively talking back to adults
   - Frequent nightmares
   - Increased eating of unhealthy foods
   - Smoking, drinking, or other drug use

6. **Voice your opinion.** Let the people who produce children's entertainment know how you feel about their products. Networks, sponsors, and game companies pay attention to letters and calls from the public. If you think a product or program is offensive, let them know about it. Encourage publishers of television guides to print ratings.

7. **Give your child other options.** Watching TV or playing video games can become a habit for your child. Help your child find other things to do with his time, such as the following:
   - Playing
   - Reading
   - Physical activity and sports
   - Learning a hobby, sport, instrument, or an art
   - Other activities with family, friends, or neighbors

8. **Set a good example.** You are the most important role model in your child's life. Limiting your own TV and movie viewing and choosing programs carefully will help your child do the same.

9. **Get more information.** The following people and places can provide you with more information:
   - **Your pediatrician.** Ask about the following brochures from the American Academy of Pediatrics (AAP):
     Television and the Family
     The Internet and Your Family
     Understanding the Impact of Media on Children and Teens
   - **Your local Parent/Teacher Association (PTA)**
   - **Public service groups** publish newsletters that review programs and games and give tips on how to make entertainment a positive experience for you and your child. Check with your pediatrician or the AAP Web site.
   - **Parents of your child's friends and classmates** can also be helpful. Talk with other parents and agree to enforce similar rules about entertainment.

For more information on the AAP Media Matters campaign, visit the AAP Web site at http://www.aap.org. Or, contact any of the following organizations:

Coin-Operated Video Games

American Amusement Machine Association (AAMA)
450 E Higgins Rd, Suite 201
Elk Grove Village, IL 60007
847/290-9088
Web site: http://www.coin-op.org

Amusement and Music Operators Association (AMOA)
450 E Higgins Rd, Suite 202
Elk Grove Village, IL 60007
847/290-5320
Web site: http://www.amoa.com

International Association of Family Amusement Centers (IAFAC)
36 Symonds Rd
Hillsboro, NH 03244
603/464-6498

Computer Games

Entertainment Software Rating Board (ESRB)
845 Third Ave
New York, NY 10022
212/759-0700
Web site: http://www.esrb.org

Internet

Recreational Software Advisory Council (RSAC)
3460 Olney-Laytonsville Rd, Suite 202
Olney, MD 20832
301/260-8669
Web site: http://www.rsac.org

Movies

Motion Picture Association of America (MPAA)
15503 Ventura Blvd
Encino, CA 91436
818/995-6600
Web site: http://www.mpaa.org

Music

Recording Industry Association of America (RIAA)
1330 Connecticut Ave NW, Suite 300
Washington, DC 20036
202/775-0101
Web site: http://www.riaa.com

Television

National Association of Broadcasters (NAB)
1771 N St NW
Washington, DC 20036
202/429-5300
Web site: http://www.nab.org

TV Parental Guidelines Monitoring Board
PO Box 14097
Washington, DC 20004
202/879-9364
Web site: http://www.tvguidelines.org

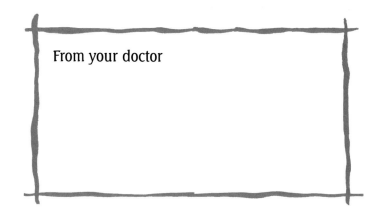

From your doctor

American Academy of Pediatrics

DEDICATED TO THE HEALTH OF ALL CHILDREN™

The American Academy of Pediatrics is an organization of 55,000 primary care pediatricians, pediatric medical subspecialists, and pediatric surgical specialists dedicated to the health, safety, and well-being of infants, children, adolescents, and young adults.

American Academy of Pediatrics
PO Box 747
Elk Grove Village, IL 60009-0747
Web site — http://www.aap.org

Sex Education:
A Bibliography of Educational Materials for Children, Adolescents, and Their Families

This bibliography was prepared by the Committee on Adolescence of the American Academy of Pediatrics to assist health professionals in recommending educational materials on sexuality for children, adolescents, and their families. This bibliography includes material thought to be factually correct and suitable for the pediatric setting. Materials listed are limited to booklets, pamphlets, and fact sheets that are free or low cost.

Sex Education Bibliography

Each publication listing includes a brief synopsis of the content and the Committee's estimation of age and/or sex suitability. Developmental levels follow these approximations:

"preteen"	= late childhood (late elementary grades)
"young teen"	= early adolescence (middle/junior high school)
"midteen"	= middle adolescence (junior/senior high school)
"older teen"	= late adolescence (senior high school/college)
"adult"	= young adults, parents (college level)

Addresses for sources and other purchasing information are found at the end of the bibliography with sources listed alphabetically.

The Committee will maintain this bibliography in a fashion that is both current and in accord with the needs of the Academy's membership. We welcome comments about the bibliography and information on new educational materials that might be included in future editions.

AIDS

Abstinence & HIV
Basic information about HIV transmission and benefits to abstinence.
Pamphlet for all teens, adults.
ETR Associates.

AIDS...What We Need to Know
Basic facts about HIV infection and AIDS.
Pamphlet for young teens, midteens (appealing style).
March of Dimes.

HIV ABC's
Facts about AIDS prevention.
Pamphlet for young teens, midteens.
ETR Associates.

HIV and AIDS—Facts for Young People
Facts about HIV infection, AIDS symptoms, and prevention.
Illustrated booklet for preteens to midteens.
Channing L. Bete Co, Inc.

HIV: Antibody Test
Basic information about many aspects of HIV.
Series of pamphlets for older teens, adults.
ETR Associates.

HIV: Think About It
Basic information in simple language.
Bilingual pamphlet for teens, adults with limited reading skills.
ETR Associates.

How to Talk to Your Children About AIDS
Basic facts; suggestions for teaching children at various ages.
Pamphlet for parents.
SIECUS.

How to Talk to Your Teens and Children About HIV/AIDS
Facts about HIV/AIDS; guidelines for teaching children at various ages.
Pamphlet for parents. (Spanish)
The National PTA.

Know the Facts about HIV and AIDS
Facts about HIV/AIDS; guidelines for teaching children at various ages.
Pamphlet for parents.
American Academy of Pediatrics.

Talking with Your Child About AIDS—From Preschool Through High School
Basic facts about HIV/AIDS; possible questions and proposed answers for developmental stages K-teens.
Pamphlet for parents.
Channing L. Bete Co, Inc.

Teens and HIV! Why Risk It?
Basic information about HIV transmission and prevention.
Pamphlet for young to mid-teens. (Spanish)
ETR Associates.

Teens Talk About HIV & AIDS
Basic facts about HIV/AIDS transmission and prevention.
Illustrated pamphlet for all teens.
Channing L. Bete Co, Inc.

What Is Safer Sex?
Basic guidelines for behaviors that reduce risk for AIDS.
Pamphlet for sexually active teens, adults.
ETR Associates.

What Young People Should Know About AIDS
Facts about transmission, symptoms, risk factors, prevention, treatment.
Illustrated booklet for midteens, older teens.
Channing L. Bete Co, Inc.

Young People Get AIDS
Facts about HIV/AIDS transmission and prevention, stresses everyone is at risk.
Illustrated pamphlet for all teens.
Channing L. Bete Co, Inc.

Breast Care

Why Now?
Illustrated guide to breast self-examination; facts about Pap test.
Pamphlet for all ages (No. 2039).
American Cancer Society.

Contraception

Birth Control Facts
Fold-out chart comparing major methods.
Pamphlet for teens, adults.
ETR Associates.

Birth Control for You and Your Partner
Basic facts about contraception.
Pamphlet for older teens, adults.
Channing L. Bete Co, Inc.

Birth Control Pills
Use, method of action, side effects, complications.
Pamphlet for midteens, older teens.
American College of Obstetricians and Gynecologists.

Birth Control: Talking With Your Daughter
Guidelines for communication about female responsibilities, best methods.
Pamphlet for parents.
ETR Associates.

Birth Control: Talking With Your Parents
Guidelines for communication about sexuality, contraception.
Pamphlet for midteens.
ETR Associates.

Birth Control: Talking With Your Partner
Guidelines for communication, self-assertiveness.
Pamphlet for teens, adults.
ETR Associates.

Birth Control: Talking With Your Son
Guidelines for communication about male responsibilities, male methods.
Pamphlet for parents.
ETR Associates.

The Condom
Facts about correct use, effectiveness.
Pamphlet for teens, adults.
ETR Associates.

Condoms: Talking With Your Partner
Guidelines for communication, responses to common objections.
Pamphlet for teens, adults.
ETR Associates.

Condoms: Think About It
Basic facts about correct condom use.
Illustrated bilingual pamphlet for young to mid-teens.
ETR Associates.

If You Are A Man...Birth Control
Facts about male responsibilities, prevention methods.
Pamphlet for teen boys, adults.
ETR Associates.

The Morning After Pill
Facts about use, method of action, side effects.
Pamphlet for all teens.
Planned Parenthood of Minnesota.

Sex and Birth Control
Basic information about birth control.
Pamphlet for midteens.
ETR Associates.

Sex Is Safer With a Condom
Facts about correct condom use.
Illustrated booklet for mid to older teens.
Channing L. Bete Co, Inc.

What Everyone Should Know About Contraception
Basic facts about conception, benefits of contraception, all methods.
Illustrated booklet for midteens.
Channing L. Bete Co, Inc.

Health Care for Men

For Men Only
Illustrated pamphlet to self-examination.
Pamphlet for all teens.
American Cancer Society.

Pregnancy and Parenting

Are You Ready? Am I Parent Material?; Babies Change Your Life!; Babies and Relationships; Pregnancy: Get Real!; The Truth About Babies; To Be Pregnant
Explains pros/cons of pregnancy, parenthood, and babies.
Series of pamphlets for all teens.
ETR Associates.

Deciding to Wait: Guidelines for Teens— Facts You Should Know About Teenage Pregnancy
Basic facts about health risks, prenatal care.
Fact sheet for midteens. (Spanish)
March of Dimes.

Making the Right Choice: Facts Young People Need to Know on Preventing Pregnancy
Offers advice to teens on how to postpone sex and avoid pregnancy.
Pamphlet for all teens.
American Academy of Pediatrics.

Pregnancy: Am I at Risk? A Birth Control Checklist
Checklist to determine risk of unplanned pregnancy, with advice on do's/don'ts.
Pamphlet for all teens.
ETR Associates.

Pregnant?
Discusses choices and feelings involved with an unplanned pregnancy.
Booklet for all teens.
ETR Associates.

Special Needs of Pregnant Teens
Detailed information about prenatal care and the special needs of pregnant teens.
Pamphlet for all teens and adults.
American College of Obstetricians and Gynecologists.

What You Should Know About Teen Parenthood
Facts about parental responsibilities, childbirth preparation, parenting skills, support services.
Illustrated booklet for midteens.
Channing L. Bete Co, Inc.

What You Should Know About Teen Pregnancy
Facts about sexual responsibility, challenges of parenthood, physiology of pregnancy, contraception, pregnancy diagnosis, and options.
Illustrated booklet for midteens.
Channing L. Bete Co, Inc.

Puberty

As Boys Grow Up
Basic facts about puberty, pregnancy.
Booklet for preteens, young teens.
Channing L. Bete Co, Inc.

As Girls Grow Up
Basic facts about puberty, pregnancy.
Booklet for preteens, young teens.
Channing L. Bete Co, Inc.

From Boy to Man—What Boys Should Know About Growing Up
Facts about puberty, pregnancy.
Illustrated booklet for preteens to young teens.
Channing L. Bete Co, Inc.

From Girl to Woman—What Girls Should Know About Growing Up
Facts about puberty, pregnancy.
Illustrated booklet for preteens to young teens.
Channing L. Bete Co, Inc.

Growing Up Boys/El Crecimiento de los Muchachos
Basic facts about puberty, sexual maturation, feelings.
Bilingual booklet for preteen boys.
Planned Parenthood of Southern Arizona.

Growing Up Girls/El Crecimiento de las Niñas
Basic facts about puberty, sexual maturation, menstruation, feelings.
Bilingual booklet for preteen girls.
Planned Parenthood of Southern Arizona.

Having Your Period
Basic facts about puberty, menstruation in simple language.
Pamphlet for preteen girls.
Planned Parenthood Federation of America.

Menstruation
Basic facts about menstruation.
Pamphlet for preteen girls.
Parlay International.

Menstruation: Talking With Your Daughter
Basic facts about menstruation.
Pamphlet for parents and preteen girls.
ETR Associates.

Puberty: Information for Girls and Boys
Discusses physical and emotional changes that occur during puberty.
Brochure for parents and preteens/young teens.
American Academy of Pediatrics.

Reproductive Health Care

The Abnormal Pap
Describes what happens in the event of an abnormal pap test and possible courses of treatment.
Pamphlet for all teens.
ETR Associates.

Pelvic Examination
Facts about the pelvic exam.
Booklet for young teen/older teen women.
Parlay International.

Pelvic Exam: Talking With Your Daughter

Facts about gynecologic examination; guidelines for parental support.
Pamphlet for parents and young teens.
ETR Associates.

The Pelvic Exam

Describes the pelvic exam procedure and answers common questions.
Brochure for parents and all teens.
American Academy of Pediatrics.

Your Pap Test

Basic facts about the pap test.
Pamphlet for all teens.
ETR Associates.

Sexual Abuse

Child Sexual Abuse Prevention Tips to Parents

Guidelines for communication, response to abuse, detection.
Pamphlet for adults. (Spanish)
National Clearinghouse on Child Abuse
and Neglect Information.

Child Sexual Abuse: What It Is and How to Prevent It—Guidelines for Parents

Detailed facts about causes, consequences, detection, prevention.
Pamphlet for adults.
American Academy of Pediatrics.

Stop It! What to Do If Someone Touches You and You Don't Like It

Facts about good touches and bad touches.
Booklet for younger children and preteens.
ETR Associates.

Touch Talk! What to Do If Someone Touches You and You Don't Like It

Facts about good touches and bad touches.
Booklet for younger children and preteens.
ETR Associates.

What Everyone Should Know About the Sexual Abuse of Children

Basic facts about nature, etiology, and consequences of sexual abuse;
guidelines for reporting, assisting child, teaching prevention.
Booklet for older teens, adults.
Channing L. Bete Co, Inc.

Sexuality: For Parents

How to Talk to Your Teen About the Facts of Life

Guidelines for communication; basic facts about puberty, menstruation, con-
traception, common parent and teen concerns; guide to other resources.
Pamphlet for parents.
Planned Parenthood Federation of America.

Sex: Talking With Your Child

Guide to early psychosexual development, common concerns; strategies
for communication.
Pamphlet for parents.
ETR Associates.

Sexual Responsibility: Talking With Your Teen

Guidelines for discussing sexuality, decision making, and responsible behavior.
Pamphlet for parents.
ETR Associates.

Talking to Adolescents About Sex

Guidelines for discussing sexuality.
Booklet for parents.
Channing L. Bete Co, Inc.

Talking With Your Child About Sex

Guidelines for communication, especially with young children.
Pamphlet for parents.
National PTA.

Talking With Your Teens About Sex

Guidelines for communication with older children and adolescents.
Pamphlet for parents.
National PTA.

Teaching Your Children About Sexuality

Guide to sexual development; guidelines for communication.
Pamphlet for parents.
American College of Obstetricians and Gynecologists.

Tips for Parents of Adolescents

Offers suggestions on communicating with teens and discussing important
issues such as dating, tobacco, and drugs.
Brochure for parents.
American Academy of Pediatrics.

Sexuality: For Teenagers

About Dealing With Sexual Pressure

Facts about sexual pressures, feelings, self-respect, with tips for
resisting pressure.
Booklet for all teens.
Channing L. Bete Co, Inc.

Abstinence: Think About It

Describes benefits to abstinence.
Bilingual pamphlet for all teens.
ETR Associates.

Being a Teenager: You and Your Sexuality

Facts about physical changes, feelings, relationships, contraception;
suggestions about decision making.
Pamphlet for midteens.
American College of Obstetricians and Gynecologists.

Deciding About Sex

Guide to decision-making process, contraception, and possible consequences.
Pamphlet for all teens.
Planned Parenthood of Minnesota.

Deciding to Wait: What You Need to Know

Explains the risks involved in sexual intercourse, the benefits of delaying sex, and how to say "no."
Brochure for all teens.
American Academy of Pediatrics.

Drinking, Drugs & Sex

Basic facts about the effects of drug use and sex.
Pamphlet for all teens.
Planned Parenthood of Minnesota.

Flirting or Harassment?

Explains how a compliment to one person can be considered an offensive remark to someone else.
Photopamphlet for all teens.
ETR Associates.

How to Be a Better Lover

Emphasizes self-respect.
Pamphlet for all teens.
USDHHS.

If You Think Saying "No" Is Tough, Just Wait 'til You Say "Yes"

Highlights consequences of sexual activity.
Pamphlet for all teens.
USDHHS.

Making Decisions About Sex

Guide to decision-making, consequences.
Booklet for all teens.
Channing L. Bete Co, Inc.

Making Decisions About Sex, Drugs and Your Health

Conversation-style information; discusses risk-taking and sex, drugs, and alcohol.
Booklet for midteens, older teens.
Krames Communications.

A Man's Guide to Sexuality

Guide to male responsibility, decision making; self-test on sexuality knowledge.
Pamphlet for midteen/older teen males.
Planned Parenthood Federation of America.

Not Everyone's Doin' It!

Sample scenario of teens deciding to wait.
Photopamphlet for all teens.
ETR Associates.

101 Ways to Say No to Sex

One hundred and one ways to help teens choose abstinence.
Pamphlets for all teens.
ETR Associates.

Rape: Am I at Risk? A Self-Protection Checklist

Checklist for determining risk of sexual assault with self-protection suggestions.
Pamphlet for all teens.
ETR Associates.

Safer Sex: Talking With Your Partner

Guidelines for communication; basic facts about AIDS prevention.
Pamphlet for older teens/adults.
ETR Associates.

Saying "No" to Sex—It Makes Sense

Emphasizes self-respect, with helpful suggestions on how to deal with sexual pressure.
Pamphlet for all teens.
Channing L. Bete Co, Inc.

Sex and Abstinence: The Decision is Yours

Describes benefits of abstinence.
Pamphlet for all teens.
ETR Associates.

Sex and You: It's Time to Start Talking

Encourages communication.
Pamphlet for all teens.
ETR Associates.

Sexual Feelings: Accepting Yourself and Others

Discusses sexual feelings and attractions, including for same sex.
Pamphlet for young teens/midteens.
ETR Associates.

Stop Acquaintance Rape

Discusses prevalence, avoidance, awareness, communication, and seeking help.
Pamphlet for midteens, older teens.
Planned Parenthood of Minnesota.

Teen Questions About Sex

Facts about puberty, sexual behaviors, contraception, pregnancy.
Booklet for midteens.
Planned Parenthood Center of Syracuse.

Teen Sex: It's Okay to Say No Way

Guidelines for decision making, saying "no."
Pamphlet with cartoon illustrations for midteens.
Planned Parenthood Federation of America.

Teen Talk
Basic facts about sexuality, feelings, relationships, pressures, decision making, supporting abstinence.
Pamphlet for all teens.
Office of Population Affairs Clearinghouse.

Teens Talk Sex
Teens of varying ages talk about their individual opinions about sex.
Pamphlet for all teens.
March of Dimes.

What is Sexual Harassment?
Teens answer questions about sexual harassment.
Photopamphlet for all teens.
ETR Associates.

What Women and Men Should Know About Date Rape
Basic facts about causes, consequences; suggestions for responsible dating behavior and self-protection.
Illustrated booklet for midteens, older teens.
Channing L. Bete Co, Inc.

Why Wait?—Two Teens Face Pressure to Have Sex
Sample scenario of teens dealing with sexual pressure.
Pamphlet for all teens.
Channing L. Bete Co, Inc.

Worth Waiting
Sample scenario of teens deciding to wait.
Photopamphlet for all teens.
ETR Associates.

You Didn't Get Pregnant. You Didn't Get AIDS. So Why Do You Feel So Bad?
Discusses the possible emotional consequences of not waiting.
Pamphlet for all teens.
USDHHS.

Sexually Transmitted Diseases

About Herpes
Basic facts about diagnosis, treatment, prevention.
Illustrated booklet for midteens.
Channing L. Bete Co, Inc.

Chlamydia
Facts about infections, complications, diagnosis, treatment.
Pamphlet for midteens, older teens, adults.
ETR Associates.

Chlamydia; Genital Herpes; Genital Warts; Sexually Transmitted Diseases
Facts about infections, complications, diagnosis, treatment.
Series of pamphlets for midteens.
Planned Parenthood of Minnesota.

Chlamydia— A Hidden Danger
Explains symptoms, transmission, treatment.
Pamphlet for all teens.
Channing L Bete Co, Inc.

Condoms and STD
Basic facts about condoms, correct use, prevention of sexually transmitted infections.
Pamphlet for teens, adults.
ETR Associates.

Condyloma
Facts about diagnosis, treatment, partner responsibilities.
Booklet for older teens (detailed color illustrations).
Krames Communications.

The Correct Use of Condoms: A Message to Teens
Basic facts about condoms, correct use, and prevention of STDs.
Pamphlet for mid to older teens and adults.
American Academy of Pediatrics.

Facts About Sexually Transmitted Diseases
Facts about six of the most common STDs, symptoms, treatment, and prevention.
Pamphlet for all teens.
Parlay International.

Find Out About STDs—It Could Save Your Life
Discusses health risks associated with sexual contact, describes some STDs, diagnosis, and treatment.
Pamphlet for all teens.
Channing L. Bete Co, Inc.

Genital Herpes
Basic facts about cause, symptoms, fetal effects, prevention.
Fact sheet for midteens.
March of Dimes.

Genital Warts; Gonorrhea; Hepatitis B; Herpes; NGU (Nongonococcal Urethritis); PID; Syphilis
Basic facts about causes, symptoms, fetal effects, prevention, and treatment.
Series of pamphlets for all teens.
ETR Associates.

Genital Warts—What You Need to Know
Explains causes, treatment, and how to avoid transmission.
Pamphlet for all teens.
Channing L Bete Co, Inc.

Herpes; Overcoming a Viral Assault
Facts about diagnosis, prevention, coping with disease.
Booklet for older teens, adults (detailed color illustrations).
Krames Communications.

How to Prevent Sexually Transmitted Diseases
Detailed information about STDs.
Pamphlet for older teens.
American College of Obstetricians and Gynecologists.

Protect Yourself From STDs

Discusses the causes and prevention of STDs.
Booklet for midteens, older teens.
Channing L. Bete Co, Inc.

Sex and STD: Are You at Risk?

Basic information about STDs and prevention.
Pamphlet for all teens.
ETR Associates.

STD: Am I at Risk? A Self-Protection Checklist

Checklist to determine risk of STD contraction, advice on do's/don'ts.
Pamphlet for all teens.
ETR Associates.

STD Facts

Basic facts in general, facts about many specific infections.
Fold-out chart. Pamphlet for teens, adults.
ETR Associates.

STD, You and Others

Basic instructions about treatment of infection, compliance with medical recommendations, and communication with partner.
Pamphlet for teens, adults.
ETR Associates.

STDs: Sexually Transmitted Diseases

Common myths and facts, typical symptoms in each sex, general risks; facts about major infections, including AIDS.
Booklet for midteens, older teens, adults (detailed color illustrations).
Krames Communications.

STD: What You Need to Know

Basic facts about symptoms and prevention.
Booklet for all teens. (Spanish)
Education Programs Associates.

What Everyone Should Know About Chlamydia

Basic facts about symptoms, complications, diagnosis, treatment, prevention.
Illustrated booklet for midteens.
Channing L. Bete Co, Inc.

What Everyone Should Know About STDs

Basic facts about STDs in general, major infections, prevention, medical care.
Illustrated booklet for midteens.
Channing L. Bete Co, Inc.

What You Should Know About Condoms and STDS

Describes various STDs and prevention.
Illustrated booklet for mid to older teens, adults. (Spanish)
Krames Communications.

What You Should Know About Genital Warts

Describes the causes, symptoms, treatments, and prevention.
Booklet for midteens, older teens.
Channing L. Bete Co, Inc.

What You Should Know About STDs

Describes the most common STDs and discusses symptoms, effects on health, and treatment.
Pamphlet for older teens, adults.
March of Dimes.

Other Resources

Child Sexual Abuse: Prevention, Education, and Treatment

An annotated bibliography of available print materials regarding child sexual abuse.
Bibliography for parents and older teens.
SIECUS.

Growing Up

An annotated bibliography of books about sexuality for children and adolescents.
Bibliography for parents.
SIECUS.

HIV/AIDS

An annotated bibliography profiling resources in HIV/AIDS.
Bibliography for older teens, adults.
SIECUS.

How to Talk to Your Children About Sexuality and Other Important Facts

An annotated bibliography for parents on available sex education materials.
Bibliography for parents.
SIECUS.

Information to Assist in Selecting and Ordering Educational Materials

Addresses are provided for all organizations whose materials are listed in this bibliography. Some quantity prices are included for comparison of anticipated costs of materials. Prices, purchasing policies, and publication availability change frequently. Free catalogs and price lists should be requested for current information about quantity purchase, shipping/handling expenses, and imprinting. Many of these catalogs list materials on other topics that would be useful for the practice setting.

American Academy of Pediatrics

PO Box 927, Elk Grove Village, IL 60009-0927.
Pamphlets at $24.95/$29.95 per 100 (members/nonmembers) plus handling;
single copies free (send a self-addressed, stamped envelope to Dept C).

American Cancer Society, Inc.

625 North Court, Suite 280, Palatine, IL 60067-8162 (800/ACS-2345).
Limited quantities free.

American College of Obstetricians and Gynecologists

Resource Center, 409 12th St, SW, Washington, DC 20024-2188. Contact the Resource Center for a current price list and list of available titles; samples free. Professional materials are also available.

Channing L. Bete Co. Inc.

200 State Rd, South Deerfield, MA 01373-0200.
Samples free; unit pricing based on total quantity ordered—call for pricing 1-800-628-7733.
Many in Spanish.

Education Programs Associates

1 W Campbell Ave, Suite 40, Campbell, CA 95008-1039. Pamphlets 1-500/$.40-$.70 each, plus shipping/handling (add 14% for orders $0-$99, add 12% for $100-$299.99, add 10% for $300-$499.99, add 8% for $501+).

ETR Associates

PO Box 1830, Santa Cruz, CA 95061-1830. Call for price information 800/321-4407. Some in Spanish.

Krames Communications

1100 Grundy Ln, San Bruno, CA 94066-3030. Booklets $1.25-$1.95 each for 25-199 plus shipping/handling; limited samples free. Some available in Spanish.

March of Dimes Birth Defects Foundation

1275 Mamaroneck Ave, White Plains, NY 10605. Packets of 50 - $4-$8/packet, plus shipping/handling, 800/367-6630; limited samples free 914/997-4720. Some in Spanish.

National Clearinghouse on Child Abuse and Neglect Information

PO Box 1182, Washington, DC 20013. Single copies free; some available for cost of reproduction. Some in Spanish.

National PTA

National PTA Orders, 330 N Wabash Ave, Suite 2100, Chicago, IL, 60611-3690 (312/670-6782). Send $1 (for shipping/handling) to receive the catalog. Members receive discounts on order.

Office of Population Affairs Clearinghouse

PO Box 30686, Bethesda, MD 20824-0686; 301/654-6190. Limited quantities free.

Parlay International

5835 Doyle Street, #111, Box 8817, Emeryville, CA 94662-0817. Packets of 50—$20/packet for 1-5, $16/packet for 6-19, $14/packet for 20-49 plus shipping/handling; samples free. 800/457-2752

Planned Parenthood Center of Syracuse, Inc.

1120 E Genesee St, Syracuse, NY 13210-1994. Booklets $.65-$.90 each for 1-9, $.50-$.75 each for 10-99, $.45-$.60 each for 100-499, $.40-$.50 each for 500-999, $.25-$.35 each for 1000 or more plus shipping/handling.

Planned Parenthood Federation of America, Inc.

Attn: Marketing, 810 Seventh Ave, New York, NY 10019. Pamphlets $34-$38 per 100 plus shipping/handling; samples $1-$3 each. Some in Spanish.

Planned Parenthood of Minnesota

The Resource Center, 1200 Lagoon Ave, Dept. 300, Minneapolis, MN 55408. Booklets $.40-$.70 each for 50-199, $.30-$.60 each for 200 or more; samples free.

Planned Parenthood of Southern Arizona, Inc.

127 S Fifth Ave, Tucson, AZ 85701-2091. Pamphlets $.35-$.95 each for 2-99, $.30-$.85 each for 100-999 plus shipping/handling. Some in Spanish.

SIECUS
(Sex Information and Education Council of the United States)

130 W 42nd St, Ste 2500, New York, NY 10036. One copy free with SAS business size envelope; $1.00/each for 2-49, $.80 each for 50-100, multiples of 100 at $.65 per hundred, multiples of 1000 at $400 per thousand.

USDHHS (US Department of Health and Human Services)

National AIDS Information Clearinghouse, PO Box 6003, Rockville, MD 20850. No cost.

COMMITTEE ON ADOLESCENCE, 1996–1997

Marianne E. Felice, MD, Chair
Suzanne Boulter, MD
David W. Kaplan, MD, MPH
Luis F. Olmedo, MD

Ellen S. Rome, MD, MPH
I. Ronald Shenker, MD
Barbara C. Staggers, MD

Liaison Representatives

Paula Hillard, MD
 American College of Obstetricians and Gynecologists
Diane Sacks, MD
 Canadian Paediatric Society
Richard Sarles, MD
 American Academy of Child and Adolescent Psychiatry

Section Liaison

Samuel Leavitt, MD
 Section on School Health

Consultant

Edward M. Gotlieb, MD

Staff

Kathleen Sanabria, MBA
Susan Wizniak

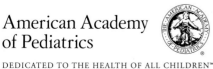

American Academy of Pediatrics

DEDICATED TO THE HEALTH OF ALL CHILDREN™

The American Academy of Pediatrics is an organization of 55,000 primary care pediatricians, pediatric medical subspecialists, and pediatric surgical specialists dedicated to the health, safety, and well-being of infants, children, adolescents, and young adults.

American Academy of Pediatrics
PO Box 747
Elk Grove Village, IL 60009-0747
Web site — http://www.aap.org

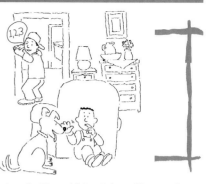

Sibling Relationships

Part I Siblings, Step-siblings, Half-siblings, and Twins

Siblings are very important to many of us. Almost 80% of children grow up with at least one brother or sister. Even though they may not get along all the time, siblings play very positive roles in each other's lives. Brothers and sisters learn their first lessons about getting along with others from one another. They are friends, playmates, and keepers of secrets. They help one another learn to relate to the outside world. They even protect and watch out for each other.

When brothers and sisters do not get along, their arguments can cause a parent to feel frustrated and angry. Each child also makes different demands on you. Your relationship with one child may lead the other to feel that you are playing favorites.

It may be hard to keep the peace in your family. This brochure offers information that may help you understand why your children get along the way they do, and how you can help them learn to live together in peace.

Why siblings get along the way they do

Many things affect relationships between brothers and sisters. Some of these are:

- Personality
- Age
- Number of years between siblings (spacing)
- Gender
- Birth order

Personality similarities and differences

Parents often wonder how children growing up in the same home with the same parents can be so different. The fact is that siblings are usually more different than alike.

Two factors affect your children's personalities—nature (what they were born with) and nurture (their experiences). Even though they have the same parents, each child's genetic makeup is different. Their experiences are also not the same. As a result, each child develops his own personality.

Some parents feel it is important to always treat each child the same way. They do not want one child to think they love the other more. Treating your children differently does not have to mean you are playing favorites. Each child is an individual, and you should treat him that way. Doing so is part of what makes each child a unique person. It is a way of showing that you appreciate how special he is.

Age, gender, birth order, and spacing

Your children's ages make a big difference in how you treat them and in how well they get along. For example, you may hug and kiss your toddler more than your school-age child. As a result, your older child may think that you love the younger sibling more. Parents should treat younger children differently than older ones, however. A toddler's needs are not the same as those of a school-age child.

Gender affects your children's relationships with each other, as well. Many parents find that children of different genders tend to get along better than do children of the same gender. Siblings of the same sex tend to compete with each other more than they do with opposite-sex siblings.

Birth order and family size also affect how children behave. The experience of an only child is different from that of a child in a larger family. Also, an older child's experience is different from a younger one's: The older child has a younger sibling, while the younger child has an older sibling. A third child has two older siblings, and so on. Because of birth order, family size, and individual experiences, no two children view the family the same way.

How your children are spaced affects how well they get along, too. Children who are less than 2 years apart often have more conflict than children who are spaced further apart. This may be because they compete over the same "turf." You might want to keep this in mind when you are planning your family.

Understanding sibling rivalry

Few things are more upsetting than children who do not get along. No matter how hard you try to keep the peace, your children are likely to fight over toys, pick on or tattle on one another, and tease and criticize each other. You may wonder, "What have I done wrong?" The answer is probably nothing. Sibling rivalry is a natural part of growing up.

Sibling rivalry between children who are under 4 years of age tends to be at its worst when they are less than 3 years apart. This is largely because preschool children still depend on their parents a great deal and have not made

---

Step-siblings and half-siblings

Step-families create another type of sibling rivalry. With current high divorce and remarriage rates, the number of step-siblings and half-siblings is growing. This creates new conflicts. When two families become one, children who barely know each other may all of a sudden share bedrooms and bathrooms. This can cause fights over toys, space, and what to watch on TV. At the same time, children are trying to get used to their parents' new marriage, new step-parents, and maybe a new house. Also, parents may decide to have more children, introducing half-siblings into the family. It is not always an easy adjustment.

Here are some ideas to cut down on problems in step-families and families with half-siblings:

- Do not expect step-siblings to spend all of their time together.
- Each child should spend some time alone with his or her own parent.
- Whenever possible, step-siblings and half-siblings should have their own rooms. If they have to share a room, however, each youngster should have her own toys and other possessions; do not force children to turn all their things into community property.
- If you and your new spouse decide to have a child together, you should be open and honest about it with your older children. Reassure them that your decision to have a child together does not mean you will love them less. Involve them in planning for the new baby as much as possible.
- Both parents should be involved in parenting each child.

friends or gotten close to other adults yet. Children who are 2 and 3 years old are also very self-centered and have a very hard time sharing their parents with siblings.

Competition between brothers and sisters can heat up as children grow older. It is often at its worst when children are between 8 and 12 years old. Siblings close in age or those who have the same interests tend to compete more.

Sometimes, especially when children are several years apart, the older one accepts and protects the younger sibling. Once the younger one grows and develops more skills and talents, however, the older child may feel "shown up" by the younger one. The older child may feel threatened or embarrassed. He may then begin to compete with the younger child, or become more aggressive toward him. The younger child, too, may become jealous about the privileges his big brother or sister gets as he or she gets older. Though you may think you know, it is often hard to tell which child is causing the problem.

In many cases, the oldest child in the family feels a greater sense of rivalry than the younger ones. A younger child may look up to his older brother or sister, but the oldest child may think his siblings disturb his privacy or threaten his special status in the family.

Preteens and teenagers can pose other problems. Younger children may resent the older ones' freedoms and privileges, and older ones may resent being asked to watch over their younger siblings. Parents should explain that there are different rules for each child based on age and degree of maturity. Although you will do your best to be fair, things may not always be *equal* for the siblings. Explain to your younger child that he will have the same privileges when he gets older. At the same time, do not make your preteen or teenager take his little brother or sister along everywhere he goes.

What parents can do about sibling rivalry

Here are some tips on managing conflict between your children:

- **Do not compare your children in front of them.** It is natural to notice differences between your children. Just try not to comment on these in front of them. It is easy for a child to think that he is not as good or as loved as his sibling when you compare them. Remember, each child is a special individual. Let each one know that.
- **As much as possible, stay out of your children's arguments.** You may have to step in and settle a spat between toddlers or preschoolers. For example, if they are arguing over blocks, you might need to split the blocks into piles for each of them. Older children will probably settle an argument peacefully if left alone. If your children try to involve you, explain that they are both responsible for creating the problem and for ending it. Do not take sides. Set guidelines on how your children can disagree and resolve their conflicts. Of course, you must get involved if the situation gets violent. Make sure your children know that you will not stand for such behavior. If there is any reason to suspect that your children may become violent, watch them closely when they are together. Preventing violence is always better than punishing after the fact, which often makes the rivalry worse. Praise your children when they solve their arguments, and reward good behavior.
- **Be fair.** Divide household chores fairly. If you must get involved in your children's arguments, listen to all sides of the story. Make a "no tattling"

rule. Give children privileges that are right for their ages, and try to be consistent. If you allowed one child to stay up until 9 o'clock at 10 years of age, the other should have the same bedtime when she is 10.

- **Respect your child's privacy.** When it is necessary to punish or scold, do it with the child alone in a quiet, private place. When possible, do not embarrass one child by scolding him in front of the others. This will only make the other child tease the one you punished.
- **Use regular family meetings for all family members to express their thoughts and feelings, as well as to plan the week's events. Give positive recognition and rewards (allowances, special privileges).**

Sibling relationships are very special. We form our earliest bonds with our brothers and sisters. No one else shares the same family history. By helping your children learn to value, love and respect their siblings, you are giving them a great gift—the gift of a lifelong friend.

Raising twins

From the very start it is important that you treat your twin babies as individuals. If they are identical, it is easy to treat them as a "package," giving them the same clothing, toys, and attention. But although they may look alike, emotionally they are very different. In order to grow up happy and secure as individuals, they need you to support their differences.

Identical and fraternal twins compete with each other and depend on each other as they grow. Sometimes one twin acts as the leader and the other the follower. Either way, most twins develop very close relationships early in life simply because they spend so much time with each other.

If you also have other children, your twin newborns may make your older children doubly jealous. Twins need huge amounts of your time and energy, and will get a lot of extra attention from friends, relatives, and strangers on the street. You can help your other children accept this by offering them "double rewards" for helping with the new babies. If you have twin newborns, it is even more important that you spend some very special time alone with the other children, doing their favorite things.

As your twins get a little older, especially if they are identical, they may choose to play only with each other. This may make their other siblings feel left out. To keep the twins from leaving other children out, urge them to play separately with other children. Also, you or their babysitter might play with just one twin, while the other plays with a sibling or friend.

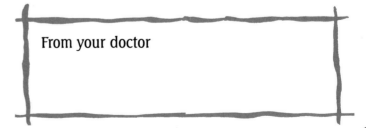

From your doctor

American Academy of Pediatrics

DEDICATED TO THE HEALTH OF ALL CHILDREN™

The American Academy of Pediatrics is an organization of 55,000 primary care pediatricians, pediatric medical subspecialists, and pediatric surgical specialists dedicated to the health, safety, and well-being of infants, children, adolescents, and young adults.

American Academy of Pediatrics
PO Box 747
Elk Grove Village, IL 60009-0747
Web site — http://www.aap.org

Copyright ©1996 American Academy of Pediatrics

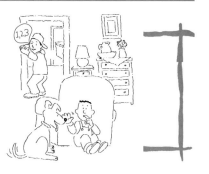

Sibling Relationships

Part II Preparing for a New Baby

Preparing your children for a new baby

A new baby brings both joys and challenges to a family. Parents are excited but they are also nervous about how their older children will react to the newborn. All sorts of questions come up: how should we tell our older children that they are going to have a baby brother or sister? Will they be jealous of the new baby? How can we make sure they will get along as they get older?

How your children react to a new baby depends largely on their ages at the time the baby is born. Knowing what to expect from each age group will make it easier to handle the changes in your family.

Ages 2 to 4

Toddlers and preschoolers may have a hard time adjusting to a new baby, especially if they are between 2 and 3 years old. At this age, your child is still very attached to you and does not yet understand about sharing you with others. Your child also may be very sensitive to changes going on around her, and may feel threatened by the idea of a new family member. Here are some suggestions for how to ease your preschooler into being a big brother or big sister.

- **Wait a while before telling your preschooler that you are going to have a baby, but do not wait too long.** A child younger than 4 will have a hard time understanding an abstract concept like an unborn baby. You should explain it to your child when you start buying nursery furniture or baby clothes, or when she starts to ask about mom's growing "stomach." Picture books for preschoolers can be very helpful. So can sibling preparation classes (ask your hospital if they offer them). Try to tell your child before she hears about the new baby from someone else.
- **Be honest.** Do not promise that things will be the same after the baby comes, because they will not be, no matter how hard you try. Explain that the baby will be cute and cuddly, but will also cry and take a lot of your time and attention. Also, make sure that your older child knows that the baby will not be an instant playmate. Let your preschooler know that you will love her just as much after the baby is born as you do now.
- **Involve your preschooler in planning for the baby.** This will make her less jealous. Let her shop with you for baby items. Show her pictures of herself as a newborn. If you are going to use some of her old baby things, let her play with them a bit before you get them ready for the new baby.
- **Do not make major changes in your preschooler's routine until after the baby is born.** You should complete making any changes such as toilet training or switching from a crib to a bed before the baby arrives. If that is not possible, put them off until after the baby is settled in at home. Otherwise, your preschooler may feel overwhelmed by trying to learn new things on top of all the changes caused by the new baby.

- **Expect your child to "regress" a little.** Do not worry too much if news that a baby is coming or if the baby's arrival makes your preschooler start acting like a baby again. For example, your toilet-trained child might suddenly start having "accidents," or she might want to take a bottle. This is normal and is your older child's way of making sure she still has your love and attention. Instead of telling her to act her age, let her have the attention she needs. Praise her when she acts more "grown-up."
- **Prepare your child for when you are in the hospital.** Toddlers and preschoolers may be confused when you leave for the hospital. Explain to your child that you will be back with the new baby in a few days.
- **Set aside some special time for your older child.** No matter how busy you are with the new baby, make sure you save some special time each day just for you and your older child. Read, play games, listen to music, or simply talk together. Show her that you want to know what she is doing, thinking, and feeling—not only about the baby but about everything else in her life. Also, make her feel a part of things by having her cuddle next to you when you feed the baby.
- **Encourage visitors to give attention to your older child.** Visitors can make such a fuss over a new baby that your older child might feel left out. Ask family and friends to spend a little time with your older child when they come to see the new baby. They might also give her a small gift when they bring gifts for the baby.
- **Have your older child spend time with dad.** A new baby presents a great opportunity for fathers to spend time alone with older children.

School-age children

Children older than 5 are usually not as threatened by a newborn as younger children are. This is particularly true if the school-age child has good self-esteem and feels loved and valued. Even so, your older child may resent the attention the baby gets. To prepare your school-age child for a new baby:

- **Tell your child about what is happening in language she can understand.** Explain what having a new brother or sister means, noting that the changes may affect her—both the good and the not-so-good. **Make your firstborn feel like a part of the process.** Have your older child help get the house ready for the new sibling by fixing up the baby's bedroom, picking out a new crib, buying diapers. If there is time, have her come to the hospital soon after the delivery so that she feels part of the growing family. Then, when you bring the baby home, make your older child feel that she has a role to play in caring for the baby. Tell her she can hold the baby, although she must ask you first. Praise her when she is gentle and loving toward the baby.

- **Make sure your older child feels listened to.** Do not overlook your older child's needs and activities. Let her know she can talk about her feelings. Tell her: "A new baby means a lot more work for me. If you ever feel that I am not spending enough time with you, let me know so I can give you plenty of extra love." Make an effort to spend some time alone with her each day; use that as a chance to make her feel like the most important person in your life.

What parents can do about sibling rivalry

It is important not to get too upset when your children are jealous of each other, especially if the older child is a preschooler. It takes time for a youngster to learn that his parents do not love him any less because they have another child to love.

Here are some tips on managing conflict between your children:

- **If your older child starts imitating the baby, do not make fun of or punish him.** Let him drink from a bottle or climb in the crib once or twice, but make it very clear that he does not have to act like a baby to get your attention. Praise him when he acts "grown up" and give him chances to be a "big brother." It should not take long for him to see that he gets more attention by acting his age than by acting like a baby.

- **If your older child is between 3 and 5 years old, try to cut down on conflicts over space by setting aside an area just for her.** Giving your older child her own space and keeping her things apart from shared ones will cut down on quarrels.

- **Do not compare your children in front of them.** It is natural to notice differences between your children. Just try not to comment on these in front of them. It is easy for a child to think that he is not as good or as loved as his sibling when you compare them. Remember, each child is a special individual. Let each one know that.

- **As much as possible, stay out of your children's arguments.** You may have to step in and settle a spat between toddlers or preschoolers. For example, if they are arguing over blocks, you might need to split the blocks into piles for each of them. Older children will probably settle an argument peacefully if left alone. If your children try to involve you, explain that they are both responsible for creating the problem and for ending it. Do not take sides. Set guidelines on how your children can disagree and resolve their conflicts. Of course, you **must** get involved if the situation gets violent. Make sure your children know that you will not stand for such behavior. If there is any reason to suspect that your children may become violent, watch them closely when they are together. Preventing violence is always better than punishing after the fact, which often makes the rivalry worse. Praise your children when they solve their arguments, and reward good behavior.

- **Be fair.** Divide household chores fairly. If you must get involved in your children's arguments, listen to all sides of the story. Make a "no tattling" rule. Give children privileges that are right for their ages, and try to be consistent. If you allowed one child to stay up until 9 o'clock at 10 years of age, the other should have the same bedtime when she is 10.

- **Respect your child's privacy.** When it is necessary to punish or scold, do it with the child alone in a quiet, private place. When possible, do not embarrass one child by scolding him in front of the others. This will only make the other child tease the one you punished.

- **Use regular family meetings for all family members to express their thoughts and feelings, as well as to plan the week's events. Give positive recognition and rewards (allowances, special privileges).**

Sibling relationships are very special. We form our earliest bonds with our brothers and sisters. No one else shares the same family history. By helping your children learn to value, love and respect their siblings, you are giving them a great gift—the gift of a lifelong friend.

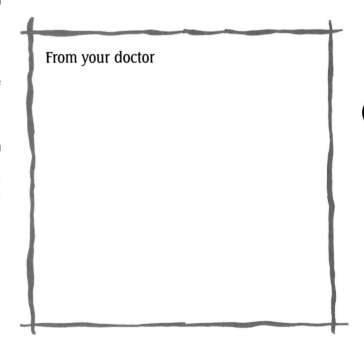

From your doctor

American Academy of Pediatrics

DEDICATED TO THE HEALTH OF ALL CHILDREN™

The American Academy of Pediatrics is an organization of 55,000 primary care pediatricians, pediatric medical subspecialists, and pediatric surgical specialists dedicated to the health, safety, and well-being of infants, children, adolescents, and young adults.

American Academy of Pediatrics
PO Box 747
Elk Grove Village, IL 60009-0747
Web site — http://www.aap.org

Copyright ©1996 American Academy of Pediatrics

Single Parenting

Part I What You Need to Know

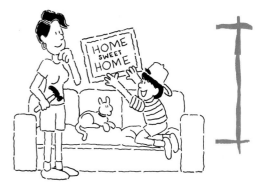

Single-parent families are more and more common in today's society. One of every four American children lives in a single-parent home. While most single-parent homes are the result of divorce, many parents are raising children alone for other reasons as well. Some parents may be alone due to the death of a spouse. Others choose to have or adopt a child without a partner. Whatever the circumstances, single parents cope with unique issues and challenges.

A death in the family

Losing a parent is one of the most traumatic events that can happen to a child. A child under 5 years of age cannot understand that death is permanent. Older children may have an understanding, but will have many questions they may be afraid to ask. Where did Daddy go when he died? Why did he die? Who will take care of me if you die? Children can react to death in many ways. Some will be quiet and sad. Others may be angry, guilty, or refuse to believe the parent is gone. It's important to accept your child's response, whatever it is. If signs of sadness or anger continue, talk to your pediatrician. He or she may recommend professional counseling to help get the healing process back on track.

Unplanned pregnancy

An unplanned pregnancy brings great change. The job of caring for a new baby is not easy, especially for single parents. Those who work may feel they aren't able to spend enough time at home with the baby. Money can be tight. Finding affordable child care might be hard. Be aware that help is available. Family, friends, and religious and community leaders are your best resources for support. If you need to find a job, employment agencies and temporary services can help. You may also qualify for government programs such as Head Start, Temporary Assistance for Needy Families (TANF), Women, Infants, and Children Supplemental Feeding Program (WIC), and Earned Income Credit (EIC).

Single-parent adoption

It is increasingly common for a single person to adopt a child on his or her own. Adoption can bring special challenges to parents. The child may be a baby just a few days old, or she could be school age. The adopted child may be of another country, race, culture, or from an abusive background. As a result, adoptive families can easily feel different from other families. The differences are real, but the rewards of working through these issues can be great. Working with your pediatrician to prevent and solve problems can be very important to your child's happiness and success.

Divorce and separation

Nearly two thirds of all single-parent families are the result of a divorce or separation. For a child, divorce can be just as hard as the death of a parent. A long period of grief and mourning can be expected. The age of the child also plays a role. A preschooler may regress in such things as toilet training, and may develop new fears or nightmares. A school-age child is more likely to show anger and feel guilty or sad. He may also do poorly in school. A teenager may worry about moving away from friends or not having money for college. No matter the age, some children feel responsible for the divorce of their parents and dream about getting them back together.

Divorce or separation often leaves parents angry with each other. During disagreements with your child's other parent, stop and ask yourself: How will this affect my child? You may disagree with each other, but try to set aside your differences for your child's sake. Use the following tips to avoid problems:

- **Never force your child to take sides.** Every child will have loyalties to both parents.
- **Don't involve your child in arguments** between the two of you.
- **Don't criticize each other in front of your child.** Even if you find out the other parent is saying bad things about you, explain to your child that people sometimes say mean things when they are angry.
- **Discuss your concerns and feelings with your child's other parent** when and where your child cannot hear.
- **Don't fight in front of the children,** especially about them.

If you are considering separation or divorce, you may find it helpful to discuss it with your pediatrician or ask for a copy of the American Academy of Pediatrics brochure *Divorce and Children*. A visit with a counselor may also help by giving you and your child a chance to talk about any problems and to plan for the changes ahead.

Talking with your child

Talking with your child is a very important way for you to help each other through tough times. Being able to share her fears, worries, and feelings with you can make your child feel safe and special. The more often you talk, the more comfortable she will feel. Be patient as you listen to her questions. You don't have to have all the answers. Sometimes just listening is more helpful than giving advice. If needed, don't hesitate to get help from your pediatrician or a family counselor. The following suggestions may be useful in talking with your child about the changes in your family.

239

- **Be honest with your child.** If your spouse has died, your young child may not understand what has happened. Be careful what you say. Young children often see death as a temporary situation. It is very important not to talk about death as "going away" or "going to sleep." Your child may believe that the deceased parent will come back, wake up, or the child may think that she will die while asleep. If you are going through a divorce, talk about it in simple terms. Try not to blame your ex-spouse or show your anger. Explain that parents sometimes choose to live separately. Give your child all the comfort she needs to feel safe and loved.

- **Make sure your child knows he is not the cause.** Children will often think that it's their fault that one parent has left. After a separation, divorce, or a death of a parent, children may blame themselves. They may feel alone, unwanted, or unloved. Let him know the changes are not his fault, that you love him and won't leave him.

- **Talk to your child about his fears.** Confusion about a parent leaving or dying can be scary for your child. In your child's mind, if one parent can leave, maybe the other one can too. He may think being away from a parent is temporary and that if he behaves, the parent will return. It is important to discuss these fears with your child, and to be as reassuring as possible.

Find good child care

Good child care is essential for your child's well-being and your peace of mind. If you are a working parent, finding quality child care may be one of the most difficult tasks you will face.

Never leave a child home alone. Find someone you trust to take care of your children while you are working. Don't rely on older brothers and sisters to babysit for younger siblings. Even the most reliable brother or sister does not have the maturity to be responsible for a younger sibling on a daily basis. Also, be careful about asking new friends or partners to watch your children, even for a short time. They may not have the patience, especially if the child's behavior becomes difficult. Children need to be cared for by an adult with proven experience in child care. The best way to make sure your child is getting good care is to visit the child care center or watch your babysitter when he or she is with your child.

Your pediatrician can offer advice on finding the best child care for your family. The local city or county government in your area may also have a list of licensed child care centers or homes. Ask your pediatrician for the brochure *Child Care: What's Best for Your Family* from the American Academy of Pediatrics. It includes a checklist of what to ask and what to look for when choosing child care services. You may also find the AAP book *Caring for Your Baby and Young Child: Birth To Age 5* helpful.

Custody

All children need a place where they can feel truly at home. Although the parent who lives with the child takes care of the day-to-day needs, the parent without custody should remain as involved as possible. He or she can still help with homework, go to athletic or other after-school events, and contribute support.

Cooperation between parents is very important for a child's long-term well-being. Remember, it's the job of both parents to stay involved in their child's life. Work together to arrange a flexible schedule for visits. Neither parent should be kept from taking part in raising the child. Make sure your child knows that it is okay to love both parents.

Dating and the single parent

Be choosy about which dates you introduce to your children. Try to form a solid relationship before bringing someone new into your home. Particularly, overnight guests may confuse your child. If you are dating someone special, you may not know how to present him or her to your child. Talk to your friend about your child before they meet. When you feel the time is right, let your child meet your new partner. Don't expect them to be close right away. Give them time to become friends.

If your new partner is new to child-rearing, he or she may feel awkward with your family. Observe how your friend gets along with your child. He or she should be patient and understanding. Before you leave your child with a new partner, be sure that he or she can be trusted.

A new life

Raising a child on your own isn't easy. Single parents face unique problems, but children in single-parent homes can grow up just as happy as children in two-parent homes. Providing a loving, supportive home for your children is the most important factor in helping them grow up well-adjusted and happy. By seeking out the information provided here, you've taken the first step to adapting to the changes in your life. Making the right choices for you and your children will help all of you live a new and rewarding life together as a family.

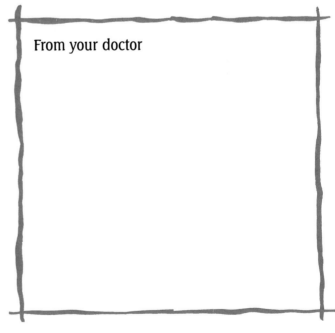

From your doctor

American Academy of Pediatrics

DEDICATED TO THE HEALTH OF ALL CHILDREN™

The American Academy of Pediatrics is an organization of 55,000 primary care pediatricians, pediatric medical subspecialists, and pediatric surgical specialists dedicated to the health, safety, and well-being of infants, children, adolescents, and young adults.

American Academy of Pediatrics
PO Box 747
Elk Grove Village, IL 60009-0747
Web site — http://www.aap.org

Single Parenting

Part II Additional Resources

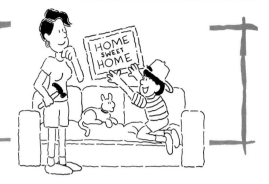

10 ways to reduce stress

Single-parenthood brings added pressure and stress to the job of raising children. With no one to share day-to-day responsibilities or decision-making, parents must provide greater support for their children while they themselves may feel alone. The following suggestions may help reduce stress in your family:

1. **Get a handle on finances.** Finances are often a problem for single parents. Learn how to budget your time and money. Know when your paycheck or other income will arrive, and keep track of household bills. If you write down monthly bills and due dates, they will be easier to manage. Do what you can to improve your finances. Contact employment and temporary agencies for help finding a job. Consider getting your high school diploma, a college degree, or other special training.

2. **Talk early and often.** Don't leave your child in the dark about the changes in the family. She will handle her problems much better by talking about her feelings. Sit quietly with your child just before bedtime. It may be a great time for her to talk with you.

3. **Find support and use it.** Don't try to handle everything by yourself. Get help whenever you can. It is difficult when a single parent must hold down a job and care for children at the same time. Try not to feel guilty about things you can't do or can't provide without a partner. You will need the support that family and friends can give. Get to know other single parents through support groups. Your pediatrician can also be a great source of help and information.

4. **Take time for family.** Working every day, fixing dinner, cleaning the house, and paying the bills can be overwhelming. Set aside some time each day to enjoy your children and your relationship with them. Spend quiet time playing, reading, working on arts-and-crafts projects, or just listening to music together. Time spent together is one of the most important things you can give to your child.

5. **Take time for yourself.** Whether you are reading, relaxing, or visiting with friends, time spent away from your children is important for you, and for them. Go to a movie. Find a hobby. Do things that interest you. Being a single parent doesn't mean you can't have an adult life.

6. **Keep a daily routine.** Making rules, setting a good example, and providing support is tough, but giving in to your child's demands will not help. Schedule meals, chores, and bedtime at regular times so that your child knows what to expect each day. A routine will help your child feel more secure.

7. **Maintain consistent discipline.** If others help in the care of your child, talk to them about your own methods of discipline. Divorced or separated parents should work together to use the same way of disciplining their children. Discipline doesn't have to mean physical punishment. You can teach a child to behave in ways that are good for both himself and those around him. Many good methods have been developed. Check your local library for helpful books on parenting. Local hospitals, the YMCA, and church groups often sponsor parenting classes. Learning good ways to handle your child's behavior will reduce stress for both of you.

8. **Treat kids like kids.** Children have a right to enjoy childhood and grow up at their own pace. Though single parenting can get lonely, resist treating your children like substitutes for a partner. Avoid expressing your frustration to them. Try not to rely on them for comfort or sympathy. As children grow older, they will be able to take on more responsibility and help around the house. Don't expect too much too soon.

9. **Stay positive.** The pain of a separation, divorce, or death will ease over time. Be aware that your children will always be affected by your mood and attitude. They will need your praise and your love through hard times. It's okay to be honest about your own feelings of sadness and loss, but let them know better times lie ahead for both of you.

10. **Take care of yourself.** This is a difficult time for you, too. Exercising regularly, maintaining a proper diet, and getting enough rest can help you better deal with stress. Visit your own doctor on a regular basis. Ask your pediatrician not only about help for your child, but also about help for yourself.

A word about...child support

In a divorce, separation, or unplanned pregnancy, both parents have a continuing financial obligation to the child. If you have custody of your child, seek child support. According to the US Department of Health and Human Services, millions of single-parent households do not receive child support. In some cases, one parent doesn't want money from the other parent. In others, the parent may not be able or willing to pay or perhaps cannot even be found. Many times, the parent with custody simply does not try to get child support.

Contact your state child support enforcement agency for guidelines on what parents must pay for child support. If your child's other parent has disappeared or won't cooperate, your state or local government may be able to help.

For more information, contact:
Department of Health and Human Services
Office of Child Support Enforcement
370 L'Enfant Promenade, SW
Washington, DC 20447
202/401-9373
Web site: www.acf.dhhs.gov/programs/cse/index.html

The information contained in this publication should not be used as a substitute for the medical care and advice of your pediatrician. There may be variations in treatment that your pediatrician may recommend based on individual facts and circumstances.

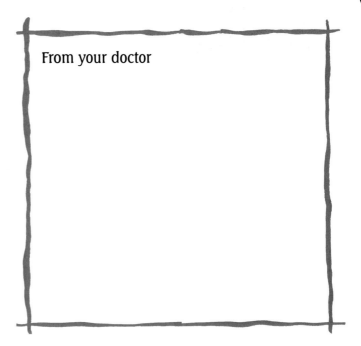

From your doctor

American Academy of Pediatrics

DEDICATED TO THE HEALTH OF ALL CHILDREN™

The American Academy of Pediatrics is an organization of 55,000 primary care pediatricians, pediatric medical subspecialists, and pediatric surgical specialists dedicated to the health, safety, and well-being of infants, children, adolescents, and young adults.

American Academy of Pediatrics
PO Box 747
Elk Grove Village, IL 60009-0747
Web site — http://www.aap.org

Sleep Problems in Children

Part I Infants, Toddlers, and Preschoolers

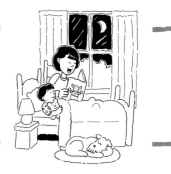

Sleep problems are very common among children during the first few years of life. Problems may include a reluctance to go to sleep, waking up in the middle of the night, nightmares, and sleepwalking. In older children, bed-wetting can also become a challenge.

Children vary in the amount of sleep they need and the amount of time it takes to fall asleep. How easily they wake up and how quickly they can resettle are also different for each child. It is important, however, that as a parent you help your child develop good sleep habits at an early age. The good news is that most sleep problems can be solved and your pediatrician can help.

Infants

Newborn infants have irregular sleep cycles, which take about 6 months to mature. While newborns sleep an average of 16 to 17 hours per day, they may only sleep 1 or 2 hours at a time. As children get older, the total number of hours they need for sleep decreases. However, different children have different needs. It is normal even for a 6 month old to wake up briefly during the night, but these awakenings should only last a few minutes and children should be able to go back to sleep on their own. Here are some suggestions that may help your baby (and you) sleep better at night:

1. **Try to keep her as calm and quiet as possible.** When feeding or changing your baby during the night, avoid stimulating her or waking her up too much so she can easily fall back to sleep.

2. **Don't let your infant sleep as long during the day.** If she sleeps for large blocks of time during the day, she will be more likely to be awake during the night.

3. **Put your baby into the crib at the first signs of drowsiness.** Ideally it is best to let the baby learn to relax and settle herself to sleep. If you make a habit of holding or rocking her until she falls asleep, she may learn to need you to get back to sleep when she wakes up in the middle of the night. This may interfere with her learning to settle herself and fall asleep alone.

4. **Try to avoid putting your baby to bed with a pacifier.** Your baby may get used to falling asleep with it and have trouble learning to settle herself without it. Pacifiers should be used to satisfy the baby's need to suck, not to help a baby sleep. If your baby falls asleep with a pacifier, gently remove it before putting her in bed.

5. **Begin to delay your reaction to infant fussing at 4 to 6 months of age.** Wait a few minutes before you go in to check her, because she will probably settle herself and fall back to sleep in a few minutes anyway. If she continues to cry, check on her, but avoid turning on the light, playing, picking up, or rocking her. If crying continues or begins to sound frantic, wait a few more minutes and then recheck the baby. If she is unable to settle herself, consider what else might be bothering her. She may be hungry, wet or soiled, feverish, or otherwise not feeling well.

6. **Ideally, by a few weeks of age a baby should sleep in a separate room from his parents.**

If your baby is ill, these suggestions should be relaxed. After she feels better, begin to reestablish sleep patterns.

Infant sleep positioning and SIDS

The American Academy of Pediatrics recommends that parents and caregivers place healthy infants on their backs when putting them down to sleep. This is because recent studies have shown an increased incidence of Sudden Infant Death Syndrome (SIDS) in infants who sleep on their stomachs. There is no evidence that sleeping on the back is harmful to healthy infants.

©2002 American Academy of Pediatrics

Toddlers and preschoolers

Many parents find their toddler's bedtime one of the hardest parts of the day. It is common for children this age to resist going to sleep, especially if there are older siblings who are still awake. However, remember toddlers and pre-schoolers usually need 10 to 12 hours of sleep each night. If your child's sleeping time does not approach this level, talk to your pediatrician.

Following are some tips to help your toddler develop good sleep habits:

1. **Make sure there is a quiet period before your child goes to bed.** Establish a pleasant routine that may include reading, singing, or a warm bath. A regular routine will help your child understand that it will soon be time to go to sleep. If parents work late hours, it may be tempting to play with their child before bedtime. However, active play just before bedtime may leave the child excited and unable to sleep. Limit television viewing and video game play before bed.

2. **Try to set a consistent schedule** for your child and make bedtime the same time every night. His sleep patterns will adjust accordingly.

3. **Allow your child to take a favorite teddy bear, toy, or special blanket to bed each night.** Such comforting objects often help children fall asleep—especially if they awaken during the middle of the night. Make sure the object is safe. A teddy bear may have a ribbon, button, or other part that may pose a choking hazard for your child. Look for sturdy construction at the seams. Stuffing or pellets inside the stuffed animal may also pose a danger of choking.

4. **Make sure your child is comfortable.** Check the temperature in your child's room. Clothes should not restrict movement. He may like to have a drink of water before bed, have a night-light left on, or the door left slightly open. Try to handle your child's needs before bedtime, so that he doesn't use them to avoid going to bed.

5. **Try to avoid letting your child sleep with you.** This will only make it harder for him to learn to settle himself and fall asleep when he is alone.

6. **Try not to return to your child's room every time he complains or calls out.** A child will quickly learn if you always give in to his requests at bedtime. When your child calls out, try the following:
   - Wait several seconds before answering. Your response time can be longer each time to give your child the message that it is time for sleep. It also gives him the opportunity to fall asleep on his own.
   - Reassure your child that you are there. If you need to go into his room, do not stimulate the child or stay too long.
   - Move farther from your child's bed every time you go to reassure him, until you can do this verbally without entering his room.

The information contained in this publication should not be used as a substitute for the medical care and advice of your pediatrician. There may be variations in treatment that your pediatrician may recommend based on individual facts and circumstances.

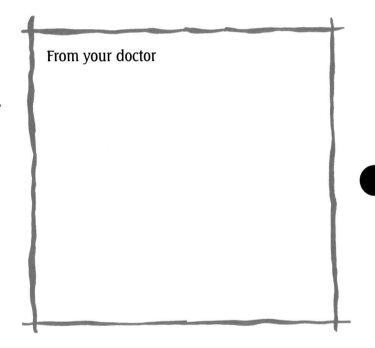

From your doctor

American Academy of Pediatrics

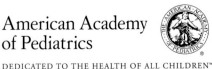

DEDICATED TO THE HEALTH OF ALL CHILDREN™

The American Academy of Pediatrics is an organization of 55,000 primary care pediatricians, pediatric medical subspecialists, and pediatric surgical specialists dedicated to the health, safety, and well-being of infants, children, adolescents, and young adults.

American Academy of Pediatrics
PO Box 747
Elk Grove Village, IL 60009-0747
Web site — http://www.aap.org

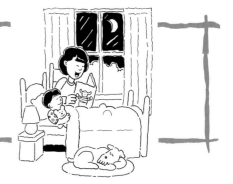

Sleep Problems in Children
Part II Common Sleep Problems

Common sleep problems

For a young child, many things can interrupt a good night's sleep. As a parent, you may be able to prevent some of them.

Nightmares

Nightmares are scary dreams that usually happen during the second half of the night, when dreaming is most intense. This may occur more than once a night. After the nightmare is over, your child may wake up and can tell you what occurred. Children may be crying or fearful after a nightmare but will be aware of your presence. They may have trouble falling back to sleep because they can remember the details of the dream.

How to handle nightmares:
- Go to the child as quickly as possible.
- Assure her that you are there and will not let anything harm her. Allow the child to have the bedroom light on for a short period to reassure her.
- If your child is fearful, comfort and calm her.
- Keep in mind that a nightmare is real to a young child. Listen to her and encourage her to tell you what happened in the dream.
- Once the child is calm, encourage her to go back to sleep.

Night terrors

Night terrors are more severe or frightening than nightmares, but not as common. They occur most often in toddlers and preschoolers. Night terrors come out of the deepest stages of sleep, usually within an hour or so after a child falls asleep. During a night terror, children usually cannot be awakened or comforted. Night terrors may also cause the following:
- Uncontrollable crying
- Sweating, shaking, and fast breathing
- A terrified, confused, and glassy-eyed appearance
- Thrashing around, screaming, kicking, or staring
- Child may not realize anyone is with him
- Child may not appear to recognize you
- Child may try to push you away, especially when you try to restrain him

Night terrors may last as long as 45 minutes, but are usually much shorter. Children seem to fall right back to sleep after a night terror, but they actually have not been awake. Like nightmares, night terrors may occur more often in times of stress or may relate to difficult feelings or fears. However, unlike a nightmare, a child will not remember a night terror.

How to handle night terrors:
- Remain calm. Night terrors are usually more frightening for the parent than for the child.
- Do not try to wake your child.
- Make sure the child does not injure himself. If the child tries to get out of bed, gently restrain him.
- Remember, after a short time, your child will probably relax and sleep quietly again.
- If your child has night terrors, be sure to explain to your baby-sitters what they are and what to do.

Keep in mind that night terrors do not always indicate serious problems. Your child will be more likely to have night terrors when he is overly tired and during periods of stress. Your child can become overly tired when he gives up a daytime nap, wakes up too early, or his nighttime sleep is interrupted. Try to keep your child on a regular sleep schedule or increase the amount of sleep he gets to prevent night terrors. Night terrors usually disappear by the time a child reaches grade school. If they do persist, talk to your pediatrician.

Sleepwalking and sleep talking

Like night terrors, sleepwalking and sleep talking happen when a child is in a deep sleep. While sleepwalking, your child may have a blank, staring face. She may not respond to others and be very difficult to awaken. When your child does wake up, she will probably not remember the episode. Sleepwalking children will often return to bed by themselves and will not even remember that they have gotten out of bed. Sleepwalking can be common, and tends to run in families. It can even occur several times in one night among older children and teenagers. If you have concerns or the condition persists, talk to your child's pediatrician.

How to handle sleepwalking and sleep talking:
- Make sure your child doesn't hurt herself while sleepwalking. Clear the bedroom area of potential hazards that your child could trip over or fall on.
- Lock outside doors so your child cannot leave the house.
- Block stairways so your child cannot go up or down.
- There is no need to try to wake your child when she is sleepwalking or sleep talking. Gently lead her back to bed and she will probably settle down on her own.

Sleepwalking and sleep talking are more likely to occur when your child is overly tired or under stress. Keeping your child's sleep schedule regular may help prevent sleepwalking and sleep talking.

Bed-wetting (also called enuresis)

Nighttime bed-wedding is normal and very common among preschoolers. It affects about 40% of 3 year olds and may run in families. The most common reasons your child may wet the bed include the following:

- A bladder that has not yet developed enough to hold urine for a full night.
- Your child may not yet be able to recognize a full bladder and wake up to use the toilet.
- Stress. Changes in the home, such as a new baby, moving, or a divorce can lead to a sudden case of bed-wetting for a child who has been dry at night in the past.

How to handle bed-wetting:

- Do not blame or punish the child for bed-wetting.
- Have your child use the toilet and avoid drinking large amounts of fluid just before bedtime.
- Until your child can stay dry during the night, put a rubber or plastic cover over the mattress to protect against wetness and odors. Keep the bedding clean.
- If your child is old enough, involve him in handling the problem. Encourage him to help change the wet sheets and covers. This will help teach responsibility and avoid the embarrassment of having other family members know about the problem every time it happens. Do not, however, use this as punishment for the child.
- Talk to your pediatrician about other approaches to bed-wetting, such as rewards for younger children or alarm devices for the older child.

Most importantly, don't pressure your child. Bed-wetting is beyond a child's control and he may only become sad or frustrated if he cannot stop. Set a "no-teasing" rule in the family. Make sure your child understands that bed-wetting is not his fault and it will get better in time.

Teeth grinding

It is also common for children to grind their teeth during the night. Though it produces an unpleasant sound, it is usually not harmful to your young child's teeth. It may be related to tension and anxiety and usually disappears in a short while. However, it may reappear with the next stressful episode.

Give it time

Handling your child's sleep problems may be a challenge and it is normal to become upset at times when a child keeps you awake at night. Try to be understanding. A negative response by a parent can sometimes make a sleep problem worse, especially if it is associated with a stressful situation like divorce, a new sibling, a tragedy in the family, problems at school, or some other recent change in your child's life.

If the problem persists, there may be a physical or emotional reason that your child cannot sleep. If you feel you need additional help, start a sleep diary and discuss the problem with your pediatrician. Keep in mind that most sleep problems are very common, and with time and your pediatrician's help, you and your child will overcome them.

Keeping a sleep diary

It may be helpful for you in preparation for discussing a sleep problem with your pediatrician to keep a sleep diary for your child.
Chart the following:

- Where your child sleeps
- How much sleep she normally gets at night
- What time she was put to bed
- What the child needs to fall asleep (favorite toy, blanket, etc)
- The time it takes for her to fall asleep
- The time that you went to bed
- The time awakened during the night
- How long it took to fall back to sleep
- What you did to comfort and console the child
- The time the child woke up in the morning
- The time and length of naps
- Any changes or stresses in the home

Keep in mind that every child is different and no two children may have the same sleep patterns or problems.

The information contained in this publication should not be used as a substitute for the medical care and advice of your pediatrician. There may be variations in treatment that your pediatrician may recommend based on individual facts and circumstances.

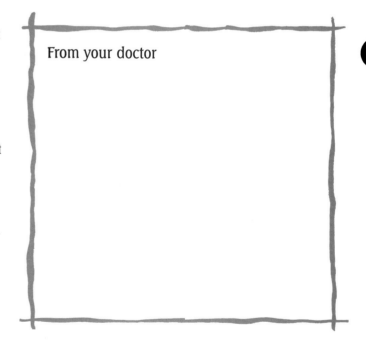

From your doctor

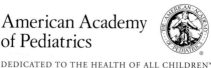

American Academy of Pediatrics

DEDICATED TO THE HEALTH OF ALL CHILDREN™

The American Academy of Pediatrics is an organization of 55,000 primary care pediatricians, pediatric medical subspecialists, and pediatric surgical specialists dedicated to the health, safety, and well-being of infants, children, adolescents, and young adults.

American Academy of Pediatrics
PO Box 747
Elk Grove Village, IL 60009-0747
Web site — http://www.aap.org

Television and the Family

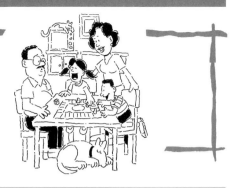

Family is the most important influence in a child's life, but television is not far behind. Television can inform, entertain, and teach us. However, some of what TV teaches may not be what you want your child to learn. TV programs and commercials often show violence, alcohol or drug use, and sexual content that are not suitable for children or teenagers. Studies show that TV viewing may lead to more aggressive behavior, less physical activity, altered body image, and increased use of drugs and alcohol. By knowing how television affects your children and by setting limits, you can help make your child's TV-watching experience less harmful, but still enjoyable.

How TV affects your child

There are many ways that television affects your child's life. When your child sits down to watch TV, consider the following:

Time

Children in the United States watch about 4 hours of TV every day. Watching movies on tape or DVD and playing video games only adds to time spent in front of the TV screen. It may be tempting to use television, movies, and video games to keep your child busy, but your child needs to spend as much time exploring and learning as possible. Playing, reading, and spending time with friends and family are much healthier than sitting in front of a TV screen.

Nutrition

Studies show that children who watch too much television are more likely to be overweight. They do not spend as much time running, jumping, and getting the exercise they need. They often snack while watching TV. They also see many commercials for unhealthy foods, such as candy, snacks, sugary cereals, and drinks. Commercials almost never give information about the foods children should eat to keep healthy. As a result, children may persuade their parents to buy unhealthy foods.

Violence

If your child watches 3 to 4 hours of noneducational TV per day, he will have seen about 8,000 murders on TV by the time he finishes grade school. Children who see violence on television may not understand that real violence hurts and kills people. They become numb to violence. If the "good guys" use violence, children may learn that it is okay to use force to solve problems. Studies show that even children's cartoons contain a significant amount of violence.

Research also shows a very strong link between exposure to violent TV and violent and aggressive behavior in children and teenagers. Watching a lot of violence on television can lead to hostility, fear, anxiety, depression, nightmares, sleep disturbances, and post-traumatic stress disorder. It is best not to let your child watch violent programs and cartoons.

A word about...TV for toddlers

Children of all ages are constantly learning new things. The first 2 years of life are especially important in the growth and development of your child's brain. During this time, children need good, positive interaction with other children and adults to develop good language and social skills. Learning to talk and play with others is far more important than watching television.

Until more research is done about the effects of TV on very young children, the American Academy of Pediatrics (AAP) does not recommend television for children younger than 2 years of age. For older children, the AAP recommends no more than 1 to 2 hours per day of quality screen time.

Sex

Television exposes children to adult behaviors, like sex. But it usually does not show the risks and results of sexual activity. On TV, sexual activity is shown as normal, fun, exciting, and without consequences. In commercials, sex is often used to sell products and services. Your child may copy what she sees on TV to feel more grown up.

Alcohol, tobacco, and other drugs

Young people today are surrounded by messages that say drinking alcohol and smoking cigarettes or cigars are normal activities. These messages do not say that alcohol and tobacco harm people and may lead to death. Beer and wine are some of the most advertised products on television. TV programs and commercials often show people who drink and smoke as healthy, energetic, sexy, and successful. It is up to you to teach your child the truth about the dangers of alcohol, tobacco, and other drugs.

Commercials

The average child sees more than 40,000 commercials each year. Commercials are quick, fast-paced, and entertaining. After seeing the same commercials over and over, your child can easily remember a song, slogan, or catchy phrase. Commercials try to convince your child that having a certain toy or eating a certain food will make him happy or popular. Older children can begin to understand how ads use pictures, music, and sound to entertain. Kids need to know that ads try to convince people to buy things they may not need.

Learning

Television affects how your child learns. High-quality, nonviolent children's shows can have a positive effect on learning. Studies show that preschool children who watch educational TV programs do better on reading and math tests than children who do not watch those programs. When used carefully, television can be a positive tool to help your child learn.

10 things parents can do

As a parent, there are many ways you can help your child develop positive viewing habits. The following tips may help:

1. Set limits

Limit your child's use of TV, movies, and video and computer games to no more than 1 or 2 hours per day. Do not let your child watch TV while doing homework. Do not put a television in your child's bedroom.

2. Plan your child's viewing

Instead of flipping through channels, use a program guide and the TV ratings to help you and your child choose shows. Turn the TV on to watch the program you chose and turn it off when the program is over.

3. Watch TV with your child

Whenever possible, watch TV with your child and talk about what you see. If your child is very young, she may not be able to tell the difference between a show, a commercial, a cartoon, or real life. Explain that characters on TV are make-believe and not real.

Some "reality-based" programs may appear to be "real," but most of these shows focus on stories that will attract as many viewers as possible. Much of their content is not appropriate for children. News broadcasts also contain violent or other inappropriate material. If your schedule prevents you from watching TV with your child, talk to her later about what she watched. Better yet, record the programs so that you can watch them *with* your child at a later time.

4. Find the right message

Even a poor program can turn out to be a learning experience if you help your child find the right message. Some television programs may portray people as stereotypes. Talk with your child about the real-life roles of women, the elderly, and people of other races that may not be shown on television. Discuss ways that people are different and ways that we are the same. Help your child learn tolerance for others. Remember, if you do not agree with certain subject matter, you can either turn off the TV or explain why you object.

5. Help your child resist commercials

Do not expect your child to be able to resist ads for toys, candy, snacks, cereal, drinks, or new TV programs without your help. When your child asks for products advertised on TV, explain that the purpose of commercials is to make people want things they may not need. Limit the number of commercials your child sees by watching public television stations (PBS). You can also record programs and leave out the commercials or buy or rent children's videos or DVDs.

6. Look for quality children's videos and DVDs

There are many quality videos and DVDs available for children that you can buy or rent. Check reviews before buying or renting programs or movies. Information is available in books, newspapers, and magazines, as well as on the Internet.

7. Give other options

Watching TV can become a habit for your child. Help your child find other things to do with his time, such as playing; reading; learning a hobby, a sport, an instrument, or an art; or spending time with family, friends, or neighbors.

TV Parental Guidelines and the v-chip

In 1996, Congress passed a law that helps parents control what their children watch on television. The law called for a rating system to be developed. The ratings, known as the TV Parental Guidelines, help parents know which programs contain sex and violence. Parents can use a computer device in their televisions called the v-chip to block programs according to these ratings. The law requires all new television sets with screens 13" or larger that were made in the United States after January 1, 2000, to have the v-chip.

The ratings apply to all TV programs except news and sports. They appear for 15 seconds at the start of a program. When the rating appears on the screen, an electronic signal sends the rating to the v-chip in your television set.

The ratings are as follows:

TV-Y   **For all children**

TV-Y7   **For children age 7 and older.** The program may contain mild violence that could frighten children younger than age 7.

TV-Y7-FV **For children age 7 and older.** The program contains fantasy violence that is glorified and used as an acceptable, effective way to solve a problem. It is more intense than TV-Y7.

TV-G   **For general audience.** Most parents would find this program suitable for all ages. There is little or no violence, no strong language, and little or no sexual content.

TV-PG   **Parental guidance is suggested.** Parents may find some material unsuitable for younger children. It may contain moderate violence, some sexual content, or strong language.

TV-14   **Parents are strongly cautioned.** The program contains some material that many parents would find unsuitable for children younger than age 14. It contains intense violence, sexual content, or strong language.

TV-MA   **For mature audience.** The program may not be suitable for children younger than age 17. It contains graphic violence, explicit sexual activity, or crude language.

Additional letters may be added to the ratings to indicate violence (V), sexual content (S), strong language (L), or suggestive dialogue (D).

This ratings system was created to help parents choose programs that are suitable for children, even without the use of the v-chip. The ratings are usually included in local TV listings. Before watching, check your local TV listings to find out if a program contains violence, sexual content, or strong language. Remember that ratings are not used for news programs, which may not be suitable for young children. Also, TVs with screens smaller than 13" will not have the v-chip.

More information is available at the following Web sites:

- www.fcc.gov/vchip
- www.vchipeducation.org

8. Set a good example

You are the most important role model in your child's life. Limiting your own TV viewing and choosing programs carefully will help your child do the same.

The Children's Television Act of 1990

The Children's Television Act ensures that TV stations pay attention to the needs of children from age 2 to 16. Under this law, stations must air at least 3 hours of educational and informational shows for children each week. They must also limit advertising during children's shows to 12 minutes per hour on weekdays and 10.5 minutes per hour on weekends. Stations that do not follow the law risk losing their license.

Keep tabs on TV stations in your community. TV stations file quarterly Children's Television Programming Reports with the Federal Communications Commission (FCC). You can access these reports on the FCC's Web site at svartifoss2.fcc.gov/prod/kidvid/prod/kidvid.htm.

You can also file complaints with the FCC. More information is available at
Federal Communications Commission
Consumer Information Bureau
Consumer Complaints
445 12th St SW
Washington, DC 20554
Phone: 888/225-5322 (toll-free)
Fax: 202/418-0232
www.fcc.gov/cib

9. Express your views

When you like or do not like something you see on television, make yourself heard. Write to the TV station, network, or the program's sponsor. Stations, networks, and sponsors pay attention to letters from the public. If you think a commercial is misleading, write down the product name, channel, and time you saw the commercial and describe your concerns. Call your local Better Business Bureau if the commercial is for a local business or product. For national advertising, send the information to

Children's Advertising Review Unit
Council of Better Business Bureau
845 Third Ave
New York, NY 10022

Encourage publishers of TV guides to print ratings and feature articles about shows that are educational for children.

10. Get more information

The following people and places can provide you with more information about the proper role of TV in your child's life:

- **Your pediatrician** may have information about TV or can help you get it through the AAP. Ask for the AAP brochures *Understanding the Impact of Media on Children and Teens* and *The Ratings Game: Choosing Your Child's Entertainment*. Information from the AAP is also available on the Internet at www.aap.org and www.medem.com.
- **Public service groups** publish newsletters that review programs and give tips on how to make TV a positive experience for you and your child.

Toppling TVs pose a hazard

Newer televisions with larger, heavier screens in smaller casings can present a danger to toddlers. Small children are being seriously injured and, in some cases, killed when these front-heavy models fall on them. More than 2,000 children end up in the emergency room each year due to injuries from falling televisions, according to the US Consumer Product Safety Commission.

The following safety tips can be used to prevent such injuries:

- Place your television set on low furniture that is the proper size and is designed to support your TV model.
- Use braces or anchors to secure televisions and supporting furniture to the wall.
- Do not place remote controls, videos, or other objects that children might try to reach on top of the television.
- Do not allow children to play with or climb on the television set.

You can also help by encouraging manufacturers to design models that are more stable and to provide methods for tethering TVs to the wall.

- **The parent organization at your child's school.**
- **Parents of your child's friends and classmates** can also be helpful. Talk with other parents and agree to enforce similar rules about TV viewing.

When used properly, television can inform, educate, and entertain you and your family. By taking an active role in your child's viewing, you can help make watching TV a positive and healthy experience.

The information contained in this publication should not be used as a substitute for the medical care and advice of your pediatrician. There may be variations in treatment that your pediatrician may recommend based on individual facts and circumstances.

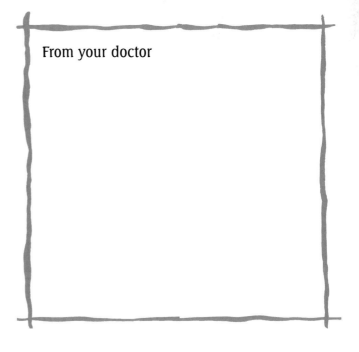

From your doctor

American Academy of Pediatrics

DEDICATED TO THE HEALTH OF ALL CHILDREN™

The American Academy of Pediatrics is an organization of 55,000 primary care pediatricians, pediatric medical subspecialists, and pediatric surgical specialists dedicated to the health, safety, and well-being of infants, children, adolescents, and young adults.

American Academy of Pediatrics
PO Box 747
Elk Grove Village, IL 60009-0747
Web site — http://www.aap.org

Temper Tantrums:
A Normal Part of Growing Up

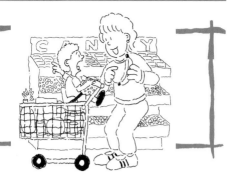

Strong emotions are hard for a young child to hold inside. When children feel frustrated, angry, or disappointed, they often express themselves by crying, screaming, or stomping up and down. As a parent, you may feel angry, helpless, or embarrassed. Temper tantrums are a normal part of your child's development as he learns self-control. In fact, almost all children have tantrums between the ages of 1 and 3. You've heard them called "the terrible twos." The good news is that by age 4, temper tantrums usually stop.

Why do children have tantrums?

Your young child is busy learning many things about her world. She is eager to take control. She wants to be independent and may try to do more than her skills will allow. She wants to make her own choices and often may not cope well with not getting her way. She is even less able to cope when she is tired, hungry, frustrated, or frightened. Controlling her temper may be one of the most difficult lessons to learn.

Temper tantrums are a way for your child to let off steam when she is upset. Following are some of the reasons your child may have a temper tantrum:

- Your child may not fully understand what you are saying or asking, and may get confused.
- Your child may become upset when others cannot understand what she is saying.
- Your child may not have the words to describe her feelings and needs. After 3 years of age, most children can express their feelings, so temper tantrums taper off. Children who are not able to express their feelings very well with words are more likely to continue to have tantrums.
- Your child has not yet learned to solve problems on her own and gets discouraged easily.
- Your child may have an illness or other physical problem that keeps her from expressing how she feels.
- Your child may be hungry, but may not recognize it.
- Your child may be tired or not getting enough sleep.
- Your child may be anxious or uncomfortable.
- Your child may be reacting to stress or changes at home.
- Your child may be jealous of a friend or sibling. Children often want what other children have or the attention they receive.
- Your child may not yet be able to do the things she can imagine, such as walking or running, climbing down stairs or from furniture, drawing things, or making toys work.

How to help prevent temper tantrums

As a parent, you can sometimes tell when tantrums are coming. Your child may seem moody, cranky, or difficult. He may start to whine and whimper. It may seem as if nothing will make him happy. Finally, he may start to cry, kick, scream, fall to the ground, or hold his breath. Other times, a tantrum may come on suddenly for no obvious reason. You should not be surprised if your child has tantrums only in front of you. This is one way of testing your rules and limits. Many children will not act out their feelings around others and are more cautious with strangers. Children feel safer showing their feelings to the people they trust.

You will not be able to prevent all tantrums, but the following suggestions may help reduce the chances of a tantrum:

- **Encourage your child to use words** to tell you how he is feeling, such as "I'm really mad." Try to understand how he is feeling and suggest words he can use to describe his feelings.
- **Set reasonable limits** and don't expect your child to be perfect. Give simple reasons for the rules you set, and don't change the rules.
- **Keep a daily routine** as much as possible, so your child knows what to expect.
- **Avoid situations that will frustrate your child,** such as playing with children or toys that are too advanced for your child's abilities.
- **Avoid long outings or visits** where your child has to sit still or cannot play for long periods of time. If you have to take a trip, bring along your child's favorite book or toy to entertain him.
- **Be prepared with healthy snacks when your child gets hungry.**
- **Make sure your child is well rested,** especially before a busy day or stressful activity.
- **Distract your child** from activities likely to lead to a tantrum. Suggest different activities. If possible, being silly, playful, or making a joke can help ease a tense situation. Sometimes, something as simple as changing locations can prevent a tantrum. For example, if you are indoors, try taking your child outside to distract his attention.
- **Be choosy about saying "no."** When you say no to every demand or request your child makes, it will frustrate him. Listen carefully to requests. When a request is not too unreasonable or inconvenient, consider saying yes. When your child's safety is involved, do not change your decision because of a tantrum.
- **Let your child choose whenever possible.** For example, if your child resists a bath, make it clear that he will be taking a bath, but offer a simple decision he can make on his own. Instead of saying, "Do you want to take a bath?" Try saying, "It's time for your bath. Would you like to walk upstairs or have me carry you?"
- **Set a good example.** Avoid arguing or yelling in front of your child.

©2002 American Academy of Pediatrics

A word about...safety

Many times, you will have to tell your child "no" to protect her from harm or injury. For example, the kitchen and bathroom can be hazardous places for your child. Your child will have trouble understanding why you will not let her play there. This is a common cause of a tantrum. "Childproof" your home and make dangerous areas or objects off-limits.

Keep an eye on your child at all times. After telling your child "no," never leave her alone in a situation that could be hazardous. Take away dangerous objects from your child immediately and replace them with something safe. It is up to you to keep your child safe and teach her how to protect herself from getting hurt. Be consistent and clear about safety.

What to do when tantrums occur

When your child has a temper tantrum, follow the suggestions listed below:

1. Distract your child by calling his attention to something else, such as a new activity, book, or toy. Sometimes just touching or stroking a child will calm him. You may need to gently restrain or hold your child. Interrupt his behavior with a light comment like, "Did you see what the kitty is doing?" or "I think I heard the doorbell." Humor or something as simple as a funny face can also help.

2. Try to remain calm. If you shout or become angry, it is likely to make things worse. Remember, the more attention you give this behavior, the more likely it is to happen again.

3. Minor displays of anger such as crying, screaming, or kicking can usually be ignored. Stand nearby or hold your child without talking until he calms down. This shows your support. If you cannot stay calm, leave the room.

4. Some temper tantrums cannot be ignored. The following behaviors should not be ignored and are not acceptable:
   - Hitting or kicking parents or others
   - Throwing things in a dangerous way
   - Prolonged screaming or yelling

   Use a cooling-off period or a "time-out" to remove your child from the source of his anger. Take your child away from the situation and hold him or give him some time alone to calm down and regain control. For children old enough to understand, a good rule of thumb for a time-out is 1 minute of time for every year of your child's age. (For example, a 4 year old would get a 4-minute time-out.) But even 15 seconds will work. If you cannot stay calm, leave the room. Wait a minute or two, or until his crying stops, before returning. Then help him get interested in something else. If your child is old enough, talk about what happened and discuss other ways to deal with it next time.

   For more information, ask your pediatrician about the American Academy of Pediatrics brochure *Discipline and Your Child*.

   You should never punish your child for temper tantrums. He may start to keep his anger or frustration inside, which can be unhealthy. Your response to tantrums should be calm and understanding. As your child grows, he will learn to deal with his strong emotions. Remember, it is normal for children to test their parents' rules and limits.

Do not give in by offering rewards

Do not reward your child for stopping a tantrum. Rewards may teach your child that a temper tantrum will help her get her way. When tantrums do not accomplish anything for your child, they are less likely to continue.

You may also feel guilty about saying "no" to your child at times. Be consistent and avoid sending mixed signals. When parents don't clearly enforce certain rules, it is harder for children to understand which rules are firm and which ones are not. Be sure you are having some fun each day with your child. Think carefully about the rules you set and don't set too many. Discuss with those who care for your child which rules are really needed and be firm about them. Respond the same way every time your child breaks the rules.

When temper tantrums are serious

Your child should have fewer temper tantrums by the middle of his fourth year. Between tantrums, his behavior should seem normal and healthy. Like every child, yours will grow and learn at his own pace. It may take time for him to learn how to control his temper. When the outbursts are severe or happen too often, they may be an early sign of emotional problems. Talk to your pediatrician if your child causes harm to himself or others during tantrums, holds his breath and faints, or if the tantrums get worse after age 4. Your pediatrician will make sure there are no serious physical or psychological problems causing the tantrums. He or she can also give you advice to help you deal with these outbursts.

It is important to realize that temper tantrums are a normal part of growing up. Tantrums are not easy to deal with, and they can be a little scary for you and your child. Using a loving and understanding approach will help your child through this part of his development.

The information contained in this publication should not be used as a substitute for the medical care and advice of your pediatrician. There may be variations in treatment that your pediatrician may recommend based on individual facts and circumstances.

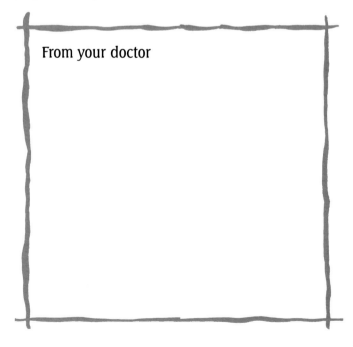

From your doctor

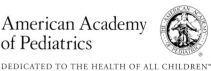

American Academy of Pediatrics

DEDICATED TO THE HEALTH OF ALL CHILDREN™

The American Academy of Pediatrics is an organization of 55,000 primary care pediatricians, pediatric medical subspecialists, and pediatric surgical specialists dedicated to the health, safety, and well-being of infants, children, adolescents, and young adults.

American Academy of Pediatrics
PO Box 747
Elk Grove Village, IL 60009-0747
Web site — http://www.aap.org

Copyright ©1989, Updated 3/99
American Academy of Pediatrics

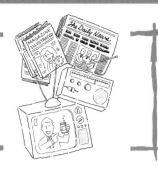

Understanding the Impact of Media on Children and Teens

In a matter of seconds, most children can mimic a movie or TV character, sing an advertising jingle, or give other examples of what they have learned from media. Sadly, these examples may include naming a popular brand of beer, striking a "sexy" pose, or play fighting. Children only have to put a movie into the VCR, open a magazine, click on a Web site, or watch TV to experience all kinds of messages. It really is that easy.

Media offer entertainment, culture, news, sports, and education. They are an important part of our lives and have much to teach. But some of what they teach may not be what we want children to learn.

This brochure gives an overview of some of the messages media send young people that could be negative or harmful to their health. You will learn how you can teach your children to better understand the media messages they see and hear in print, over airwaves, on networks, and on-line.

The power of media messages

Sometimes you can see the impact of media right away, such as when your child watches superheros fighting and then copies their moves during play. But most of the time the impact is not so immediate or obvious. It occurs slowly as children see and hear certain messages over and over, such as the following:

- Fighting and other violence used as a way to "handle" conflict
- Cigarettes and alcohol shown as cool and attractive, not unhealthy and deadly
- Sexual action with no negative results, such as disease or unintended pregnancy

Media messages: good or bad?

Whatever form they take (ads, movies, computer games, music videos), messages can be good or bad for your child. Just as you would limit certain foods in your child's diet that may be unhealthy, you also should limit her media diet of messages. Some examples of these follow.

Use of cigarettes and alcohol

Messages about tobacco and alcohol are everywhere in media. Kids see characters on screen smoking and drinking. They see signs for tobacco and alcohol products at concerts and sporting events. Advertising and movies send kids the message that smoking and drinking make a person sexy or cool and that "everyone does it." Advertising also sways teens to smoke and drink. Teens who see a lot of ads for beer, wine, liquor, and cigarettes admit that it influences them to want to drink and smoke. It is not by chance that the three most advertised cigarette brands are also the most popular ones smoked by teens.

Advertisers of tobacco and alcohol purposely leave out the negative information about their products. As a result, young people often do not know what the health risks are when they use these products. Sometimes TV broadcasts and print articles do the same thing. For example, a magazine might do a story about the common causes of cancer but not mention smoking as a top cause. Does your child know why? The answer may be that the magazine publisher takes money to publish tobacco ads or even owns another company that makes cigarettes.

Fatty foods and thin bodies

Media heavily promote unhealthy foods while at the same time telling people they need to lose weight and be thin. Heavy media use can also take time away from physical activity.

Studies show that girls of all ages worry about their weight. Many of them are starting to diet at early ages. Media can promote an unrealistic image of how people look. Often, the thin and perfect-looking person on screen or in print is not even one whole person but parts of several people! This "person" is created by using body doubles, airbrushing, and computer-graphics techniques.

Violence

Children learn their attitudes about violence at a very young age and these attitudes tend to last. Although TV violence has been studied the most, researchers are finding that violence in other media impacts children and teens in many of the same harmful ways.

- From media violence children learn to behave aggressively toward others. They are taught to use violence instead of self-control to take care of problems or conflicts.
- Violence in the "media world" may make children more accepting of real-world violence and less caring toward others. Children who see a lot of violence from movies, TV shows, or video games may become more fearful and look at the real world as a mean and scary place.

Although the effects of media on children might not be apparent right away, children are being negatively affected. Sometimes children may not act out violently until their teen or young-adult years.

Media education basics

Parents need to set limits and be actively involved with the TV shows, computer games, magazines, and other media that children use. But this is only one step in helping media play a positive role in children's lives. Because media surround us and cannot always be avoided, one way to filter their messages is to develop the skills to question, analyze, and evaluate them. This is called *media literacy* or *media education*.

Just as a print-literate child learns to be critical of the things he reads, he should also be able to do the same with moving pictures and sounds. Your child can learn to understand both the obvious and hidden messages in all media. Once children learn media education skills, they will begin to ask questions and think about the media messages they watch, read, and hear. And they usually will enjoy doing it!

Following are basic media education points your child should know:

- **People create media messages.** Any media message, whether it's a magazine article or a TV talk show, is created by a team of people. Those people write it, decide what pictures to use, and what to leave out. All of these things give the message a purpose.

- **Each media form uses its own language.** Newspapers make headlines large to attract readers to certain stories. Media with sound may use music to make people feel a range of emotions. When children learn about these techniques they are able to understand how a message is delivered instead of only being affected by it.

- **No two people experience the same media message in exactly the same way.** How a person interprets a message depends on things unique to that person's life. These can include age, values, memories, and education.

- **Media messages have their own values and points of view.** These are built into the message itself. Children should compare the promoted values against their own values. It is important for children to learn that they have a *choice* in whether to accept the values that are being promoted in any media message.

Everyday media education ideas

Besides asking how and why media messages are created, children of various ages can do everyday activities with you or other adults to help build media education skills. Make a game out of the following:

- Play "Spot the Commercials." Help your child learn to tell the difference between a regular program and the commercials that support it. This may be tricky during children's shows because many commercials advertise toys based on TV characters.

- Do a taste test to compare a heavily advertised brand with a generic or other nonadvertised brand. Try products such as cereals or soft drinks. See whether your child and his friends can tell the difference and whether advertising influenced their guesses.

- Look at the headlines, photos, and placements of articles in a newspaper. How do these affect which stories your child wants to read? Read a few stories and compare their content with their headlines and photos.

- When you see a movie, video, or video game with your child, talk about whether what happens on screen would happen in the "real" world. For example, would a person *really* be able to drive a car super fast, down narrow streets, without crashing?

- While shopping, compare products with advertisements your child has seen. Look at the ingredients, label, or packaging. Is any of this information in the ad? Does the ad give any specific information about the product itself? How is the product different than it seemed from the ad or packaging?

- How many brands of beer, cigarettes, or other such products can your child name? If she can name even one, this is a great way to begin talking about the power of advertising. Discuss the health risks of using these products and how the ads leave out that information.

- Watch a music video with your child. What stories are the pictures telling? Does the story on screen match the meaning of the words in the song? How does the video make your child feel? Can your child note any stereotypical, violent, or sexual images in the video? Is there any tobacco, alcohol, or drug use? Watch a music video with the sound off and see how it is different.

How a media message is created

The exercise that follows is a fun way for older children to think about who puts together a media message and why.

Have your child choose a media message and then answer the following questions about it. Television commercials are easy to practice with because they are short and often contain powerful words, images, and music. You could also pick a video game, the packaging for a children's toy, or a music video. The choices are endless.

1. **Describe the kinds of people involved in creating the message.** These can include writers, photographers, designers, special effects people, or stunt people.

2. **Depending on the media message you choose, talk about the visual effects that were used** (lighting, camera angles, computer-generated images, etc). Also discuss the sound (the words that are spoken, who says them, music, special effects, and other sounds). How do these different things affect the power and meaning of the message?

3. **Discuss the purpose of the message.** Are the people who made the message trying to give you information? Do they want you to do something (such as buy a product)? Or is the message just to entertain you? Many times the true meaning of a message is hidden below the surface—it is not always stated in the message. As children gain more experience questioning how messages are put together, they will be able to get at the true meaning of any message.

4. **What does your child think about the message?** Does she agree with it or disagree with it, and why? One reason to accept or reject a message could be to decide whether it is realistic or agrees with her values.

Set the home stage for media education

Starting when children are very young, most of their media use takes place in the home. Parents can help their children make better use of media by doing the following:

Make a media plan. Schedule media times and choices in advance, just as you would other activities. A media plan helps everyone to choose and use media carefully.

Set media time limits. Limit children's total screen time. This includes time watching TV and videotapes, playing video and computer games, and surfing the Internet. One way to do this is to use a timer. When the timer goes off, your child's media time is up, no exceptions. The American Academy of Pediatrics recommends no more than 1 to 2 hours of quality TV and videos a day for older children and no screen time for children under the age of 2.

Set family guidelines for media content. Help children and teens choose shows, videos, and video games that are appropriate for their ages and interests. Get into the habit of checking the content ratings and parental advisories for all media. Use these ratings to decide what media are suitable for your child.

Be clear and consistent with children about media rules. If you do not approve of their media choice, explain why and help them choose something more appropriate.

Keep TV sets, VCRs, video games, and computers out of children's bedrooms. Instead, put them where you can be involved and monitor children's use. If children or teens are allowed to have a TV set or other media in their bedrooms, know what media they are using and supervise their media choices. If you have Internet access, supervise your children while they are on-line.

Make media a family activity. Whenever possible, use media with your children and discuss what they see, hear, and read. When you share your children's media experiences, you can help them analyze, question, and challenge the meaning of messages for themselves. During a media activity, help children "talk back," or question what they see. Do this during a violent act, an image or message that is misleading, or an advertisement for an unhealthy product.

"Talking back," or asking questions about media messages, builds the lifelong skills your child needs to be a critical media consumer. Discuss how the media messages compare with the values you are teaching your child.

Look for media "side effects." Unless they come clearly labeled as containing violence, sex, or graphic language, parents often overlook the messages children are getting from media. Instead, be aware of the media children and teens use and the impact it could be having. This is especially important if your child shows any of the following behaviors:

- Poor school performance
- Hitting or pushing other kids often
- Aggressively talking back to adults
- Frequent nightmares
- Increased eating of unhealthy foods
- Smoking, drinking, or drug use

Talk to your child's pediatrician about any behavior that is a concern. Your pediatrician may take a media history of your child. This can help uncover whether certain behavioral problems exist or could develop based on how much and what kind of media your child uses. If there are problems or you think they could develop, work with your child to change his media use.

Voice your opinion. Let people who profit from the media and set guidelines about content know how you feel about media messages.

- In a phone call, letter, or e-mail message, tell companies and advertisers what you like and what you do not like. Have your kids voice their opinions too. One letter or call can make a difference.
- When media content and advertisers do not support your family's values, voice your opinion with your buying power. Do not buy their products, and tell them why.
- Support media literacy education in your child's school.

It's up to parents like you. You can learn more about media's impact by talking with your child's pediatrician and reading about media education. Schools, hospitals, and community groups may hold free workshops on topics such as taking control of kids' TV watching.

You can make a difference in the way media impacts your kids. If you limit, supervise, and share media experiences with children, they have much to gain. When you help your children understand how their media choices affect them, they actively control their media use rather than giving in to the influence of media without thinking about it.

Visiting the on-line world

Spend time with your child on the Internet and monitor where she goes and who she "talks" to on-line. Children need to be protected on-line. They are "clicks" away from being exploited by advertisers and exposed to violence, sex, adult language, and substance use.

Check for on-line ratings to help you assess violence, sex, language, and "adult" material. Use Internet-blocking programs as one way to protect your child on-line.

Make it a rule to never give out personal information on-line. This includes your child's name, address, phone number, school name or location, facts about parents and siblings, or favorite products.

The information contained in this publication should not be used as a substitute for the medical care and advice of your pediatrician. There may be variations in treatment that your pediatrician may recommend based on individual facts and circumstances.

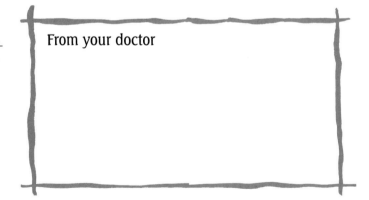

From your doctor

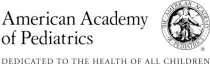

American Academy of Pediatrics

DEDICATED TO THE HEALTH OF ALL CHILDREN™

The American Academy of Pediatrics is an organization of 55,000 primary care pediatricians, pediatric medical subspecialists, and pediatric surgical specialists dedicated to the health, safety, and well-being of infants, children, adolescents, and young adults.

American Academy of Pediatrics
PO Box 747
Elk Grove Village, IL 60009-0747
Web site — http://www.aap.org

Copyright ©1999   American Academy of Pediatrics

SECTION SIX

Developmental Issues

Helping Your Child Learn to Read

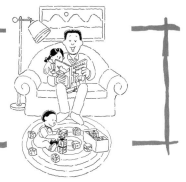

Does your child listen closely during story time? Does your child like to look through books and magazines? Does your child like learning the names of letters? If the answer is "yes" to any of these questions, your child may have already learned some important early reading skills and may be ready to learn some of the basics of reading. This brochure gives tips on how to make reading a family tradition and how to help your child develop a love of learning.

Reading tips

The following are a few tips to keep in mind as your child learns to read:

- Set aside time every day to read together. Many children like to have stories read to them at bedtime. This is a great way to wind down after a busy day and get ready for sleep.
- Leave books in your child's room for her to enjoy on her own. Make sure her room is reading-friendly with a comfortable bed or chair, bookshelf, and reading lamp.
- Read books that your child enjoys. After a while, your child may learn the words to her favorite book. When this happens, let your child complete the sentences or take turns reciting the words.
- Do not drill your child on letters, numbers, colors, shapes, or words. Instead, make a game out of it and find ways to encourage your child's curiosity and interests.

Start the process early

A child as young as 6 months of age can begin to enjoy books. The following are some age-by-age activities to help your young child learn language and begin to make the connection between words and meaning:

Birth to 1 year of age

- Play frequently with your baby. Talk, sing, recite rhymes, and do finger plays. This helps your baby learn spoken language and builds a strong foundation for reading.
- Talk with your baby, making eye contact. Allow time for your baby to respond before moving on to the next idea.
- Give your baby board books or soft books to look at, chew on, or bang on the table.
- Look at picture books with your baby and name the objects that he sees. Say things like "See the baby!" or "Look at the puppy!"
- Snuggle with your baby on your lap and read aloud to him. He may not understand the story, but he will love to hear the sound of your voice and the rhythm of the language.

1 to 3 years of age

- Read to your child every day. Allow your child to pick which books he wants, even if he picks the same one time and time again!
- Let your child "read" to you by naming objects in the book or making up a story.

- Make regular trips to the library with your child. Most children find it very exciting to get a library card. Make this moment something to celebrate.
- Continue to talk, sing, recite rhymes, and play with your child.

3 to 5 years of age

- By 3 to 5 years of age, most children are just beginning to learn the alphabet—singing their ABCs, knowing the letters of their names. Read alphabet books with your child and point out letters as you read.
- Help your child recognize whole words as well as letters. Learning and remembering what words look like are the first steps to learning to read. Point out common, everyday things like the letters on a stop sign or the logo on a favorite restaurant.
- As you read together, ask your child to make up his own story about what is happening in the book. Keep reading a part of your child's bedtime routine.
- Some educational television shows, videos, and computer programs can help your child learn to read. They can also make learning fun. But you need to be involved, too. If your child is watching *Mr. Rogers' Neighborhood* or *Sesame Street,* for example, sit and talk about what the program is trying to teach. Limit screen time to no more than 1 or 2 hours per day of educational, nonviolent programs.
- If possible, give your child a subscription to a children's magazine. Children love getting mail, and it is something they can read as well!
- Provide opportunities for your child to use written language for many purposes. Write shopping lists together. Compose letters to send to friends or relatives.

Reading aloud with your child

Reading books aloud is one of the best ways you can help your child learn to read. This can be fun for you, too. The more excitement you show when you read a book, the more your child will enjoy it. The most important thing to remember is to let your child set her own pace and have fun at whatever she is doing. Do the following when reading to your child:

- Run your finger under the words as you read to show your child that the print carries the story.
- Use funny voices and animal noises. Do not be afraid to ham it up! This will help your child get excited about the story.
- Stop to look at the pictures; ask your child to name things she sees in the pictures. Talk about how the pictures relate to the story.
- Invite your child to join in whenever there is a repeated phrase in the text.
- Show your child how events in the book are similar to events in your child's life.
- If your child asks a question, stop and answer it. The book may help your child express her thoughts and solve her own problems.
- Keep reading to your child even after she learns to read. A child can listen and understand more difficult stories than she can read on her own.

Listening to your child read aloud

Once your child begins to read, have him read out loud. This can help build your child's confidence in his ability to read and help him enjoy learning new skills. Take turns reading with your child to model more advanced reading skills.

If your child asks for help with a word, give it right away so that he does not lose the meaning of the story. Do not force your child to sound out the word. On the other hand, if your child wants to sound out a word, do not stop him.

If your child substitutes one word for another while reading, see if it makes sense. If your child uses the word "dog" instead of "pup," for example, the meaning is the same. Do not stop the reading to correct him. If your child uses a word that makes no sense (such as "road" for "read"), ask him to read the sentence again because you are not sure you understand what has just been read. Recognize your child's energy limits. Stop each session at or before the earliest signs of fatigue or frustration.

Most of all, make sure you give your child lots of praise! You are your child's first, and most important, teacher. The praise and support you give your child as he learns to read will help him enjoy reading and learning even more.

Learning to read in school

Most children learn to read by 6 or 7 years of age. Some children learn at 4 or 5 years of age. Even if a child has a head start, she may not stay ahead once school starts. The other students most likely will catch up during the second or third grade. Pushing your child to read before she is ready can get in the way of your child's interest in learning. Children who really enjoy learning are more likely to do well in school. This love of learning cannot be forced.

As your child begins elementary school, she will begin her formal reading education. There are many ways to teach children to read. One way emphasizes word recognition and teaches children to understand a whole word's meaning by how it is used. Learning which sounds the letters represent—phonics—is another way children learn to read. Phonics is used to help "decode" or sound out words. Focusing on the connections between the spoken and written word is another technique. Most teachers use a combination of methods to teach children how to read.

Reading is an important skill for children to learn. Most children learn to read without any major problems. Pushing a child to learn before she is ready can make learning to read frustrating. But reading together and playing games with books make reading fun. Parents need to be involved in their child's learning. Encouraging a child's love of learning will go a long way to ensuring success in school.

The American Academy of Pediatrics gratefully acknowledges the assistance of the Reach Out and Read program in the development of this brochure. Reach Out and Read is a pediatric early literacy program that makes literacy promotion and giving out books part of pediatric primary care. This program is endorsed by the American Academy of Pediatrics. For more information about Reach Out and Read, please contact the program at

Reach Out and Read
National Center
29 Mystic Ave
Somerville, MA 02145
617/629-8042
www.reachoutandread.org

Dyslexia

Does your child reverse letters or numbers or see them upside down? Does he read very slowly, really struggle to decode words, or continually misspell fairly simple words?

Most children have these problems when they are first learning to read. However, if no improvements are made over several years, these problems may be a sign of *dyslexia*, a reading disorder. Today, dyslexia is easier to identify than other learning problems. Talk to your pediatrician if, by 7 years of age, your child often does the following:

- Confuses the order of letters in words
- Does not look carefully at all the letters in a word, guessing what the word is from the first letter
- Loses his place on a page while reading, sometimes in the middle of a line
- Reads word by word, struggling with almost every one of them
- Reads very slowly and tires easily from reading

The information contained in this publication should not be used as a substitute for the medical care and advice of your pediatrician. There may be variations in treatment that your pediatrician may recommend based on individual facts and circumstances.

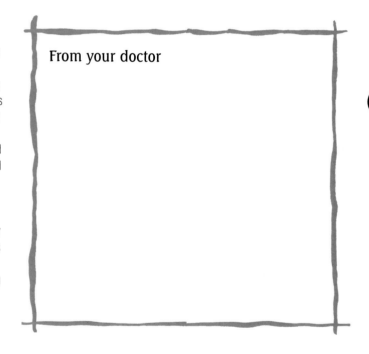

From your doctor

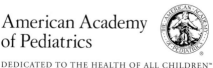

American Academy of Pediatrics

DEDICATED TO THE HEALTH OF ALL CHILDREN™

The American Academy of Pediatrics is an organization of 55,000 primary care pediatricians, pediatric medical subspecialists, and pediatric surgical specialists dedicated to the health, safety, and well-being of infants, children, adolescents, and young adults.

American Academy of Pediatrics
PO Box 747
Elk Grove Village, IL 60009-0747
Web site — http://www.aap.org

Copyright ©1999, Updated 1/02   American Academy of Pediatrics

Learning Disabilities and Children

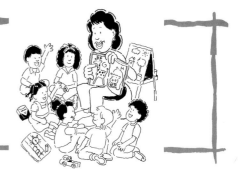

What is a learning disability?

During the preschool years, children undergo rapid change and growth—physically, mentally, and emotionally. And they do this at different rates. So it is important to know whether they are ready and able to succeed in school. There are many reasons why they may not be able to learn, such as:

- hearing problems
- poor motivation
- emotional problems
- mental retardation

Some school-age children with none of the above problems still have trouble in a school setting. These children may have normal, near normal, or above normal intelligence. This inability to reach their full potential is called a **learning disability.**

In many cases, the cause of a learning disability is not known. Experts believe that children with learning disabilities have a problem with the way the brain handles information. This hinders the normal learning process. Learning disabilities often make children feel bad about themselves. Parents need to understand this and provide their children with love and support.

The problem they are going through is similar to a distorted television picture caused by "technical problems" at the station. There is nothing wrong with the TV camera at the station or the TV set in your home. Yet, the picture is not clear. Something in the internal workings of the TV station prevents it from presenting a good picture.

There may be nothing wrong with the way children with learning disabilities take in information. Their senses of sight and sound are fine. The problem occurs in the brain **after** the eyes or ears have done their job. For example, it is easy to blame reading difficulties on the eyes. But, **visual problems do not cause learning disabilities.** Children with learning disabilities have no greater rate of eye problems than the rest of the population.

This problem in brain function delays the normal learning process. For this reason, it requires special teaching methods. A learning disability is not just a minor problem that simply goes away as children mature. A learning disability must be identified and treated early. If it is, there's a greater chance that children with learning disabilities will reach their potential. If it isn't, it could lead to major emotional problems causing depression and withdrawal. Both factors are linked to school failure.

Learning disabilities are not uncommon. They appear to be more common in boys than girls. More than 1 out of 10 public school students may be in need of special education. Of these, about half have some type of learning disability.

What are the causes of learning disabilities?

Some children are born into families with a history of learning disabilities. Others have risk factors that may make them more likely to have learning disabilities. These risk factors include:

- low birth weight
- stress before or after birth
- treatment for cancer or leukemia
- infections of the central nervous system
- severe head injuries

What are some common problems these children experience?

At an early age, children with potential learning disabilities may define and translate symbols differently. They often do not understand what they see or hear. Some cannot grasp how letters make up words, how words make up sentences, and how sentences make up thoughts. Structured writings appear foreign. Experts use the term **perceptual disability** to describe these problems. Perceptual problems may affect how children follow oral instructions, copy from the blackboard, or recall what a teacher or parent has said. These children may often have problems organizing their assignments at school and at home.

What are the warning signs?

It may not be easy to detect learning disabilities in children. This type of problem does not reveal itself in a day or a week. There are warning signs, however, that can help parents know if their children have a learning disability. Parents should note if any of the situations listed below are present in their preschool children:

Delays in language development. By 2 1/2 years old, children should be able to put sentences together.

Trouble with speech. By 3 years old, parents and others should understand what children say more than half of the time.

Trouble with coordination. Just before kindergarten, children should be able to tie shoes, button, hop, and cut.

Short attention span. Between 3 and 5 years old, children should be able to sit still while being read a short story. (Attention span should increase with age during this period.)

Regard these signs as risk factors only. Remember that no child develops in the same manner or at the same pace. These signs may not always reveal a learning disability. If you have any questions about the proper activities for your child's age, talk to your pediatrician.

When is the best time to diagnose/identify a learning disability?

The sooner it is detected, the sooner these children can receive special attention and treatment. In past generations, learning disabilities often were not recognized. Many people struggled and few learned to adjust to their weaknesses. Those who weren't able to adjust suffered frustration and endured a series of life-long failures. This sometimes led to school dropout, delinquency, and unemployment.

Children with undiagnosed learning disabilities could become angry and frustrated. This can lead to severe emotional problems. They often think they are dumb, although their intelligence is often above normal. Aggressive behavior, withdrawal, or depression could result. This, in turn, could worsen the existing trouble with reading, writing, spelling, or math.

Early treatment and special education can have a good effect on these children. Family love and support play major roles in helping children live with their learning disability. Such caring by parents helps children feel better about themselves. It also gives children a greater sense of confidence and inner strength. They need this now as well as later in life.

Who is most likely to suspect a learning disability?

The people who have the most contact with the children are parents, preschool teachers, or pediatricians. Doctors or teachers can give screening tests to see if a problem exists. The pediatrician can help the parents decide if further evaluation is needed. This may include an eye exam by a doctor (ophthalmologist), a psychological exam by a psychologist, an ear exam by an ear/nose/throat doctor, or a language assessment by a speech and language clinician. Federal laws require that schools test and help all children with language and/or learning disabilities. These tests are at no cost to parents. New laws ensure diagnostic and remedial services to all children from birth to 21 years of age.

Are there cures for learning disabilities?

There is no cure for a learning disability. Despite the many frustrations, proper help from a number of professionals can make the difference. Children may learn to achieve and lead a fruitful life in spite of their disability.

There are people and groups who offer simple answers or solutions for learning disabilities. Be cautious of these claims. Some allege that visual treatments can help although **no data support this theory**. Others believe in special diets and exercise. Still others claim certain vitamins will provide children's bodies with a needed balance and cure the problem. Keep in mind there is no guidance to support any of these treatments. There are no quick fixes for a learning disability. Dealing with this problem is tough. It's often a lifelong battle.

What's the outlook like today for children with a learning disability?

Early identification and treatment cannot be stressed enough. With the proper help, children with learning disabilities can become quite successful later in life. Famous Americans with learning disabilities include: inventor Thomas Edison, Vice President Nelson Rockefeller, scientist Albert Einstein, and athlete Bruce Jenner. These people rose above their disability and went on to achieve great personal and national goals.

People who learn to overcome their disability can do great things in life. For children with a learning disability, nothing can replace a good educational program and proper medical management. As important are loving and supportive parents, family, and friends.

The information contained in this publication should not be used as a substitute for the medical care and advice of your pediatrician. There may be variations in treatment that your pediatrician may recommend based on individual facts and circumstances.

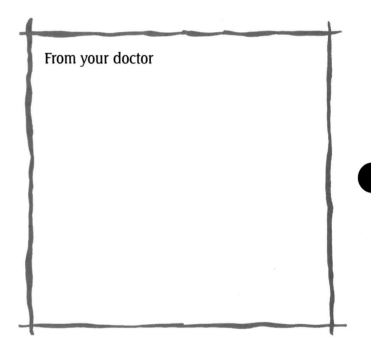

From your doctor

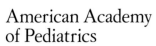

American Academy of Pediatrics

DEDICATED TO THE HEALTH OF ALL CHILDREN™

The American Academy of Pediatrics is an organization of 55,000 primary care pediatricians, pediatric medical subspecialists, and pediatric surgical specialists dedicated to the health, safety, and well-being of infants, children, adolescents, and young adults.

American Academy of Pediatrics
PO Box 747
Elk Grove Village, IL 60009-0747
Web site — http://www.aap.org

Learning Disabilities and Young Adults

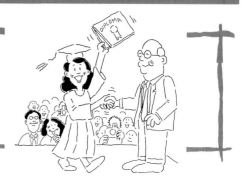

Experts estimate that as many as 12 percent of all school-aged youths in elementary, junior high and high school have some type of learning problem. These students may have emotional problems, poor hearing or vision problems; they also could be developmentally delayed. Other young people who do not face these obvious stumbling blocks still fail to do well in school or at work. These teens and young adults may have an unrecognized learning disability.

This brochure explains some of the different types of learning disabilities and how to help your learning-disabled teen or young adult cope with these problems. It also explains the training and education options that are available so your son or daughter can learn valuable job skills and work around a disability.

What is a learning disability?

Experts say that learning disabilities are due to problems with the way the brain handles information. Having a disability means that learning is difficult despite a person's best attempts. The good news is that many of these problems can be overcome by using different skills. Many learning-disabled people have made their mark in science, the arts and other fields. Albert Einstein is a good example. He learned new skills to solve problems.

Many learning-disabled youths may have normal or above-average intelligence. However, these teens may have a hard time working with written figures, spoken ideas, or certain letters and words. A student may have a hard time knowing how letters make up words, how words combine to create sentences and how sentences express thoughts. This can lead to problems with reading, spelling, writing and math.

What causes a learning disability?

A number of different factors may lead to a learning disability, such as inherited (genetic) health problems, low birth weight in ill babies or harmful environmental conditions. However, the causes are often unknown. Despite these problems, children with a disability can lead a normal life.

Experts look for early signals of a disability, including:
- failing to follow directions and appearing to "forget" what a parent or teacher says
- constant daydreaming or taking an unusually long time to finish a task
- problems organizing work at home and school

Some learning-disabled people may have several disabilities that combine to worsen the problem. For example, these students may:
- fail to learn facts and information
- handle assignments poorly
- have problems relating with peers
- not understand jokes, subtle responses or facial expressions
- have trouble paying attention or may be overactive
- feel bad about themselves

As a result, they could become unsure or uneasy in school. On the job, these workers may:
- fail to finish projects that require reading or math skills
- seem to "forget" what people say
- not understand a request
- clash with other workers

If your teen or young adult has problems like these, you should contact teachers, your pediatrician or other professionals who can help. Experts can identify the problem and find ways to help.

Building on strengths

Your teen has special talents as well as weaknesses. He may be good at math, music or sports, or he could be skilled at art or working with tools. Finding special strengths, and learning to use them, is hard work. It may be difficult for him to accept and work around a weak point. Encourage your son to use his strengths to explore and meet new challenges. This can help him develop new skills.

Developing social skills

The teen years are an awkward time of change. A learning disability can make growing up even harder, because being like other youths is important for your teen. Disabilities combined with the pain of growing up can make your teen sad, angry or withdrawn. Talking about the problem may be difficult.

In groups, a learning-disabled worker or student may be shy. Many learning-disabled youths have above average intelligence and special skills that others may not have. Your family can help by pointing out that a learning disability is not tied to how smart she is. Family members also can help by finding clubs and teams that stress friendship and fun, instead of just winning.

Your teen's pediatrician can help with tests that identify a disability. The doctor also may refer your teen to other medical specialists. Depending on what your teen's needs are, she may be referred to a pediatric neurologist, a behavioral pediatrician, a psychiatrist, a psychologist or an educator. Look for local groups in your state for support and information on learning disabilities.

Look for opportunities

Start planning for adulthood. Your child must make career and education choices during the school years. Most schools have special classes to teach your learning-disabled youth the right skills for the work force and/or higher education.

Find a specialist who can help. Teachers, employers, and college and job counselors can encourage your son or daughter to tap into special skills and cope with weak points.

Look for career search programs. These programs teach the skills that are necessary for teens to succeed in the workplace. Many career search programs include aptitude tests to help youths find the right talents and choose a career. A good program teaches useful job skills and also shows the value of self-esteem and decision-making skills.

Vocational programs. These programs teach young people how to apply for a job, accept directions, and get along with family, friends and coworkers.

Some high schools and colleges have programs to help learning-disabled students learn new skills. Counselors can direct students to tutors, study groups or graduate assistants who are willing to help.

Types of learning disabilities

Dyslexia is a term that describes serious problems with reading. With this problem, your child may not understand letters, groups of letters, sentences or paragraphs.

At the beginning of first grade, children may occasionally reverse and rotate the letters they read and write. This may be normal when first learning to read. By the middle of first grade (and with maturity) these problems disappear.

However, a young student with dyslexia (reading disabilities) may not overcome these problems. The difficulty can continue as the student gets older.

- To her, a "b" may look like a "d."
- She may write "on," when she really means "no."
- Your daughter may reverse a "6" to make "9."

This is not a vision problem. The problem involves how the brain interprets the information it "sees."

Dysgraphia is a term for problems with writing. With this problem, your teen may not form letters correctly, and there is difficulty writing within a certain space. Writing neatly takes time and effort. But despite the extra effort, handwriting still may be hard to read.

A teacher may say that a learning-disabled student can't finish written tests and assignments on time. Supervisors may find that written tasks are always late or incomplete.

Dyscalculia is a term for problems doing math. With this problem, your teen may not grasp math concepts. He may do well in history and language, but he may fail tests involving fractions and percentages. Math is difficult for many students. But with dyscalculia, a young person may have a much more difficult time doing math than others his age. Dyscalculia may prevent your teen from solving basic math problems that others his age complete with no difficulty.

Auditory memory and processing disabilities is a term for problems understanding and remembering words or sounds. Your daughter may hear normally, but she may not remember key facts because her memory does not store and interpret facts correctly. This is not caused by a hearing problem. It happens when the brain fails to understand words or sounds the right way.

Parents, teachers and pediatricians usually detect learning disabilities during the school years, but a problem may not surface until the teen years. It's important to remember that it's never too late to get help.

Communication is the key that opens the door to the working world. You can help your young adult land that first job by helping him practice for interviews, choose the right clothes to wear and maintain a positive point of view. With a little coaching, he can build self-esteem and become a successful worker.

Coping on the job

Choose the right career. Your young adult can find and hold a good job. Landing the right job increases her chance of success—especially if the work is rewarding. Handling on-the-job tasks will help her deal with problem situations and build self-esteem.

Ask for help. Hiding a disability can make a situation worse. It pays to ask questions. When your teen asks at work—and a supervisor is willing to help—a job can open new doors of opportunity.

It's the law. Federal law forbids discrimination against disabled persons in the workplace. Some employers know that it's good business to provide the help that learning-disabled people need. During an interview, an employer may ask to see written proof of a disability from a pediatrician or some other professional.

Continuing education

Learning disabilities are not tied to intelligence, which is why some learning-disabled students can perform well in high school and college. If your teen has not completed high school, he should try to obtain the Graduate Equivalency Diploma (GED). Ask a counselor for help. A counselor may be able to recommend a tutor who works with the learning disabled. Passing the GED test will make a learning-disabled youth confident during job interviews and help him land a good job. Some young adults choose to attend a trade school or junior college after high school. Other students may complete a two-year community college program and then move on to a four-year school. Many learning-disabled students can meet the entrance requirements for a four-year college. These schools usually expect all young adults to meet the same standards. This includes high school grade point averages and ACT and/or SAT scores.

Some colleges have special testing and admissions policies for the learning disabled, such as SAT or ACT tests that are not timed. To apply to special college programs, students usually need written proof of a disability and recommendations from teachers and counselors.

College is hard work. Your young adult can meet this challenge by carefully arranging schedules and asking others for help. Tutors usually are available for specific classes, and more and more colleges have writing clinics to help students develop communications skills.

It's also very important to notify the admissions counselor if your son or daughter has a disability. Ask about special classes for the learning disabled. Many community colleges have programs aimed at skills, such as aviation technology, auto mechanics, computer technology, electronics and cosmetology. In these programs, students learn valuable skills that help them find a job. With all the facts, a student can decide if the college has the right programs and services for him or her.

Support from friends and family is vital

Whether at work or school, it's important to praise your son or daughter for doing a good job. But if he or she fails, coaching and support from family and friends is very important.

Coping with a learning disability is a lifelong job. It's a full-time job for your teen's friends and family members, too. With the right support from friends and family, your teen can build a positive self-esteem despite the occasional setbacks. Without support, a learning disability is much harder to cope with.

Friends and family can help by working on new solutions, providing new challenges, offering praise when it is due and encouraging learning disabled teens.

Written reminders, quiet study areas and scheduled study times are great ways to learn the right skills for the workplace.

Hard work leads to success

People from all walks of life have overcome disabilities to become very successful. Some of the success stories include singer/actress Cher; actors Harry Anderson and Tom Cruise; inventor Thomas Edison; former Vice President Nelson Rockefeller; baseball pitcher Nolan Ryan; Olympic diver Greg Louganis; and former British Prime Minister Winston Churchill.

Your pediatrician, together with educators and other professionals, can help with early detection of a learning disability. Contact a pediatrician if you have other questions, and remember the following tips:

- Promote a positive self-image.
- Emphasize your teen's best assets.
- Work with your child to help him/her develop compensation skills.
- Be patient, and never demand that your teen complete a task that is too difficult for him/her.
- Work with useful aids such as calculators, word processors, tape recorders and typewriters.
- Know what kind of help is available through schools and employers.
- Practice skills at home.
- Find a tutor or a training program
- Seek a quiet, distraction-free place to study.
- Talk to counselors and set reasonable goals.
- Learn what rights a disabled person has under the law.
- Don't be afraid to ask questions or find help; it's never too late.

For more information on learning disabilities, refer to the following resources:

- Learning Disabilities Association of America
  4156 Library Rd
  Pittsburgh, PA 15234
  412/341-1515
- HEATH Resource Center
  (The National Clearinghouse on
  Postsecondary Education for Individuals With Disabilities)
  One Dupont Circle
  Suite 800
  Washington, DC 20036
  800/544-3284
- National Information Center for Children and Youths With Disabilities (NICHCY)
  PO Box 1492
  Washington, DC 20013
  800/999-5599
- Mangrum CT, Strichart SS, Peterson's Guide to Colleges With Programs for Learning-Disabled Students, Peterson's Guide, Inc., Princeton, NJ: 1988.

The information contained in this publication should not be used as a substitute for the medical care and advice of your pediatrician. There may be variations in treatment that your pediatrician may recommend based on individual facts and circumstances.

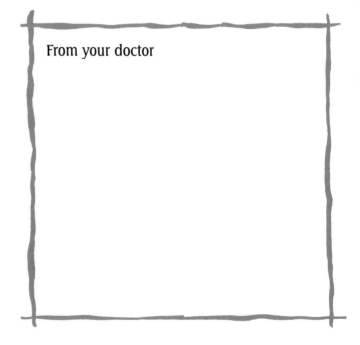

From your doctor

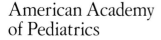

American Academy of Pediatrics

DEDICATED TO THE HEALTH OF ALL CHILDREN™

The American Academy of Pediatrics is an organization of 55,000 primary care pediatricians, pediatric medical subspecialists, and pediatric surgical specialists dedicated to the health, safety, and well-being of infants, children, adolescents, and young adults.

American Academy of Pediatrics
PO Box 747
Elk Grove Village, IL 60009-0747
Web site — http://www.aap.org

Your Child's Growth:
Developmental Milestones

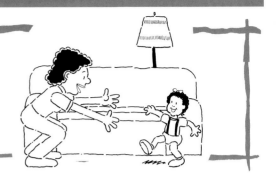

Watching a young child grow is a wonderful and unique experience for a parent. Learning to sit up, walk, and talk are some of the more major developmental milestones your child will achieve. But your child's growth is a complex and ongoing process. Young bodies are constantly going through a number of physical and mental changes.

Although no two children develop at the same rate, they should be able to do certain things at certain ages. As a parent, you are in the best position to note your child's development, and you can use the milestones described in this brochure as guidelines.

At the ages noted in this brochure, observe your child for 1 month. (This lets you take into account any days when your child may be acting differently because she is sick or upset.) Use the milestones listed for each age to see how your child is developing.

Remember, a "No" answer to any of these questions does not necessarily mean that there is a problem. Every child develops at his own pace and may sometimes develop more slowly in certain areas than other children the same age. Keep in mind these milestones should be used only as guidelines.

Plan to talk about these guidelines with your pediatrician during your next office visit if you note the following:

• Major differences between your child's development and the milestones.
• Your child does not yet do many of the things usually done at her age.

3 Months

When your baby is lying on his back, does he move each of his arms equally well? Check "No" if your baby makes jerky or uncoordinated movements with one or both of his arms or legs, or uses only one arm all the time. ❏ Yes ❏ No

Does your baby make sounds such as gurgling, cooing, babbling, or other noises besides crying? ❏ Yes ❏ No

Does your baby respond to your voice? ❏ Yes ❏ No

Are your baby's hands frequently open? ❏ Yes ❏ No

When you hold your baby in the upright position, can she support her head for more than a moment? ❏ Yes ❏ No

6 Months

Have you seen your baby play with his hands by touching them together? ❏ Yes ❏ No

Does your baby turn her head to sounds that originate out of her immediate area? ❏ Yes ❏ No

Has your baby rolled over from his stomach to his back or from back to stomach? ❏ Yes ❏ No

When you hold your baby under her arms, can she bear some weight on her legs? Check "Yes" only if she tries to stand on her feet and support some of her weight. ❏ Yes ❏ No

When your baby is on his stomach, can he support his weight on outstretched hands? ❏ Yes ❏ No

Does your baby see small objects such as crumbs? ❏ Yes ❏ No

Does your baby produce a string of sounds? ❏ Yes ❏ No

Does she react to the emotions of others? ❏ Yes ❏ No

Does your baby begin to relax when you read him a bedtime story? ❏ Yes ❏ No

Does your baby notice herself and her actions in a mirror? ❏ Yes ❏ No

Does your baby reach out for you to pick him up? ❏ Yes ❏ No

9 Months

When your baby is playing and you come up quietly behind her, does she sometimes turn her head as though she hears you? (Loud sounds do not count.) Check "Yes" only if you have seen her respond to quiet sounds or whispers. ❏ Yes ❏ No

Can your baby sit without support and without holding up his body with his hands? ❏ Yes ❏ No

Does your baby crawl or creep on her hands and knees? ❏ Yes ❏ No

Does your baby hold his bottle? ❏ Yes ❏ No

Does your baby deliberately drop or throw toys? ❏ Yes ❏ No

Does she bang, strike, and shake her toys? ❏ Yes ❏ No

When you show your baby a book, does he get excited, then try to grab and taste it? ❏ Yes ❏ No

Is your baby wary of unfamiliar people? ❏ Yes ❏ No

Does your baby make sounds that use vowels and consonants? ❏ Yes ❏ No

12 Months

When you hide behind something or around a corner and then reappear, does your baby look for you and eagerly plan for you to reappear? ❏ Yes ❏ No

Does your baby pull up to stand? ❏ Yes ❏ No

Does your baby walk holding on to furniture? ❏ Yes ❏ No

Does your baby make "ma-ma" or "da-da" sounds? Check "Yes" if she makes either sound. ❏ Yes ❏ No

Does your baby say at least one word? ❏ Yes ❏ No

Is your baby able to locate sounds by turning his head? ❏ Yes ❏ No

Does your baby imitate familiar adult behavior, such as using a cup or telephone? ❏ Yes ❏ No

Does your baby turn her books face up, but turn several pages at once? ❏ Yes ❏ No

Does your baby look for and find toys? ❏ Yes ❏ No

Does your baby eagerly explore objects and spaces? ❏ Yes ❏ No

18 Months

Can your child hold a regular cup or glass without help and drink from it without spilling? ❏ Yes ❏ No

Can your child walk all the way across a large room without falling or wobbling from side to side? ❏ Yes ❏ No

Does your child take off his shoes by himself? ❏ Yes ❏ No

Does your child feed herself? ❏ Yes ❏ No

Does your child clearly look to his parents in stressful situations? ❏ Yes ❏ No

Does your child have temper tantrums? ❏ Yes ❏ No

Does your child say at least 4 to 10 words? ❏ Yes ❏ No

Does your child point to a picture that you name in a book? ❏ Yes ❏ No

Does your child pretend to talk? ❏ Yes ❏ No

2 Years

Can your child say things like "all gone," "go bye-bye," or other two-word sentences? ❏ Yes ❏ No

Does your child say about 50 words? ❏ Yes ❏ No

Can your child take off clothes such as pajamas (tops or bottoms) or pants? (Diapers, hats, and socks do not count.) ❏ Yes ❏ No

Does your child run without falling? ❏ Yes ❏ No

Does your child look at pictures in a picture book? ❏ Yes ❏ No

Does your child carry around a favorite book and pretend to read it to you? ❏ Yes ❏ No

Does your child tell you what she wants? ❏ Yes ❏ No

Does your child repeat words others say? ❏ Yes ❏ No

Does your child point to at least one named body part? ❏ Yes ❏ No

Does your child participate in play with other children? ❏ Yes ❏ No

Does your child show increasing independence, wanting to do things his way? ❏ Yes ❏ No

Does your child like to collect or hoard things? ❏ Yes ❏ No

3 Years

Can your child name at least one picture when you look at animal books together? ❏ Yes ❏ No

Does your child enjoy sitting together for at least 5 minutes for story time? ❏ Yes ❏ No

Can your child answer "what" questions about the story that you have just read together? ❏ Yes ❏ No

Can your child throw a ball overhand (not sidearm or underhand) toward your stomach or chest from a distance of 5 feet? ❏ Yes ❏ No

Is your child easily understood by most adults? ❏ Yes ❏ No

Does your child help put things away? ❏ Yes ❏ No

Can your child answer the question, "Are you a boy or girl?" ❏ Yes ❏ No

Can your child name at least one color? ❏ Yes ❏ No

Does your child talk in three-word sentences most of the time? ❏ Yes ❏ No

4 Years

Can your child pedal a tricycle at least 10 feet forward? ❏ Yes ❏ No

Does your child play hide-and-seek, cops-and-robbers, or other games where she takes turns and follows rules? ❏ Yes ❏ No

Does your child turn paper pages in a book one at a time? ❏ Yes ❏ No

Does your child retell stories that are familiar? ❏ Yes ❏ No

Can your child tell you what action is taking place in a picture? ❏ Yes ❏ No

Does your child use action words (verbs)? ❏ Yes ❏ No

Does your child play pretend games, such as with toys, dolls, animals, or even an imaginary friend? ❏ Yes ❏ No

Can your child copy a circle? ❏ Yes ❏ No

Does your child pretend to write, making marks on a page that only he can read? ❏ Yes ❏ No

Does your child mostly use four-word or five-word sentences when talking? ❏ Yes ❏ No

5 Years

Can your child button some of her clothing or her doll's clothes? (Snaps do not count.) ❏ Yes ❏ No

Does your child react well when you leave him with a friend or sitter? ❏ Yes ❏ No

Can your child name at least three colors? ❏ Yes ❏ No

Can your child walk down stairs alternating her feet? ❏ Yes ❏ No

Can your child jump with his feet apart (broad jump)? ❏ Yes ❏ No

Can your child point while counting at least three different objects? ❏ Yes ❏ No

Can your child name a coin correctly? ❏ Yes ❏ No

Does your child like to relax together with you for 10 to 20 minutes of story time? ❏ Yes ❏ No

Can your child copy a square? ❏ Yes ❏ No

Can your child name at least some letters of the alphabet when she sees them? ❏ Yes ❏ No

Can your child identify and print the first letter in his name? ❏ Yes ❏ No

Can your child recognize and name several single numbers? ❏ Yes ❏ No

Does your child recognize common street and store signs (eg, "Stop," "Open")? ❏ Yes ❏ No

6 Years

Can your child tie her shoes? ❏ Yes ❏ No

Can your child dress himself completely without help? ❏ Yes ❏ No

Can your child catch a small bouncing ball, such as a tennis ball, using only her hands? (Large balls do not count.) ❏ Yes ❏ No

Can your child skip with both feet? ❏ Yes ❏ No

Can your child tell his age correctly? ❏ Yes ❏ No

Can your child repeat at least four numbers in the proper sequence? ❏ Yes ❏ No

Can your child recognize and name at least 10 letters in the alphabet? ❏ Yes ❏ No

Does your child know the sounds of most letters of the alphabet? ❏ Yes ❏ No

Can your child recognize and read 15 or more common words? ❏ Yes ❏ No

Can your child copy a few simple words from a book? ❏ Yes ❏ No

As a parent, you are in the best position to note these subtle aspects of your child's behavior. These clues signal that your child's development is on schedule or that something might be wrong. A "No" answer to any of the questions may be a warning sign. Make sure to bring it to your pediatrician's attention. Remember, these milestones are an aid, not a test.

If you have any questions, plan to discuss them with your pediatrician. Pediatricians are trained to detect and treat developmental problems in children. Many problems, if detected early, can be treated by your pediatrician and successfully managed.

Copyrighted information used in this brochure was granted courtesy of William Frankenburg, MD, and Josiah Dodds, MD.

The information contained in this publication should not be used as a substitute for the medical care and advice of your pediatrician. There may be variations in treatment that your pediatrician may recommend based on individual facts and circumstances.

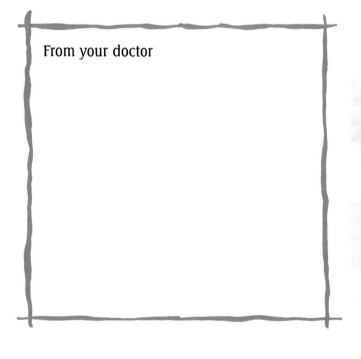

From your doctor

American Academy of Pediatrics

DEDICATED TO THE HEALTH OF ALL CHILDREN™

The American Academy of Pediatrics is an organization of 55,000 primary care pediatricians, pediatric medical subspecialists, and pediatric surgical specialists dedicated to the health, safety, and well-being of infants, children, adolescents, and young adults.

American Academy of Pediatrics
PO Box 747
Elk Grove Village, IL 60009-0747
Web site — http://www.aap.org

Copyright ©1990, Updated 6/01   American Academy of Pediatrics

SECTION SEVEN

Safety and Prevention

Air Bag Safety

An air bag can save your life. However, air bags and young children do not mix. The following information will help keep you and your children safe.

- The safest place for *all* infants and children under 12 years of age to ride is in the back seat.
- *Never* put an infant under 1 year of age in the front seat of a car with an air bag.
- Infants must always ride in rear-facing car seats in the back seat until they are at least 20 pounds AND 1 year of age.
- All children should be properly secured in car safety seats, booster seats, or shoulder/lap belts correct for their size.
- Seat belts must be worn correctly at all times by all passengers to provide the best protection.

What Parents Can Do

- Eliminate potential risks of air bags to children by buckling them in the *back* seat for every ride.
- Plan ahead so that you do not have to drive with more children than can be safely restrained in the backseat.
- For most families, installation of air bag on/off switches is not necessary. Air bags that are turned off provide no protection to older children, teens, parents, or other adults riding in the front seat.
- Air bag on/off switches should only be used if your child has special health care needs, your pediatrician recommends constant observation during travel, and no other adult is available to ride in the back seat with your child.

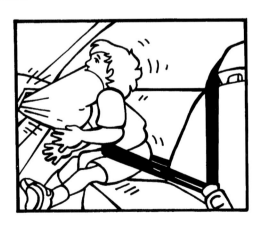

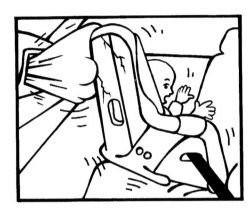

- If no other arrangement is possible and an older child *must* ride in the front seat, move the vehicle seat back as far as it can go, away from the air bag. Be sure the child is properly buckled. Keep in mind that your child may still be at risk for injuries from the air bag. The back seat is the safest place for children to ride.

The information contained in this publication should not be used as a substitute for the medical care and advice of your pediatrician. There may be variations in treatment that your pediatrician may recommend based on individual facts and circumstances.

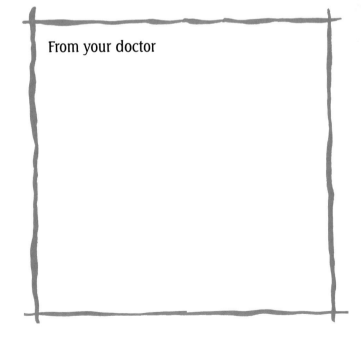

From your doctor

American Academy
of Pediatrics

DEDICATED TO THE HEALTH OF ALL CHILDREN™

The American Academy of Pediatrics is an organization of 55,000 primary care pediatricians, pediatric medical subspecialists, and pediatric surgical specialists dedicated to the health, safety, and well-being of infants, children, adolescents, and young adults.

American Academy of Pediatrics
PO Box 747
Elk Grove Village, IL 60009-0747
Web site — http://www.aap.org

Anesthesia and Your Child

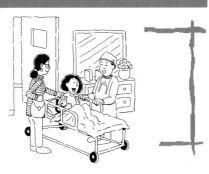

Any time a child requires a hospital visit, it can cause anxiety—for both parent and child. This especially may be the case when the visit involves any type of procedure that might require anesthesia. Examples of such procedures are surgery, some types of x-rays, and certain tests to examine the stomach or intestines.

The purpose of anesthesia is to enable your child's surgery, medical test, or treatment to occur without pain, memory, or movement.

Your child's comfort and safety are very important. The person(s) providing your child's anesthesia will monitor heart rate, blood pressure, breathing, temperature, and the oxygen level in the blood before, during, and after anesthesia. Your child's unique needs, the procedure involved, and your child's health will help determine the type of anesthesia.

Most anesthesia providers work as a team. Anesthesiologists (doctors), residents (doctors-in-training), certified registered nurse anesthetists (CRNAs), physician's assistants, and nurses may all be part of this team.

Preparing for anesthesia

Before having anesthesia, your child will need a physical examination. At this time, either your pediatrician or a member of the anesthesia care team will review your child's current health and medical history. You will answer questions about your child's health. This may take place on the day of the surgery, test, or treatment, or in the days just before it occurs.

It is important to tell the doctor about any of the following that apply to your child:

- Allergies, including allergies to food, drugs, or latex (rubber).
- All medications that your child is taking, including herbal or natural types and inhaled (breathed in) medications.
- Breathing problems, including asthma, croup or wheezing, snoring, and apnea (periods when breath is held during sleep).
- Any recent illnesses, especially bad colds.
- Any problems that your child had as a newborn, such as premature birth, breathing problems such as croup or asthma, or birth defects.
- Heart problems, including holes between the heart chambers, valve problems, heart murmurs, or irregular heartbeats.
- Any other medical problems that your child has or has had, especially if they required visits to a doctor or a stay in the hospital.
- Any previous surgery or procedure using anesthesia.
- Previous problems with anesthesia or surgery, such as airway problems, problems going to sleep or waking up from anesthesia, or problems with nausea and vomiting after surgery.
- Any family history (both sides of the family) of problems with anesthesia.
- Family history of bleeding problems.
- Whether your child or anyone in the household smokes.
- If your child has any loose teeth. (Sometimes loose teeth must be removed for your child's safety.)
- Whether your child may be pregnant.

Your child may need blood tests prior to anesthesia. Other tests, such as x-rays, are needed sometimes. Most of the time few, if any, tests are required.

What is a pediatric anesthesiologist?

A *Pediatric Anesthesiologist* has the experience and training to help ensure a successful surgery, test, or treatment for your child.

A pediatric anesthesiologist is a fully trained anesthesiologist who has completed at least 1 year of specialized training in anesthesia care of infants and children. Most pediatric surgeons deliver care to children in the operating room along with a pediatric anesthesiologist. Many children who need surgery have complex medical problems that affect many parts of the body. The pediatric anesthesiologist has special training and experience to evaluate these complex problems and to plan a safe anesthetic for each child.

What are the risks of anesthesia for my child?

Minor side effects of anesthesia, such as a sore throat, nausea, and vomiting, are common. Major problems are rare. Ask the anesthesiologist to explain the specific risks for your child.

What do I tell my child about anesthesia?

Begin talking about the hospital visit 5 to 6 days in advance for older children, and 2 or 3 days ahead for toddlers. Be honest with your child. Depending on your child's age, use familiar words such as "sore" for pain or "taking a nap" for being put under anesthesia.

Explain that the sleep from anesthesia is different from sleep at home. During anesthesia a person does not feel pain. Your child will not wake up in the middle of the procedure. At the end of the surgery, test, or treatment, the anesthesiologist will take away the medicine that provides this type of "sleep" and your child will awaken and return to his family.

Children between the ages of 3 and 12 may not be ready to hear about the risks of surgery or anesthesia. Often, they understand enough to be scared, but not enough to be reassured. Your anesthesiologist may want to tell you about the risks when your child is not present.

If your child becomes worried when you talk about what anesthesia will be like, explain that it is OK to be scared. Point out that the anesthesia care team will work hard to make your child feel safe and comfortable. You can help keep your child's fears to a minimum by being calm and reassuring.

Some hospitals offer special programs that explain the anesthesia and surgery process to children and families. Ask for books and videotapes that can help you prepare your child and yourself.

What if my child gets sick just before the scheduled time?

Call your anesthesia care team and your doctor if your child becomes ill near the time scheduled for the procedure. If your child develops a cold or other illness, the surgery, test, or treatment may have to be rescheduled because the risk of added problems may increase. If your child is exposed to chickenpox within 3 weeks of the procedure, it may be rescheduled because of the risk to other patients. Your child may be able to spread chickenpox before skin spots develop.

The day of the procedure

Can my child eat, drink, or take medicine on the day of anesthesia?

Except for emergencies, your child's stomach should be empty when anesthesia is started. This helps to prevent vomiting, which may cause food or stomach acid to get into the lungs. It is important to check with your surgeon or anesthesiologist prior to your child's anesthesia for specific guidelines for your child. The following are general recommendations:

Infants younger than 1 year of age may have

- Solid food until 8 hours before anesthesia (NOTE: baby food and cereal are solid foods)
- Infant formula until 6 hours before anesthesia
- Breast milk until 4 hours before anesthesia
- Clear liquids until 2 to 4 hours before anesthesia

Children of all ages may have

- Solid food until 8 hours before anesthesia (NOTE: baby food and cereal are solid foods). In general, no solid foods are allowed after a certain time the evening before anesthesia.
- Clear liquids (eg, apple juice, clear soda, Popsicles, or a prepared electrolyte solution) until 2 hours before anesthesia (NOTE: orange juice with pulp, milk, and baby formula are not clear liquids).

Remember, each health care facility has its own guidelines for eating and drinking prior to anesthesia. Check with your anesthesia care team to learn the instructions for your child. Failing to follow your health care facility's guidelines may result in the delay of your child's procedure.

In addition, ask your anesthesiologist which, if any, of your child's routine medications may be taken on the day of anesthesia. Some medications may be given on the morning of anesthesia with small sips of water, but not mixed with solids such as applesauce. However, other medications, including herbal and natural types, may interact with drugs used for anesthesia and must be stopped prior to anesthesia.

On the morning that your child is to receive anesthesia

- Be sure to follow the fasting (not eating) instructions.
- Dress your child in loose-fitting, comfortable clothes.
- Give any medications (that your anesthesiologist has approved) with a sip of water.
- Bring a favorite comfort object such as a blanket, stuffed animal, or toy.
- Be a calm and reassuring parent for your child.

What will my child do while waiting for anesthesia?

Most large hospitals have a special waiting area with space and toys for play. If you have not done so already, you will meet the anesthesia care team at this time. They will review your child's records, briefly examine your child, tell you how they will keep your child safe, discuss the risks, and answer any remaining questions or concerns.

Will my child be worried?

A calm and supportive family can provide the most help in ensuring that your child will not be overly worried or upset. As mentioned, a special blanket, stuffed animal, or toy also may provide comfort.

Often, sedatives (medications to help your child relax) are given before the start of anesthesia to help reduce fear and worry. The choice of whether to provide a sedative will depend on your child's age, level of anxiety, medical condition, and your hospital's practices. Sedatives may be given through the mouth, nose, or rectum (the anal opening), or as an injection.

How will anesthesia be given to my child?

Most children get to choose one of the following ways for anesthesia to be started:
- By breathing anesthetic gases through a mask
- Through a needle that is put into a vein (IV)
- Through a needle that is put into a muscle (an injection)

When a mask is used, there is no need for shots and no pain is involved. However, some children do not like having masks placed on their faces. An injection can be briefly painful and frightening to a child. However, it is quick and does not require your child to remain still. If an IV is used, the use of local anesthetic (numbing medicine) at the IV site will make this less painful.

If a mask will be used to start anesthesia, talk to your child about this before the day of the surgery, test, or treatment. Explain that the mask contains special air that helps children feel sleepy. The mask may be treated with a special smell to make the process more comfortable. This method may not be used in certain cases, such as for some emergencies, in the case of stomach or bowel problems, or if your child has eaten recently.

Once a child reaches about 10 years of age, anesthesia usually is started by IV. No matter how anesthesia is started, your child will be kept comfortable and asleep with a combination of gas and IV anesthetics. Your child will not awaken during the surgery, test, or treatment. She will awaken once the procedure is completed, unless there is a need for intensive care at that time. If your child needs this type of care, your anesthesiologist will explain this to you.

Can I be with my child when anesthesia is started?

Some hospitals allow 1 support person (usually a parent) to go with the child into the operating room or other area where your child is to receive anesthesia. Check on the policy at your hospital ahead of time. Your child's anesthesiologist will make the final decision.

Many anesthesiologists feel that giving children sedatives makes separation much easier and that parents do not need to be present. Whatever the decision, remember that the anesthesia care team has a lot of experience with helping children stay calm during these moments.

If you are able to be present for the start of anesthesia, ask the anesthesiologist beforehand what you should expect to see and how your child might react. Understanding what is to happen will make you feel more comfortable.

It is important to realize that even if you are allowed to be with your child for the start of anesthesia, it is no guarantee that your child will not get upset before going to sleep. This depends on your child's age, temperament, and past experiences.

After the procedure

Where will my child go after the procedure?

Your child will go to a recovery room or an intensive care unit, depending on the type of surgery, test, or treatment, and your child's medical condition. Usually, parents are allowed to be present once their child is admitted to these areas and the child's condition is stable. After a routine procedure, the recovery stay is usually 30 minutes to 2 hours. Then your child may go to a regular hospital bed or a short-stay unit, or be discharged and able to go home.

How will my child behave after the procedure?

Children come out of anesthesia in different ways. Some are alert and calm right away. Others may remain groggy for a longer period of time. Infants and toddlers may be irritable until the effects of the anesthesia have worn off. If this is the case, your child may need more sedative medication while "sleeping off" the remaining effects of anesthesia.

Will my child feel pain?

One of the main goals of anesthesia is to prevent pain during and after the procedure. If your child is in pain in the recovery room, he may get more pain medicine. Pain medication comes in many different forms and can be given in many different ways. Your child's doctors will discuss the options with you and your child ahead of time.

Will nausea and vomiting be a problem?

Nausea and vomiting are very common after anesthesia and may be due to your child's condition, the procedure, or the side effects of anesthesia. If your child is vomiting a lot, she may need to stay in the hospital longer. Sometimes an unplanned overnight stay in the hospital is needed. There are medications that can be given to your child during or after anesthesia to reduce the chance that this will be a problem.

   Discuss your questions or concerns with your anesthesia care team and your pediatrician or other doctor(s) who are involved. These health care professionals are trained to ensure your child's comfort and safety throughout the process.

The information contained in this publication should not be used as a substitute for the medical care and advice of your pediatrician. There may be variations in treatment that your pediatrician may recommend based on individual facts and circumstances.

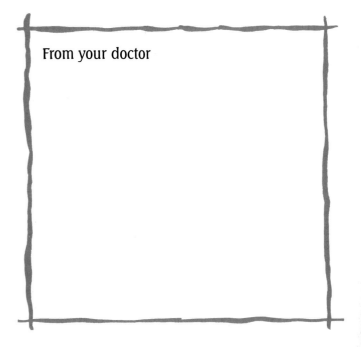

From your doctor

You can reach someone from your anesthesia care team at

_____.

   Be sure to keep your anesthesia care team informed about your child's health just before the procedure. Call this number and/or the doctor who is performing the procedure if your child develops a cold or other illness or has been exposed to chickenpox within 3 weeks of the procedure.

American Academy of Pediatrics

DEDICATED TO THE HEALTH OF ALL CHILDREN™

The American Academy of Pediatrics is an organization of 55,000 primary care pediatricians, pediatric medical subspecialists, and pediatric surgical specialists dedicated to the health, safety, and well-being of infants, children, adolescents, and young adults.

American Academy of Pediatrics
PO Box 747
Elk Grove Village, IL 60009-0747
Web site — http://www.aap.org

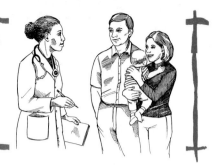

Car Seat Shopping Guide for Children With Special Needs
Guidelines for Parents

All children must be transported as safely as possible. However, because of certain health problems, not all children can ride in many of the car seats commonly found in stores. Children with breathing problems, casts, or other health care needs may need to use special car seats. This information from the American Academy of Pediatrics will introduce you to some child restraint options available for children with special health care needs.

General guidelines

When transporting a child with special needs, keep the following in mind:

- Talk to your pediatrician about your child's transportation needs. Some children with special health care needs may be able to use standard child restraints.
- Check the label on the seat and make sure it states that the seat meets or exceeds federal safety standards.
- Never try to alter a car seat to fit a child with special health care needs. Never use a car seat that has been changed unless it has been crash tested with the modification.
- New child restraints are being developed every year. Keep up-to-date on what might be available for your child.
- Car seats for children with special needs are often expensive. Check with your pediatrician, local children's hospital, or the National Easter Seal Society (800/221-6827) to find out if there are any car seat loan programs in your area. If not, check to see if your insurance will help cover the cost.

Using the seat

- Read the instructions for both the child restraint **and** your vehicle. Both sets of instructions will be necessary to make sure your child is secure in the seat and the seat is correctly installed in your vehicle.
- The back seat is the safest place for all children to ride. **Never** put a rear-facing infant in front of a passenger-side air bag. In a crash, the air bag inflates very quickly and with great force. The child safety seat could be hit by the air bag and cause serious injuries or even death to the child (see illustration below).
- Never place anything under or behind a child in a child restraint.

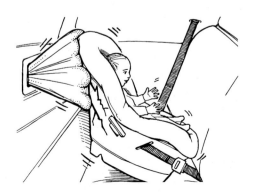

Travel suggestions

- If you have portable equipment (walkers, crutches, oxygen tanks, monitors, etc), make sure they are safely stored and secured during travel so that they do not become flying objects in the event of a crash or sudden stop.
- Make sure any equipment that uses batteries has enough power for at least double the length of your trip.
- Depending on your child's condition, you may want to limit the amount of car travel.
- Make frequent stops if your trip is long.
- Whenever possible, an adult should ride in the back seat next to your child to watch him closely.

Premature and low birth weight infants

If your baby was born prematurely or is very small, the following information will help you transport your child safely.

- Select a car seat that will fit your tiny baby. Seats that have less than 5½ inches from the crotch strap to the seat back will help keep your baby from slouching forward. Seats that have less than 10 inches from the lowest harness strap position to the seat bottom will keep the harness from crossing over your baby's ears.
- Do not use a car seat with a shield or tray. In a crash or sudden stop, these could injure your infant's neck or head.
- Make sure the harness of the car seat fits over your infant's shoulders and holds your baby in the seat.
- Place rolled receiving blankets on both sides of your baby to center her in the car seat. Place a rolled diaper or washcloth between your child's diaper area and the crotch strap to keep your baby from slipping down (see illustration below).

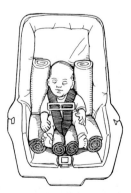

Some premature infants have breathing problems when they sit semi-upright in a car seat. Make sure your baby is observed and monitored in a car seat by hospital staff before going home. Your child may need to use a car bed if she experiences any of the following while in a car seat:

- a decrease in oxygen levels
- slow heart rate
- apnea

Car beds

There are many reasons why children need to travel lying down in a car bed, including:

- Trouble breathing when sitting upright or semi-upright
- Poor muscle control
- Bones that break very easily
- Recent surgery on the spine
- Wearing a cast

At this time there is one car bed available for infants. The Ultra Dream Ride by Cosco is designed for infants who weigh up to 20 pounds and are up to 26 inches long.

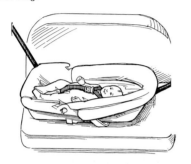

Infants and toddlers with tracheostomies

Most children with a tracheostomy will fit in a standard car seat. Avoid using child restraints with a tray or shield. In a crash, these could come in contact with the tracheostomy, and injure your child or block his airway.

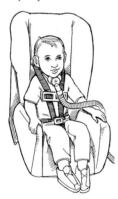

Infants and toddlers in hip spica casts

Hip spica casts and other orthopedic devices, such as splints, can make it impossible for a child to sit in a standard car seat. The Spelcast convertible car seat has been designed for children in casts. It is used rear-facing for infants up to 20 pounds and forward-facing for toddlers up to 40 pounds and 40 inches. An optional tether is available for use forward-facing.

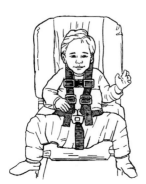

Older children in hip spica casts

The modified E-Z-On Vest is designed for children 2 years and older who weigh up to 100 pounds. It allows a child to lie down in the back seat of the vehicle (see illustration below). It requires two seat belts for installation.

Never use a reclined vehicle seat to transport a child. In a crash, the child can slip out of position and not be protected by the seat belt.

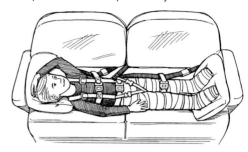

Children who can sit up in their casts

Children who can sit up in their casts may be able to use a standard car seat. Make sure the cast does not get in the way of the buckle or hit the sides of the restraint. A Spelcast car seat can be useful for children in broomstick casts whose legs are spread widely apart.

If an older child is in a cast and can sit up, she may be able to use a booster seat or a seat belt. Make sure she is using the booster seat or seat belt properly and has enough leg room. The lap belt should be worn low and snug across the hips. The shoulder belt should be across the chest, never behind the back or under the arm. Put padding or blankets on the floor so that the child's legs will be better supported.

Larger children and child restraints

Some children still need the support of a child restraint even after they have outgrown a standard car seat. This would include children with cerebral palsy, poor head/neck control, and various neuromuscular disorders. There are seats available that fit children who weigh up to 105 pounds (see illustration). These car seats come with extra pads and accessories to help position the child in the seat. Work with an occupational or physical therapist to position your child in these types of seats. These child restraints also come with an extra strap called a tether. The tether, along with the vehicle seat belt, must be used to install the restraint correctly.

If your older child does not need a larger car seat but has difficulty sitting still in a vehicle or gets out of his seat belt, an upright vest is available from E-Z-On Products. It is installed in the car with the vehicle seat belts and a tether. In a bus, it must be installed with the seat belt and a special strap called a cam wrap.

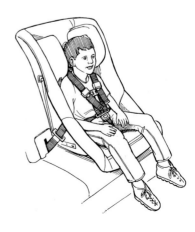

Tether straps

Many child restraints designed for children with special health care needs must be installed with a tether strap and a seat belt. A tether strap attaches to the restraint and is bolted into your car (see illustration). The tether strap and hardware come from the car seat manufacturer and limit forward movement of the car seat in the vehicle. Some cars come with holes already drilled for tethers. Others need to have holes drilled for installation. If your car seat requires a tether, be sure to take your vehicle to a dealer who can help you find the hole or drill one for you. Never drill a hole yourself. You could puncture the gas line or damage your vehicle.

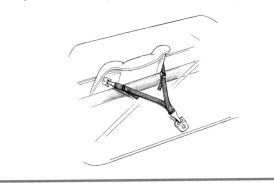

Older children and belt-positioning boosters or seat belts

If your child is able to sit up unassisted and is too large for a standard car seat, a belt-positioning booster car seat should be used until your child is large enough to use a seat belt. A belt-positioning booster seat will help position the seat belts on your child's body and will fit your child until she weighs about 60–80 pounds. There are different kinds of belt-positioning boosters and it is important you get the type that will fit your child and work with the seat belts in your car.

Belt-positioning booster seats raise a child up so that the lap and shoulder belts fit properly (see illustration). This helps protect the upper body and head. These seats must be used with a lap/shoulder belt. Some come with additional harnesses that can be used for children at lower weights.

When your child is ready to wear a seat belt, make sure it fits properly. Remember, lap belts need to be worn low and snug on the hips. Shoulder belts should be worn across the chest. Never place a shoulder belt behind a child's back or under a child's arms. This could result in injury to the child.

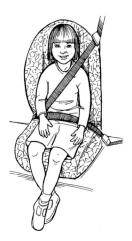

Children and wheelchairs

Most wheelchairs are not crash tested. Whenever possible, buckle your child in a car seat, booster, or use seat belts depending on the child's size and development. If you transport your child in a wheelchair, install it in a forward-facing position with four-point tie-down devices attached to the main frame of the wheelchair (see illustration). Then restrain your child separately with a shoulder/lap belt. Positioning belts used with wheelchairs are not safety restraints. Lap trays attached to the wheelchair should be removed and secured separately during transport. If a child is going to school and has an Individual Education Plan (IEP), he should be evaluated for any special transportation needs. Discuss this with the child's therapist or school transport personnel.

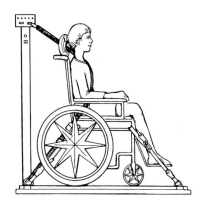

Medical equipment

If your child must travel with medical equipment, the equipment will also need to be secured in the vehicle. At this time, there is no single product available to secure medical equipment. Recommendations include wedging the equipment on the vehicle floor with pillows or securing it with bungee cords or seat belts not being used by a passenger.

©2002 American Academy of Pediatrics

For additional information

American Academy of Pediatrics
141 Northwest Point Blvd
PO Box 927
Elk Grove Village, IL 60009-0927
847/228-5005

Automotive Safety for Children Program
Riley Hospital for Children
575 West Drive, Room 004
Indianapolis, IN 46202
317/274-2977

Kids Are Riding Safe/Special Kids Are
    Riding Safe
National Easter Seal Society
230 W. Monroe
11th Floor
Chicago, IL 60606
800/221-6827

Mobile Teaching School Bus Project
Department of Community Education
Riley Hospital for Children
575 West Drive, Room 008
Indianapolis, IN 46202
317/278-0506

The information contained in this publication should not be used as a substitute for the medical care and advice of your pediatrician. There may be variations in treatment that your pediatrician may recommend based on individual facts and circumstances.

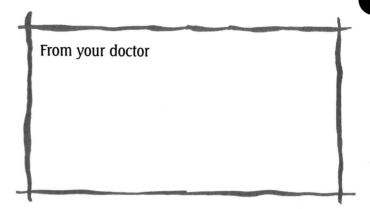

From your doctor

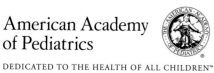

American Academy
of Pediatrics

DEDICATED TO THE HEALTH OF ALL CHILDREN™

The American Academy of Pediatrics is an organization of 55,000 primary care pediatricians, pediatric medical subspecialists, and pediatric surgical specialists dedicated to the health, safety, and well-being of infants, children, adolescents, and young adults.

American Academy of Pediatrics
PO Box 747
Elk Grove Village, IL 60009-0747
Web site — http://www.aap.org

Choking Prevention and First Aid for Infants and Children

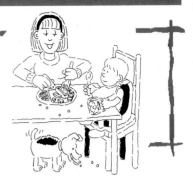

When children begin crawling, or eating table foods, parents must be aware of the dangers and risks of choking. Older infants and children less than 5 years of age can easily choke on food and small objects.

Choking occurs when food or small objects get caught in the throat and block the airway. This prevents oxygen from getting to the lungs and the brain. When the brain goes without oxygen for more than 4 minutes, brain damage or even death may occur. Many children die from choking each year. Most children who choke to death are younger than 5 years of age. Two thirds of choking victims are infants younger than 1 year of age.

Balloons, balls, marbles, pieces of toys, and foods cause the most choking deaths.

The American Academy of Pediatrics believes that parents and other caregivers can prevent choking. The Academy offers the following choking prevention and first aid information for parents and caregivers of infants and children.

Dangerous foods

Do not feed children younger than 4 years of age any round, firm food unless it is chopped completely. Round, firm foods are common choking dangers. When infants and young children do not grind or chew their food well, they may attempt to swallow it whole. The following foods can be choking hazards:

- Hot dogs
- Nuts and seeds
- Chunks of meat or cheese
- Whole grapes
- Hard, gooey, or sticky candy
- Popcorn
- Chunks of peanut butter
- Raw vegetables
- Raisins
- Chewing gum

Dangerous household items

Keep the following household items away from infants and children:

- Latex balloons
- Coins
- Marbles
- Toys with small parts
- Toys that can be compressed to fit entirely into a child's mouth
- Small balls
- Pen or marker caps
- Small button-type batteries
- Medicine syringes

What you can do to prevent choking

- *Learn cardiopulmonary resuscitation (CPR)* (basic life support).
- *Be aware that balloons pose a choking risk* to children of any age.
- *Keep the above foods from children* until 4 years of age.
- *Insist that children eat at the table,* or at least while sitting down. They should never run, walk, play, or lie down with food in their mouths.
- *Cut food for infants and young children* into pieces no larger than one-half inch and teach them to chew their food well.
- *Supervise mealtime* for infants and young children.
- *Be aware of older children's actions.* Many choking incidents occur when older brothers or sisters give dangerous foods, toys, or small objects to a younger child.
- *Avoid toys with small parts* and keep other small household items out of reach of infants and young children.
- *Follow the age recommendations on toy packages.* Age guidelines reflect the safety of a toy based on any possible choking hazard as well as the child's physical and mental abilities at various ages.
- *Check under furniture and between cushions* for small items that children could find and put in their mouths.
- *Do not let infants and young children play with coins.*

First aid for the child who is choking

Make a point to learn the instructions on the reverse side of this brochure. Post the chart in your home. However, these instructions should *not* take the place of an approved class in basic first aid, CPR, or emergency prevention. Contact your local American Red Cross office or the American Heart Association to find out about classes offered in your area. Most of the classes teach basic first aid, CPR, and emergency prevention along with what to do for a choking infant or child. Your pediatrician also can help you understand these steps and talk to you about the importance of supervising mealtime and identifying dangerous foods and objects.

The information contained in this publication should not be used as a substitute for the medical care and advice of your pediatrician. There may be variations in treatment that your pediatrician may recommend based on individual facts and circumstances.

From your doctor

American Academy of Pediatrics

DEDICATED TO THE HEALTH OF ALL CHILDREN™

The American Academy of Pediatrics is an organization of 55,000 primary care pediatricians, pediatric medical subspecialists, and pediatric surgical specialists dedicated to the health, safety, and well-being of infants, children, adolescents, and young adults.

American Academy of Pediatrics
PO Box 747
Elk Grove Village, IL 60009-0747
Web site — http://www.aap.org

CHOKING/CPR

LEARN AND PRACTICE CPR

IF ALONE WITH A CHILD WHO IS CHOKING...

1. SHOUT FOR HELP.   2. START RESCUE EFFORTS FOR 1 MINUTE.   3. CALL 911 OR AN EMERGENCY NUMBER.

YOU SHOULD START FIRST AID FOR CHOKING IF...	DO NOT START FIRST AID FOR CHOKING IF...
• The child cannot breathe at all (the chest is not moving up and down). • The child cannot cough, talk, or make a normal voice sound. • The child is found unconscious. (Go to CPR.)	• The child can breathe, cry, talk, or make a normal voice sound. • The child can cough, sputter, or move air at all. The child's normal reflexes are working to clear the airway.

FOR INFANTS LESS THAN 1 YEAR OF AGE

INFANT CHOKING

Begin the following if the infant is choking and is unable to breathe. However, if the infant is coughing, crying, speaking, or able to breathe at all, DO NOT do any of the following. Depending on the infant's condition, call 911 or the pediatrician for further advice.

1 FIVE BACK BLOWS

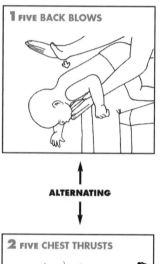

ALTERNATING

2 FIVE CHEST THRUSTS

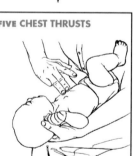

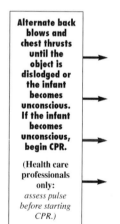

Alternate back blows and chest thrusts until the object is dislodged or the infant becomes unconscious. If the infant becomes unconscious, begin CPR.

(Health care professionals only: *assess pulse before starting CPR.*)

INFANT CPR (Cardiopulmonary Resuscitation)

To be used when the infant is unconscious or when breathing stops.

1 OPEN AIRWAY
- **Look** for movement of the chest and abdomen.
- **Listen** for sounds of breathing.
- **Feel** for breath on your cheek.
- **Open** airway as shown.
- **Look** for a foreign object in the mouth. **If you can see** an object in the infant's mouth, sweep it out carefully with your finger. **Do not** try a finger sweep if the object is in the infant's throat, because it could be pushed further into the throat.

2 RESCUE BREATHING
- **Position** head and chin with both hands as shown — head gently tilted back, chin lifted.
- **Seal** your mouth over the infant's mouth and nose.
- **Blow gently,** enough air to make chest rise and fall 2 times.

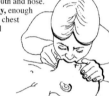

If no rise or fall, repeat 1 & 2. If no response, treat for blocked airway. (See "INFANT CHOKING" steps 1 & 2 at left.)

3 ASSESS RESPONSE
- Place your ear next to the infant's mouth and look, listen, and feel for **normal breathing** or **coughing**.
- Look for **body movement**.

If you cannot see, hear, or feel signs of normal breathing, coughing, or movement, start chest compressions.

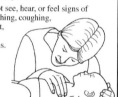

4 CHEST COMPRESSIONS
- **Place** 2 fingers of one hand over the lower half of the chest. Avoid the bottom tip of the breastbone.
- **Compress** chest 1/2" to 1" deep.
- **Alternate** 5 compressions with 1 breath.
- **Compress** chest 100 times per minute.

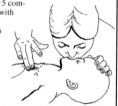

Check for signs of normal breathing, coughing, or movement every minute.

If at any time an object is coughed up or the infant/child starts to breathe, call 911 or the pediatrician for further advice.

Ask the pediatrician for information on Choking/CPR instructions for children older than 8 years of age and on an approved first aid course or CPR course in your community.

CHOKING/CPR

LEARN AND PRACTICE CPR

IF ALONE WITH A CHILD WHO IS CHOKING...
1. SHOUT FOR HELP.   2. START RESCUE EFFORTS FOR 1 MINUTE.   3. CALL 911 OR AN EMERGENCY NUMBER.

YOU SHOULD START FIRST AID FOR CHOKING IF...	DO NOT START FIRST AID FOR CHOKING IF...
• The child cannot breathe at all (the chest is not moving up and down). • The child cannot cough, talk, or make a normal voice sound. • The child is found unconscious. (Go to CPR.)	• The child can breathe, cry, talk, or make a normal voice sound. • The child can cough, sputter, or move air at all. The child's normal reflexes are working to clear the airway.

FOR CHILDREN 1 TO 8 YEARS OF AGE

CHILD CHOKING

Begin the following if the child is choking and is unable to breathe. However, if the child is coughing, crying, speaking, or able to breathe at all, DO NOT do any of the following, but call the pediatrician for further advice.

CONSCIOUS

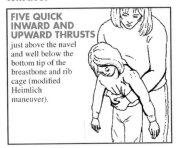

FIVE QUICK INWARD AND UPWARD THRUSTS just above the navel and well below the bottom tip of the breastbone and rib cage (modified Heimlich maneuver).

If the child becomes unconscious, begin CPR.

CHILD CPR (Cardiopulmonary Resuscitation)

To be used when the child is UNCONSCIOUS or when breathing stops.

1 OPEN AIRWAY
- **Look** for movement of the chest and abdomen.
- **Listen** for sounds of breathing.
- **Feel** for breath on your cheek.
- **Open** airway as shown.
- **Look** for a foreign object in the mouth. **If you can see** an object in the child's mouth, sweep it out carefully with finger. **Do not** try a finger sweep if the object is in the child's throat because it could be pushed further into the throat.

2 RESCUE BREATHING
- **Position** head and chin with both hands as shown.
- **Seal** your mouth over child's mouth.
- **Pinch** child's nose.
- **Blow** enough air to make child's chest rise and fall 2 times.

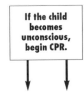

2A HEALTH CARE PROFESSIONALS ONLY:
- *Use abdominal thrusts to try to remove an airway obstruction.*
- *Continue steps 1, 2, and 2A until the object is retrieved or rescue breaths are effective.*
- *Assess pulse before starting CPR.*

If no rise or fall, repeat 1 & 2. If still no rise or fall, continue with step 3 (below).

3 ASSESS RESPONSE
- Place your ear next to the child's mouth and look, listen, and feel for **normal breathing** or **coughing.**
- Look for **body movement.**

If you cannot see, hear, or feel signs of normal breathing, coughing, or movement, start chest compressions.

4 CHEST COMPRESSIONS
- **Compress** chest 1" to 1½".
- **Alternate** 5 compressions with 1 breath.
- **Compress** chest 100 times per minute.

Press with the heel of 1 hand on the lower half of the chest. Lift fingers to avoid ribs. Do not press near the bottom tip of the breastbone.

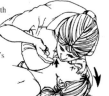

Be sure someone calls 911 as soon as possible, and by 1 minute after starting rescue efforts.

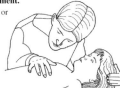

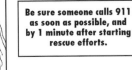

If at any time an object is coughed up or the infant/child starts to breathe, call 911 or the pediatrician for further advice.

Ask the pediatrician for information on Choking/CPR instructions for children older than 8 years of age and on an approved first aid course or CPR course in your community.

Environmental Tobacco Smoke: A Danger to Children

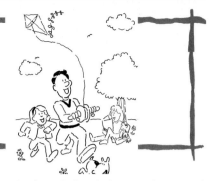

Smoking is the leading cause of preventable death in the United States. It causes almost 20% of all the deaths in this country each year. People who are around smokers can't help breathing in the smoke that comes from cigarettes, pipes, or cigars. Researchers have now found that breathing in someone else's smoke is very dangerous, especially for children. The American Academy of Pediatrics offers parents the followings information to help them create a "tobacco-free environment" for their children.

What is Environmental Tobacco Smoke (ETS)?

Environmental Tobacco Smoke, or ETS, is the smoke that is breathed out by a smoker. ETS also includes the smoke that comes from the tip of a burning cigarette. Exposure to ETS happens any time someone breathes in the smoke that comes from a cigarette, pipe, or cigar. ETS contains many dangerous chemicals that have been proven to cause cancer. It is estimated that ETS causes 3,000 lung cancer deaths each year to people who don't even smoke!

ETS and children

ETS has almost 4,000 chemicals in it that infants and children breathe in whenever someone smokes around them. Children who breathe in ETS are at risk for many serious health problems.

When a mother smokes during pregnancy, she has a higher risk of having a premature baby or a baby who is not fully developed. When a mother smokes during her pregnancy or around her newborn, the infant has a higher risk of Sudden Infant Death Syndrome (SIDS). Children who breathe in someone else's cigarette smoke (especially children under 2 years of age) have a higher risk of getting other serious medical problems or making them worse, including the following:

- Ear infections and hearing problems
- Upper respiratory infections
- Respiratory problems such as bronchitis and pneumonia
- Asthma

Children of smokers also cough and wheeze more and have a harder time getting over colds. In addition, ETS can cause a stuffy nose, headaches, sore throat, eye irritation, hoarseness, dizziness, nausea, loss of appetite, lack of energy, or fussiness.

Children with asthma are especially sensitive to ETS. ETS can actually increase the number and severity of asthma attacks, which may require trips to the hospital. Also, exposure to the smoke of as few as 10 cigarettes per day raises a child's chances of getting asthma even if that child has never had any symptoms.

In addition, ETS can cause problems for children later in life including:

- Lung cancer
- Heart disease
- Cataracts (eye disease)

With all of these dangers, it's easy to understand why children should not be exposed to ETS.

Inhaling the smoke from the cigarettes of others is dangerous for pregnant women, too. Pregnant women should stay away from smoking areas and ask smokers not to smoke around them.

Smoking During Pregnancy

When a woman smokes during her pregnancy, her unborn child is exposed to the chemicals in the smoke. This can be very harmful to the child and can lead to many serious health problems including:

- Miscarriage
- Prematurity (having a baby that is not fully developed)
- Low birth weight - therefore a less healthy baby
- Sudden Infant Death Syndrome (SIDS)
- Some childhood cancers

These risks go up the longer a mother smokes and the more cigarettes she smokes during her pregnancy. Quitting anytime during the pregnancy will help—of course, the sooner the better.

How parents can protect their children from ETS

If you are a smoker—quit! It's one of the most important things you can do for the health of your children and the best way to prevent your child from being exposed to ETS. If you are having trouble quitting smoking, ask your doctor for help. Also, contact your local chapter of the American Lung Association, American Heart Association, the American Cancer Society, or other groups that sponsor stop-smoking classes.

As a parent, you are a role model. Children watch what their parents do. If your child sees you smoking, he or she may want to try smoking and grow up to become a smoker as well. Cigarette smoking by children and adolescents causes the same health problems that affect adults.

Tobacco-free environments for children

Parents need to be aware of the many places where their children can be exposed to ETS. Even if there are no smokers in your home, your children can still be exposed to ETS in other places, including:

- In the car or on a bus
- In a restaurant
- At a friend's or relative's house
- At the mall
- At the babysitter's house
- At sports events or pop music concerts

How do you avoid being around smokers? One way is to ask people not to smoke around your children or remove your child from places where there are smokers. The following tips may help you keep your children from being exposed to ETS:

- Don't let people smoke in your house. Don't put out any ashtrays—this will discourage people from lighting up. Remember, air flows throughout a house, so smoking in even one room allows smoke to go everywhere.
- Don't let people smoke in your car. Opening windows is not enough to clear the air.
- Choose a babysitter who doesn't allow smoking in the house.
- Avoid crowded, smoky restaurants when you are with your child.
- When you are with your child in public places-shopping malls, restaurants, bowling alleys—sit in "nonsmoking" sections.
- Help get your child's school to be smoke-free. Get your children involved in this effort as well.

Almost 50% of the homes in the United States have at least one smoker living there. This means that millions of children in the United States are breathing in ETS in their own homes. If you smoke around your child or allow your child to be exposed to ETS in other places, you may be putting him or her into more danger than you realize.

Parents need to make every effort to keep their children away from smokers and ETS. Parents who smoke should think about quitting, not just for their own sake, but for the health of their children.

For additional information for parents and teens on tobacco use, see the following handouts by the American Academy of Pediatrics:
Smoking: Straight Talk for Teens and
Tobacco Use: A Message to Parents and Teens.

Smoking and Children—A Fire Hazard

In addition to the dangers of ETS, smoking around children can also pose fire and burn dangers. Children can get burned if they play with lit cigarettes, cigars, or with lighters or matches. Keep the following guidelines in mind to keep your child safe from injury:

- Never smoke while you are holding your baby.
- Never leave a lit cigarette, cigar, or pipe unattended.
- Keep matches and lighters out of your child's reach.

Cigarette lighters are especially dangerous. Cigarette lighters can be found in almost 30 million homes in the United States. Each year children under 5 years old playing with lighters cause more than 5,000 home fires resulting in about 150 deaths and more than 1,000 injuries. The Consumer Product Safety Commission (CPSC) now requires that butane cigarette lighters be made child-resistant. This new rule will prevent hundreds of deaths and fire-related injuries to children each year. But remember, lighters can be made child-resistant, not childproof. It is still very important to keep lighters and matches away from children.

The information contained in this publication should not be used as a substitute for the medical care and advice of your pediatrician. There may be variations in treatment that your pediatrician may recommend based on individual facts and circumstances.

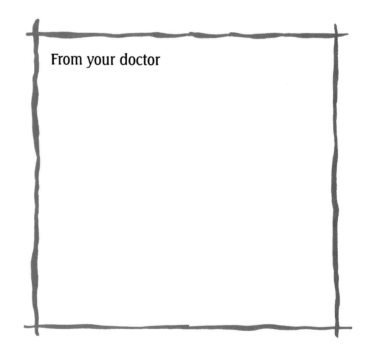

From your doctor

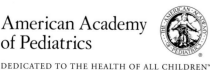

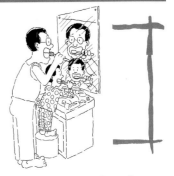

A Guide to Children's Dental Health

The road to a bright smile begins long before the first tooth breaks through the gum. Parents play a big part in helping their children develop healthy teeth. Early monitoring by a pediatrician is important. Regular care by a dental professional, getting enough fluoride, and eating right are all steps to good dental health. By following these steps and teaching them to your children, you can help your children grow up to have healthy teeth and winning smiles.

When do teeth start to form?

Teeth start forming under the gums even before a child is born. During pregnancy, a woman can get her child's teeth off to a healthy start by following her doctor's advice and eating a well-balanced diet. A child's first tooth generally breaks through the gum at about 5 or 6 months of age, but this can vary quite a bit. Some children already have a tooth when they are born. It may be a real tooth or an extra tooth. To find out, your pediatrician may have your child see a pediatric dentist. Other children may not get their first tooth until after 1 year of age.

What can I expect when my child starts teething?

When teething begins, your child's gum may be swollen in the spot where a tooth is about to break through. To ease the sensation of teething, you can give infants a one-piece teething ring or pacifier to suck on. (Teething rings and pacifiers made up of more than one piece may become unattached and may cause choking.) You should never give infants pacifiers that have been dipped in sweet liquids. Sugar from such liquids stays on the teeth and provides food for bacteria that can cause tooth decay.

When they are several months old, infants begin to produce more saliva than they are able to swallow, which causes them to drool. Also at about the same age they begin to put objects in their mouths and bite or chew on them. Drooling and chewing on objects (or rubbing them against the gum) are a natural part of an infant's development and may or may not signify teething.

Why are baby teeth important?

Baby teeth, or primary teeth, help children chew food, speak clearly, and retain space for their permanent teeth that start to come in at about 5 or 6 years of age.

It is important to get children into the habit of good dental care at an early age. Children who begin to take care of their teeth at a young age are more likely to have good dental habits as adults.

What is fluoride and why is it important?

Your toothpaste and drinking water may have fluoride in them, but you may not know what fluoride is or why it is important. Fluoride is a natural chemical that can be added to drinking water. It strengthens enamel, the hard outer coating on teeth. Enamel production occurs before teeth break through; so even before teeth actually appear, fluoride helps prevent decay. Fluoride also helps repair early damage to teeth. The fluoride content of local water supplies varies. Water that has low levels of fluoride can be a problem for infants who get very little fluoride from breast milk or formula. Check with your local water department to find out the exact water-fluoride level in your area. Then talk with your pediatrician to see if your child needs additional fluoride. Infants who are not getting enough fluoride should start taking additional amounts at 6 months of age. These children should continue to take additional fluoride until they are at least 16 years old.

When should I start cleaning my child's teeth?

Daily dental cleaning should start as soon as your infant's first tooth appears. Wipe the teeth with a piece of gauze or a damp cloth. Switch to a toothbrush with a fluoride toothpaste as the child gets older. Fluoride in toothpaste absorbs into the tooth enamel and helps prevent tooth decay. Because children tend to swallow toothpaste, put only a small (pea-sized) amount of fluoride toothpaste on your child's toothbrush. Ingesting too much fluoride while brushing can result in bright white tooth staining (mottling).

Also check the teeth for early signs of decay. These appear as white, yellow, or brown spots on the teeth. Some children may develop decay in spite of the best preventive efforts. This may be because it runs in their family. Genetic influence also plays a role in a person's overall dental health.

Does thumb sucking hurt teeth?

Thumb sucking is normal in infants and young children and should cause no permanent problems if not continued past the age of 5. Likewise, it is harmless for infants to use pacifiers. Children who suck their thumbs past the age of 5 may need a referral to a pediatric dentist to determine if problems are developing.

Can putting children in bed with a bottle harm their teeth?

Infants put to bed with a bottle filled with milk or juice have a higher risk of developing "baby bottle tooth decay" or "nursing bottle decay." When these infants fall asleep, they can end up with a small pool of liquid in their mouths. The sugar in milk or juice creates a breeding ground for bacteria, which damage their teeth. This process may lead to severe decay. Toddlers who carry around and suck on a bottle filled with milk, juice, or other sugary liquids can also develop baby bottle tooth decay.

There are some steps parents can take to avoid baby bottle tooth decay:
- Do not put children to bed with a bottle.
- Do not use a bottle of milk or juice as a pacifier during the day. This means you should not let a child walk around with the bottle.
- Teach children to drink from a cup as soon as they are old enough to hold one. Most children can do this well before their first birthday.

Are there other eating habits that are bad for a child's teeth?

Sweets like candy or cookies can lead to tooth decay. Starchy foods such as crackers and sticky foods such as raisins, tend to stay on the teeth long. These foods are also more likely to lead to tooth decay. Sugar from fruits and fruit juices left on the teeth for long periods of time is also not healthy for teeth. Starches and fruits, however, are a necessary part of any child's diet. To avoid tooth decay, give children these foods only at mealtime (before the teeth have been brushed), not at bedtime. For healthy teeth, offer children a well-balanced diet with a variety of foods.

When should children be seen by a dentist?

Before the age of 3, your child's basic dental care can be handled by your pediatrician. During regular well-child visits, your pediatrician will check your child's teeth and gums to make sure they are healthy. However, if dental problems do arise, your pediatrician may refer your child to a dental professional. A pediatric dentist (pedodontist) specializes in the care of children's teeth, but some general dentists are interested in treating children's dental needs and will also see children.

Situations in which a pediatrician may wish to refer a child to a dental professional before age 3 include:

- If the child chips or injures a tooth or has an injury to the face or mouth.
- If the teeth show any signs of discoloration. This could be a sign of tooth decay.
- If a tooth is painful or is sensitive to hot or cold foods or liquids. This could also be a sign of decay.

Most mouth pain in children is not dental in origin. It could be a sign of infection. A pediatrician can rule out medical conditions that are not related to a child's dental health.

Prevention

Children should get regular dental checkups after age 3 or when all 20 baby teeth have come in. Parents might prefer to take their children to a pediatric dentist for these regular checkups. As previously noted, some children may need earlier visits to the dentist.

Regular dental checkups, a balanced diet, fluoride, injury prevention, and brushing are all important for healthy teeth. Starting children off with good dental habits now will help them grow up with healthy smiles.

The information contained in this publication should not be used as a substitute for the medical care and advice of your pediatrician. There may be variations in treatment that your pediatrician may recommend based on individual facts and circumstances.

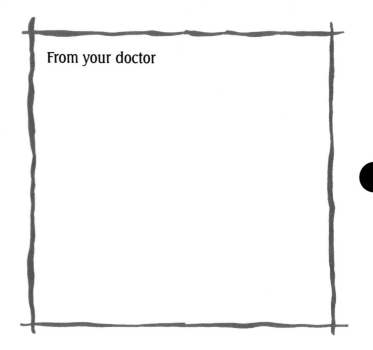

From your doctor

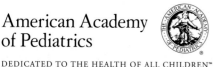

American Academy of Pediatrics

DEDICATED TO THE HEALTH OF ALL CHILDREN™

The American Academy of Pediatrics is an organization of 55,000 primary care pediatricians, pediatric medical subspecialists, and pediatric surgical specialists dedicated to the health, safety, and well-being of infants, children, adolescents, and young adults.

American Academy of Pediatrics
PO Box 747
Elk Grove Village, IL 60009-0747
Web site — http://www.aap.org

Copyright ©1991, Updated 1/96
American Academy of Pediatrics

Home Safety Checklist

Use this checklist to help ensure that your home is safer for your child. A "full-house survey" is recommended at least every 6 months. Every home is different, and no checklist is complete and appropriate for every child and every household.

Your Child's Bedroom

- ☐ Is there a safety belt on the changing table to prevent falls?

- ☐ Is the baby powder out of baby's reach during diaper changing? Inhaled powder can injure a baby's lungs. Use cornstarch rather than talcum powder.

- ☐ Are changing supplies within your reach when baby is being changed?

- ☐ Never leave a child unattended on a changing table, even for a moment.

- ☐ Is there a carpet or a nonskid rug beneath the crib and changing table?

- ☐ Are drapery and blind cords out of the baby's reach from the crib and changing table? They can strangle children if they are left loose.

- ☐ Have bumper pads, toys, pillows, and stuffed animals been removed from the crib by the time the baby can pull up to stand? If large enough, these items can be used as a step for climbing out.

- ☐ Have all crib gyms, hanging toys, and decorations been removed from the crib by the time your baby can get up on his hands and knees? Children can get tangled in them and become strangled.

- ☐ Make sure the crib has no elevated corner posts or decorative cutouts in the end panels. Loose clothing can become snagged on these and strangle your baby.

- ☐ Does the mattress in the crib fit snugly, without any gaps, so your child cannot slip in between the crack and the crib side?

- ☐ The slots on the crib should be no more than 2⅜ inches apart. Widely spaced slots can trap an infant's head.

- ☐ Are all screws, bolts, and hardware, including mattress supports, in place to prevent the crib from collapsing?

- ☐ Make sure there are no plastic bags or other plastic material in or around the crib that might cause suffocation.

- ☐ Check the crib for small parts and pieces that your child could choke on.

- ☐ Make sure the night-light is not near or touching drapes or a bedspread where it could start a fire. Buy only "cool" night-lights that do not get hot.

- ☐ Is there a smoke detector in or near your child's bedroom?

- ☐ Make sure that window guards are securely in place to prevent a child from falling out the window. Never place a crib, playpen, or other children's furniture near a window.

- ☐ Are there plug protectors in the unused electrical outlets? These keep children from sticking their fingers or other objects into the holes.

- ☐ Make sure a toy box does not have a heavy, hinged lid that can trap your child. (It is safer with no lid at all.)

- ☐ To keep the air moist, use a cool mist humidifier (not a vaporizer) to avoid burns. Clean it frequently and empty it when not in use to avoid bacteria and mold from growing in the still water.

- ☐ To reduce the risk of SIDS (Sudden Infant Death Syndrome), put your baby to sleep on her back in a crib with a firm, flat mattress and no soft bedding underneath her.

Your Bedroom

- ☐ Do not keep a firearm anywhere in the house. If you must, lock up the gun and the bullets separately.

- ☐ Check that there are no prescription drugs, toiletries, or other poisonous substances accessible to young children.

- ☐ If your child has access to your bedroom, make sure drapery or blind cords are well out of reach. Children can get tangled in them and become strangled.

- ☐ Is there a working smoke detector in the hallway outside of the bedroom?

The Bathroom

- ☐ Is there a nonskid bath mat on the floor to prevent falls?

- ☐ Is there a nonskid mat or no-slip strips in the bathtub to prevent falls?

- ☐ Are the electrical outlets protected with Ground Fault Circuit Interrupters to decrease the risk of electrical injury?

- ☐ Are medications and cosmetics stored in a locked cabinet well out of your child's reach?

- ☐ Are hair dryers, curling irons, and other electrical appliances unplugged and stored well out of reach? They can cause burns or electrical injuries.

- ☐ Are there child-resistant safety latches on all cabinets containing potentially harmful substances (cosmetics, medications, mouthwash, cleaning supplies)?

- ☐ Are there child-resistant caps on all medications, and are all medications stored in their original containers?

- ☐ Is the temperature of your hot water heater 120°F or lower to prevent scalding?

- ☐ Do you need a doorknob cover to prevent your child from going into the bathroom when you are not there? Teach adults and older children to put the toilet seat cover down and to close the bathroom door when done—to prevent drowning.

- ☐ Remember, supervision of young children is essential in the bathroom, especially when they are in the tub—to prevent drowning.

The Kitchen

- ☐ Make sure that vitamins or other medications are kept out of your child's reach. Use child-resistant caps.

- ☐ Keep sharp knives or other sharp utensils well out of the child's reach (using safety latches or high cabinets).

- ☐ See that chairs and step stools are away from counters and the stove, where a child could climb up and get hurt.

- ☐ Use the back burners and make sure pot handles on the stove are pointing inward so your child cannot reach up and grab them.

- ☐ Make sure automatic dishwasher detergent and other toxic cleaning supplies are stored in their original containers, out of a child's reach, in cabinets with child safety latches.

☐ Keep the toaster out of your child's reach to prevent burns or electrical injuries.

☐ Keep electrical appliances unplugged from the wall when not in use, and use plug protectors for wall outlets.

☐ Are appliance cords tucked away so that they cannot be pulled on?

☐ Make sure that your child's high chair is sturdy and has a seat belt with a crotch strap.

☐ Is there a working fire extinguisher in the kitchen? Do all adults and older children know how to use it?

The Family Room

☐ Are edges and corners of tables padded to prevent injuries?

☐ Are houseplants out of your child's reach? Certain houseplants may be poisonous.

☐ Are televisions and other heavy items (such as lamps) secure so that they cannot tip over?

☐ Are there any unnecessary or frayed extension cords? Cords should run behind furniture and not hang down for children to pull on them.

☐ Is there a barrier around the fireplace or other heat source?

☐ Are the cords from drapes or blinds kept out of your child's reach to prevent strangulation?

☐ Are plug protectors in unused electrical outlets?

☐ Are matches and lighters out of reach?

Miscellaneous Items

☐ Are stairs carpeted and protected with non-accordion gates?

☐ Are the rooms in your house free from small parts, plastic bags, small toys, and balloons that could pose a choking hazard?

☐ Do you have a plan of escape from your home in the event of a fire? Have you reviewed and practiced the plan with your family?

☐ Does the door to the basement have a self-latching lock to prevent your child from falling down the stairs?

☐ Do not place your child in a baby walker with wheels. They are very dangerous, especially near stairs.

☐ Are dangerous products stored out of reach (in cabinets with safety latches or locks or on high shelves) and in their original containers in the utility room, basement, and garage?

☐ If your child has a playpen, does it have small-mesh sides (less than ¾ inch mesh) or closely spaced vertical slats (less than 2⅜ inches)?

☐ Are the numbers of the Poison Control Center and your pediatrician posted on all phones?

☐ Do your children know how to call 911 in an emergency?

☐ Inspect your child's toys for sharp or detachable parts. Repair or throw away broken toys.

The Playground

☐ Are the swing seats made of something soft, not wood or metal?

☐ Is the surface under playground equipment energy absorbent, such as rubber, sand, sawdust (12 inches deep), wood chips, or bark? Is it well maintained?

☐ Is your home playground equipment put together correctly and does it sit on a level surface, anchored firmly to the ground?

☐ Do you check playground equipment for hot metal surfaces such as those on slides, which can cause burns? Does your slide face away from the sun?

☐ Are all screws and bolts on your playground equipment capped? Do you check for loose nuts and bolts periodically? Be sure there are no projecting bolts, nails, or s-links.

☐ Do you watch your children when they are using playground equipment—to prevent shoving, pushing, or fighting?

☐ Never let a child play on playground equipment with dangling drawstrings on a jacket or shirt.

The Pool

☐ Never leave your child alone in or near the pool, even for a moment.

☐ Do you have a 4-foot fence around all sides of the pool that cannot be climbed by children and that separates the pool from the house?

☐ Do fence gates self-close and self-latch, with latches higher than your child's reach?

☐ Does your pool cover completely cover the pool so that your child cannot slip under it?

☐ Do you keep rescue equipment (such as a shepherd's hook or life preserver) and a telephone by the pool?

☐ Does everyone who watches your child around a pool know basic lifesaving techniques and CPR?

☐ Does your child know the rules of water and diving safety?

The Yard

☐ Do you use a power mower with a control that stops the mower if the handle is let go?

☐ Never let a child younger than 12 years of age mow the lawn. Make sure your older child wears sturdy shoes (not sandals or sneakers) while mowing the lawn and that objects such as stones and toys are picked up from the lawn before it is mowed.

☐ Do not allow young children in the yard while you are mowing.

☐ Teach your child to never pick and eat anything from a plant.

☐ Be sure you know what is growing in your yard so, if your child accidentally ingests a plant, you can give the proper information to your local Poison Control Center.

The information contained in this publication should not be used as a substitute for the medical care and advice of your pediatrician. There may be variations in treatment that your pediatrician may recommend based on individual facts and circumstances.

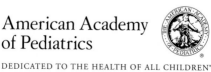

American Academy of Pediatrics

DEDICATED TO THE HEALTH OF ALL CHILDREN™

The American Academy of Pediatrics is an organization of 55,000 primary care pediatricians, pediatric medical subspecialists, and pediatric surgical specialists dedicated to the health, safety, and well-being of infants, children, adolescents, and young adults.

American Academy of Pediatrics
PO Box 747
Elk Grove Village, IL 60009-0747
Web site — http://www.aap.org

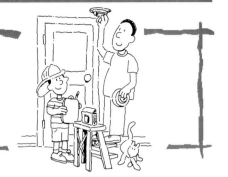

Keep Your Family Safe:

Fire Safety and Burn Prevention at Home

Fires and burns cause more than 4,000 deaths and more than 50,000 hospitalizations every year. Winter is an especially dangerous time, as space heaters, fireplaces, and candles get more use in the home. It is no surprise that most fires in the home occur between December and February. However, you might be surprised at how easy it is to reduce the risk of fire in your home. Follow these suggestions to keep your home and family safe from fire all year round.

Smoke alarms save lives

Most fatal fires in the home happen while people are sleeping. One of the most important steps you can take to protect your family against fire is to install smoke alarms and keep them in good working order. Smoke alarms are available at most home and hardware stores and often cost $10 or less. Check with your fire department to see if they give out and install free smoke alarms.

- Install smoke alarms outside every bedroom or any area where someone sleeps. Be sure there is at least one alarm on every level of your home or at each end of a mobile home.
- Place smoke alarms away from the kitchen and bathroom. False alarms can occur while cooking or even showering.
- Test smoke alarms every month by pushing the test button.
- Change the batteries when they get low, or at least once a year such as when you change your clocks back in the fall.
- Replace smoke alarms every 10 years.
- Never paint a smoke alarm.
- Clean smoke alarms monthly by dusting or vacuuming.
- Smoke alarms with a flashing light and an alarm should be used in homes with hard-of-hearing or deaf children or adults.

Prevention around the home

Take a careful look at each room of your home. Use the following checklists and safety tips to reduce the risk of fire:

- ☐ Make an escape plan. Practice it every 6 months. Every member of the family should know at least two exits from each room and where to meet outside.
- ☐ Inspect and replace any electrical cords that are worn, frayed, or damaged. Never overload outlets. Avoid running electrical cords under carpet or furniture as they can overheat and start a fire.
- ☐ Make sure doors and windows are easy to open.
- ☐ Automatic home fire sprinkler systems are affordable and practical for many homes.
- ☐ Wood stoves usually cannot be safely installed in mobile homes. If one is present, it should be inspected by the local fire department to be sure it is safely vented.
- ☐ Avoid using alternative heating sources such as kerosene heaters and electric space heaters. If they must be used, keep them away from clothing, bedding, and curtains, and unplug them at night. If kerosene heaters must be used, make sure there is adequate ventilation to prevent carbon monoxide poisoning.

Bedrooms

- ☐ Check the labels of your child's pajamas. Children should always wear flame-retardant and/or close-fitting sleepwear.
- ☐ If a bedroom is on an upper floor, make sure there is a safe way to reach the ground, such as a noncombustible escape ladder.
- ☐ In the event of a fire, test any closed doors with the back of your hand for heat. Do not open the door if you feel heat or see smoke. Close all doors as you leave each room to keep the fire from spreading.

- ❖ *Never smoke in bed or when you are drowsy or have been drinking. Tobacco and smoking products, matches, and lighters are the most common cause of fatal fires in the home.*

Living and family rooms

- ☐ Make sure all matches, lighters, and ashtrays are out of your child's sight and reach. Better yet, keep them in a locked cabinet.
- ☐ Use large, deep ashtrays that won't tip over, and empty them often. Fill ashtrays with water before dumping ashes in the wastebasket.
- ☐ Give space heaters plenty of space. Keep heaters *at least* 3 feet from anything that might burn, like clothes, curtains, and furniture. Always turn space heaters off and unplug them when you go to bed or leave the home.
- ☐ Have fireplaces and chimneys cleaned and inspected once a year.
- ☐ Use a metal screen or glass doors in front of the fireplace.

- ❖ *Never leave children alone in a room with candles, heaters, or with a burning fireplace.*

Kitchen

- ☐ Keep your stove and oven clean and free of anything that could catch fire. Do not place pot holders, curtains, or towels near the burners.
- ☐ Install a portable fire extinguisher in the kitchen, high on a wall, and near an exit. (Choose a multipurpose, dry chemical extinguisher). Adults should know how to use it properly when the fire is small and contained, such as in a trash can. Call your fire department for information on how to use fire extinguishers.

- ❖ *Never leave cooking food unattended.*
- ❖ *Never pour water on a grease fire.*
- ❖ *If a fire starts in your oven, keep the oven door closed and call the fire department.*

Garage, storage area, and basement

- ☐ Have your furnace inspected at least once a year.
- ☐ Do not store anything near a heater or furnace. Remove trash from the home.
- ☐ Clean your dryer vent after every use. Lint buildup can start a fire.
- ☐ Check to make sure paint and other flammable liquids are stored in their original containers, with tight-fitting lids. Store them in a locked cabinet if possible, out of your child's reach, and away from appliances, heaters, pilot lights, and other sources of heat or flame.
- ☐ Never use flammable liquids near a gas water heater.
- ☐ Store gasoline, propane, and kerosene outside the home in a shed or detached garage. Keep them tightly sealed and labeled in approved safety containers.

- ❖ *Gasoline should be used only as a motor fuel, never as a cleaning agent.*
- ❖ *Never smoke near flammable liquids.*

Outdoors

☐ Move barbecue grills away from trees, bushes, shrubs, or anything that could catch fire. *Never* use grills indoors, on a porch, or on a balcony.

☐ Place a barrier around open fires, fire pits, or campfires. *Never* leave a child alone around the fire. Always be sure to put the fire out completely before leaving or going to sleep.

❖ *Do not start lawnmowers, snowblowers, or motorcycles near gasoline fumes. Let small motors cool off before adding fuel.*

❖ *Be very careful with barbecue grills. Never use gasoline to start the fire. Do not add charcoal lighter fluid once the fire has started.*

Know what to do in a fire

- **If you get trapped by smoke or flames,** close all doors. Stuff towels or clothing under the doors to keep out smoke. Cover your nose and mouth with a damp cloth to protect your lungs. If there is no phone in the room, wait at a window and signal for help with a light-colored cloth or flashlight.

- **Crawl low under smoke.** Choose the safest exit. If you must escape through a smoky area, remember that cleaner air is always near the floor. Teach your child to crawl on her hands and knees, keeping her head less than 2 feet above the floor, as she makes her way to the nearest exit.

- **Don't stop. Don't go back.** In case of fire, do not try to rescue pets or possessions. Once you are out, do not go back in for any reason. Firefighters have the best chance of rescuing people who are trapped. Let firefighters know right away if anyone is missing.

- **Stop, drop, and roll! Cool and call.** Make sure your child knows what to do if his clothes catch fire.
  Stop! — Do not run.
  Drop! — Drop to the ground right where you are.
  Roll! — Roll over and over to put out the flames. Cover your face with your hands.
  Cool — Cool the burned area with water.
  Call — Call for help.

Fire and children

A child's curiosity about fire is natural and in most cases is no cause for concern. However, when a child begins to use fire as a weapon, it can be very dangerous. Almost half of all people arrested for arson are under the age of 18. Fire setting by children may be a call for help or a way to oppose authority. A child who sets fires may have depression, stress, anger, or a sense of failure or may be acting out against abuse. Use the following tips when talking to your child about preventing fires:

- Teach your child that matches and lighters are tools for grown-ups only.
- Older children should be taught to use fire properly, and only in the presence of an adult.

If you suspect that your child is setting even very small fires, address the problem right away. Discuss any problems in the child's life that may be causing the behavior. Listen carefully to what your child says. Some children may have trouble talking openly with a parent. Consult your pediatrician, who can suggest ways to help. Many schools and fire departments offer programs to help children who play with fires or set fires.

For your sitters

When you are away from home and someone else cares for your children, take the following steps to ensure that your children and the sitter will be just as safe as when you are there.

- Let your sitter know where the safest exits are from your home. Discuss the family's escape plan.
- Tell the sitter where the outside meeting place is that the family has agreed upon in case of fire.

Fire drills — be prepared!

Even preschool-aged children (3 and older) can begin to learn what to do in case of a fire.

1. **Install at least one smoke alarm** on every level of your home.
2. **Have an escape plan** and practice it with your family. This will help you and your family reach safety when it counts. When a fire occurs, there will be no time for planning an escape.
3. **Draw a floor plan of your home.** Discuss with your family two ways to exit every room. Make sure everyone knows how to get out and that doors and windows can be easily opened. *If you live in an apartment building, never use an elevator during a fire. Use the stairs!*
4. **Agree on a meeting place.** Choose a spot outside your home near a tree, street corner, fence, or mailbox where everyone can gather after escaping. Teach your children that the sound of a smoke alarm means to go outside right away and meet at the designated place.
5. **Know how to call the fire department.** The fire department should be called from outside using a portable phone or from a neighbor's home. Whether the number is 911 or a regular phone number, everyone in the family should know it by heart. Make sure your children know your home address too. Teach your children that firefighters are friends and never to hide from them.
6. **Practice, practice, practice.** Practice your exit drill at least twice a year. Remember that fire drills are not a race. Get out quickly, but calmly and carefully. Try practicing realistic situations. Pretend that some exits or doorways are blocked or that the lights are out. The more prepared your family is, the better your chances of surviving a fire.

Note: Parents of children with special needs should consider a safety plan that fits their child's needs and abilities. For example, a child who is hard-of- hearing or deaf may need a smoke alarm with a flashing strobe-light feature.

- Remind sitters *never* to leave the children alone.
- In case of fire, instruct the sitter to leave the house immediately with the children and call the fire department from a neighbor's house or an outside telephone.
- Remind sitters that you do not allow smoking in or around your home and children and not to bring matches or lighters into the home.
- Make sure to leave a list of emergency information near the phone. Include the following:
  ❖ Local fire and police department phone numbers
  ❖ Poison control center phone number
  ❖ Your pediatrician's name and phone number
  ❖ Where you can be reached
  ❖ Children's full names
  ❖ Your full home address and phone number (and, if you live in a rural area, any fire identifiers)
  ❖ Neighbor's name and phone number
  ❖ Any special instructions
- Provide your sitter with a copy of this brochure to read.

Burn prevention

Most burn injuries happen in the home. For a young child, there are many ordinary places in the home that can be dangerous. Hot bath water, radiators, and even food that is too hot can cause burns. The following tips and suggestions will help you avoid the possibility of burn injury to your child:

- Keep matches, lighters, and ashtrays out of the reach of children.
- Childproof all electrical outlets with plastic plugs.
- Do not allow your child to play close to fireplaces, radiators, or space heaters.
- Replace all frayed, broken, or worn electrical cords.
- Never leave barbecue grills unattended.

- Teach your children that irons, curling irons, grills, radiators, and ovens can get very hot and are dangerous to touch or play near. Never leave any of these items unattended with children near. Unplug all appliances after using them.

Kitchen concerns

- *Never* leave a child alone in the kitchen when food is cooking.
- Enforce a "kid-free" zone 3 feet around the oven or stove while you are cooking. Use a playpen, high chair, or other stationary device to keep your child from getting too close.
- Never leave a hot oven door open.
- Use back burners if possible. When using front burners, turn pot handles inward. Never let them stick out where a child could grab them.
- Do not leave spoons or other utensils in pots while cooking.
- Turn off burners and ovens when they are not being used.
- Do not use wet pot holders, as they may cause steam burns.
- Carefully place wet foods into a deep fryer or frying pan containing grease rather than tossing them in. The reaction between hot oil and water will splatter.
- Remove pot lids carefully to avoid being burned by steam. Remember, steam is hotter than boiling water.
- In case of a small pan fire, carefully slide a lid over the pan to smother the flames, turn off the burner, and wait for the pan to cool completely.
- Never carry your child and hot liquids at the same time.
- Never leave hot liquids, like a cup of coffee, where children can reach them. Don't forget that a child can get burned from hot liquids by pulling on hanging tablecloths.
- Wear tight-fitting or rolled-up sleeves when cooking to reduce the risk of your clothes catching on fire.
- In microwave ovens, use only containers that are made for microwaves. Test microwaved food for heat and steam before giving it to your child. (Never warm a bottle in the microwave. It can heat the liquid unevenly and burn your child.)
- Avoid letting appliance cords hang over the side of countertops, where children could pull on them.

Hot water

- Lower the thermostat on your water heater so that the temperature at the tap is less than 120°F to prevent scalding.
- When using tap water, always turn on the cold water first, then add hot. When finished, turn off the hot water first.
- Test the temperature of bath water with your forearm or the back of your hand before placing your child in the water.
- Use a cool-mist vaporizer to treat upper-respiratory illnesses, as hot water vaporizers can cause steam burns or can spill on your child.
- Never leave children alone in the bathroom for any reason. They are at risk of burns and drowning.

First aid for burns

For severe burns, immediately call 911 or your local emergency number. Until help arrives, follow these steps

1. Cool the burn.
For 1st and 2nd degree burns, cool the burned area with cool running water for 10 minutes. This helps stop the burning process, numbs the pain, and prevents or reduces swelling. *Do not use ice on a burn. It may delay healing.*

Different degrees of burns

Following are the four different levels of burns and the symptoms of each:

- **1st degree burns are minor and heal quickly.** Symptoms are redness, tenderness, and soreness (like most sunburns).
- **2nd degree burns are serious injuries.** First aid and medical treatment should be given as soon as possible. Symptoms are blistering (like a severe sunburn), pain, and swelling.
- **3rd degree burns are severe injuries.** Medical treatment is needed right away. Symptoms are white, brown, or charred tissue often surrounded by blistered areas. There may be little or no pain at first.
  - ❖ Deep 2nd and 3rd degree burns are called *full-thickness burns* and are very serious.
- **4th degree burns are severe injuries that involve both skin and underlying structures, such as muscle and bone.** These often occur with electrical burns and may be more severe than they appear. They may cause serious complications and should be seen by a doctor immediately.

Remember to call your pediatrician if your child suffers anything more than a minor burn. ALL electrical burns and any burn on the hand, foot, face, or genitals should receive medical attention right away.

Also, do not rub a burn, it can increase blistering.
For 3rd degree burns, cool the burn with wet, sterile dressings until help arrives.

2. Remove burned clothing.
Lay the person flat on her back and take off the burned clothing that isn't stuck to the skin. Remove any jewelry or tight-fitting clothing from around the burned area before swelling begins. If possible, elevate the injured area.

3. Cover the burn.
After the burn has cooled, apply a clean, dry gauze pad to the burned area. Do not break any blisters. This could allow germs into the wound.
Never put grease (including butter or medical ointments) on the burn. Grease holds in heat, which may make the burn worse.

4. Treat for shock.
Keep the person's body temperature normal. Cover unburned areas with a dry blanket.

Adapted from material provided by the National Fire Protection Association (NFPA). For more information, call 617/770-3000, or visit the NFPA Web site at www.nfpa.org or its family Web site at www.sparky.org.

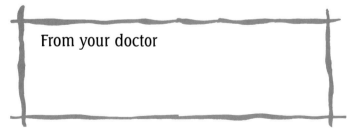

From your doctor

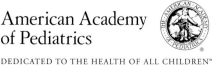

American Academy of Pediatrics

DEDICATED TO THE HEALTH OF ALL CHILDREN™

The American Academy of Pediatrics is an organization of 55,000 primary care pediatricians, pediatric medical subspecialists, and pediatric surgical specialists dedicated to the health, safety, and well-being of infants, children, adolescents, and young adults.

American Academy of Pediatrics
PO Box 747
Elk Grove Village, IL 60009-0747
Web site — http://www.aap.org

Keep Your Family Safe from Firearm Injury

American Academy of Pediatrics and Center to Prevent Handgun Violence

One out of five pediatricians nationwide has treated a young gunshot victim.

American Academy of Pediatrics, 1994

A Message from Your Pediatrician

Whether you have an infant or a teenager, keeping a gun at home poses a very real danger to your family. As a parent, you are already familiar with safety measures such as seat belts, bicycle helmets, window guards, and locking up medicines and poisons. This brochure provides easy steps you can take now to reduce the risk of gun injury–steps that can save you and your family considerable pain later.

The safest thing is to not have a gun in your home, especially not a handgun. If you already own one or plan to keep one in your home, please read this brochure very carefully. It may be vital to your family's health and safety.

Simplest Steps that Can Save Lives

A gun at home is 43 times more likely to be used to kill (including suicides) a family member or friend than to kill in self-defense.[1]

If You Keep a Gun, Empty It Out, Lock It Up!

- Always keep your gun unloaded and locked up.
- Lock and store bullets in a separate location.
- Make sure children don't have access to the keys.
- Ask police for advice on safe storage and gun locks.
- The best way to reduce gun risks is to remove the gun from your home.

Even If You Don't Own a Gun...

- Talk with your children about the risk of gun injury outside the home in places where they may visit and play.
- Tell your children to steer clear of guns when they are in the homes of their friends.
- Speak with the parents of your children's friends to find out if they keep a gun at home.
- If they do, urge them to empty it out and lock it up.
- Pass along this brochure to them.

Recognizing And Reducing The Risks To Your Family

Toddlers and Young Children

- Because even the most well-behaved children are curious by nature and will eagerly explore their environment, the safest thing is to not keep a gun at home.

- Explain to your children that guns are dangerous and that children should never touch guns.
- Tell your children that gun violence on TV and in the movies is not real. Explain that in real life, children are hurt and killed with guns.
- Children gradually learn and often forget and test the rules, so periodically repeat the message to stay away from guns.

Preteens and Teenagers

- Talk to your children about ways to solve arguments and fights without guns or violence.
- Keep in mind that teenagers don't always follow the rules. Also remember that preteens and teens are attracted to guns as symbols of power. Since you cannot always count on teens to stay away from guns, you have to keep guns away from them.
- Depressed preteens and teens commit suicide with guns more often than with any other method. No longer children and not yet adults, they may consider suicide if they're sad, angry, not being taken seriously, or if they feel ignored.
- Be extremely cautious about allowing children to participate in shooting activities.

Important Numbers

If you or your teenager is troubled or having personal problems, you can call:
1-800-448-3000
Boys Town National Hotline

To receive free information on how you and your family can work to prevent violence in your community, call:
1-800-WE-PREVENT
Crime Prevention Coalition

The above numbers are included with the permission of Boys Town and the National Crime Prevention Council, Secretariat to the Crime Prevention Coalition.

For more information, write to:

Center to Prevent Handgun Violence
1225 Eye Street, N.W., Suite 1100
Washington D.C. 20005

1. Kellerman AL and Reay DT, 1986.

The information contained in this publication should not be used as a substitute for the medical care and advice of your pediatrician. There may be variations in treatment that your pediatrician may recommend based on individual facts and circumstances.

American Academy of Pediatrics

DEDICATED TO THE HEALTH OF ALL CHILDREN™

The American Academy of Pediatrics is an organization of 55,000 primary care pediatricians, pediatric medical subspecialists, and pediatric surgical specialists dedicated to the health, safety, and well-being of infants, children, adolescents, and young adults.

American Academy of Pediatrics
PO Box 747
Elk Grove Village, IL 60009-0747
Web site — http://www.aap.org

Lawn Mower Safety

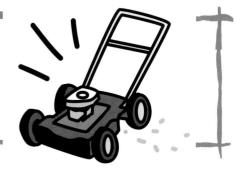

Each year many children are injured severely by lawn mowers. Power mowers can be especially dangerous. However, most lawn mower-related injuries can be prevented by following these safety guidelines.

When is my child old enough to mow the lawn?

Before learning how to mow the lawn, your child should show the maturity, good judgment, strength and coordination that the job requires. In general, the American Academy of Pediatrics recommends that children should be at least

- 12 years of age to operate a walk-behind power mower or hand mower safely
- 16 years of age to operate a riding lawn mower safely

It is important to teach your child how to use a lawn mower. Before you allow your child to mow the lawn alone, spend time showing him or her how to do the job safely. Supervise your child's work until you are sure that he or she can manage the task alone.

Before mowing the lawn:

1. Make sure that children are indoors or at a safe distance well away from the area that you plan to mow.
2. Read the lawn mower operator's manual and the instructions on the mower.
3. Check conditions
   - Do not mow during bad weather, such as during a thunderstorm.
   - Do not mow wet grass.
   - Do not mow without enough daylight.
4. Clear the mowing area of any objects such as twigs, stones, and toys, that could be picked up and thrown by the lawn mower blades.
5. Make sure that protective guards, shields, the grass catcher, and other types of safety equipment are placed properly on the lawn mower and that your mower is in good condition.
6. If your lawn mower is electric, use a ground fault circuit interrupter to prevent electric shock.
7. Never allow children to ride as passengers on ride-on lawn mowers or garden tractors.

While mowing:

1. Wear sturdy closed-toe shoes with slip-proof soles, close-fitting clothes, safety goggles or glasses with side shields, and hearing protection.
2. Watch for objects that could be picked up and thrown by the mower blades, as well as hidden dangers. Tall grass can hide objects, holes or bumps. Use caution when approaching corners, trees or anything that might block your view.
3. If the mower strikes an object, stop, turn the mower off, and inspect the mower. If it is damaged, do not use it until it has been repaired.
4. Do not pull the mower backwards or mow in reverse unless absolutely necessary, and carefully look for children behind you when you mow in reverse.
5. Use extra caution when mowing a slope.
   - When a walk-behind mower is used, mow across the face of slopes, not up and down, to avoid slipping under the mower and into the blades.
   - With a riding mower, mow up and down slopes, not across, to avoid tipping over.
6. Keep in mind that lawn trimmers also can throw objects at high speed.
7. Remain aware of where children are and do not allow them near the area where you are working. Children tend to be attracted to mowers in use.

Stop the engine and allow it to cool before refueling.

Always turn off the mower and wait for the blades to stop completely before

- Crossing gravel paths, roads or other areas
- Removing the grass catcher
- Unclogging the discharge chute
- Walking away from the mower

The information contained in this publication should not be used as a substitute for the medical care and advice of your pediatrician. There may be variations in treatment that your pediatrician may recommend based on individual facts and circumstances.

This information is based on the American Academy of Pediatrics' policy statement *Lawn Mower Injuries to Children*, published in June 2001. *Parent Pages* offers parents relevant facts that explain current policies about children's health.

The information contained in this publication should not be used as a substitute for the medical care and advice of your pediatrician. There may be variations in treatment that your pediatrician may recommend based on individual facts and circumstances.

American Academy of Pediatrics

DEDICATED TO THE HEALTH OF ALL CHILDREN™

The American Academy of Pediatrics is an organization of 55,000 primary care pediatricians, pediatric medical subspecialists, and pediatric surgical specialists dedicated to the health, safety, and well-being of infants, children, adolescents, and young adults.

American Academy of Pediatrics
PO Box 747
Elk Grove Village, IL 60009-0747
Web site — http://www.aap.org

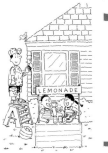
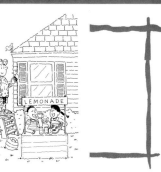

Lead Poisoning: Prevention and Screening

Of all the health problems caused by the environment, lead poisoning is the most preventable. Despite this, almost 1 million children in the United States have elevated levels of lead in their blood. Any child can be at risk for lead poisoning. This brochure has been developed by the American Academy of Pediatrics to inform parents about the risks of lead poisoning and how to prevent it. The brochure also discusses lead screening and treatment for lead poisoning.

How can lead hurt my child?

You may have heard that children can be harmed by the lead in pencils. This is not true. There is no actual lead in pencils and there is no lead in the paint on the outside of pencils.

Children *can* be harmed by lead by:

- Getting lead dust from old paint on their hands or toys and then putting their hands in their mouths
- Breathing in lead dust from old paint
- Eating chips of old paint or dirt that contain lead
- Drinking water from pipes lined or soldered with lead

Once lead enters the body, it travels through the bloodstream and is stored mainly in the bones where it can remain for a lifetime. Very high levels of lead in the body may cause many long-term problems, including:

- Kidney problems
- Anemia
- Hearing loss
- Developmental delays
- Growth problems
- Seizures and coma

Most children with high lead levels in their blood show no obvious symptoms until they reach school age. At that point, some may show learning and behavioral problems.

Where can lead be found?

Lead is most often found in the following places:

- Dust and paint chips from old paint
- Homes built before 1950, particularly those that are in need of repair or are in deteriorating condition
- Soil that has lead in it
- Hobby materials such as stained glass, paints, solders, fishing weights, and buckshot
- Folk remedies
- Workplace dust brought home on the clothing of people who have jobs that use lead, such as battery manufacturers or smelting companies
- Food stored in some ceramic dishes (especially if made in another country)
- Older painted toys and antique furniture such as cribs
- Tap water in homes that have lead pipes
- Mini-blinds manufactured outside the United States before July 1996

Prevention—what you can do

- If your home was built before 1950, ask your pediatrician to test your child for lead.
- If your home was built before 1978, talk to your pediatrician or health department about safe ways to remodel *before* any work is done.
- Know your state's laws regarding lead removal. Some states do not allow home owners to remove lead, only certified de-leaders.
- Clean and cover any chalking, flaking, or chipping paint with a new coat of paint, duct tape, or contact paper. It is important to check for paint dust or flaking paint at window areas where children often play.
- Repair areas where paint is dusting, chipping, or peeling before placing cribs, playpens, beds, or highchairs next to them.
- Encourage your children to wash their hands frequently, especially before eating.
- Check your home or apartment for possible lead contamination before moving in. Keep in mind that landlords are legally responsible for removing any lead found on their property.
- If you work around lead or have hobbies that involve lead, change clothes and shoes before entering your home. Keep clothes at work or wash work clothes as soon as possible.
- Check with your pediatrician or health department to see if your area has a problem with lead in the water.
- If you have lead pipes, run the first morning tap water for 2 minutes before using it for drinking or cooking. Do not use hot tap water for mixing formula, drinking, or cooking.

You can also reduce the risks of lead by making sure your child eats a well-balanced diet. Give your child nutritious, low-fat foods that are high in calcium and iron, like meat, beans, spinach, and low-fat dairy products. Calcium and iron in particular reduce the amount of lead absorbed by the body.

Lead screening

The only way to know for sure if your child has been exposed to lead is to have your pediatrician test your child's blood. Lead screening tests use either a small amount of blood from a finger prick or a larger sample of blood from a vein in the arm. These tests measure the amount of lead in the blood.

Treatment

For children with *low* levels of lead in their blood, identify and eliminate the sources of lead to avoid future health problems. Children with *high* levels of lead in their blood usually need to take a drug that binds the lead in the blood and helps the body get rid of it. This treatment is often done in the hospital and usually is given as a series of shots. Some children with lead poisoning need more than one type of treatment and several months of close follow-up. If the damage is severe, the child may need special schooling and therapy.

Most young children put things other than food into their mouths. They chew on toys, taste the sand at the park, and eat cat food if given the chance. This rarely causes any harm, as long as poisons and sharp objects are kept out of reach. Lead, however, can be very dangerous to children. Infants and toddlers can get sick by putting their fingers in their mouths after touching lead dust, eating lead paint chips, or breathing in lead dust. Lead poisoning can cause learning disabilities, behavioral problems, anemia, or damage to the brain and kidneys. Talk to your pediatrician about getting a blood test, especially if your child is under 3 years of age. Take the steps listed in this brochure to make sure your child does not come into contact with lead.

Should my child be screened for lead?

If you can answer "yes" to any of the following questions, especially numbers 1, 2, and 3, your child may need to be screened for lead. Talk to your pediatrician about lead screening for your child.

1. Does your child live in or regularly visit a house that was built before 1950? This includes a home child care center or the home of a relative.
2. Does your child live in or regularly visit a house built before 1978 that has been remodeled in the last 6 months? Are there any plans to remodel?
3. Does your child have a brother, sister, housemate, or playmate who is being treated for lead poisoning?
4. Have you ever been told that your child has high levels of lead in his or her blood or lead poisoning?
5. Does your child live with an adult whose job or hobby involves exposure to lead?
6. Does your child live near an active lead smelter, battery recycling plant, or other industry likely to release lead into the environment?
7. Does your child live within one block of a major highway or busy street?
8. Do you use hot tap water for cooking or drinking?
9. Has your child ever been given home remedies (azarcon, greta, pay looah)?
10. Has your child ever lived outside the United States?
11. Does your family use pottery or ceramics for cooking, eating, or drinking?
12. Have you seen your child eat paint chips?
13. Have you seen your child eat soil or dirt?
14. Have you been told your child has low iron?

The information contained in this publication should not be used as a substitute for the medical care and advice of your pediatrician. There may be variations in treatment that your pediatrician may recommend based on individual facts and circumstances.

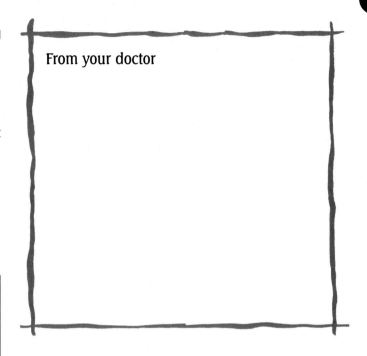

From your doctor

American Academy of Pediatrics

DEDICATED TO THE HEALTH OF ALL CHILDREN™

The American Academy of Pediatrics is an organization of 55,000 primary care pediatricians, pediatric medical subspecialists, and pediatric surgical specialists dedicated to the health, safety, and well-being of infants, children, adolescents, and young adults.

American Academy of Pediatrics
PO Box 747
Elk Grove Village, IL 60009-0747
Web site — http://www.aap.org

Copyright ©1998   American Academy of Pediatrics

Minor Head Injuries in Children

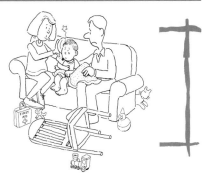

Almost all children bump their heads every now and then. While these injuries can be upsetting, most head injuries are minor and do not cause serious problems. In very rare cases, problems can occur after a minor bump on the head. This brochure, developed by the American Academy of Pediatrics, will help parents understand the difference between a head injury that needs only a comforting hug and one that requires immediate medical attention.

The information in this brochure is intended for children who
- Were well *before* the injury
- Act normally *after* the injury
- Have no cuts on the head or face (this is called a closed head injury)
- Have no other injuries to the body

The information in this brochure is *not* intended for children who
- Are younger than 2 years of age
- Have possible neck injuries
- Already have nervous system problems, such as seizures or movement disorders
- Have difficulties or delays in their development
- Have bleeding disorders or bruise easily
- Are victims of child abuse

Children with these conditions may have more serious problems after a mild head injury.

What should I do if my child has a head injury but does not lose consciousness?

For anything more than a light bump on the head, you should call your pediatrician. Your pediatrician will want to know when and how the injury happened and how your child is feeling.

If your child is alert and responds to you, the head injury is mild and usually no tests or X-rays are needed. Your child may cry from pain or fright, but this should last no longer than 10 minutes. You may need to apply a cold compress for 20 minutes to help the swelling go down and then watch your child closely for a period of time.

If there are any changes in your child's condition, call your pediatrician right away. You may need to bring your child to the pediatrician's office or directly to the hospital. The following are signs of a more serious injury:
- a constant headache that gets worse
- slurred speech
- dizziness that does not go away or happens repeatedly
- extreme irritability or other abnormal behavior
- vomiting more than two times
- clumsiness or difficulty walking
- oozing blood or watery fluid from the nose or ears
- difficulty waking up

- unequal size of the pupils (the dark center part) of the eyes
- unusual paleness that lasts for more than an hour
- convulsions (seizures)

What if my child loses consciousness?

If your child loses consciousness, call your pediatrician. Special tests may need to be done as soon as possible so that your pediatrician can find out how serious the injury is.

If the test results are normal, your pediatrician will want you to watch your child closely for a period of time. Your pediatrician will let you know if this can be done at home or in the hospital. If you take your child home and her condition changes, call your pediatrician right away since more care may be needed.

What kinds of tests may be needed? Where are they done?

A CAT scan is a special type of X-ray that gives a view of the brain and the skull. It is painless. Not every hospital can do CAT scans. Your child may need to go to a hospital or clinic that can do the scan.

What is the difference between a head X-ray and CAT scan?

- *Head X-rays* can show fractures (bone breaks) of the skull, but do not show if there is a brain injury.
- *CAT scans* can show brain injury and may be helpful in deciding the seriousness of the injury. They can even show very minor injuries that may not need treatment.

What happens if the CAT scan or head X-ray shows a problem?

More tests will probably be needed and your pediatrician may want a head injury specialist to examine your child.

What should I do if my child needs to be observed at home?

You or another responsible adult should stay with your child for the first 24 hours and be ready to take your child back to the pediatrician or hospital if there is a problem. Your child may need to be watched carefully for a few days because there could be a delay in signs of a more serious injury.

It is okay for your child to go to sleep. However, your pediatrician may recommend that you check him every 2 to 3 hours to make sure he moves normally, wakes enough to recognize you, and responds to you.

If your pediatrician prescribes medicines, follow the directions carefully. Do not give pain medication, except for acetaminophen, unless your pediatrician says it is okay. Your pediatrician will let you know if your child can eat and drink as usual.

What if my child gets worse?

If your child gets worse, your pediatrician will need to examine him again. If a CAT scan has not been done, your pediatrician may order one. Your pediatrician also may talk with a specialist or admit your child to the hospital for closer observation.

Call your pediatrician or return to the hospital if your child experiences any of the following:

- Vomits more than twice
- Cannot stop crying
- Looks sicker
- Has a hard time walking, talking, or seeing
- Is confused or not acting normally
- Becomes more and more drowsy, or is hard to wake up
- Seems to have abnormal movements or seizures or any behaviors that worry you

Will my child have any permanent damage from a minor head injury?

If your child does well through the observation period, there should be no long-lasting problems. Remember, most head injuries are mild. However, be sure to talk with your pediatrician about any concerns or questions you might have.

The information contained in this publication should not be used as a substitute for the medical care and advice of your pediatrician. There may be variations in treatment that your pediatrician may recommend based on individual facts and circumstances.

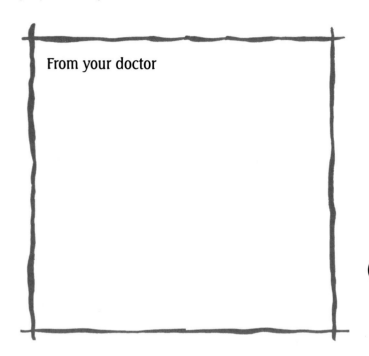

From your doctor

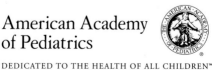

American Academy
of Pediatrics

DEDICATED TO THE HEALTH OF ALL CHILDREN™

The American Academy of Pediatrics is an organization of 55,000 primary care pediatricians, pediatric medical subspecialists, and pediatric surgical specialists dedicated to the health, safety, and well-being of infants, children, adolescents, and young adults.

American Academy of Pediatrics
PO Box 747
Elk Grove Village, IL 60009-0747
Web site — http://www.aap.org

A Parent's Guide to Water Safety

Part I Infants and Preschoolers

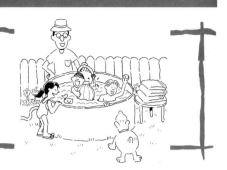

In many parts of the United States, drowning is the number one cause of death in children under age 5. Children drown in pools, rivers, bathtubs, toilets, and even large buckets of water. Any amount of water—even a few inches in a bathtub—can be dangerous to a child. This brochure has been developed by the American Academy of Pediatrics to help you keep your children safe around water.

Infants (0–1 year of age)—home hazards

Infants and toddlers are not able to protect themselves from drowning, even in a few inches of water. Children this age are most at risk of drowning in bathtubs or by falling into large buckets found around the house. Many bathtub drownings happen when a parent leaves a small child alone or with another young child. Remember, *never* leave a young child alone in a bathtub—even for a few seconds. Even supporting devices, such as bath rings, are not enough to keep your child from drowning. Children must be watched by an adult *at all times* while in the bathtub.

Toilets, 5-gallon buckets, and other large containers commonly found in the home (like large coolers with melted ice in them) are also very dangerous for a child of this age. Every year there are reports of children who have leaned forward while looking into an open toilet or large bucket, tipped into the toilet or bucket, and drowned. Since the head is the heaviest part of a small child's body, he or she can easily fall into these containers. Also, when large containers are filled with liquid, they weigh more than the child and will not tip over to allow the child to get out. Parents need to keep a close eye on their children, especially as they learn to crawl. Make sure to:

- Empty all buckets and any other large containers after each use.
- Never leave a small child alone in a bathroom.
- Keep bathroom doors closed at all times. Install a hook-and-eye latch, a doorknob cover on the outside of the door, or reverse the doorknob so that the lock is on the outside.
- Keep toilets closed or use toilet locks to keep small children from falling into them.

Preschoolers (1–5 years of age)—swimming pools

Parents should not put a swimming pool in their yard until their child is over 5 years of age. Swimming pools are the number one drowning risk for preschool-age children. A child can drown in her own backyard pool or spa even while an adult is there. In most cases, though, tragedy happens when a young child wanders away from the house and into the pool without a parent knowing it. A child can easily slip into the water without making a sound or splash. It is not until a parent notices the child missing that she is found in the water.

Swimming lessons

Though swimming lessons are widely available, they are not recommended for children under age 3. There are two reasons:
- Parents may get a false sense of security because they think their child can swim.
- Young children have a higher risk of getting infections from dirty water or getting sick from swallowing too much water.

If you want to put your small child in a swimming program, choose one that does not require your child to put his or her head under water. Also, find a program that allows you to be involved in all activities. Once your child is ready (usually around 5 years old), enroll him or her in swimming lessons. This will help your child to feel more comfortable in and around water. Remember, teaching your child to swim DOES NOT mean he or she is safe in the water. Even a child who knows how to swim may drown a few feet from safety if he or she gets confused or scared. Also remember that even a child who knows how to swim needs to be watched at all times. No one, adult or child, should ever swim alone.

CPR: life-giving breath

CPR (cardiopulmonary resuscitation) can save a child's life and help reduce injury after a near-drowning. Anyone watching a small child around a pool should learn and regularly review CPR for infants and children. In an emergency, CPR should be given immediately at poolside. Studies have found that the sooner CPR is given, the greater a victim's chances of survival. CPR training is available through the American Red Cross, the American Heart Association, and your local hospital or fire department.

Besides CPR training, here are some other ways to be ready for an emergency:
- Always have a phone near the pool and post the telephone numbers for the emergency medical services (usually 911) in your area.
- Post safety and CPR instructions at poolside.
- Make sure all rescue equipment (shepherd's hook, safety ring, rope) is nearby.

In the event of an emergency:
- Yell for help. Carefully lift the child out of the water.
- Start CPR right away. Have someone call the emergency medical service (911).
- Even if the child seems normal when revived, see your pediatrician right away.

Rules for pool safety

There are several other things you can do to keep your small child safe around a pool. Watch him or her closely when near pools or spas. Never leave a small child alone in or near a pool, even for a moment. Keep toys away from the pool so that your child is not tempted to reach for them. Empty blow-up pools and put them away after each use. The following rules will also help keep your child safe around water:

- Never swim alone.
- Do not use a diving board in a pool that is not approved for it.
- Avoid pool slides; they are very dangerous.
- Prevent shock hazards by keeping electrical appliances away from the pool.
- Do not allow tricycles or wagons at poolside.
- Keep a phone at poolside for emergency use.

It may not be possible to watch a child every second. For this reason, there should be a fence around the pool or spa that:

- completely separates the pool from the house and play area of the yard
- has four sides—not including the wall of the house
- is at least 48 inches tall
- does not have more than 4 inches between slats (in chain-link fences, the diamond shape should not be bigger than 1¾ inches)
- has a self-closing and self-latching gate that is in good working order. The latches should be higher than a child can reach
- has a gate that opens away from the pool so that, if unlatched, it closes when a toddler leans against it

Combined with the watchful eyes of an adult, a fence is the best way to protect not only your child, but other children who may visit or live in the neighborhood. Automatic pool covers (motorized covers operated by a switch), door alarms, or pool alarms also can be helpful when used with a four-sided fence. When using pool covers, cover the pool completely so that your child cannot slip under the pool cover. Make sure there is no standing water on top of the pool cover. Be aware that floating solar covers are not safety covers.

Life jackets and life preservers

If your family enjoys boating, sailing, and canoeing on lakes, rivers, and streams, make sure everyone wears the correct life jacket. Many young people think life jackets are hot, bulky, and ugly. However, today's models look better, feel better, and provide better protection. Many states require the use of life jackets and life preservers, and they must be present on all boats traveling in bodies of water supervised by the US Coast Guard. Parents should choose life jackets that are appropriate for their child's weight and age and are approved by the US Coast Guard.

Use only life jackets that have been tested by Underwriters Laboratory (UL). If they have been tested, they will have a label that says so. Life jackets are also labeled as to whether they are for a child or adult. Remember, unless your child uses a life jacket, he or she is not protected. Also, a life jacket should not be used in place of adult supervision.

Keep the following tips in mind:

- Your child should wear a life jacket at all times when on boats or near bodies of water.
- Teach your child how to put on his or her own life jacket.
- Make sure your child is comfortable wearing a life jacket and knows how to use it.
- Make sure the life jacket is the right size for your child. The jacket should not be loose. It should always be worn as instructed with all straps belted.
- Blow-up water wings, toys, rafts, and air mattresses should never be used as life jackets or life preservers. They are not safe.

The information contained in this publication should not be used as a substitute for the medical care and advice of your pediatrician. There may be variations in treatment that your pediatrician may recommend based on individual facts and circumstances.

WRONG!

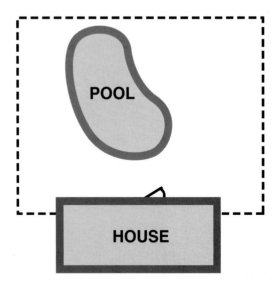

RIGHT!

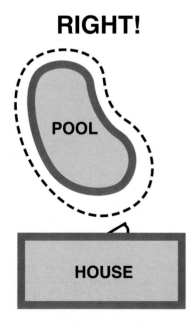

American Academy
of Pediatrics

DEDICATED TO THE HEALTH OF ALL CHILDREN™

The American Academy of Pediatrics is an organization of 55,000 primary care pediatricians, pediatric medical subspecialists, and pediatric surgical specialists dedicated to the health, safety, and well-being of infants, children, adolescents, and young adults.

American Academy of Pediatrics
PO Box 747
Elk Grove Village, IL 60009-0747
Web site — http://www.aap.org

A Parent's Guide to Water Safety

Part II School-age Children and Adolescents

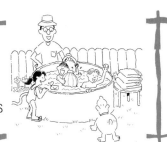

School-age children (5–12 years of age)—outdoor hazards

Swimming and water sports are great fun and good exercise for children this age. However, many drownings of school-age children occur in oceans, lakes, rivers, and streams. Never let your child swim in any body of water without an adult watching. Also, do not let your child water-ski, scuba dive, or snorkel without instructions from a qualified teacher.

Other water hazards found near many homes include ditches, post holes, wells, fish ponds, and fountains. Watch your child closely if he is playing near any of these areas.

Rules for swimming safety

Teach your child the following safety rules and make sure they are obeyed:
- Never swim alone.
- Never dive into water unless given the okay by an adult who knows the depth of the water.
- Always use a life vest when boating, fishing, waterskiing, or playing in a river or stream.
- Never swim around anchored boats, in motorboat lanes, or where people are waterskiing.
- Never swim during electrical storms.
- Never push or hold another person under water, or call for help in fun. A cry for help should only be made in a true emergency.
- If you should swim or drift far from shore, stay calm, and tread water or float on your back until help arrives. Keep your hands under the surface of the water for better body position, balance, and floating.
- Do not let your child use blow-up toys or mattresses in water that is above her waist. Remember, water wings and other blow-up swimming aids should not be used in place of life vests. In fact, they often give a false sense of security and can even be dangerous if they deflate suddenly or if your child slips out of them.

Adolescents (12–18 years old)—diving and swimming while intoxicated

Older children and teenagers are also at risk from drowning even though they are more likely to have had swimming lessons. Children in this age group often drown while swimming in unsupervised places such as water-filled quarries, rivers, or ponds. Often the swimmer thinks he can swim better than he actually can, and does not understand the water currents or the depth of the water. Adolescents are also at risk of drowning as a result of serious injury from diving or swimming while drinking alcohol or using other drugs.

Diving

Many swimmers are seriously injured each year from diving mishaps. Serious spinal cord injuries, brain damage, and death can occur to swimmers who:
- dive into shallow areas of lakes, ponds, streams, or swimming pools where the depth of the water is not known
- dive into aboveground pools
- hit the bottom of a pool as it slopes toward the shallow end
- spring upward from the diving board and hit it on the way down

Avoid getting hurt by following these simple common-sense rules:
- Never swim or dive while drinking alcohol or using other drugs.
- Check the depth of the water—go into the water feet first, especially when going in the water for the first time.
- Never dive into aboveground pools because they are usually not deep enough.
- Never dive into the shallow end of a pool.
- Never dive through inner tubes or other pool toys.
- Learn how to dive properly by taking classes.

CPR: life-giving breath

CPR (cardiopulmonary resuscitation) can save a child's life and help reduce injury after a near-drowning. Anyone watching a small child around a pool should learn and regularly review CPR for infants and children. In an emergency, CPR should be given immediately at poolside. Studies have found that the sooner CPR is given, the greater a victim's chances of survival. CPR training is available through the American Red Cross, the American Heart Association, and your local hospital or fire department.

Besides CPR training, here are some other ways to be ready for an emergency:
- Always have a phone near the pool and post the telephone numbers for the emergency medical services (usually 911) in your area.
- Post safety and CPR instructions at poolside.
- Make sure all rescue equipment (shepherd's hook, safety ring, rope) is nearby.

In the event of an emergency:
- Yell for help. Carefully lift the child out of the water.
- Start CPR right away. Have someone call the emergency medical service (911).
- Even if the child seems normal when revived, see your pediatrician right away.

Alcohol

Among teenagers, drowning is often the result of risky behavior, alcohol, or both. Drinking alcohol or using other drugs while swimming, diving, and playing water sports puts swimmers at serious risk of drowning. These activities require clear thinking, coordination, and the ability to judge distance, depth, speed, and direction. Alcohol affects the part of the brain that allows a person to stay in control and impairs all of these skills.

Encourage your teen to take swimming, diving, and water safety or rescue classes. This will give him or her the skills needed to swim and dive safely. Your teen will also be less likely to act recklessly.

Children are naturally curious about water—whether it be in a pool, lake, or large bucket. However, each year, too many young children die or are left brain damaged because of preventable drowning injuries. By following simple safety precautions, your family can enjoy the water and prevent these tragedies.

Life jackets and life preservers

If your family enjoys boating, sailing, and canoeing on lakes, rivers, and streams, make sure everyone wears the correct life jacket. Many young people think life jackets are hot, bulky, and ugly. However, today's models look better, feel better, and provide better protection. Many states require the use of life jackets and life preservers, and they must be present on all boats traveling in bodies of water supervised by the US Coast Guard. Parents should choose life jackets that are appropriate for their child's weight and age and are approved by the US Coast Guard.

Use only life jackets that have been tested by Underwriters Laboratory (UL). If they have been tested, they will have a label that says so. Life jackets are also labeled as to whether they are for a child or adult. Remember, unless your child uses a life jacket, he or she is not protected. Also, a life jacket should not be used in place of adult supervision.

Keep the following tips in mind:

- Your child should wear a life jacket at all times when on boats or near bodies of water.
- Teach your child how to put on his or her own life jacket.
- Make sure your child is comfortable wearing a life jacket and knows how to use it.
- Make sure the life jacket is the right size for your child. The jacket should not be loose. It should always be worn as instructed with all straps belted.
- Blow-up water wings, toys, rafts, and air mattresses should never be used as life jackets or life preservers. They are not safe.

The information contained in this publication should not be used as a substitute for the medical care and advice of your pediatrician. There may be variations in treatment that your pediatrician may recommend based on individual facts and circumstances.

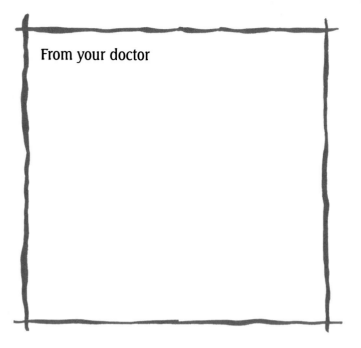

From your doctor

Playground Safety

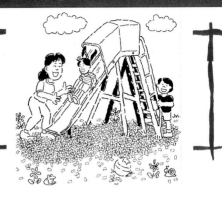

Each year about 250,000 children ages 15 and younger get hurt on playground equipment and are treated for their injuries in emergency rooms. Between 10 and 20 children die each year from playground injuries. About one-fourth of all playground injuries happen on home equipment, but most occur at school and public playgrounds.

This brochure can help you determine whether playground equipment—at your home, your child's school, or in your neighborhood—is as safe as possible.

How are children injured?

Falls cause about 75% of playground injuries. Children:
- Fall off equipment
- Fall from heights, especially from climbing structures (such as monkey bars)
- Trip over equipment

Other playground injuries are caused by:
- Blows from equipment, especially swings
- Cuts from sharp edges, hardware, or loose or exposed nails and screws

Types of Injuries

Many injuries, such as cuts, scrapes, and bruises, are not serious. However, some head injuries can be serious or even fatal. Other common playground injuries—many of which can be prevented—are broken bones, sprains, and injuries to the teeth and mouth.

Preventing Playground Injuries

Most important:
- The best way to prevent serious head injuries is to have a surface that will absorb impact when children land on it. This is especially needed under and around swings, slides, and other equipment. (See "What are safer surfaces?").
- To prevent injuries from falls, platforms should not be higher than 8 feet above the ground and should have guard rails (38 inches high).
- Vertical and horizontal spaces should be less than 3 1/2 inches wide or more than 9 inches wide. This is to keep a small child's head from getting trapped.
- Objects that stick out (bolts, nails, etc.), hooks that are not closed all the way ("S" hooks), sharp edges, and pinch points also cause many playground injuries. Equipment must be free of these hazards.
- Even with these measures children still need to be watched closely while they are playing.

Also important:
- Carefully maintain all equipment. Be sure that it has been installed exactly according to the manufacturer's directions.
- Swings should be clear of other equipment by a distance equal to twice the height of the swing, measured from the center of the swing while it is at rest. Swing seats should be made of soft materials such as rubber, plastic, or canvas. Children under 5 years of age should use chair swings. Make sure open hooks , or "S" hooks, on swing chains are closed to form a figure "8."
- Make sure equipment is the right size for the children playing on it. For example, smaller swings are meant for smaller children and can break if larger children use them.
- Make sure children cannot reach any moving parts that might pinch or trap any body part.
- Play equipment should be installed at least 6 feet from any barrier, such as a wall or fence, and should be securely anchored to prevent tipping. The concrete anchors should be buried below the surface of the dirt and beneath the full depth of the ground cover of absorbent material. Some equipment, such as swings and slides, requires a larger "fall zone" around it.
- Wood fences and equipment should be free of splinters; all fences and equipment should be free of nails that stick out.
- Metal slides exposed to direct sunlight can burn children's hands and legs. Plastic slides are less likely to cause burn injuries. Position slides in the shade or face them away from the afternoon sun.
- Slides should have a platform with rails at the top for children to hold. The sides of the slide should be 4 inches high.
- Make sure there are no rocks, pieces of glass, sticks, toys, debris, or other children at the base of a slide. These could get in the way of a child landing safely. The cleared and safer-surfaced area should extend from the exit of the slide a distance equal to the height of the slide plus 4 feet.

The Danger of Drawstrings

Drawstrings can strangle a child if they get caught on playground equipment. One way to prevent this it to take the drawstrings off the hoods and collars of your child's jackets, shirts, and hats and shorten the drawstrings around the bottom of coats and jackets.

If you want to leave the drawstrings, you can either:
- Cut all the ends just short enough so that they tie
- Sew a seam at the middle of the hood, collar, or waistband to prevent either side from pulling out if caught on an object

The best way to prevent drawstrings from getting caught on anything is to choose clothing that does not have them.

What are safer surfaces?

Did you know that even a 1-foot fall onto asphalt or concrete can cause a fatal head injury? Or that a 4-foot fall onto packed earth or grass can also cause serious injury or death?

Safer surfaces make a serious or fatal head injury less likely to occur if a child falls. This is because such surfaces absorb the impact of a fall. Some examples of "safer surfaces" include:

- Sand (10 inches deep)
- Wood chips (12 inches deep)
- Rubber outdoor mat (follow manufacturers' instructions)

Sand and wood chips, which absorb impact, should be raked at least weekly to keep them soft. They also need refilling often to keep the correct depth.

No surface is totally safe. Many injuries are preventable, but they will sometimes occur even at the safest playgrounds-and even with the best supervision. Be prepared to handle an injury if it does occur.

For more information... about playground safety, "safer surfaces," or to get a copy of the *Handbook for Public Playground Safety,* contact the US Consumer Product Safety Commission, Washington, DC. 20207.

The information contained in this publication should not be used as a substitute for the medical care and advice of your pediatrician. There may be variations in treatment that your pediatrician may recommend based on individual facts and circumstances.

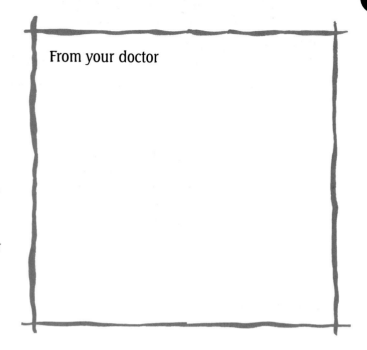

From your doctor

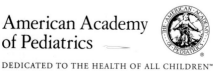

American Academy
of Pediatrics

DEDICATED TO THE HEALTH OF ALL CHILDREN™

The American Academy of Pediatrics is an organization of 55,000 primary care pediatricians, pediatric medical subspecialists, and pediatric surgical specialists dedicated to the health, safety, and well-being of infants, children, adolescents, and young adults.

American Academy of Pediatrics
PO Box 747
Elk Grove Village, IL 60009-0747
Web site — http://www.aap.org

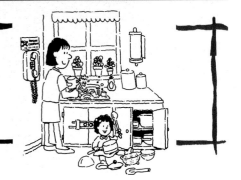

Protect Your Child From Poison
Part I Prevention and Treatment

Children can get very sick if they come in contact with medications, household pesticides, chemicals, cosmetics, or plants. This can happen at any age and can cause serious reactions. However, most children who come in contact with poison are *not* permanently harmed if they are treated right away. This brochure has been developed by the American Academy of Pediatrics to inform parents how to prevent poisonings and what to do if their child has been poisoned.

Prevention

Young children are poisoned most commonly by things in the home such as:
- drugs and medications (iron medications are one of the most common causes of poisonings in children under age 5)
- cleaning products
- plants
- cosmetics
- pesticides
- paints and solvents

Most poisonings occur when parents are not paying close attention. If you are ill or stressed, you may not watch your child as closely as usual. The hectic routine of getting dinner on the table causes so many lapses in parental attention that late afternoon is known as "the arsenic hour" by poison center personnel.

In addition, children like to put things into their mouths and taste things. This is a natural way for children to learn about the world around them. Children also copy adults without knowing what they are doing.

The best way to prevent poisonings is to lock up all toxic substances where your child cannot get to them. Also, watch your child even more closely whenever you are somewhere that is not childproofed. Be especially attentive when your child is visiting another home, or a grandparent's home, where childproofing may not have been done.

Treatment

Swallowed poison

If you find your child with an open or empty container of a toxic substance, your child may have been poisoned. Stay calm and act quickly.

First, get the poison away from your child. If there is still some in your child's mouth, make him spit it out, or remove it with your fingers. Keep this material along with any other evidence that might help determine what was swallowed.

Next, check for these signs:
- severe throat pain
- breathing difficulty
- sudden behavior changes, such as unusual sleepiness, irritability, or jumpiness
- unexplained nausea or vomiting
- stomach cramps without fever
- burns on your child's lips or mouth
- unusual drooling, or odd odors on your child's breath
- unexplained stains on your child's clothing
- convulsions or unconsciousness (only in very serious cases)

If your child has any of these signs, call 911 right away. Take the poison container with you to help the doctor determine what was swallowed. *Do not make your child vomit,* as this may cause further damage. Also, *do not follow instructions about poisoning on the label* of the container, as these are often out of date.

If your child does not have these symptoms, call your regional poison center or pediatrician. They will need the following information in order to help you:
- Your name and phone number.
- Your child's name, age, and weight.
- Any medical conditions your child may have.
- Any medications your child may be taking.
- The name of the substance your child swallowed. Read it off the container and spell it.
- The ingredients of the substance your child swallowed if they are listed on the label. If your child has swallowed a prescription medicine, give all the information on the label including the name of the drug. If the name of the drug is not on the label, give the name and phone number of the pharmacy, and the date of the prescription.
- What the pill looked like (if you can tell) and if it had any printed numbers on it. If your child swallowed another substance, such as a part of a plant, describe it as much as you can to help identify it.
- The time your child swallowed the poison (or when you found your child), and the amount you think was swallowed.

If the poison is extremely dangerous, or if your child is very young, you may be told to make him vomit and take him directly to the nearest hospital. Otherwise, you will be given instructions to follow at home.

Syrup of ipecac

If you are told to make your child vomit, give him syrup of ipecac in the recommended dose. Encourage your child to drink a glass of water as well.

Place your child over your lap, face down, the head lower than the hips. Get ready to catch the vomit in a large bowl so that it can be inspected or until your pediatrician or the poison center tells you to throw it away. If your child vomits for more than 2 hours after taking the syrup of ipecac, or shows any of the symptoms described earlier, call your pediatrician. If your child does not vomit within 20 minutes after taking the syrup of ipecac, repeat the dose once.

In some cases vomiting may be dangerous, so never make a child vomit unless the poison center tells you to do so. Strong acids (such as toilet bowl cleaner) or strong alkalies (such as lye, drain or oven cleaner, or dishwasher detergent) can burn the throat—and vomiting will only make the damage worse. In such cases you probably will be told to have the child drink milk or water.

> ### Recommended dosage schedule for syrup of ipecac:
> - 1 month to 1 year—check with your pediatrician or poison center
> - 1 year to 10 years—½ ounce (1 tablespoon or 3 teaspoons or 15 milliliters) followed by two glasses of water

Poison on the skin

If your child spills a dangerous chemical on her body, remove her clothes and rinse the skin with lukewarm—not hot—water. If the area shows signs of being burned, continue rinsing for at least 15 minutes, no matter how much your child may protest. Then call the poison center for further advice. Do not use ointments or grease.

Poison in the eye

Flush your child's eye by holding the eyelid open and pouring a steady stream of lukewarm water into the inner corner. A young child is sure to object to this, so get another adult to hold your child while you rinse the eye. If that is not possible, wrap your child tightly in a towel and clamp him under one arm. This way you will have one hand free to hold the eyelid open and the other to pour in the water. Continue flushing the eye for 15 minutes. Then call the poison center for further instructions. Do not use an eyecup, eyedrops, or ointment unless the poison center tells you to do so.

Poison fumes

In the home, poisonous fumes can come from:
- a car running in a closed garage
- leaky gas vents
- wood, coal, or kerosene stoves that are not working properly

If your child is exposed to fumes or gases, get her into fresh air right away. If she is breathing, call the poison center for further instructions. If she has stopped breathing, start CPR and do not stop until she breathes on her own or someone else can take over. If you can, have someone call 911 right away. If you are alone, wait until your child is breathing or, after 1 minute of CPR, call 911.

Be prepared

Be prepared for a poisoning emergency by posting the poison center phone number by every phone in your home. To locate the nearest poison center, call 202/362-7217, or write to the American Association of Poison Control Centers, 3201 New Mexico Avenue, NW, Suite 310, Washington, DC 20016.

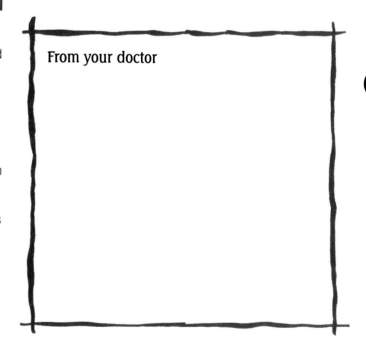

From your doctor

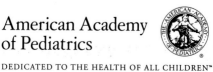

American Academy of Pediatrics

DEDICATED TO THE HEALTH OF ALL CHILDREN™

The American Academy of Pediatrics is an organization of 55,000 primary care pediatricians, pediatric medical subspecialists, and pediatric surgical specialists dedicated to the health, safety, and well-being of infants, children, adolescents, and young adults.

American Academy of Pediatrics
PO Box 747
Elk Grove Village, IL 60009-0747
Web site — http://www.aap.org

Protect Your Child From Poison

Part II Poison Proofing Your Home

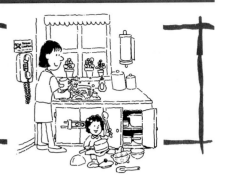

Poison-proofing your home

- Keep all drugs, medications, household cleaning products, and cosmetics locked up and out of your child's reach.
- Use safety latches on drawers and cabinets that contain objects that might be dangerous to your child.
- Keep a small bottle of *syrup of ipecac* on hand with your other medicines—out of children's reach. It is available without prescription at most pharmacies. Use it only with instructions from the poison center or your pediatrician.
- Post the poison center and other emergency numbers near every phone in your home. Be sure that your babysitter knows how to use these numbers.

In the kitchen

- Store cleaners, lye, furniture polish, dishwasher soap, and other dangerous products in a locked cabinet.
- If you must store items under the sink, use safety latches that lock every time you close the cabinet (most hardware and department stores have them).
- Never put dangerous substances into containers that look as if they might hold things your child usually eats or drinks.

In the bathroom

- Buy and keep all medicines in containers with safety caps. Remember, however, that these caps are *child-resistant*, not *childproof*, so store them in a locked cabinet.
- Throw away any leftover prescription medicines.
- Do not keep toothpaste, soaps, shampoos, and other frequently used items in the same cabinet as dangerous products.
- Do not take medicine in front of small children; they may try to copy you.
- Never say that a medicine is candy in order to get your child to take it.
- Check the label every time you give medication. This will help you to be sure you are giving the right medicine in the right amounts. Mistakes are more common in the middle of the night, so always turn on a light when handling any medication.

In the garage and basement

- Keep paints, varnishes, thinners, pesticides, and fertilizers in a locked cabinet in their original, labeled containers.
- Read labels on all household products before you buy them. Try to find the least toxic ones for the job. Buy only what you need to use right away.
- Never put poisonous or toxic products in containers that were once used for food, especially empty drink bottles, cans, or cups.
- Never run your car in a closed garage. Be sure that coal, wood, or kerosene stoves are in good working order. If you smell gas, turn off the stove or gas burner, leave the house, and call the gas company.

The information contained in this publication should not be used as a substitute for the medical care and advice of your pediatrician. There may be variations in treatment that your pediatrician may recommend based on individual facts and circumstances.

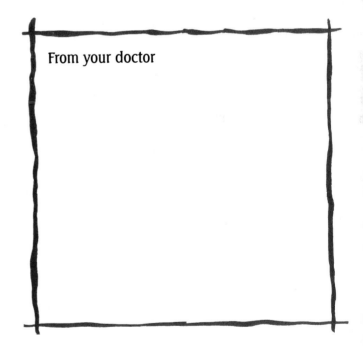

From your doctor

American Academy of Pediatrics

DEDICATED TO THE HEALTH OF ALL CHILDREN™

The American Academy of Pediatrics is an organization of 55,000 primary care pediatricians, pediatric medical subspecialists, and pediatric surgical specialists dedicated to the health, safety, and well-being of infants, children, adolescents, and young adults.

American Academy of Pediatrics
PO Box 747
Elk Grove Village, IL 60009-0747
Web site — http://www.aap.org

Raising Children to Resist Violence
What You Can Do

Research has shown that violent or aggressive behavior is often learned early in life. However, parents, family members, and others who care for children can help them learn to deal with emotions without using violence. Parents and others can also take steps to reduce or minimize violence. This brochure is designed to help parents work within the family, school, and community to prevent and reduce youth violence.

Suggestions for Dealing With Children

Parents play a valuable role in reducing violence by raising children in safe and loving homes. Here are suggestions that can help. You may not be able to follow each one exactly, but if you do your best, it will make a difference in your children's lives.

Give your children consistent love and attention.

Every child needs a strong, loving relationship with a parent or other adult to feel safe and secure and to develop a sense of trust. Without a steady bond to a caring adult, a child is at risk for becoming hostile, difficult, and hard to manage. Behavior problems and delinquency are less likely to develop in children whose parents are involved in their lives, especially at an early age.

It's not easy to show love to a child all the time. It can be even harder if you are a young, inexperienced, or single parent, or if your child is sick or has special needs. If your baby seems unusually difficult to care for and comfort, discuss this with your child's pediatrician, another physician, a psychologist, or a counselor. He or she can give you advice and direct you to local parenting classes that teach positive ways to handle the difficulties of raising children.

It is important to remember that children have minds of their own. Their increasing independence sometimes leads them to behave in ways that disappoint, anger, or frustrate you. Patience and a willingness to view the situation through children's eyes, before reacting, can help you deal with your emotions. Do your best to avoid responding to your children with hostile words or actions.

Make sure your children are supervised.

Children depend on their parents and family members for encouragement, protection, and support as they learn to think for themselves. Without proper supervision, children do not receive the guidance they need. Studies report that unsupervised children often have behavior problems.

- Insist on knowing where your child is at all times and who their friends are. When you are unable to watch your children, ask someone you trust to watch them for you. Never leave young children home alone, even for a short time.
- Encourage your school-aged and older children to participate in supervised after-school activities such as sports teams, tutoring programs, or organized recreation. Enroll them in local community programs, especially those run by adults whose values you respect.

- Accompany your children to supervised play activities and watch how they get along with others. Teach your children how to respond appropriately when others use insults or threats or deal with anger by hitting. Explain to your children that these are not appropriate behaviors, and encourage them to avoid other children who behave that way.

Show your children appropriate behaviors by the way you act.

Children often learn by example. The behavior, values, and attitudes of parents and siblings have a strong influence on children. Values of respect, honesty, and pride in your family and heritage can be important sources of strength for children, especially if they are confronted with negative peer pressure, live in a violent neighborhood, or attend a rough school.

Most children sometimes act aggressively and may hit another person. Be firm with your children about the possible dangers of violent behavior. Remember also to praise your children when they solve problems constructively without violence. Children are more likely to repeat good behaviors when they are rewarded with attention and praise.

You can teach your children non-aggressive ways to solve problems by:
- Discussing problems with them,
- Asking them to consider what might happen if they use violence to solve problems, and
- Talking about what might happen if they solve problems without violence.

This kind of "thinking out loud" together will help children see that violence is not a helpful solution.

Parents sometimes encourage aggressive behavior without knowing it. For example, some parents think it is good for a boy to learn to fight. Teach your children that it is better to settle arguments with calm words, not fists, threats, or weapons.

Help your children learn constructive, nonviolent ways to enjoy their free time. Teach them your favorite games, hobbies, or sports, and help them develop their own talents and skills. Read stories to younger children, take older children to the library, or tell family stories about admired relatives who have made the world a better place.

Don't hit your children.

Hitting, slapping, or spanking children as punishment shows them that it's okay to hit others to solve problems and can train them to punish others in the same way they were punished.

Physical punishments stop unwanted behavior only for a short time. Even with very harsh punishment, children may adapt so that it has little or no effect. Using even more punishment is equally ineffective.

Nonphysical methods of discipline help children deal with their emotions and teach them nonviolent ways to solve problems. Here are some suggestions:

- Giving children "time out"—making children sit quietly, usually 1 minute for each year of age (this is not appropriate for very young children),
- Taking away certain privileges or treats, and
- "Grounding"—not allowing children to play with friends or take part in school or community activities (this is only appropriate for older children or adolescents).

Punishment that involves taking away privileges or "grounding" should be consistently applied for realistic, brief periods.

Children need to feel that if they make mistakes, they can correct them. Show them how to learn from their errors. Help them figure out what they did wrong and how they can avoid making similar mistakes in the future. It is especially important not to embarrass or humiliate your children at these times. Children always need to feel your love and respect.

A positive approach to changing behaviors is to emphasize rewards for good behavior instead of punishments for bad behavior. Remember that praise and affection are the best rewards.

Be consistent about rules and discipline.

When you make a rule, stick to it. Children need structure with clear expectations for their behavior. Setting rules and then not enforcing them is confusing and sets up children to "see what they can get away with."

Parents should involve children in setting rules whenever possible. Explain to your children what you expect, and the consequences for not following the rules. This will help them learn to behave in ways that are good for them and for those around them.

Make sure your children do not have access to guns.

Guns and children can be a deadly combination. Teach your children about the dangers of firearms or other weapons if you own and use them. If you keep a gun in your home, unload it and lock it up separately from the bullets. Never store firearms, even if unloaded, in places where children can find them.

Don't carry a gun or a weapon. If you do, this tells your children that using guns solves problems.

Try to keep your children from seeing violence in the home or community.

Violence in the home can be frightening and harmful to children. Children need a safe and loving home where they do not have to grow up in fear. Children who have seen violence at home do not always become violent, but they may be more likely to try to resolve conflicts with violence.

Work toward making home a safe, nonviolent place, and always discourage violent behavior between brothers and sisters. Keep in mind as well that hostile, aggressive arguments between parents frighten children and set a bad example for them.

If the people in your home physically or verbally hurt and abuse each other, get help from a psychologist or counselor in your community. He or she will help you and your family understand why violence at home occurs and how to stop it.

Sometimes children cannot avoid seeing violence in the street, at school, or at home, and they may need help in dealing with these frightening experiences. A psychologist or counselor at school or a religious leader are among those who can help them cope with their feelings.

Try to keep your children from seeing too much violence in the media.

Seeing a lot of violence on television, in the movies, and in video games can lead children to behave aggressively. As a parent, you can control the amount of violence your children see in the media.

Here are some ideas:
- Limit television viewing time to 1 to 2 hours a day.
- Make sure you know what TV shows your children watch, which movies they see, and what kinds of video games they play.
- Talk to your children about the violence that they see on TV shows, in the movies, and in video games.Help them understand how painful it would be in real life and the serious consequences for violent behaviors.
- Discuss with your children ways to solve problems without violence.

Teach your children ways to avoid becoming victims of violence.

It is important that you and your children learn to take precautions against becoming the victims of a violent crime. Here are some important steps that you can take to keep yourself and your children safe:
- Teach your children safe routes for walking in your neighborhood.
- Encourage them to walk with a friend at all times and only in well-lighted, busy areas.
- Stress how important it is for them to report any crimes or suspicious activities they see to you, a teacher, another trustworthy adult, or the police. Show them how to call 911 or the emergency service in your area.
- Make sure they know what to do if anyone tries to hurt them: Say "no," run away, and tell a reliable adult.
- Stress the dangers of talking to strangers. Tell them never to open the door to or go anywhere with someone they don't know and trust.

Help your children stand up against violence.

Support your children in standing up against violence. Teach them to respond with calm but firm words when others insult, threaten, or hit another person. Help them understand that it takes more courage and leadership to resist violence than to go along with it.

Help your children accept and get along with others from various racial and ethnic backgrounds. Teach them that criticizing people because they are different is hurtful, and that name-calling is unacceptable. Make sure they understand that using words to start or encourage violence—or to quietly accept violent behavior—is harmful. Warn your child that bullying and threats can be a setup for violence.

An Extra Suggestion for Adults:

Take care of yourself and your community.

Stay involved with your friends, neighbors, and family. A network of friends can offer fun, practical help, and support when you have difficult times. Reducing stress and social isolation can help in raising your children.

Get involved in your community and get to know your neighbors. Try to make sure guns are not available in your area as well. Volunteer to help in your neighborhood's anticrime efforts or in programs to make schools safer for children. If there are no programs like this nearby, help start one!

Let your elected officials know that preventing violence is important to you and your neighbors. Complain to television stations and advertisers who sponsor violent programs.

Encourage your children to get involved in groups that build pride in the community, such as those that organize cleanups of litter, graffiti, and run-down buildings. In addition to making the neighborhood a safer place, these groups provide a great opportunity for parents, children, and neighbors to spend time together in fun, safe, and rewarding activities.

Potential Warning Signs

Parents whose children show the signs listed below should discuss their concerns with a professional, who will help them understand their children and suggest ways to prevent violent behavior.

Warning Signs in the Toddler and Preschool Child:

- Has many temper tantrums in a single day or several lasting more than 15 minutes, and often cannot be calmed by parents, family members, or other caregivers;
- Has many aggressive outbursts, often for no reason;
- Is extremely active, impulsive, and fearless;
- Consistently refuses to follow directions and listen to adults;
- Does not seem attached to parents, for example, does not touch, look for, or return to parents in strange places;
- Frequently watches violence on television, engages in play that has violent themes, or is cruel toward other children.

Warning Signs in the School-aged Child:

- Has trouble paying attention and concentrating;
- Often disrupts classroom activities;
- Does poorly in school;
- Frequently gets into fights with other children in school;
- Reacts to disappointments, criticism, or teasing with extreme and intense anger, blame, or revenge;
- Watches many violent television shows and movies or plays a lot of violent video games;
- Has few friends, and is often rejected by other children because of his or her behavior;
- Makes friends with other children known to be unruly or aggressive;
- Consistently does not listen to adults;
- Is not sensitive to the feelings of others;
- Is cruel or violent toward pets or other animals;
- Is easily frustrated.

Warning Signs in the Preteen or Teenaged Adolescent:

- Consistently does not listen to authority figures;
- Pays no attention to the feelings or rights of others;
- Mistreats people and seems to rely on physical violence or threats of violence to solve problems;
- Often expresses the feeling that life has treated him or her unfairly;
- Does poorly in school and often skips class;
- Misses school frequently for no identifiable reason;
- Gets suspended from or drops out of school;
- Joins a gang, gets involved in fighting, stealing, or destroying property;
- Drinks alcohol and/or uses inhalants or drugs.

This brochure is a collaborative project of the American Psychological Association and the American Academy of Pediatrics. Many experts from both of these professional groups contributed to the development of the material presented here.

American Psychological Association
750 First St. NE
Washington, DC 20002-4242

This information should not be used as a substitute for professional health and mental health care or consultation. Based on individual facts and circumstances, a psychologist or pediatrician may recommend varied approaches to child-rearing and violence prevention or treatment options for serious or chronic problems.

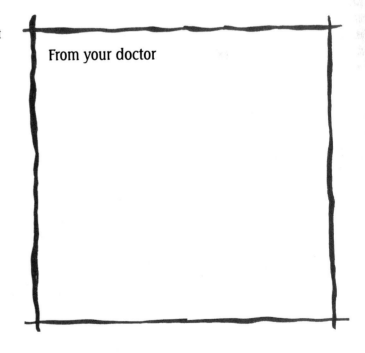

From your doctor

American Academy of Pediatrics

DEDICATED TO THE HEALTH OF ALL CHILDREN™

The American Academy of Pediatrics is an organization of 55,000 primary care pediatricians, pediatric medical subspecialists, and pediatric surgical specialists dedicated to the health, safety, and well-being of infants, children, adolescents, and young adults.

American Academy of Pediatrics
PO Box 747
Elk Grove Village, IL 60009-0747
Web site — http://www.aap.org

Sports and Your Child

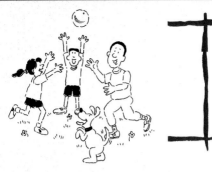

From the backyard to the playground, more American children than ever are playing games and competing in sports. Close to 6 million high school boys and girls take part in team sports on courts, in pools, on fields, and in gyms. Another 20 million join in recreational or competitive sports out of school.

Sports help boys and girls in many ways. When a body is fit, it looks and feels better. But even more important is that fit people stay healthier longer. With the right guidance, sports activities can promote a sense of personal satisfaction in young people—and that can lead to increased social acceptance.

Your pediatrician plays a vital role in making sure that your child's sports program—whether in or out of school—gets the right results. Each young athlete presents a unique picture of health, growth, physical maturity, and knowledge of basic skills. A complete medical exam will highlight your child's physical strengths and weaknesses. This "physical" may help your young athlete choose the sport that will be most rewarding for him or her.

Your doctor can counsel you in many other aspects of safe and enjoyable sports participation for your child, such as proper diet and injury prevention. Make sure that your young athlete gets the best guidance possible. Here are answers to questions that parents often ask their pediatricians.

At what age should a child get started in sports?

Infant exercise programs are unnecessary because these programs do nothing to improve your baby's physical fitness. It is a good idea to wait until your child is 6 years old before beginning team sports, since children do not understand the concept of teamwork until this age. Free play is advised until then. Although the age just mentioned is a good guideline, remember that all children are different. Two children the same age may grow and mature at different rates. A child's build also determines his or her ability to perform certain tasks. When children reach the teen years, there are many different levels of maturity.

A study of Little League World Series players revealed that almost half had already passed through puberty, although all were younger than 13 years old. Age, weight, and size should not be the only measures when deciding whether to compete in a sport at a certain level. A young teenager's physical and emotional development also are important. In puberty, boys gain more muscle mass and, therefore, more strength. Two wrestlers who are the same weight and age will not be equally matched if one athlete is mature and the other is not. This puts the less-developed boy at a disadvantage and may increase his chance of injury.

Late-developing teens should delay contact sports until their bodies have caught up with their more mature peers. A child should not be pushed into a sport that he or she is not physically or emotionally ready to handle. But if the child has a strong interest in a sport, then it may be proper to allow participation—so long as common sense prevails.

Should boys and girls play in sports together?

In recent years, sports participation for girls has been encouraged as strongly as sports activities for boys. This welcome trend pays off in many ways. By having the chance to take part in sports, girls gain self-confidence and a healthy respect for physical fitness.

Until the onset of puberty, boys and girls can compete together because boys and girls are almost the same size and weight. Girls generally enter puberty between 10 and 12 years of age, about 2 years before boys do. After puberty, boys gain an advantage in both strength and size. Therefore, safety and fairness dictate that boys and girls should no longer compete against each other in most sports. However, if there is no team for girls in a certain sport, some laws state that a girl must be allowed to compete for a position on the boys' team.

What are the risks of injury in various sports?

Despite safety measures, such as protective padding and helmets, the risk of injury is present in all sports. Some sports pose a greater risk than others, with football leading the list. Children and parents should be aware of the risks involved with each sports activity.

The chance of injury increases with the degree of contact in a sport. Football produces many times the number of injuries as the next group of sports with significant injuries: wrestling, gymnastics, soccer, basketball, and track/running. Knee injuries are the most common serious injury in major sports. Boxing involves a high risk of brain damage; therefore, no young person should participate in this sport.

Most sports injuries involve the soft tissues of the body, not the bony skeleton. Only about 5% of sports injuries involve fractures. By far the greatest number of injuries—two thirds of the total—are sprains and strains. Sprains are injuries to the ligaments, which connect one bone to another. Strains are injuries to the muscles.

If players wear protective equipment, many sports injuries can be prevented. You should urge your young athlete to use protective gear and teach your child that this equipment will increase long-term enjoyment of the sport.

What if a child wants to quit a sports program?

A child has the right to share in the decision to end his or her involvement in a sport. If a child confronts you with a desire to quit a sports program, gather as many facts as you can. Talk with the child. Ask why he or she wants to quit. There may be a blunt and simple reason, such as not getting along with a coach, or the frustration of being "benched" and never playing in any games.

Observe your child. Are there any signs of stress related to sports participation, such as vomiting, loss of appetite, or headache? Does the child appear depressed—sleeping more often than usual, acting lethargic or withdrawn? These symptoms may suggest that the degree of stress is great enough to warrant withdrawing from the sport.

Base your decision on what your child says and what you observe. Remember, children also must learn not to "quit." Your child might have won a place on the team, preventing another child from playing in that sport. Simply quitting may waste an opportunity for your child and other young athletes. However, "sticking it out" is not always in the child's best interest when tough problems crop up. You may want to work with your child's pediatrician or coach to solve the problem.

How can sports-related stress be prevented?

The main source of stress in the young athlete is the pressure to win. Sadly, many coaches and parents place winning above the values of play and learning. Measure your child's performance by the yardstick of effort; a young athlete should set goals and then strive to reach them. He or she will respond better to rewards for trying hard, or for gaining skills, than to punishment and criticism for losing.

In sports, stress can be managed through a number of simple steps. Children should be placed in groups that maintain a narrow range of age levels and degrees of skill. Only players of similar height, weight, ability, and maturity should be matched as opponents in contact sports. The rules of a sport can be changed to make it fairer for all to play. For instance, a basketball net could be lowered or a race could be shortened.

Learning to cope with stress is an important part of growing up. Children can develop stress-related symptoms from other sources besides sports, including family problems, peer conflicts, school pressures, and changes in residence. The degree of stress caused by sports often is minor compared to these other sources. Actually, sports can teach the skills for coping with stress caused by any problem. This is one reason why pediatricians encourage participation in athletics.

Should bad grades keep a child from sports?

There is no simple answer to this question. A child having trouble in the classroom still needs all the benefits of exercise, competition, and a sense of accomplishment. Sports may be the only avenue of success in a child's life, and it could be harmful to take it away.

Parents should look for other causes of poor classroom performance. Conflicts with a job or other duties might be one problem; too much TV watching might be another cause. In some cases the family and school may decide that the child is not studying enough. In this situation it is reasonable to make sports involvement dependent upon achieving better grades. Ask your child what you can do to help him or her improve at school.

Your pediatrician is the right coach to have on your team when you have concerns about your child and sports. Questions about your child's health and fitness for playing a sport can best be answered by a trained doctor who specializes in children and young people. Make sure your child gets a complete physical exam before starting a sports program. Ask your pediatrician for advice. To ensure that sports are fun for your child, keep them safe.

Physical fitness is just one important part of preventive health care for children. The American Academy of Pediatrics, representing the nation's pediatricians, is dedicated to working toward a better future for our children. Join us by making sure your children receive proper health care.

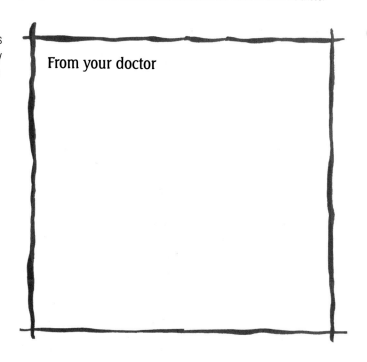

From your doctor

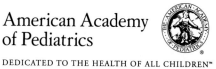

American Academy of Pediatrics

DEDICATED TO THE HEALTH OF ALL CHILDREN™

The American Academy of Pediatrics is an organization of 55,000 primary care pediatricians, pediatric medical subspecialists, and pediatric surgical specialists dedicated to the health, safety, and well-being of infants, children, adolescents, and young adults.

American Academy of Pediatrics
PO Box 747
Elk Grove Village, IL 60009-0747
Web site — http://www.aap.org

Toy Safety

Part I Guidelines for Parents

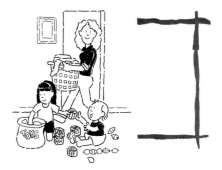

Few things make a child happier than a new toy or game. However, what seems to be harmless fun could result in a serious injury. Due to tough government regulations and efforts by US toy makers to test products, most toys on the market today are safe. Still, thousands of children suffer toy-related injuries every year. By knowing what to look for when buying toys and practicing a few simple ideas for safe use, you can often prevent problems before they occur.

How children are injured

Although most toy-related injuries are minor cuts, scrapes, and bruises, children can sometimes be seriously injured or even killed by dangerous toys or misuse of toys. Some common causes of injury are:

- **Abuse and misuse of toys.** Throwing toys, jumping on them, or taking them apart can be dangerous. When a toy breaks, sharp or pointed edges may be exposed that cause a serious injury. Something as innocent as a doll or teddy bear may quickly become a hazard when your child pulls off an eye, removes a button, or exposes a sharp edge.
- **Small, loose, or broken toys and parts.** A small toy or part can easily become lodged in a child's ear, nose, or throat. Children can be seriously injured or killed from inhaling, swallowing, or choking on objects such as marbles, small balls, toy parts, or balloons. Small toys and parts intended for older children are also involved in choking deaths among toddlers.
- **Loose string, rope, ribbons, or cord.** These items can easily become tangled around your child's neck and strangle her. Dangling objects such as crib mobiles can be deadly if your child becomes entangled in them. Loose or long pieces of clothing, such as hood cords, can also strangle your child when the cords get tangled or caught on playground equipment. Strings or cords tied to pacifiers have been involved in numerous strangulation deaths in young children as well.
- **Toy guns.** Eye injuries often result from toys that shoot plastic objects or other flying pieces. Arrows, darts, or pellets can also be choking hazards. Very loud snapping or machine-gun noises can damage hearing. "Caps" are a hazard when used indoors or closer than 12 inches from your child's ear.
- **Riding toys.** Injuries are caused not only when children fall off riding toys, but also when they ride them in the street when traffic is present or into swimming pools, ponds, and lakes.
- **Beach and pool toys** are usually not approved flotation devices. Never leave your child unattended at any time near a pool, beach, or pond. It only takes a few moments for a child to drown, even in very shallow water.
- **Electric plug-in toys.** Even if the label on a toy says it is UL-approved, burns and shocks can still result from frayed cords, misuse, or prolonged use of the toy.
- **Chemistry sets and hobby kits.** These kits can cause fires, explosions, or poisoning. They may contain chemicals that are often poisonous if swallowed, and they can catch fire or explode, causing serious burns and eye injuries.

- **Toy chests and other storage containers.** Toy chests can pinch, bruise, or break tiny fingers and hands if a lid closes suddenly. Death can even occur when a heavy lid without a safety support hinge traps and strangles a small child. Your child can also suffocate if trapped inside a toy chest. Open containers without lids are safest for toy storage.

Although children may like to play by themselves, injuries often occur when there is no proper supervision. Young children are more interested in having fun than in safety. As a result, improper play could lead to a serious toy-related injury. Proper supervision and teaching safe play are very important. Always supervise your child.

A word about...toy guns

It has been shown that toy guns can cause serious or fatal injuries to children. This is especially true for pellet and BB guns. Although these are often thought of as toys, they can be high-powered, lethal devices. Parents should also be aware that studies in recent years have raised questions about the effect playing with toy firearms has on a child's developing personality. Playing with toy weapons and firearms may cause more aggressive, violent behavior in some children. Playing with toy firearms may also make it easier for a child to mistake a real firearm for a toy.

Tips for buying toys

Use the following guidelines to choose safe and appropriate toys for your child.

1. **Read the label** before buying the toy. Warning labels provide important information about how to use a toy, what ages the toy is safe for, and whether adult supervision is recommended. Be sure to show your child how to use the toy properly.
2. **Think LARGE** when it comes to choosing toys. Make sure all toys and parts are larger than your child's mouth to prevent choking. Avoid small toys intended for older children that could fit into your child's mouth. This will decrease the risk of choking.
3. **Avoid toys that shoot small objects into the air.** They can cause serious eye injuries or choking.
4. **Avoid toys that make loud or shrill noises** to help protect your child's hearing. Ask to try the toy in the store. Check the loudness of the sound it makes. Don't buy toys that may be too loud for your child's sensitive hearing.
5. **Look for sturdy toy construction.** When buying a soft toy or stuffed animal, make sure the eyes, the nose, and any other small parts are secured tightly. Make sure it is machine washable. Check to see that seams and edges are secure. Remove loose ribbons or strings to avoid strangulation. Avoid toys containing small bean-like pellets or stuffing that can cause choking or suffocation if swallowed.

Age recommendations

Age recommendations printed on toy packages are very important. They reflect the safety of a toy based on four categories. These include:

- The safety aspects of the toy and any possible choking hazards
- The physical ability of the child to play with the toy
- The ability of a child to understand how to use a toy
- The needs and interests at various levels of a child's development

These recommendations are based on general developmental levels of each age group. However, every child is different. What is right for one child may not suit the skills and needs of another. Match the toy to your child's abilities. A toy that is too advanced or too simple for your child may be misused, which could lead to an injury.

6. **Watch out for sharp points or edges** and toys made from thin plastic or other material that may break easily. Don't buy toys with metal parts for a baby or toddler. If your older child plays with darts or arrows, make sure they have blunt tips made of soft rubber or flexible plastic. Tips should be securely fastened.

7. **Avoid toxic items and materials** that could cause poisoning. Look for paint sets, crayons, and markers that are labeled nontoxic. Small batteries are not only toxic, they also can pose a choking or swallowing hazard.

8. **Avoid hobby kits and chemistry sets** for any child younger than 12 years old. If these kits are purchased for older children (12 to 15 years of age), make sure you provide proper supervision and store them out of reach of young children.

9. **Electric toys should be "UL Approved"** Check the label to make sure the toy is approved by the Underwriters Laboratories.

10. **Be careful when buying crib toys.** Strings or wires that hang in a crib should be kept short. They may pose a serious strangulation hazard when a child begins to crawl or stand. Remove crib gyms and mobiles as soon as your child can push up on her hands and knees.

11. **Choose a toy chest carefully.** Look for smooth, finished edges that are nontoxic. If it has a lid, make sure it is sturdy, with locking supports and safe hinges. It should stay open in any position and hinges should not pinch your child's skin. The chest should also have ventilation holes to prevent suffocation if your child becomes trapped inside. The best toy chest is a box or basket without a lid.

How to prevent toy injuries

Use the following guidelines to keep your child safe:

Supervise your child's play

Injuries can happen despite your best efforts to choose the safest toy for your child. Supervision is the best way to prevent injuries.

- Keep all toys with small parts away from your young child until she learns not to put them in her mouth, usually by about the age of 5 years.
- Do not allow your child to play with a toy that was intended for an older child. Watch older children too, as they might put things in a smaller child's mouth.

- Keep uninflated and broken balloons away from children of all ages, as they are a serious choking hazard. When a child tries to inflate a balloon, he can easily inhale it. Also, never allow a child to place an inflated balloon in his mouth.
- To prevent injuries, stop reckless or improper play. Make sure your child never plays with toys near stairs, traffic, or swimming pools.

Store toys properly

- Store toys on a shelf or in a toy chest. They should be out of the way and off the floor, to avoid being stepped on or tripped over. A toy designed for an older child should be stored far out of reach of a curious toddler.
- Teaching your child to pick up and put toys away will help her learn to become responsible for her belongings.
- Never store a toy in its original packaging. Staples can cause cuts and plastic wrap can lead to choking or suffocation. To avoid injuries, immediately discard toy packaging before giving a new toy to your baby or toddler.

Keep toys in good condition

- Make sure you examine toys regularly. Look for damaged or broken parts that may pose a hazard. Look for splinters on wooden toys, loose eyes or small parts on dolls, rips or exposed wires in stuffed animals, or rust on metal toys.
- Never leave metal toys outside overnight. Rain, snow, or even dew may cause them to rust. Repair or replace any broken parts.
- If you're ever in doubt about a toy's safety, throw it away.

Playtime should be fun...and safe

Playing with toys is an important part of your child's development and growth. Choosing toys carefully will assure that playtime is educational, fun, and, most importantly, safe. By using the guidelines listed above, you can help prevent toy-related injuries. If you're not sure about a toy's safety or proper use, call the manufacturer. Your child's pediatrician can also help you decide which toys are safe and appropriate for your infant, toddler, or young child.

The information contained in this publication should not be used as a substitute for the medical care and advice of your pediatrician. There may be variations in treatment that your pediatrician may recommend based on individual facts and circumstances.

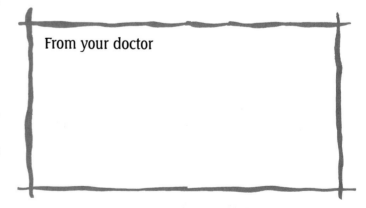

From your doctor

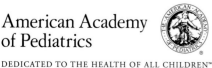

American Academy of Pediatrics

DEDICATED TO THE HEALTH OF ALL CHILDREN™

The American Academy of Pediatrics is an organization of 55,000 primary care pediatricians, pediatric medical subspecialists, and pediatric surgical specialists dedicated to the health, safety, and well-being of infants, children, adolescents, and young adults.

American Academy of Pediatrics
PO Box 747
Elk Grove Village, IL 60009-0747
Web site — http://www.aap.org

Copyright ©1994, Updated 12/98
American Academy of Pediatrics

Toy Safety

Part II Age-Appropriate Toys and Toys to Avoid

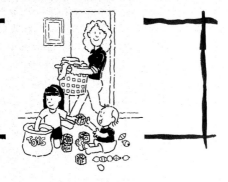

Age-appropriate toys

The following is a list of toys that the American Academy of Pediatrics recommends for specific age groups. Use these recommendations when shopping for toys. Keep in mind, these are only guidelines. All toys can be dangerous when they are not used properly or are in poor condition. Parents should continue to watch out for mislabeled toys and always provide proper supervision for young children.

Newborn to 1-year-old baby

Choose brightly-colored, lightweight toys that appeal to your baby's sight, hearing, and touch.

1. Cloth, plastic, or board books with large pictures
2. Large blocks of wood or plastic
3. Pots and pans
4. Rattles
5. Soft, washable animals, dolls, or balls
6. Bright, movable objects that are out of baby's reach
7. Busy boards
8. Floating bath toys
9. Squeeze toys

1 to 2-year-old toddler

Toys for this age group should be safe and be able to withstand a toddler's curious nature.

1. Cloth, plastic, or board books with large pictures
2. Sturdy dolls
3. Kiddy cars
4. Musical tops
5. Nesting blocks
6. Push and pull toys (remember—no long strings)
7. Stacking toys
8. Toy telephones (without cords)

2 to 5-year-old preschooler

Toys for this age group can be creative or imitate the activity of parents and older children.

1. Books (short stories or action stories)
2. Blackboard and chalk
3. Building blocks
4. Crayons, non-toxic finger paints, clay
5. Hammer and bench
6. Housekeeping toys
7. Outdoor toys: sandbox (with a lid), slide, swing, playhouse
8. Transportation toys (tricycles, cars, wagons)
9. Tape or record player

10. Simple puzzles with large pieces
11. Dress-up clothes
12. Tea party utensils

5 to 9-year-old children

Toys for this age group should help your child develop new skills and creativity.

1. Blunt scissors, sewing sets
2. Card games
3. Doctor and nurse kits
4. Hand puppets
5. Balls
6. Bicycles with helmets
7. Crafts
8. Electric trains
9. Paper dolls
10. Jump ropes
11. Roller skates with protective gear
12. Sports equipment
13. Table games

10 to 14-year-old boys and girls

Hobbies and scientific activities are ideal for this age group.

1. Computer games
2. Sewing, knitting, needlework
3. Microscopes/telescopes
4. Table and board games
5. Sports equipment
6. Hobby collections

Toys to avoid

Infants and toddlers should never be given toys with the following:

- Parts that could pull off and/or fit into a child's mouth, nose, or ear
- Exposed wires and parts that get hot
- Lead paint
- Toxic materials
- Breakable parts
- Sharp points or edges
- Glass or thin parts
- Springs, gears, or hinged parts that could pinch tiny fingers or become caught in your child's hair

To check whether a toy is unsafe or to report a toy-related injury, call the Consumer Product Safety Commission at 800/638-2772 or visit their Web site at www.cpsc.gov

The information contained in this publication should not be used as a substitute for the medical care and advice of your pediatrician. There may be variations in treatment that your pediatrician may recommend based on individual facts and circumstances.

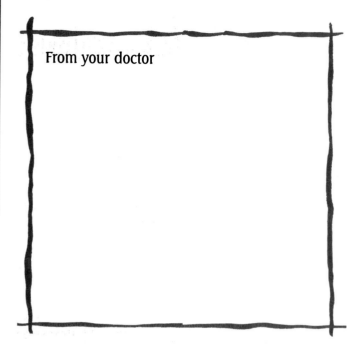

From your doctor

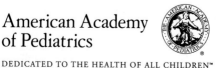

American Academy of Pediatrics

DEDICATED TO THE HEALTH OF ALL CHILDREN™

The American Academy of Pediatrics is an organization of 55,000 primary care pediatricians, pediatric medical subspecialists, and pediatric surgical specialists dedicated to the health, safety, and well-being of infants, children, adolescents, and young adults.

American Academy of Pediatrics
PO Box 747
Elk Grove Village, IL 60009-0747
Web site — http://www.aap.org

Trampolines

Trampolines often are described as fun for kids and a way to get exercise. However, an estimated 100,000 people were injured on trampolines in 1999. That is almost triple the number of people injured in 1991. Most of these injuries happened on home trampolines.

The American Academy of Pediatrics recommends that trampolines *never* be used at home, in routine gym classes, or on playgrounds.

Trampolines can be very dangerous

Almost two thirds of the people injured from trampolines are children ages 6 through 14 years. Common injuries include the following:

- Broken bones (sometimes needing surgery)
- Concussions and other head injuries
- Sprains/strains
- Bruises, scrapes, and cuts
  Neck and spinal cord injuries that can result in permanent paralysis or death also occur.

How children are hurt

Children can be hurt on trampolines in many ways. Most injuries result from the following:

- Landing wrong while jumping
- Attempting stunts
- Colliding with another person on the trampoline
- Falling or jumping off the trampoline
- Landing on the springs or frame of the trampoline
  Adult supervision will not adequately prevent injuries on home trampolines. Trampolines should be used only in supervised training programs for gymnastics, diving, or other competitive sports. A professional trained in trampoline safety should always supervise the use of trampolines.

Don't risk it! Parents should find out if their children's friends have trampolines before sending their children over to play. Children and teenagers should never use trampolines at their home or another person's home, in routine gym classes, or on the playground!

The information contained in this publication should not be used as a substitute for the medical care and advice of your pediatrician. There may be variations in treatment that your pediatrician may recommend based on individual facts and circumstances.

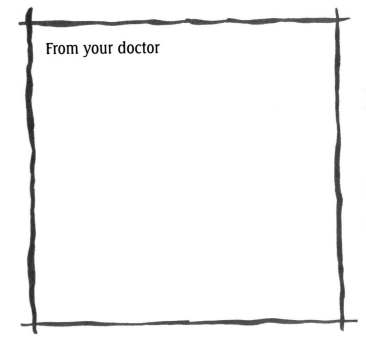

From your doctor

American Academy of Pediatrics

DEDICATED TO THE HEALTH OF ALL CHILDREN™

The American Academy of Pediatrics is an organization of 55,000 primary care pediatricians, pediatric medical subspecialists, and pediatric surgical specialists dedicated to the health, safety, and well-being of infants, children, adolescents, and young adults.

American Academy of Pediatrics
PO Box 747
Elk Grove Village, IL 60009-0747
Web site — http://www.aap.org

When Your Child Needs Emergency Medical Services

It is rare for children to become seriously ill with no warning. Based on your child's symptoms, you should usually contact your pediatrician's office for advice. Timely treatment of symptoms can prevent an illness from getting worse or turning into an emergency.

What is a true emergency?

A true emergency is when you believe a severe injury or illness is threatening your child's life or may cause permanent harm. In these cases, a child needs emergency medical treatment right away.

Discuss with your child's pediatrician in advance what you should do in case of a true emergency.

Many true emergencies involve sudden injuries. These injuries are often caused by the following:

- Bicycle or car crashes, falls, or other violent impacts
- Poisoning
- Burns or smoke inhalation
- Choking
- Near drowning
- Firearms or other weapons
- Electric shocks

Other true emergencies can result from either medical illnesses or injuries. You can often tell that these emergencies are happening if you observe your child showing any of the following:

- Acting strangely or becoming more withdrawn, less alert
- Increasing trouble with breathing
- Bleeding that does not stop
- Skin or lips that look blue or purple (or gray for darker-skinned children)
- Rhythmical jerking and loss of consciousness (a seizure)
- Unconsciousness
- Very loose or knocked-out teeth, or other major mouth or facial injuries
- Increasing or severe persistent pain
- A cut or burn that is large or deep
- Any loss of consciousness, confusion, a bad headache, or vomiting several times after a head injury
- Decreasing responsiveness when you talk to your child

Call your child's pediatrician or poison control center at once if your child has swallowed a suspected poison or another person's medication, even if your child has no signs or symptoms.

Always call for help if you are concerned that your child's life may be in danger or that your child is seriously hurt.

In case of a true emergency

- Stay calm.
- If it is needed and you know how, start rescue breathing or CPR (cardiopulmonary resuscitation).
- If you need immediate help call "911." (If you do not have "911" service in your area, call your local emergency ambulance service or county emergency medical service. Otherwise, call your pediatrician's office and state clearly that you have an emergency.
- If there is bleeding, apply continuous pressure to the site with a clean cloth.
- If your child is having a seizure, place her on a carpeted floor with her head turned to the side, and stay with your child until help arrives.

After you arrive at the emergency department, make sure you tell the emergency staff the name of your child's pediatrician. Your pediatricians can work closely with the emergency department and can provide them with additional information about your child. Bring any medication your child is taking and his immunization record with you to the hospital. Also bring any suspected poisons or other medications your child might have taken.

Important Emergency Phone Numbers

Keep the following numbers handy by taping them on or near your phone:

Your home phone and address _____

_____

Your child's pediatrician: # _____

Emergency medical services:
(ambulance/911 in most areas) # _____

Police (911 in most areas) # _____

Fire department (911 in most areas) # _____

Poison control center # _____

Hospital # _____

Dentist # _____

It is important that sitters know where to find emergency phone numbers. If you have "911" service in your area, make sure your sitter knows to dial "911" in case of an emergency. Be sure your sitter knows your home address and phone number, since an emergency operator would ask for this information. Always leave your sitter the phone number and address where you can be located.

Remember, for any emergency always call your child's pediatrician or EMS. If your child is seriously ill or injured, it may be safer for your child to be transported by emergency medical services.

The information contained in this publication should not be used as a substitute for the medical care and advice of your pediatrician. There may be variations in treatment that your pediatrician may recommend based on individual facts and circumstances.

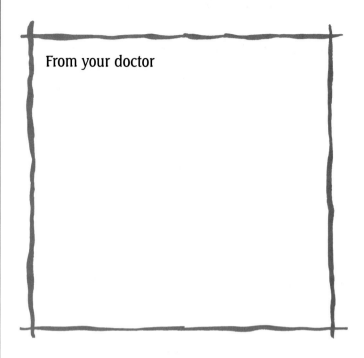

From your doctor

American Academy of Pediatrics

DEDICATED TO THE HEALTH OF ALL CHILDREN™

The American Academy of Pediatrics is an organization of 55,000 primary care pediatricians, pediatric medical subspecialists, and pediatric surgical specialists dedicated to the health, safety, and well-being of infants, children, adolescents, and young adults.

American Academy of Pediatrics
PO Box 747
Elk Grove Village, IL 60009-0747
Web site — http://www.aap.org

Your Child and the Environment

Guidelines for Parents

Part I Where Children Live

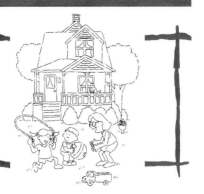

Children can be exposed to a number of environmental hazards where they live, in their food, and where they learn and play. Children are growing and, per pound of weight, drink more water, eat more food, and breathe more air than adults. Because of this, they are at higher risk for these hazards. In addition, children are more likely to put things into their mouths, and often spend more time close to the ground where many hazards are found. Environmental hazards cannot be avoided completely. However, there are many ways parents can reduce their children's exposure to them. This brochure has been developed by the American Academy of Pediatrics to help parents protect their children from environmental hazards.

Where children live

Children spend a good part of each day at home where they eat, sleep, and play. For most children, home is where they feel secure and comfortable. But there can also be things in the home that are harmful to children. Some of these things are in the air they breathe, or in the dust and dirt found in homes and yards.

Air pollution *inside* the home can be harmful to children. Indoor air pollution is caused by a buildup of gas or other chemicals inside a building. Some examples include:

- environmental tobacco smoke (ETS)
- carbon monoxide
- radon
- household products
- molds
- on-the-job hazards brought into the home
- asbestos

Environmental Tobacco Smoke (ETS)

ETS is the smoke that is breathed out by a smoker. ETS is also the smoke that comes from the tip of a lit cigarette. Exposure to ETS happens any time someone breathes in the smoke that comes from a lit cigarette, pipe or cigar. ETS contains many dangerous chemicals that have been proven to cause cancer. ETS exposure has been linked to 3,000 lung cancer deaths each year in people who don't even smoke!

What You Can Do

- If you are a smoker—quit!
- Don't let people smoke in your house or car.
- Choose a babysitter who doesn't allow smoking in the house.
- Talk to your pediatrician about ETS and ask to see the AAP brochure, *Environmental Tobacco Smoke: A Danger to Children.*

Carbon monoxide

Carbon monoxide is a toxic gas that has no taste, no color, and no odor. It is produced by appliances or heaters that burn gas, oil, wood, propane, or kerosene. Carbon monoxide can get trapped inside the home when:

- appliances do not work properly
- a stove or furnace is not working properly due to a clogged chimney or vent
- a car is left running in an attached garage
- a charcoal grill is used in a closed area

Carbon monoxide poisoning is very dangerous. This is especially true for children because they are smaller and they need more oxygen than adults. Be aware of flu-like symptoms (headache, fatigue, nausea), especially if they affect everyone in your house at the same time or go away when you leave the house. If left unchecked, exposure to carbon monoxide can lead to memory loss, personality changes, brain damage, and death.

What You Can Do

- Install carbon monoxide detectors in your home, especially near bedrooms.
- Never leave a car running in an attached garage, even if the garage door is open.
- Never use a charcoal grill inside the home or in a closed space.
- Have furnaces, wood stoves, fireplaces, hot water heaters, ovens, ranges, and clothes dryers serviced and inspected at least every year.
- Never use the oven to heat your home.

Radon

Radon is a gas that comes from the breakdown of uranium in rock and soil. Radon can also be found in water, building materials, and natural gas. Radon can seep into a home through cracks in the foundation, floors, and walls. High levels of radon have been found in homes in many parts of the United States.

Breathing in radon does not cause health problems right away. However, over long periods of time, it can increase the risk of lung cancer. Radon is believed to be the second most common cause of lung cancer (after smoking) in the United States.

What You Can Do

- Check with your health department to see if radon levels are high in your area.
- Test your home for radon. This is easy and inexpensive using radon detectors. The results of these tests can be analyzed by a certified laboratory. You cannot test yourself or your child for radon exposure.
- If radon levels in your home are too high, contact the Environmental Protection Agency and ask about their booklets on reducing radon risk or call the Radon Hotline at 800/767-7236.

Household products

Many homes contain products that can be environmental hazards like cleaning products, drain cleaner, antifreeze. These common household products give off dangerous fumes or leave residues. Many can be harmful if they are not thrown away properly (for example, if they are left in the garage).

What You Can Do

- Only use these products when necessary.
- Always use adequate ventilation.
- Store them in a safe place.
- Dispose of empty containers through your local hazardous waste disposal center.

Molds

Molds grow almost anywhere and can be found in any part of a home. Common places where molds grow include:

- damp basements
- closets
- shower stalls and bathtubs
- refrigerators
- air conditioners and humidifiers
- garbage pails
- mattresses
- carpeting (especially if it got wet)

Molds can cause health problems in children. Children who live in moldy places are more likely to develop allergies, asthma, and other health problems.

What You Can Do

- Keep the surfaces in your home dry.
- Wet items (such as carpeting that cannot be dried) should be thrown away.
- Keep air conditioners and humidifiers clean and in good working order.
- Use exhaust fans in the kitchen and the bathroom to help keep the air dry.
- Avoid using items that are likely to get moldy like foam rubber pillows and mattresses.

On the job hazards brought into the home

Sometimes a parent's job can create environmental hazards to children. This can happen when lead, chemicals, and fumes from the workplace are brought into the home on skin, hair, clothes, or shoes. People who work in the following areas are most at risk for bringing chemicals into the home:

- painting and construction sites
- auto body or repair shops
- auto battery and radiator factories
- shipyards
- area in which the person comes into contact with harmful metals or chemicals

What You Can Do

- Find out if you are exposed to lead, asbestos, mercury, or chemicals on your job.
- If so, shower and change out of work clothes and shoes before coming home.
- Wash the work clothes separately from other laundry.

Asbestos

Asbestos is a natural fiber that was commonly used in schools and homes for fireproofing, insulation, and soundproofing between the 1940s and 1970s. Asbestos is not dangerous unless it becomes crumbly. If that happens, asbestos fibers can be released into the air and breathed into the lungs. Breathing in asbestos fibers can cause chronic health problems, including a rare form of lung cancer. Schools are required by law to either remove asbestos or make sure that children are not exposed. Asbestos can still be found in certain older homes, particularly as insulation around pipes.

What You Can Do

- Do not allow children to play around exposed or deteriorating materials that may contain asbestos.
- If you think there is asbestos in your home, have a professional inspect it.
- If your home has asbestos in poor condition, use a **certified contractor** to help solve the problem. You could have more problems if the asbestos is not removed safely.

The information contained in this publication should not be used as a substitute for the medical care and advice of your pediatrician. There may be variations in treatment that your pediatrician may recommend based on individual facts and circumstances.

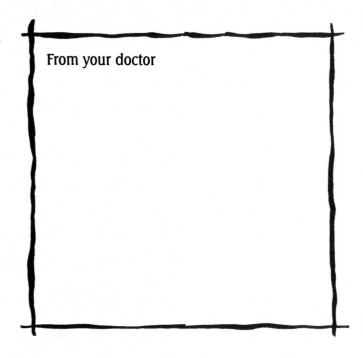

From your doctor

American Academy of Pediatrics

DEDICATED TO THE HEALTH OF ALL CHILDREN™

The American Academy of Pediatrics is an organization of 55,000 primary care pediatricians, pediatric medical subspecialists, and pediatric surgical specialists dedicated to the health, safety, and well-being of infants, children, adolescents, and young adults.

American Academy of Pediatrics
PO Box 747
Elk Grove Village, IL 60009-0747
Web site — http://www.aap.org

Copyright ©1996   American Academy of Pediatrics

Your Child and the Environment

Guidelines for Parents   Part II What Children Eat and Drink

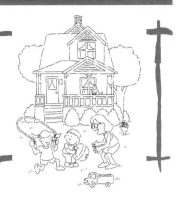

What children eat and drink

Lead

Of all the problems caused by our environment, lead poisoning is one of the most serious. Infants and toddlers can get sick by putting their fingers in their mouths after touching lead dust, eating lead paint chips, or breathing in lead dust. Lead poisoning can cause learning disabilities, behavioral problems, anemia, or damage to the brain and kidneys.

Where can lead be found?

Lead is most often found in:

- paint that is on the inside and outside of homes built before 1978
- dust and paint chips from old paint
- soil that has lead in it
- hobby materials such as paints, solders, fishing weights, and buckshot
- food stored in certain ceramic dishes (especially if dishes were made in another country)
- older painted toys and furniture such as cribs
- tap water, especially in homes that have lead pipes
- mini-blinds manufactured outside the United States before July 1996

Children who have elevated lead levels may not look or act sick. The only way to know if your child has been exposed to lead is to have your pediatrician test your child's blood.

What You Can Do

- If your home was built before 1978, consider testing the paint for lead before beginning any work.
- If lead paint is found, learn about safe ways to handle it before any work is done.
- Clean and cover any peeling, flaking, or chipping paint with a new coat of paint, duct tape, or contact paper. It is important to check for flaking paint at window areas where children often play.
- Repair areas where paint is chipped or peeling before placing cribs, playpens, beds, or highchairs next to them.
- Check with your health department to see if lead in water is a problem in your area.
- Do not use hot tap water for mixing formula, drinking, or cooking.
- Ask your pediatrician about testing your child for lead. A blood test is the only accurate way to test for lead.
- Encourage your children to wash their hands frequently, especially before eating.
- Give your child a healthy diet that includes food high in iron and calcium.
- Before moving into a home or apartment, check with your landlord or realtor for possible lead contamination.

Pesticides

Children can be exposed to pesticides in the food they eat and the water they drink. They are used by farmers as well as in home lawn and garden care. Although they are designed to kill insects, weeds, and fungi, many pesticides are toxic to the environment and to people, especially children. Too much exposure to pesticides can cause a wide range of health problems.

What You Can Do

- Keep all pesticides out of children's reach to avoid accidental poisoning.
- Wash all fruits and vegetables with water.
- Use in-season produce as they are less likely to be heavily sprayed.
- If possible, eat foods that are grown without the use of chemical pesticides.
- Use non-chemical pest control methods in your home and garden.
- Notify neighbors before any outdoor spraying.

Drinking water

Children drink 5 to 10 times more water for their size than adults. Most of this water is tap water. The quality of tap water in most areas is protected by law. Small water supplies such as those from private wells in small trailer parks or seasonal holiday communities are not.

Many people use bottled water because they think it is better than tap water. Some brands of bottled water are better than tap water. However, other brands of bottled water may only be tap water that is bottled and sold separately. Bottled water is much more expensive than tap water, but may be necessary in some areas.

A number of possible contaminants in drinking water can make children sick. These include:

- germs
- nitrates
- heavy metals
- man-made chemicals
- radioactive particles
- by-products of the disinfecting process

Some of these contaminants are more likely to be found in surface water (water from lakes and rivers). Others are more likely to be found in ground water (water from wells and underground sources). Where you live and where your drinking water comes from have a lot to do with the kind of contaminants you need to be concerned about in your water.

The quality of water in the United States is among the best in the world, but problems do still occur. County health departments and state environmental agencies are the best sources of information about water quality in your community.

What You Can Do

- Find out the source of your water.
  - If you are on a municipal water supply, the water company is required to tell you what is in the water.
  - If your water is not regulated, have it tested yearly. Many states have laws that protect renters from water supplies that are not in good working order.
  - If you have a well, make sure your water is tested yearly and that your pump is in good working order.
- Always drink and cook with **cold** water. Contaminants can build up in hot water heaters.
- If you are not sure of your plumbing, run the water for 2 minutes each morning before using water for drinking or cooking. This flushes the pipes and reduces the chances of a contaminant getting into your water.
- If you have well water and a baby under 1 year of age, have your water tested for nitrates **before** giving it to your baby. Breastfeeding, using ready-to-feed formulas, or using bottled water is wise until you know if your water is safe. If you have questions, call your health department.

If you think your water may be contaminated with germs, you can kill most of them by boiling the water and letting it cool before use. Do not boil water for longer than 1 minute. This can cause a buildup of chemicals that may be in the water.

To learn more

Environmental Protection Agency Public Information Center
Room 311 West Towers, Mail Code 3406
401 M Street, SW
Washington, DC 20460
202/260-7751

Food and Drug Administration Consumer Affairs
Room 16-75, Mail Code HFE88
5600 Fishers Lane
Rockville, MD 20857
800/532-4440

National Coalition Against the Misuse of Pesticides
701 E Street, SE
Washington, DC 20003
202/543-5450

American Lung Association
1740 Broadway
New York, NY 10019-4374
800/LUNG-USA

Agency for Toxic Substances and Disease Registry
Public Information Office
1600 Clifton Road, NE
Atlanta, GA 30333
404/639-0501

Pesticide Hotline
800/858-7378

EMF Hotline
800/363-2383

Safe Drinking Water Hotline
800/426-4791

Lead Hotline
800/LEAD-FYI

The information contained in this publication should not be used as a substitute for the medical care and advice of your pediatrician. There may be variations in treatment that your pediatrician may recommend based on individual facts and circumstances.

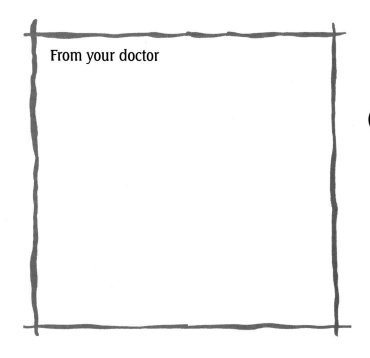

From your doctor

American Academy of Pediatrics

DEDICATED TO THE HEALTH OF ALL CHILDREN™

The American Academy of Pediatrics is an organization of 55,000 primary care pediatricians, pediatric medical subspecialists, and pediatric surgical specialists dedicated to the health, safety, and well-being of infants, children, adolescents, and young adults.

American Academy of Pediatrics
PO Box 747
Elk Grove Village, IL 60009-0747
Web site — http://www.aap.org

Your Child and the Environment

Guidelines for Parents
Part III Where Children Learn and Play

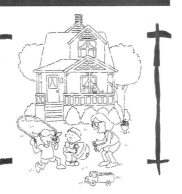

Where children learn and play

Sun

Warm, sunny days are wonderful. But what may seem harmless can be very bad for you and your child. The sun is the main cause of skin cancer, the most common form of cancer in the United States. A child's skin is very delicate and can burn easily. Sunburns can be very painful and can cause a child to become sick. The sun's rays can also cause damage to the eyes.

What You Can Do
- Keep babies under 6 months of age out of direct sunlight.
- Choose a sunscreen made for children with a sun protection factor (SPF) of at least 15.
- Use hats and sunglasses to protect your child's head and eyes from the sun.
- Encourage the use of shaded areas for your child's outdoor activities between 10 am and 4 pm when the sun's rays are strongest.
- Dress your child in lightweight clothing that covers as much of the body as possible and practical.

Outdoor air pollution

There are a number of things in the air that can be harmful to children. One serious type of air pollution is ozone. Ozone is a colorless gas that is harmful when near the ground. Ozone levels are highest in summer, in the late afternoon. It may be particularly hazardous to children because they spend so much time running and playing outdoors. Ozone pollution can cause breathing problems in children with asthma.

What You Can Do
- Restrict your child's outdoor activities when health advisories or smog alerts have been issued.
- Whenever possible, take public transportation, carpool, walk, or ride a bike instead of driving. This will help reduce the amount of air pollution caused by cars.

Insect repellent

Outdoor activities are a great way for children to have fun and exercise. But these types of activities often include insects. Be careful about the insect repellents you use on your child. Most insect repellents include a chemical called DEET (diethyltoluamide). This chemical is absorbed into the skin and can be harmful to children.

What You Can Do
- Choose an insect repellent that is made for children.
- Be sure any insect repellent used on your child contains a low level DEET (no more than 10%).
- Apply insect repellent to clothing when possible, rather than directly on the skin.

Lawn and garden fertilizers

Some common lawn and garden fertilizers can be harmful if children come in contact with them while playing in the yard. Many of these products are made with chemicals (pesticides) that are known to cause health problems, especially in children.

What You Can Do
- Use these chemicals only when needed.
- Read and follow the instructions carefully.
- Do not let your child play on a treated lawn until it has been watered twice and the odor of the pesticides has gone away.

Art supplies

Arts and crafts projects are a fun way for children to learn. However, some art supplies can cause heath problems in children who use them. While older children can usually use these products safely, most younger children and some children with disabilities cannot. Harmful art supplies can include:
- rubber cement
- permanent felt-tip markers
- pottery glazes
- enamels
- spray fixatives
- prepackaged papier mâché

What You Can Do
- Use only "nontoxic" art supplies.
- Read and follow all instructions carefully.
- Always use products in a well-ventilated room.
- Look for the ACMI "nontoxic" seal or other information on the label that says the product is safe for children.
- Talk to your school to make sure only safe art supplies are being used.

Whether it is inside or outside, children love to explore their environment. This natural curiosity is an important way for children to learn. Be aware of the possible hazards that your child may face. Keep in mind that not all environmental hazards can be avoided completely and do what you can to reduce your child's exposure.

Electric and magnetic fields—another environmental hazard?

All electric appliances like microwave ovens, computers, and TV's produce electric and magnetic fields (EMF's) when they are used. There is some concern that exposure to these fields may cause health problems, including cancer. However, research is still being done and a definite link between cancer and EMF's has not been made. Until more is known about EMF's, you can reduce your child's exposure by:

- keeping your child away from microwaves while they are in use
- having your child sit at least 3 feet from the TV screen
- moving electrical clocks, radios, and baby monitors away from your child's bed
- not using electric bedding (blankets, mattress pads, heating pads, and waterbed heaters)

To learn more

Environmental Protection Agency Public Information Center
Room 311 West Towers, Mail Code 3406
401 M Street, SW
Washington, DC 20460
202/260-7751

Food and Drug Administration Consumer Affairs
Room 16-75, Mail Code HFE88
5600 Fishers Lane
Rockville, MD 20857
800/532-4440

National Coalition Against the Misuse of Pesticides
701 E Street, SE
Washington, DC 20003
202/543-5450

American Lung Association
1740 Broadway
New York, NY 10019-4374
800/LUNG-USA

Agency for Toxic Substances and Disease Registry
Public Information Office
1600 Clifton Road, NE
Atlanta, GA 30333
404/639-0501

Pesticide Hotline
800/858-7378

EMF Hotline
800/363-2383

Safe Drinking Water Hotline
800/426-4791

Lead Hotline
800/LEAD-FYI

The information contained in this publication should not be used as a substitute for the medical care and advice of your pediatrician. There may be variations in treatment that your pediatrician may recommend based on individual facts and circumstances.

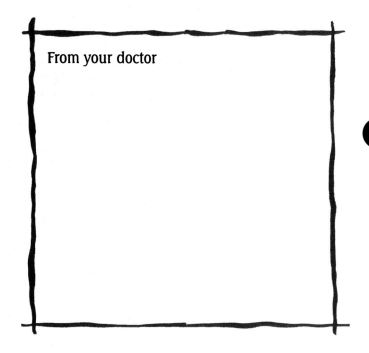

From your doctor

American Academy of Pediatrics

DEDICATED TO THE HEALTH OF ALL CHILDREN™

The American Academy of Pediatrics is an organization of 55,000 primary care pediatricians, pediatric medical subspecialists, and pediatric surgical specialists dedicated to the health, safety, and well-being of infants, children, adolescents, and young adults.

American Academy of Pediatrics
PO Box 747
Elk Grove Village, IL 60009-0747
Web site — http://www.aap.org

SECTION EIGHT

TIPP® Bicycle Safety

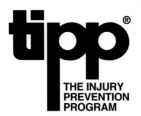

About Bicycle Helmets

tipp®
THE INJURY PREVENTION PROGRAM

About Bicycle Helmets

How can I tell if a helmet will keep my child safe?

You should only buy a helmet that meets the bicycle helmet safety standards of the Consumer Product Safety Commission (CPSC). Any helmet meeting these standards is labeled. Check the inside.

Do all helmets meet these standards?

All helmets manufactured or imported for use after March 1999 must comply with a mandatory safety standard issued by the CPSC. Older helmets certified by the American Society for Testing and Materials (ASTM) or Snell Memorial Foundation may continue to be used.

Can other kinds of helmets be used for bicycling?

Each type of helmet is designed for protection in specific conditions and may not offer enough protection in bike accidents or falls. Bike helmets are very protective in head-first falls at fairly high speeds, and are light and well ventilated for comfort and acceptability. A multisport helmet, certified to meet the CPSC standard for bicycle helmets, also is acceptable.

Where can I get a helmet?

Helmets meeting CPSC safety standards are available at bicycle shops and at some discount, department, and toy stores in adult, toddler, and children's sizes and styles. Do not resell, donate, or buy a used bike helmet because it may be too old to provide protection or may have been in a crash.

What are the various merits of the 2 types of helmets, hard shell and soft shell?

The essential part of the helmet for impact protection is a thick layer of firm polystyrene, plastic foam, that crushes on impact, absorbing the force of the blow. All helmets require a chin strap to keep them in place in a crash.

Hard-shell helmets also have a hard outer shell of plastic or fiberglass that provides a shield against penetration by sharp objects and holds the polystyrene together if it cracks in a fall or crash. These helmets are more sturdy, but tend to be heavier and warmer than the soft-shell models.

Soft-shell helmets have no hard outer shell but are made of an extra-thick layer of polystyrene covered with a cloth cover or surface coating. The cloth cover is an essential part of many soft-shell helmets. If the helmet comes with a cover, the cover must always be worn to hold the helmet together if the polystyrene cracks on impact. Both types meet CPSC standards; the main difference is style and comfort.

Although there is no consensus on the relative safety of the 2 types, models of both types have passed the CPSC test. The soft-shell helmets are lighter than the hard-shell versions but may be less durable.

(over)

American Academy of Pediatrics
DEDICATED TO THE HEALTH OF ALL CHILDREN™

SUPPORTED BY A GRANT FROM PFIZER CONSUMER HEALTHCARE, MAKERS OF **NEOSPORIN**®

How should a helmet fit?

A helmet should be worn squarely on top of the head, covering the top of the forehead. If it is tipped back, it will not protect the forehead. The helmet fits well if it doesn't move around on the head or slide down over the wearer's eyes when pushed or pulled. The chin strap should be adjusted to fit snugly.

Are there helmets for infants?

Yes. Many infant-sized helmets are of the soft-shell variety. They are light, an important consideration for small children whose necks may not be strong enough to comfortably hold a hard-shell helmet. Babies younger than 1 year have relatively weak neck structure. Neither helmets nor bike traveling is recommended for them.

How long will a child's helmet fit?

An infant's or child's helmet should fit for several years. Most models have removable fitting pads that can be replaced with thinner ones as the child's head grows.

Can a helmet be reused after an accident?

In general, a helmet that has been through a serious fall or accident should be retired with gratitude. It has served its purpose and may not provide adequate protection in another crash. If you are uncertain whether the helmet is still usable, throw it away.

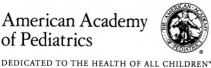

American Academy
of Pediatrics

DEDICATED TO THE HEALTH OF ALL CHILDREN™

The American Academy of Pediatrics is an organization of 55,000 primary care pediatricians, pediatric medical subspecialists, and pediatric surgical specialists dedicated to the health, safety, and well-being of infants, children, adolescents, and young adults.

American Academy of Pediatrics
PO Box 747
Elk Grove Village, IL 60009-0747
Web site — http://www.aap.org

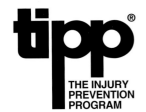

**THE INJURY
PREVENTION
PROGRAM**

Bicycle Safety: Myths and Facts

Learning to ride a bike is a developmental milestone in the life of a child. The bicycle, a child's first vehicle, is a source of pride and a symbol of independence and freedom. Yet all too often children are seriously injured, or even killed, when they fail to follow basic bicycle safety rules. The following is a list of common bicycle safety myths, coupled with the correct information you need to teach your children about safe bike riding. These facts will help you and your children make every bike ride safe.

Myth: My child doesn't need to wear a helmet on short rides around the neighborhood.

Fact: Your child needs to wear a helmet on every bike ride, no matter how short or how close to home. Many accidents happen in driveways, on sidewalks, and on bike paths, not just on streets. In fact, most bike crashes happen near home. A helmet protects your child from serious injury, and should always be worn. And remember, wearing a helmet at all times helps children develop the helmet habit.

Myth: A football helmet will work just as well as a bicycle helmet.

Fact: Only a bicycle helmet is made specifically to protect the head from any fall that may occur while biking. Other helmets or hard hats are made to protect the head from other types of injury. Never allow your child to wear another type of helmet when riding a bike, unless it is a multisport helmet certified for bicycle use by the Consumer Product Safety Commission (CPSC).

Myth: I need to buy a bicycle for my child to grow into.

Fact: Oversized bikes are especially dangerous. Your child does not have the skills and coordination needed to handle a bigger bike and may lose control. Your child should be able to sit on the seat, with hands on the handlebars, and place the balls of both feet on the ground. Your child's first bike should also be equipped with footbrakes because your child's hand muscles and coordination are not mature enough to control hand brakes.

Myth: It's safer for my child to ride facing traffic.

Fact: Your child should always ride on the right, with traffic. Riding against traffic confuses or surprises drivers. Almost one fourth of bicycle-car collisions result from bicyclists riding against traffic.

Myth: Children shouldn't use hand signals, because signaling may cause them to lose control of their bikes.

Fact: Hand signals are an important part of the "Rules of the Road" and should be taught to all children before they begin to ride in the street. They are an important communication link between cyclists and motorists. Any child who does not have the skills necessary to use hand signals without falling or swerving shouldn't be riding in the street. Many crashes involving older children occur when they fail to signal motorists as to their intended actions.

(over)

American Academy of Pediatrics

DEDICATED TO THE HEALTH OF ALL CHILDREN™

SUPPORTED BY A GRANT FROM PFIZER CONSUMER HEALTHCARE, MAKERS OF **NEOSPORIN**®

Myth: Bike reflectors and a reflective vest will make it safe for my child to ride at night.

Fact: It's never safe for your child to ride a bike at night. Night riding requires special skills and special equipment. Few youngsters are equipped with either. Never allow your child to ride at dusk or after dark.

Myth: I don't need to teach my child all of this bicycle safety stuff. I was never injured as a child. Biking is just meant to be fun.

Fact: Riding a bike is fun — if it's done safely. Unfortunately, most people don't realize hundreds of thousands of children are seriously injured each year in bicycle falls. Worse still, hundreds of children die from them each year. Although you may have been lucky enough to survive childhood without a serious bicycle-related injury, you shouldn't count on luck to protect your child.

Teach your child these basic safety rules

1. Wear a helmet.
2. Ride on the right side, with traffic.
3. Use appropriate hand signals.
4. Respect traffic signals.

Basic safety measures like these can keep bicycle riding enjoyable and safe for your child.

American Academy of Pediatrics

DEDICATED TO THE HEALTH OF ALL CHILDREN™

The American Academy of Pediatrics is an organization of 55,000 primary care pediatricians, pediatric medical subspecialists, and pediatric surgical specialists dedicated to the health, safety, and well-being of infants, children, adolescents, and young adults.

American Academy of Pediatrics
PO Box 747
Elk Grove Village, IL 60009-0747
Web site — http://www.aap.org

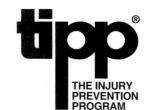

**THE INJURY
PREVENTION
PROGRAM**

The Child as Passenger on an Adult's Bicycle

A young passenger on an adult's bike makes the bike unstable and increases the braking time. A mishap at any speed easily attained during casual riding, could cause significant injury to the child. Following these guidelines decreases, but does not eliminate, the risk of injury.

Preferably, children should ride in a bicycle-towed child trailer.

1. Only adult cyclists should carry young passengers.

2. Preferably ride with passengers in parks, on bike paths, or on quiet streets. Avoid busy thoroughfares and bad weather, and ride with maximum caution and at a reduced speed.

3. Infants younger than 12 months are too young to sit in a rear bike seat and should not be carried on a bicycle. Do not carry infants in backpacks or frontpacks on a bike.

4. Children who are old enough (12 months to 4 years) to sit well unsupported and whose necks are strong enough to support a lightweight helmet may be carried in a child-trailer or rear-mounted seat.

5. A rear-mounted seat must

    a. Be securely attached over the rear wheel

    b. Have spoke guards to prevent feet and hands from being caught in the wheels

    c. Have a high back and a sturdy shoulder harness and lap belt that will support a sleeping child

6. A lightweight infant bike helmet should always be worn by a young passenger to prevent or minimize head injury. Small styrofoam helmets that meet Consumer Product Safety Commission (CPSC) standards are available.

7. The child must be strapped into the bike seat with a sturdy harness.

8. Remember, the risk of serious injury still exists when you carry a young child on your bicycle.

(over)

American Academy of Pediatrics

DEDICATED TO THE HEALTH OF ALL CHILDREN™

SUPPORTED BY A GRANT FROM PFIZER CONSUMER HEALTHCARE, MAKERS OF **NEOSPORIN®**

The Child as Passenger on an Adult's Bicycle

Dear Parent:

Your child is old enough to learn how to prevent injuries. The picture below is designed to help him or her think about safety. Read the message with your child and talk about it. Then take this safety sheet home and post it where everyone can see it.

It takes time to form a safety habit. Remind each other about these safety messages. Make safety a big part of your lives.

Get Ahead on Bike Safety...Wear a Helmet!

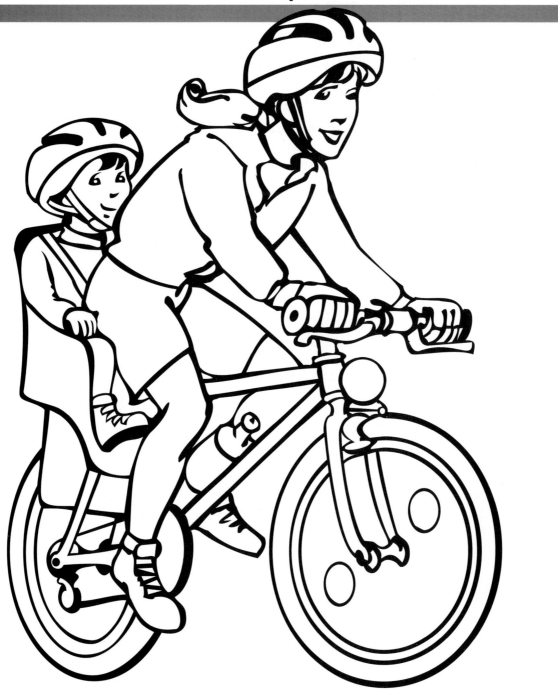

The information in this publication should not be used as a substitute for the medical care and advice of your pediatrician. There may be variations in treatment that your pediatrician may recommend based on the individual facts and circumstances.

HE0082
© 1994 American Academy of Pediatrics

American Academy of Pediatrics

DEDICATED TO THE HEALTH OF ALL CHILDREN™

The American Academy of Pediatrics is an organization of 55,000 primary care pediatricians, pediatric medical subspecialists, and pediatric surgical specialists dedicated to the health, safety, and well-being of infants, children, adolescents, and young adults.

American Academy of Pediatrics
PO Box 747
Elk Grove Village, IL 60009-0747
Web site — http://www.aap.org

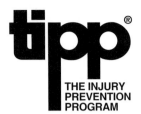

**THE INJURY
PREVENTION
PROGRAM**

Choosing the Right Size Bicycle for Your Child

A bicycle of the wrong size may cause your child to lose control and be injured. **Any bike must be the correct size for the child for whom it is bought.** To keep your child safe, the American Academy of Pediatrics recommends the following:

1. Do not push your child to ride a 2-wheeled bike until he or she is ready, at about age 5 or 6. Consider the child's coordination and desire to learn to ride. Stick with coaster brakes until your child is older and more experienced.

2. Take your child with you when you shop for the bike, so that he or she can try it out. The value of a properly fitting bike far outweighs the value of surprising your child with a new bike.

3. Buy a bike that is the right size, not one your child has to "grow into." Oversized bikes are especially dangerous.

4. How to test any style of bike for proper fit

   a. Sitting on the seat with hands on the handlebar, your child must be able to place the balls of both feet on the ground.

   b. Straddling the center bar, your child should be able to stand with both feet flat on the ground with about a 1-inch clearance between the crotch and the bar.

   c. When buying a bike with hand brakes for an older child, make sure that the child can comfortably grasp the brakes and apply sufficient pressure to stop the bike.

5. A helmet should be standard equipment. Whenever buying a bike, be sure you have a Consumer Product Safety Commission (CPSC)-approved helmet for your child.

(over)

American Academy of Pediatrics

DEDICATED TO THE HEALTH OF ALL CHILDREN™

SUPPORTED BY A GRANT FROM PFIZER CONSUMER HEALTHCARE, MAKERS OF **NEOSPORIN**®

Dear Parent:

Your child is old enough to start learning how to prevent accidents. The games below are designed to help him or her think about safety. Read the messages with your child and talk about them. Then take this safety sheet home and post it where all can see it.

It takes time to form a safety habit. Remind each other about these safety messages. Make safety a big part of your lives.

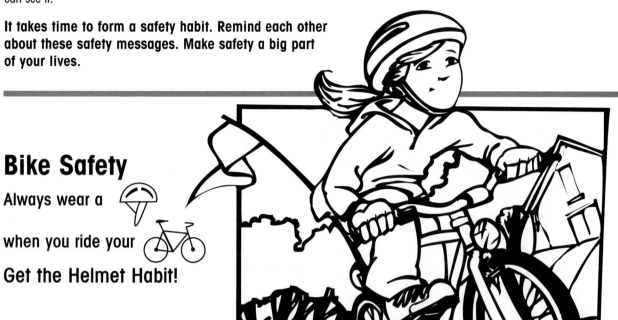

Bike Safety

Always wear a

when you ride your

Get the Helmet Habit!

Directions: Color Mary's helmet. Draw a smile on Mary's face because she is being safe.

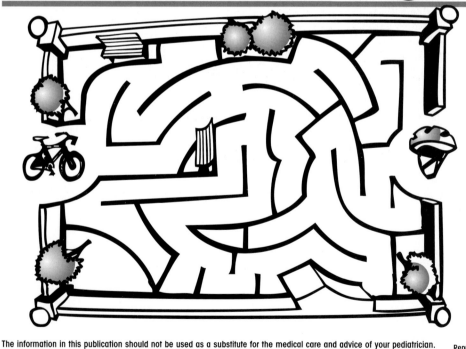

Bike Safety

Always wear a

when you ride your

Get the Helmet Habit!

Directions: Find your way through this maze. Connect the helmet with the bicycle.

The information in this publication should not be used as a substitute for the medical care and advice of your pediatrician. There may be variations in treatment that your pediatrician may recommend based on the individual facts and circumstances.

HE0080
Reproduced from TIPP 5 - and 6 - year Safety Sheets
© 1994 American Academy of Pediatrics

American Academy of Pediatrics

DEDICATED TO THE HEALTH OF ALL CHILDREN™

The American Academy of Pediatrics is an organization of 55,000 primary care pediatricians, pediatric medical subspecialists, and pediatric surgical specialists dedicated to the health, safety, and well-being of infants, children, adolescents, and young adults.

American Academy of Pediatrics
PO Box 747
Elk Grove Village, IL 60009-0747
Web site — http://www.aap.org

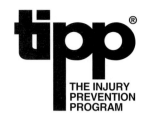

THE INJURY PREVENTION PROGRAM

Safe Bicycling Starts Early

When a child receives his or her first tricycle or bicycle, a lifelong pattern of vehicle operation is begun. A bike is not just a toy, but a vehicle that is a speedy means of transportation, subject to the same laws as motor vehicles.

Training Children in Proper Use of Their Bicycles

1. Parents should set limits on where children may ride, depending on their age and maturity. Most serious injuries occur when the bicyclist is hit by a motor vehicle.

   a. Young children should ride only with adult supervision and off the street.

   b. The decision to allow older children to ride in the street should depend on traffic patterns, individual maturity, and an adequate knowledge and ability to follow the "Rules of the Road."

2. Children must be provided with helmets (approved by the Consumer Product Safety Commission [CPSC]) and taught to wear them properly on every ride, starting when they get their first bike or tricycle.

3. The most important "Rules of the Road" for them to learn are

   a. Ride with traffic.
   b. Stop and look both ways before entering the street.
   c. Stop at all intersections, marked and unmarked.
   d. Before turning, use hand signals and look all ways.

4. Children should never ride at dusk or in the dark. This is extremely risky for children and adults. Your child should be told to call home for a ride rather than ride a bike.

5. Children should receive training in bicycle riding, including "Rules of the Road", and should have their privilege with the bike withheld if they ignore safety rules or don't wear a helmet.

6. Children should learn how to keep their bikes in good repair, with parents checking the tires, brakes, and seat and handlebar height annually.

(over)

American Academy of Pediatrics

DEDICATED TO THE HEALTH OF ALL CHILDREN™

SUPPORTED BY A GRANT FROM PFIZER CONSUMER HEALTHCARE, MAKERS OF **NEOSPORIN®**

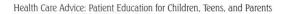

Dear Parent:

Your child is old enough to start learning how to prevent injuries. The games below are designed to help him or her think about safety. Read the messages with your child and talk about them. Then take this safety sheet home and post it where everyone can see it.

It takes time to form a safety habit. Remind each other about these safety messages. Make safety a big part of your lives.

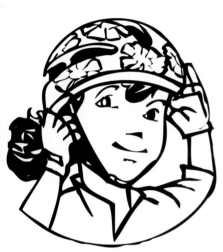

Bike Safety
Always wear a

when you ride your

Get the Helmet Habit!

```
E  H  T  E  M  L  E  H
H  E  L  E  M  H  E  T
E  L  E  H  M  E  T  M
T  M  M  T  H  L  E  L
E  E  H  E  L  M  E  T
M  T  E  M  L  E  H  H
L  H  E  L  M  T  T  E
E  M  H  E  L  M  E  T
H  E  L  H  H  E  T  M
```

Directions: Can you find the word "HELMET" in 9 different places (any direction)?

"Rules of the Road"
teaches you to ride your bike safely.

Directions: Here are seven important "Rules of the Road." Draw a line from the first part of the rule to the correct ending to complete the sentence. The first one is done for you.

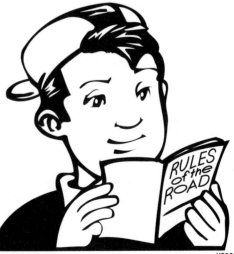

1. When turning or stopping,

2. LOOK both ways,

3. Always ride

4. Always stop at

5. When you ride on the sidewalk

6. Smart riders always

at street corners and driveways.

STOP signs and the curb.

wear their helmet.

watch out for people.

always use hand signals.

with the traffic, to the right.

The information in this publication should not be used as a substitute for the medical care and advice of your pediatrician. There may be variations in treatment that your pediatrician may recommend based on the individual facts and circumstances.

HE0081
Reproduced from TIPP 8 - years Safety Sheet
© 1994 American Academy of Pediatrics

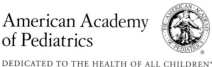

American Academy of Pediatrics

DEDICATED TO THE HEALTH OF ALL CHILDREN™

The American Academy of Pediatrics is an organization of 55,000 primary care pediatricians, pediatric medical subspecialists, and pediatric surgical specialists dedicated to the health, safety, and well-being of infants, children, adolescents, and young adults.

American Academy of Pediatrics
PO Box 747
Elk Grove Village, IL 60009-0747
Web site — http://www.aap.org

Tips for Getting Your Children to Wear Bicycle Helmets

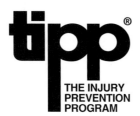

tipp® THE INJURY PREVENTION PROGRAM

Tips for Getting Your Children to Wear Bicycle Helmets

Establish the helmet habit early.

Have your children wear helmets as soon as they start to ride tricycles and if they are a passenger on the back of an adult's bike. If they learn to wear helmets whenever they ride tricycles and bikes, it becomes a habit for a lifetime. It's never too late, however, to get your children into helmets. Allow your child to participate in choosing their helmet. They'll be able to let you know if it is comfortable. And if they like the design, they are more likely to wear it.

Wear a helmet yourself.

Children learn best by observing you. Whenever you ride your bike, put on your helmet. Plan bicycle outings during which all family members wear their helmets to further reinforce the message. The most important factor influencing children to wear helmets is riding with an adult who wears a helmet.

Talk to your children about why you want them to protect their heads.

There are many things you can tell your children to convince them of the importance of helmet use.

1. Bikes are vehicles, not toys.
2. You love and value them and their intelligence, and need to protect them.
3. They can permanently hurt their brains or even die of head injuries.

Most professional athletes use helmets when participating in sports. Bicycle racers are now required to use them when racing in the United States and in the Olympics.

Reward your kids for wearing helmets.

Praise them; give them special treats or privileges when they wear their helmets without having to be told to.

Don't let children ride their bikes unless they wear their helmets.

Be consistent. If you allow your children to ride occasionally without their helmets, they won't believe that helmet use really is important. Tell your children they have to find another way to get where they are going if they don't want to use their helmets.

Encourage your children's friends to wear helmets.

Peer pressure can be used in a positive way if several families in the neighborhood start making helmet use a regular habit at the same time.

How should a helmet fit?

A helmet should be worn squarely on top of the head, covering the top of the forehead. If it is tipped back, it will not protect the forehead. The helmet fits well if it doesn't move around on the head or slide down over the wearer's eyes when pushed or pulled. The chin strap should be adjusted to fit snugly.

(over)

American Academy of Pediatrics

DEDICATED TO THE HEALTH OF ALL CHILDREN™

SUPPORTED BY A GRANT FROM PFIZER CONSUMER HEALTHCARE, MAKERS OF **NEOSPORIN**®

REMEMBER:
Head injuries can occur on sidewalks, on driveways, on bike paths, and in parks as well as on streets. You cannot predict when a fall from a bike will occur. It's important to wear a helmet on every ride.

Dear Parent:
Your child is old enough to start learning how to prevent injuries. The games below are designed to help him or her think about safety. Read the messages with your child and talk about them. Then take this safety sheet home and post it where everyone can see it.

It takes time to form a safety habit. Remind each other about these safety messages. Make safety a big part of your lives.

DIRECTIONS: Circle the signs that belong to "Rules of the Road."
Be a smart and safe rider. Learn the "Rules of the Road."

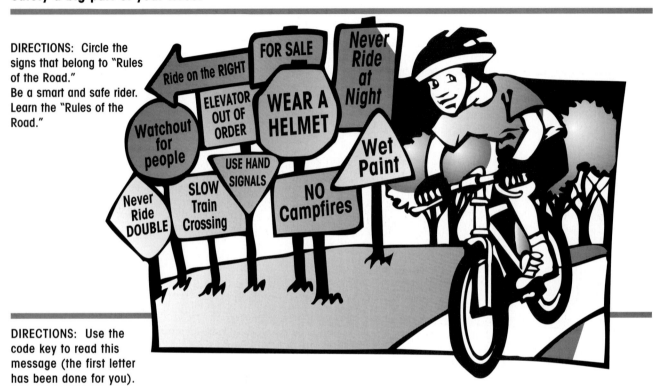

DIRECTIONS: Use the code key to read this message (the first letter has been done for you).

CODE KEY

NEVER RIDE AT NIGHT
Always put your bike away when the sun goes down.

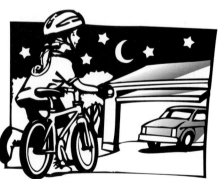

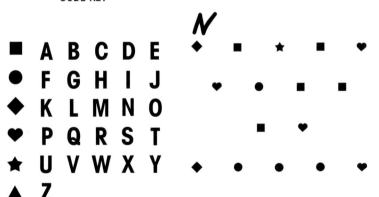

HE0079
Reproduced from 10 years Safety Sheet
© 1994 American Academy of Pediatrics

American Academy of Pediatrics
DEDICATED TO THE HEALTH OF ALL CHILDREN™

The American Academy of Pediatrics is an organization of 55,000 primary care pediatricians, pediatric medical subspecialists, and pediatric surgical specialists dedicated to the health, safety, and well-being of infants, children, adolescents, and young adults.

American Academy of Pediatrics
PO Box 747
Elk Grove Village, IL 60009-0747
Web site — http://www.aap.org

©2002 American Academy of Pediatrics

SECTION NINE

Immunization Information

The Chickenpox Vaccine:
What Parents Need to Know

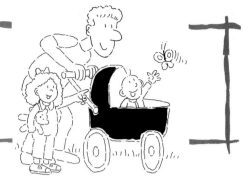

Chickenpox (varicella) is a disease affecting most children in the United States before their 10th birthday. Until recently it could not be prevented, only treated. Today, parents can have their children immunized against chickenpox. Vaccinations are an important part of your child's total health care. The chickenpox vaccine can protect your child against a severe case of chickenpox and prevent the discomfort and possible serious complications the disease can cause.

What is this disease?

Chickenpox is one of the most common childhood diseases. It is usually mild and not life-threatening to healthy children. The most obvious sign of chickenpox is a skin rash that develops on your child's scalp and body, then spreads to the face, arms, and legs over a period of 3 to 4 days. The rash forms between 250 to 500 itchy blisters that dry up into scabs 2 to 4 days later. School-age children often get a mild fever for 1 or 2 days before the rash appears. Other symptoms of chickenpox are:

- coughing
- fussiness
- loss of appetite
- headaches

Chickenpox can easily be spread in any of the following ways:
- by direct contact with an infected person, usually through fluid from broken blisters
- through the air when an infected person coughs or sneezes
- through direct contact with lesions (sores) from a person with shingles (see section on shingles)

A person with chickenpox is contagious from 1 to 2 days before the rash starts and for up to 5 days after the rash appears. A child will have to stay home from child care or school until she is no longer contagious. An adult or child who has never had chickenpox is at risk of getting it and may not show symptoms for 10 to 21 days after being exposed to the virus. Within households, 80% to 90% of at-risk persons will develop chickenpox if they are exposed to a family member who has it.

Who gets chickenpox?

Before the vaccine became available, there were about 4 million cases of chickenpox in the United States each year. Anyone can get chickenpox at any age, but it occurs most frequently in children from ages 6 to 10.

Chickenpox can occur at any time of the year. Peak times are in the winter and early spring, especially in moderate climates.

What is the treatment for chickenpox?

You may remember how itchy chickenpox was when you were a child. If your child scratches the blisters before they are able to heal, they can become infected, turn into small sores, and possibly leave scars. Discourage your child from scratching and keep his fingernails trimmed short just in case.

Oatmeal baths can help relieve itching and acetaminophen may help reduce your child's fever. Acetaminophen is a substitute for aspirin. Do not give your child aspirin or salicylate (a compound found in aspirin). They have been associated with Reye's syndrome, a disease that affects the liver and brain. If your child's fever lasts longer than 4 days, rises above 102° F after the third day of having chickenpox, or your child becomes dehydrated, call your pediatrician. Also let your pediatrician know if the rash gets very red, warm, or tender. It may mean your child has an infection and needs other treatment.

The drug acyclovir can help make a case of chickenpox less severe. Acyclovir is most often used for patients who are at risk of developing severe chickenpox, such as adolescents; children with certain skin or lung diseases; and children taking other prescribed medications, such as steroids. To be effective, acyclovir must be given within the first 24 hours of the onset of the chickenpox rash. You may want to discuss the use of acyclovir with your pediatrician.

Can chickenpox cause complications?

Most healthy children who get chickenpox won't have any complications from the disease. However, each year in the United States, about 9,000 people are hospitalized for chickenpox and about 90 people die from the disease.

The most common complication from chickenpox is a bacterial infection of the skin. The next most common problems are pneumonia and encephalitis, an infection of the brain. The following groups of people are at higher risk of developing these problems:

- people who have weak immune systems or low resistance to disease
- infants under 1 year of age
- adolescents and adults
- newborns whose mothers had chickenpox around the time of delivery
- premature infants whose mothers have not had chickenpox
- children with eczema and other skin conditions
- children receiving therapy with salicylate (a compound found in aspirin)

When an adult gets chickenpox, the disease is usually more severe, often developing into pneumonia. Adults are almost 10 times more likely to be hospitalized for chickenpox than children under 14 years of age, and adults are more than 20 times more likely to die from the disease. If a pregnant woman gets chickenpox, her unborn baby may have complications.

What is "shingles"?

Once someone has had chickenpox, the virus stays in the body of the infected person permanently. Later in life, the virus can reappear and cause shingles. Shingles can occur at any age, but usually occur after a person is 50 years old. About 10% to 20% of all people who have had chickenpox develop shingles. People with shingles typically feel numbness and itching or severe pain in the skin areas where the affected nerve roots are. Within 3 to 4 days, clusters of blister-like sores develop and last for 2 to 3 weeks.

When should my child get the chickenpox vaccine?

The American Academy of Pediatrics recommends a single dose of the chickenpox vaccine for all children between 12 and 18 months of age who have not had chickenpox. Older children should be immunized at the earliest opportunity, also with a single dose. For healthy children older than 13 who have not had chickenpox and have never been immunized against the disease, two doses of the vaccine are required, 4 to 8 weeks apart.

What are the benefits of vaccinating my child against chickenpox?

Although chickenpox is usually mild, vaccinating all children at age 1 can prevent serious medical problems and reduce the costs related to the disease. Chickenpox can be expensive and inconvenient. Parents may have to miss work while their children are home from school or child care. In the average household, a child with chickenpox misses 8 or 9 days of school, and adult caretakers lose up to 2 days of work.

Immunization with the chickenpox vaccine will prevent most children from getting chickenpox. If vaccinated children do get chickenpox, they generally have a much milder form of the disease. They have fewer skin lesions (15 to 32), a lower fever, and recover more quickly. In fact, the disease may be so mild that the skin lesions look like insect bites. Even so, vaccinated children with a mild case of chickenpox can still infect others at risk of getting chickenpox.

Currently, revaccination with the chickenpox vaccine is not recommended. However, studies are underway to determine how long protection from the vaccine lasts and whether a person will need revaccination in the future.

Is the vaccine safe?

Before becoming available, a chickenpox vaccine was tested in over 9,400 healthy children and over 1,600 adults in the United States. Since the chickenpox vaccine was licensed in 1995, several million doses of vaccine have been given to children in the United States. Studies continue to show the vaccine to be safe and effective.

Side effects from the chickenpox vaccine generally are mild and include:

- redness
- stiffness
- soreness
- tiredness
- fussiness
- fever
- nausea
- swelling where the shot was given

Also, in a small percentage of people who are vaccinated, 7%–8%, a rash of several small bumps or pimples may develop at the spot where the shot was given or on other parts of the body. This can occur up to 1 month after immunization and can last for several days.

Your child can get the chickenpox vaccine at the same time he or she gets the measles-mumps-rubella (MMR) vaccine. *If your pediatrician doesn't give your child the chickenpox and MMR vaccines at the same time, your child should wait at least 1 month between each vaccine.* Otherwise, your child can get the vaccine for chickenpox at the same time or at any time before or after vaccines for diphtheria, tetanus, pertussis (DTP), polio, hepatitis B, and *Haemophilus influenzae type b.*

Who should NOT receive the vaccine?

Although the chickenpox vaccine is approved for use in healthy children, there are certain groups of people who should not receive it, such as:

- children with a weakened immune system
- children with a life-threatening allergy to gelatin or the antibiotic neomycin
- pregnant women

Talk to your pediatrician about whether your child falls into any of the high-risk categories and should not be vaccinated against chickenpox.

The information contained in this publication should not be used as a substitute for the medical care and advice of your pediatrician. There may be variations in treatment that your pediatrician may recommend based on individual facts and circumstances.

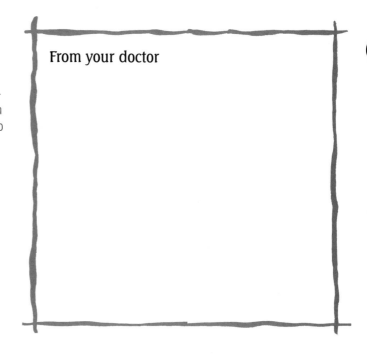

From your doctor

American Academy of Pediatrics

DEDICATED TO THE HEALTH OF ALL CHILDREN™

The American Academy of Pediatrics is an organization of 55,000 primary care pediatricians, pediatric medical subspecialists, and pediatric surgical specialists dedicated to the health, safety, and well-being of infants, children, adolescents, and young adults.

American Academy of Pediatrics
PO Box 747
Elk Grove Village, IL 60009-0747
Web site — http://www.aap.org

CHICKENPOX VACCINE

WHAT YOU NEED TO KNOW

1 | Why get vaccinated?

Chickenpox (also called varicella) is a common childhood disease. It is usually mild, but it can be serious, especially in young infants and adults.

- The chickenpox virus can be spread from person to person through the air, or by contact with fluid from chickenpox blisters.

- It causes a rash, itching, fever, and tiredness.

- It can lead to severe skin infection, scars, pneumonia, brain damage, or death.

- A person who has had chickenpox can get a painful rash called shingles years later.

- About 12,000 people are hospitalized for chickenpox each year in the United States.

- About 100 people die each year in the United States as a result of chickenpox.

Chickenpox vaccine can prevent chickenpox.

Most people who get chickenpox vaccine will not get chickenpox. But if someone who has been vaccinated *does* get chickenpox, it is usually very mild. They will have fewer spots, are less likely to have a fever, and will recover faster.

2 | Who should get chickenpox vaccine and when?

✔ **Children should get 1 dose of chickenpox vaccine between 12 and 18 months of age**, or at any age after that if they have never had chickenpox.

People who do not get the vaccine until 13 years of age or older should get **2 doses**, 4-8 weeks apart.

Ask your doctor or nurse for details.

Chickenpox vaccine may be given at the same time as other vaccines.

3 | Some people should not get chickenpox vaccine or should wait

- People should not get chickenpox vaccine if they have ever had a life-threatening allergic reaction to **gelatin**, the antibiotic **neomycin**, or (for those needing a second dose) **a previous dose of chickenpox vaccine**.

- People who are moderately or severely ill at the time the shot is scheduled should usually wait until they recover before getting chickenpox vaccine.

- Pregnant women should wait to get chickenpox vaccine until after they have given birth. Women should not get pregnant for 1 month after getting chickenpox vaccine.

- Some people should check with their doctor about whether they should get chickenpox vaccine, including anyone who:
  - Has HIV/AIDS or another disease that affects the immune system
  - Is being treated with drugs that affect the immune system, such as steroids, for 2 weeks or longer
  - Has any kind of cancer
  - Is taking cancer treatment with x-rays or drugs

- People who recently had a transfusion or were given other blood products should ask their doctor when they may get chickenpox vaccine.

Ask your doctor or nurse for more information.

4 · What are the risks from chickenpox vaccine?

A vaccine, like any medicine, is capable of causing serious problems, such as severe allergic reactions. The risk of chickenpox vaccine causing serious harm, or death, is extremely small.

Getting chickenpox vaccine is much safer than getting chickenpox disease.

Most people who get chickenpox vaccine do not have any problems with it.

Mild Problems
- Soreness or swelling where the shot was given (about 1 out of 5 children and up to 1 out of 3 adolescents and adults)
- Fever (1 person out of 10, or less)
- Mild rash, up to a month after vaccination (1 person out of 20, or less). It is possible for these people to infect other members of their household, but this is *extremely* rare.

Moderate Problems
- Seizure (jerking or staring) caused by fever (less than 1 person out of 1,000).

Severe Problems
- Pneumonia (very rare)

Other serious problems, including severe brain reactions and low blood count, have been reported after chickenpox vaccination. These happen so rarely experts cannot tell whether they are caused by the vaccine or not. If they are, it is extremely rare.

5 · What if there is a moderate or severe reaction?

What should I look for?

Any unusual condition, such as a serious allergic reaction, high fever or behavior changes. Signs of a serious allergic reaction can include difficulty breathing, hoarseness or wheezing, hives, paleness, weakness, a fast heart beat or dizziness within a few minutes to a few hours after the shot. A high fever or seizure, if it occurs, would happen 1 to 6 weeks after the shot.

What should I do?

- Call a doctor, or get the person to a doctor right away.
- Tell your doctor what happened, the date and time it happened, and when the vaccination was given.
- Ask your doctor, nurse, or health department to file a Vaccine Adverse Event Reporting System (VAERS) form, or call VAERS yourself at **1-800-822-7967.**

6 · The National Vaccine Injury Compensation Program

In the rare event that you or your child has a serious reaction to a vaccine, a federal program has been created to help you pay for the care of those who have been harmed.

For details about the National Vaccine Injury Compensation Program, call **1-800-338-2382** or visit the program's website at **http://www.hrsa.dhhs.gov/bhpr/vicp**

7 · How can I learn more?

- Ask your doctor or nurse. They can give you the vaccine package insert or suggest other sources of information.

- Call your local or state health department's immunization program.

- Contact the Centers for Disease Control and Prevention(CDC):
  - Call **1-800-232-2522**(English)
  - Call **1-800-232-0233** (Español)
  - Visit the National Immunization Program's website at **http://www.cdc.gov/nip**

American Academy of Pediatrics

 CDC

U.S. DEPARTMENT OF HEALTH & HUMAN SERVICES
Centers for Disease Control and Prevention • National Immunization Program

Reprinted by the American Academy of Pediatrics
Additional copies are available for purchase in pads of 100. To order, contact:
American Academy of Pediatrics
Division of Publications
141 Northwest Point Blvd
PO Box 747
Elk Grove Village, IL 60009-0747
Web site — http://www.aap.org
Minimum Order 100

Vaccine Information Statement   Varicella (12/16/98)   42 U.S.C. § 300-aa-26
HE0270   (Rep 7/99)

DIPHTHERIA, TETANUS, AND PERTUSSIS VACCINES

WHAT YOU NEED TO KNOW

1 Why get vaccinated?

Diphtheria, pertussis, and tetanus are serious diseases.

Diphtheria

- Diphtheria causes a thick covering in the back of the throat.
- It can lead to breathing problems, paralysis, heart failure, and even death.

Tetanus (Lockjaw)

- Tetanus causes painful tightening of the muscles, usually all over the body.
- It can lead to "locking" of the jaw so the person cannot open his mouth or swallow. Tetanus can lead to death.

Pertussis (Whooping cough)

- Pertussis causes coughing spells so bad that it is hard for infants to eat, drink, or breathe. These can last for weeks.
- It can lead to pneumonia, seizures (jerking and staring spells), brain damage, and death.

Diphtheria, tetanus, and pertussis vaccines prevent these diseases. Most children who get all their shots will be protected during childhood. Many more children would get these diseases if we stopped vaccinating.

2 Diphtheria, tetanus, and pertussis vaccines

DTP vaccine

- Protects against diphtheria, tetanus, and pertussis
- Used for many years

DTaP vaccine

- Protects against diphtheria, tetanus, and pertussis
- Newer than DTP

The Centers for Disease Control and Prevention (CDC) recommends DTaP over DTP. This is because DTaP is less likely to cause reactions than DTP.

Related vaccines

- Combinations: To reduce the number of shots a child must get, DTP or DTaP may be available in combination with other vaccines.
- DT protects against diphtheria and tetanus, *but not* pertussis. It only is recommended for children who should not get pertussis vaccine.

3 What are the risks from these vaccines?

- As with any medicine, vaccines carry a small risk of serious harm, such as a severe allergic reaction or even death.
- If there are reactions, they usually start within 3 days and don't last long.
- Most people have no serious reactions from these vaccines.

Possible reactions to these vaccines.

Mild Reactions (common)

- Sore arm or leg
- Fussy
- Tired
- Fever
- Less appetite
- Vomiting

Mild reactions are much-less likely after **DTaP** than after DTP.

Moderate to Serious Reactions (uncommon)

Moderate to serious reactions have been uncommon with DTP vaccine:

- Non-stop crying (3 hours or more) ..... 100 of every 10,000 doses
- Fever of 105 or higher .... 30 of every 10,000 doses
- Seizure (jerking or staring) .... 6 of every 10,000 doses
- Child becomes limp, pole, less alert ...... 6 of every 10,000 doses

With DTaP vaccine, these reactions are much less likely to happen.

Severe Reactions (very rare)

There are two kinds of serious reactions:

- Severe allergic reaction (breathing difficulty, shock)
- Severe brain reaction (long seizure, coma or lowered consciousness)

Is there lasting damage?

- Experts disagree on whether pertussis vaccines cause lasting brain damage.
- If they do, it is very rare.

Most experts believe serious reactions will be *more rare* after DTaP than after DTP.

4 When should my child get vaccinated?

Most children should get a dose at these ages:

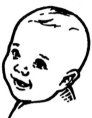

2 Months

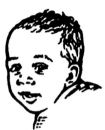

4 Months

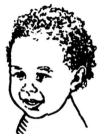

6 Months

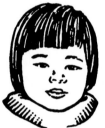

12–18 Months

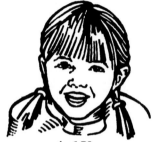

4–6 Years

At 11–12 years of age and every 10 years after that you should get a booster to prevent diphtheria and tetanus.

5 What can be done to reduce possible fever and pain after this vaccine?

Give your child an *aspirin-free* pain reliever for 24 hours after the shot.

This is important if your child has had a seizure or has a parent, brother, or sister who has had a seizure.

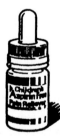

6 Some children should not get these vaccines or should wait

Tell your doctor or nurse if your child:
- Ever had a moderate or serious reaction after getting vaccinated
- Ever had a seizure
- Has a parent, brother, or sister who has had a seizure
- Has a brain problem that is getting worse
- Now has a moderate or severe illness

Your doctor or nurse has information on what to do in this case (for example, give one of these vaccines, wait, give medicine to prevent fever).

7 What if there is a moderate to severe reaction?

What should I look for?
- Any unusual conditions, such as those in item 3

What should I do?
- Call a doctor or get the child to a doctor right away.
- Tell your doctor what happened, the date and time it happened, and when the vaccination was given.
- Ask your doctor, nurse, or health department to file a Vaccine Adverse Event Report (VAERS) form, or call VAERS yourself at: 1-800-822-7967.

8 The National Vaccine Injury Compensation Program

The National Vaccine Injury Compensation Program is a federal program that helps pay for the care of those seriously injured by vaccines.

For details call 1-800-338-2382 or visit the program's website at **http://www.hrsa.dhhs.gov/bhpr/vicp/new.htm**

9 How can I learn more?

- Ask your doctor or nurse. They can give you the vaccine package insert or suggest other sources of information.
- Call your local or state health department. They can give you the *Parents Guide to Childhood Immunization* or other information.
- Contact the Centers for Disease Control and Prevention (CDC); Call 1-800-232-2522 (English) OR Call 1-800-232-0233 (Spanish) OR Visit the CDC website at **http://www.cdc.gov/nip**

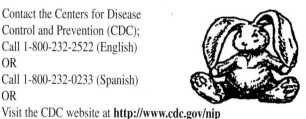

American Academy of Pediatrics
DEDICATED TO THE HEALTH OF ALL CHILDREN™

U.S. DEPARTMENT OF HEALTH & HUMAN SERVICES
Centers for Disease Control and Prevention • National Immunization Program

Reprinted by the American Academy of Pediatrics
Additional copies are available for purchase in pads of 100. To order, contact:
American Academy of Pediatrics
Division of Publications
PO Box 747
Elk Grove Village, IL 60009-0747
Web site - http://www.aap.org
Minimum Order 100

DTP/DTaP/DT(8/15/97)
Vaccine Information Statement
42 U.S.C 300aa-26
HE0113   4/98
(reprint 4/99)

Haemophilus influenzae type b

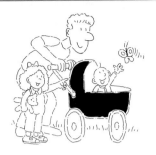

The continued occurance of preventable childhood diseases emphasizes the necessity of vaccination for all children. Regular medical care includes vaccinations, which are an important part of your child's total health care.

This brochure explains why it's important to make sure your child is vaccinated on time. Without protection provided by the Hib conjugate vaccines (*Haemophilus influenzae* type b conjugate vaccines), your child could suffer from serious illnesses that could have been prevented.

What is this disease?

Haemophilus influenzae type b is a germ (or bacterium) that can cause several kinds of dangerous infections in children. It is very different from the "flu" (influenza virus).

Why are the H influenzae vaccines so important for infants?

These vaccines provide protection during the first years of life, when it is easiest for your child to get *H influenzae* type b infection. When children are fully immunized with the *H influenzae* type B vaccine, they are protected against the illnesses caused by the *H influenzae* type b germ.

Without timely immunizations, your child faces the risk of becoming very sick with serious diseases such as:

- Meningitis, a serious infection of the covering of the brain and spinal cord. Before the vaccine was used, *H influenzae* type b was the most common cause of bacterial meningitis in the United States. It caused about 12,000 cases of meningitis each year in children younger than 5 years of age—especially in babies 6 to 12 months old. Of those children infected, 1 in 20 died from this disease, and 1 in 4 developed permanent brain damage.
- Epiglottitis, a dangerous throat infection that can cause a child to choke to death if not treated immediately.
- Pneumonia and serious infections in the blood, bones, joints, skin, and the covering of the heart.

When should my child get the Hib conjugate vaccines?

The immunization schedule will vary depending on which vaccine your child receives and at what age the series was started. The American Academy of Pediatrics (AAP) recommends that your child receive two or three doses of the vaccine between 2 to 6 months of age and a booster dose at 12 to 15 months. Your child's pediatrician will tell you about the different Hib vaccines available and the recommended immunization schedule for each.

Are there side effects to Hib conjugate vaccines?

Most children have no side effects with the Hib conjugate vaccines. There have been no serious reactions linked to these vaccines. Those side effects that sometimes occur are mild and temporary. The possible side effects include:

- Soreness, swelling, or redness where the shot was given
- A mild to moderate fever
- Fussiness

These symptoms may begin within 24 hours after the shot is given and usually go away within 48 to 72 hours.

Talk to your pediatrician about the possible reactions to these immunizations and when to call his or her office for more details. As with any medical problems, call your doctor promptly if you are concerned.

Other information...

H influenzae type b infection is one of ten childhood diseases your child needs to be vaccinated against. Your pediatrician can tell you more about other vaccines to protect against measles, mumps, rubella (German measles), diphtheria, tetanus, pertussis (whooping cough), polio, hepatitis B, and varicella (chicken pox).

Immunizations have provided protection for children for years—but the vaccines only work if you make sure your child gets immunized.

Remember…your child's health depends on it!

Immunization is just one important part of preventive health care for children. The American Academy of Pediatrics, representing the nation's pediatricians, is dedicated to working toward a better future for our children. Join us by making sure your children receive the best possible health care.

The information contained in this publication should not be used as a substitute for the medical care and advice of your pediatrician. There may be variations in treatment that your pediatrician may recommend based on individual facts and circumstances.

From your doctor

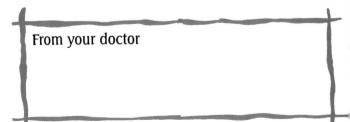

American Academy of Pediatrics

DEDICATED TO THE HEALTH OF ALL CHILDREN™

The American Academy of Pediatrics is an organization of 55,000 primary care pediatricians, pediatric medical subspecialists, and pediatric surgical specialists dedicated to the health, safety, and well-being of infants, children, adolescents, and young adults.

American Academy of Pediatrics
PO Box 747
Elk Grove Village, IL 60009-0747
Web site — http://www.aap.org

Haemophilus Influenzae Type b (Hib) Vaccine

W H A T   Y O U   N E E D   T O   K N O W

1 | What is Hib disease?

Haemophilus influenzae **type b (Hib) disease is a serious disease caused by a bacteria.** It usually strikes children under 5 years old.

Your child can get Hib disease by being around other children or adults who may have the bacteria and not know it. The germs spread from person to person. If the germs stay in the child's nose and throat, the child probably will not get sick. But sometimes the germs spread into the lungs or the bloodstream, and then Hib can cause serious problems.

Before Hib vaccine, Hib disease was the leading cause of bacterial meningitis among children under 5 years old in the United States. Meningitis is an infection of the brain and spinal cord coverings, which can lead to lasting brain damage and deafness. Hib disease can also cause:

- pneumonia
- severe swelling in the throat, making it hard to breathe
- infections of the blood, joints, bones, and covering of the heart
- death

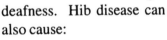

Before Hib vaccine, about 20,000 children in the United States under 5 years old got severe Hib disease each year and nearly 1,000 people died.

Hib vaccine can prevent Hib disease.
Many more children would get Hib disease if we stopped vaccinating.

2 | Who should get Hib vaccine and when?

Children should get Hib vaccine at:
- ✓ 2 months of age
- ✓ 4 months of age
- ✓ 6 months of age*
- ✓ 12-15 months of age

* Depending on what brand of Hib vaccine is used, your child might not need the dose at 6 months of age. Your doctor or nurse will tell you if this dose is needed.

If you miss a dose or get behind schedule, get the next dose as soon as you can. There is no need to start over.

Hib vaccine may be given at the same time as other vaccines.

Older Children and Adults
Children over 5 years old usually do not need Hib vaccine. But some older children or adults with special health conditions should get it. These conditions include sickle cell disease, HIV/AIDS, removal of the spleen, bone marrow transplant, or cancer treatment with drugs. Ask your doctor or nurse for details.

3 | Some people should not get Hib vaccine or should wait

- People who have ever had a life-threatening allergic reaction to a previous dose of Hib vaccine should not get another dose.

- Children less than 6 weeks of age should not get Hib vaccine.

- People who are moderately or severely ill at the time the shot is scheduled should usually wait until they recover before getting Hib vaccine.

Ask your doctor or nurse for more information.

4 | What are the risks from Hib vaccine?

A vaccine, like any medicine, is capable of causing serious problems, such as severe allergic reactions. The risk of Hib vaccine causing serious harm or death is extremely small.

Most people who get Hib vaccine do not have any problems with it.

Mild Problems

- Redness, warmth, or swelling where the shot was given (up to 1/4 of children)
- Fever over 101°F (up to 1 out of 20 children)

If these problems happen, they usually start within a day of vaccination. They may last 2-3 days.

5 | What if there is a moderate or severe reaction?

What should I look for?

Any unusual condition, such as a serious allergic reaction, high fever or behavior changes. Signs of a serious allergic reaction can include difficulty breathing, hoarseness or wheezing, hives, paleness, weakness, a fast heart beat, or dizziness within a few minutes to a few hours after the shot.

What should I do?

- Call a doctor, or get the person to a doctor right away.
- Tell your doctor what happened, the date and time it happened, and when the vaccination was given.
- Ask your doctor, nurse, or health department to file a Vaccine Adverse Event Reporting System (VAERS) form, or call VAERS yourself at **1-800-822-7967.**

6 | The National Vaccine Injury Compensation Program

In the rare event that you or your child has a serious reaction to a vaccine, a federal program has been created to help you pay for the care of those who have been harmed.

For details about the National Vaccine Injury Compensation Program, call **1-800-338-2382** or visit the program's website at **http://www.hrsa.gov/bhpr/vicp**

7 | How can I learn more?

- Ask your doctor or nurse. They can give you the vaccine package insert or suggest other sources of information.

- Call your local or state health department's immunization program.

- Contact the Centers for Disease Control and Prevention (CDC):
  - Call **1-800-232-2522** (English)
  - Call **1-800-232-0233** (Español)
  - Visit the National Immunization Program's website at **http://www.cdc.gov/nip**

American Academy of Pediatrics
DEDICATED TO THE HEALTH OF ALL CHILDREN™

U.S. DEPARTMENT OF HEALTH & HUMAN SERVICES
Centers for Disease Control and Prevention • National Immunization Program

Reprinted by the American Academy of Pediatrics. Additional copies are available for purchase in pads of 100. To order, contact:

American Academy of Pediatrics
PO Box 747
Elk Grove Village, IL 60009-0747

Web site - http://www.aap.org
Minimum Order 100

Vaccine Information Statement
Hib (12/16/98)　　　　　42 U.S.C. § 300aa-26

HE0268　　　　　　　　　　　　　　　　3-70/rev0801

Hepatitis B

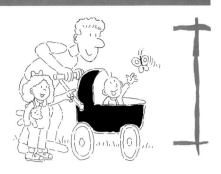

Recent outbreaks of preventable childhood diseases emphasize the necessity of vaccination for all children. Regular medical care includes vaccinations, which are an important part of your child's total health care.

This brochure explains why it's important to make sure your child is vaccinated on time. Without protection provided by the hepatitis B vaccine, your child could suffer from a serious illness that could have been prevented.

What is this disease?

Hepatitis B (HBV), or serum hepatitis virus, can cause infection at any age. It may lead to chronic infection of the liver and serious disease, especially if it is acquired during infancy or childhood. However, a child may not show signs of infection until years later when he or she develops liver failure and/or liver cancer.

HBV is transmitted in several ways, including being passed from mother to infant at the time of birth. Young children may be infected by someone living in the same household who is infected, even if that person does not appear to be sick (a carrier of HBV).

Finally, HBV can spread through sexual intercourse or through contact with infected blood, such as when drug users share needles.

It is important that your child be protected by the hepatitis B vaccine, because infection acquired during early life is most likely to cause chronic liver disease. More than 95 percent of children who receive all the recommended doses of the hepatitis B vaccine are protected against the illnesses caused by the hepatitis B virus.

When should my child get the hepatitis B vaccine?

According to the American Academy of Pediatrics, your child needs three doses of hepatitis B vaccine to be fully protected against hepatitis B infection. Ordinarily, the first vaccination will be given at birth, the second dose at 1 to 4 months, and a third dose at 6 to 18 months of age.

The first dose of the vaccine is delayed for many premature babies (and those with other illnesses during the first days of life). Newborns who have not received a vaccine dose at birth should receive three hepatitis B vaccine doses by 18 months of age.

However, if the mother tests positive for hepatitis B, the child must receive the first vaccine dose as well as hepatitis B immune globulin (HBIG) at or shortly after birth. The child also requires a second dose at 1 month and the final vaccine dose by 6 months of age.

Children and adolescents who have not previously received 3 doses of hepatitis B vaccine should start or complete the series during their 11–12 year-old check-up.

Older children, adolescents, and others living with infected household members also should receive a three-dose series to protect against hepatitis B.

Talk to your child's pediatrician if you have questions about this vaccination or about other circumstances when this vaccine is used. He or she can answer any questions you may have about when your child should receive the hepatitis B vaccine.

Are there side effects to hepatitis B vaccine?

No serious reactions have been linked to this vaccine, and most children have no side effects. Those side effects that sometimes occur—fussiness and soreness—are usually mild and temporary. These symptoms may begin within 24 hours after the shot is given and usually go away within 48 to 72 hours.

Your pediatrician can tell you more about other vaccines your child needs to stay healthy.

Immunizations have provided protection for children for years—but the vaccines only work if you make sure your child gets immunized.

Remember…your child's health depends on it!

Immunization is just one important part of preventive health care for children. The American Academy of Pediatrics, representing the nation's pediatricians, is dedicated to working toward a better future for our children. Join us by making sure your children receive the best possible health care.

The information contained in this publication should not be used as a substitute for the medical care and advice of your pediatrician. There may be variations in treatment that your pediatrician may recommend based on individual facts and circumstances.

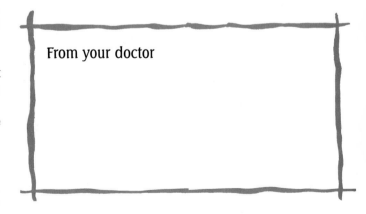

From your doctor

American Academy of Pediatrics

DEDICATED TO THE HEALTH OF ALL CHILDREN™

The American Academy of Pediatrics is an organization of 55,000 primary care pediatricians, pediatric medical subspecialists, and pediatric surgical specialists dedicated to the health, safety, and well-being of infants, children, adolescents, and young adults.

American Academy of Pediatrics
PO Box 747
Elk Grove Village, IL 60009-0747
Web site — http://www.aap.org

HEPATITIS B VACCINE

WHAT YOU NEED TO KNOW

1 Why get vaccinated?

Hepatitis B is a serious disease.

The hepatitis B virus (HBV) can cause short-term (acute) illness that leads to:

- loss of appetite
- tiredness
- pain in muscles, joints, and stomach
- diarrhea and vomiting
- jaundice (yellow skin or eyes)

It can also cause long-term (chronic) illness that leads to:

- liver damage (cirrhosis)
- liver cancer
- death

About 1.25 million people in the U.S. have chronic HBV infection.

Each year it is estimated that:

- 80,000 people, mostly young adults, get infected with HBV
- More than 11,000 people have to stay in the hospital because of hepatitis B
- 4,000 to 5,000 people die from chronic hepatitis B

Hepatitis B vaccine can prevent hepatitis B. It is the first anti-cancer vaccine because it can prevent a form of liver cancer.

2 How is hepatitis B virus spread?

Hepatitis B virus is spread through contact with the blood and body fluids of an infected person. A person can get infected in several ways, such as:

- by having unprotected sex with an infected person
- by sharing needles when injecting illegal drugs
- by being stuck with a used needle on the job
- during birth when the virus passes from an infected mother to her baby

About 1/3 of people who are infected with hepatitis B in the United States don't know how they got it.

Hepatitis B   7/11/2001

3 Who should get hepatitis B vaccine and when?

1) Everyone 18 years of age and younger
2) Adults over 18 who are at risk

Adults at risk for HBV infection include:

- people who have more than one sex partner in 6 months
- men who have sex with other men
- sex contacts of infected people
- people who inject illegal drugs
- health care and public safety workers who might be exposed to infected blood or body fluids
- household contacts of persons with chronic HBV infection
- hemodialysis patients

If you are not sure whether you are at risk, ask your doctor or nurse.

✓ **People should get 3 doses of hepatitis B vaccine according to the following schedule.** *If you miss a dose or get behind schedule, get the next dose as soon as you can. There is no need to start over.*

Hepatitis B Vaccination Schedule		WHO?		
		Infant whose mother is infected with HBV	Infant whose mother is *not* infected with HBV	Older child, adolescent, or adult
W H E N ?	First Dose	Within 12 hours of birth	Birth - 2 months of age	Any time
	Second Dose	1 -2 months of age	1 - 4 months of age (at least 1 month after first dose)	1 - 2 months after first dose
	Third Dose	6 months of age	6 - 18 months of age	4 - 6 months after first dose

- The second dose must be given at least 1 month after the first dose.
- The third dose must be given at least 2 months after the second dose and at least 4 months after the first.
- The third dose should *not* be given to infants under 6 months of age, because this could reduce long-term protection.

Adolescents 11 to 15 years of age may need only two doses of hepatitis B vaccine, separated by 4-6 months. Ask your health care provider for details.

Hepatitis B vaccine may be given at the same time as other vaccines.

4 | Some people should not get hepatitis B vaccine or should wait

People should not get hepatitis B vaccine if they have ever had a life-threatening allergic reaction to **baker's yeast** (the kind used for making bread) or to **a previous dose of hepatitis B vaccine.**

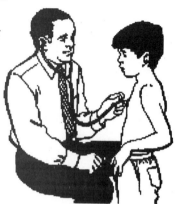

People who are moderately or severely ill at the time the shot is scheduled should usually wait until they recover before getting hepatitis B vaccine.

Ask your doctor or nurse for more information.

5 | What are the risks from hepatitis B vaccine?

A vaccine, like any medicine, is capable of causing serious problems, such as severe allergic reactions. The risk of hepatitis B vaccine causing serious harm, or death, is extremely small.

Getting hepatitis B vaccine is much safer than getting hepatitis B disease.

Most people who get hepatitis B vaccine do not have any problems with it.

Mild problems

- soreness where the shot was given, lasting a day or two (up to 1 out of 11 children and adolescents, and about 1 out of 4 adults)
- mild to moderate fever (up to 1 out of 14 children and adolescents and 1 out of 100 adults)

Severe problems

- serious allergic reaction (very rare)

6 | What if there is a moderate or severe reaction?

What should I look for?

Any unusual condition, such as a serious allergic reaction, high fever or unusual behavior. Serious allergic reactions are extremely rare with any vaccine. If one were to occur, it would be within a few minutes to a few hours after the shot. Signs can include difficulty breathing, hoarseness or wheezing, hives, paleness, weakness, a fast heart beat or dizziness.

What should I do?

- Call a doctor or get the person to a doctor right away.
- Tell your doctor what happened, the date and time it happened, and when the vaccination was given.
- Ask your doctor, nurse, or health department to file a Vaccine Adverse Event Reporting System (VAERS) form, or call VAERS yourself at **1-800-822-7967.**

7 | The National Vaccine Injury Compensation Program

In the rare event that you or your child has a serious reaction to a vaccine, a federal program has been created to help you pay for the care of those who have been harmed.

For details about the National Vaccine Injury Compensation Program, call **1-800-338-2382** or visit the program's website at **http://www.hrsa.gov/bhpr/vicp**

8 | How can I learn more?

- Ask your doctor or nurse. They can give you the vaccine package insert or suggest other sources of information.

- Call your local or state health department's immunization program.

- Contact the Centers for Disease Control and Prevention (CDC):
    - Call **1-800-232-2522** or **1-888-443-7232** (English)
    - Call **1-800-232-0233** (Español)
    - Visit the National Immunization Program's website at **http://www.cdc.gov/nip** or CDC's Division of Viral Hepatitis website at **http://www.cdc.gov/hepatitis**

U.S. DEPARTMENT OF HEALTH & HUMAN SERVICES
Centers for Disease Control and Prevention
National Immunization Program

Vaccine Information Statement
Hepatitis B (7/11/01)   42 U.S.C. § 300aa-26

Reprinted by the American Academy of Pediatrics. Additional copies are available for purchase in pads of 100. To order, contact:

American Academy of Pediatrics
PO Box 747
Elk Grove Village, IL 60009-0747

Web site - http://www.aap.org
Minimum Order 100

American Academy of Pediatrics
DEDICATED TO THE HEALTH OF ALL CHILDREN™

HE0269

3-11/rev0901

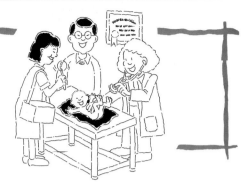

Immunizations and Your Child

Immunizations have been protecting children from serious diseases for more than 50 years.

When your child is immunized, he receives a vaccine to prevent a certain disease. Vaccines usually are given as shots. The vaccine makes your child's body produce antibodies. These antibodies make him immune to this disease should he ever come in contact with it.

Your child should receive most of her immunizations during the first 2 years of life, starting at birth. Infants and young children are more at risk of being harmed by serious diseases. That is why it is important to begin immunizations early. Your child also will need immunizations before starting school. In addition, she will need to receive vaccines as an older child and teenager.

Today children receive more immunizations than in the past because now we can protect them from more serious diseases than ever before. Most vaccines used for routine childhood immunizations can be given safely at the same time.

Your child needs the following immunizations to stay healthy:

Hepatitis B vaccine

This protects against a virus that may cause serious liver disease, as well as cancer.

Your child needs to receive doses of hepatitis B vaccine at
- Birth to 2 months of age
- 1 to 4 months of age
- 6 to 18 months of age

Any older child or teen who has not received this vaccine can begin the series of immunizations at any time.

DTaP vaccine

This protects against diphtheria (a potentially fatal throat and windpipe infection), tetanus (lockjaw), and pertussis (whooping cough).

Most children should receive this vaccine at ages
- 2 months.
- 4 months.
- 6 months.
- 15 to 18 months.
- 4 to 6 years.
- 11 to 16 years, Td (tetanus and diphtheria) only. Routine Td boosters are needed every 10 years after that.

H. influenzae type b (Hib) vaccine

This protects against *Haemophilus influenzae* type b. This bacterium is a major cause of spinal meningitis, pneumonia, and other serious infections.

Your child should receive
- Two or three doses of the Hib vaccine between 2 and 6 months of age
- A booster dose at 12 to 15 months of age

Your pediatrician can tell you about different types of the Hib vaccine that are available.

Inactivated Polio (IPV) vaccine

This protects against polio, which can cause paralysis or death. This type of polio vaccine is given as a shot and is recommended for almost everyone.

Your child should receive doses of polio vaccine at ages
- 2 months
- 4 months
- 6 to 18 months
- 4 to 6 years

Under certain circumstances your pediatrician may recommend that your child receive the oral polio vaccine, which is given by mouth.

Pneumococcal Conjugate vaccine

This protects against the pneumococcal bacteria, which can cause meningitis, pneumonia, and serious infections in the brain, bloodstream, and ears.

Your child needs this vaccine at ages
- 2 months
- 4 months
- 6 months
- 12 to 15 months

Some children between the ages of 2 and 5 years also may need this vaccine.

Measles, Mumps, Rubella (MMR) vaccine

This protects against measles, mumps, and rubella (German measles).

Your child needs to receive doses of the MMR vaccine at ages
- 12 to 15 months
- 4 to 6 years

Children who do not get the second dose on schedule should receive it at the earliest opportunity.

Varicella vaccine

This protects against chickenpox, which can cause serious complications such as bacterial skin infections, pneumonia, and infections of the brain.

If your child has not had chickenpox, he should receive
- A single dose of the varicella vaccine between the ages of 12 and 18 months
- A single dose at the earliest opportunity if he is an older child (but younger than 13 years) and has not been immunized
- Two doses of the vaccine at least 4 weeks apart, if he is older than 13 years of age and has never been immunized

Under certain conditions your child may need the following immunization:

Hepatitis A vaccine

This protects against a virus that causes liver disease. Hepatitis A virus can be spread from person to person or through contaminated food or water. Hepatitis A vaccine may be given to children 2 years of age and older. If your child needs this vaccine, your pediatrician will recommend the appropriate immunization schedule for your child.

Make sure your child is protected

It is important to keep track of your child's immunizations and make sure that your child receives each vaccine on time. Children who lag behind on getting their shots are at risk of getting very sick. They also may spread serious diseases to other people.

Keep a chart that shows each immunization that your child has received. Put that chart in a safe place where you can refer to it.

Vaccine doses that are not given at the recommended age should be given as a "catch-up" immunization at a later time. Ask your pediatrician if your child's immunizations are up-to-date.

There are some groups of people who should not receive certain vaccines. Those groups may include people with certain allergies or weakened immune systems. Your pediatrician can tell you which vaccines your child should have.

Immunizations are one of the most important ways you can protect your child against serious diseases. Much information is available about immunizations. Your pediatrician can tell you the facts.

Talk with your pediatrician about the vaccines your child needs to stay healthy.

Immunizations are safe and effective

Reactions to vaccines may occur, but they are usually mild. Severe reactions to vaccines are very rare. Children are much more likely to be harmed by serious diseases than by immunizations.

Your pediatrician may recommend acetaminophen for common side effects such as irritability and fever. If you have questions about possible reactions, call your pediatrician.

The information contained in this publication should not be used as a substitute for the medical care and advice of your pediatrician. There may be variations in treatment that your pediatrician may recommend based on individual facts and circumstances.

These guidelines are based on the Recommended Childhood Immunization Schedule—United States, January–December 2001.

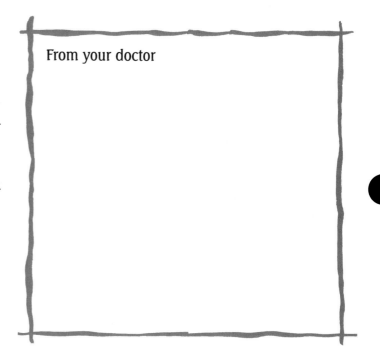

From your doctor

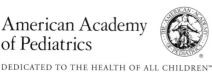

American Academy of Pediatrics

DEDICATED TO THE HEALTH OF ALL CHILDREN™

The American Academy of Pediatrics is an organization of 55,000 primary care pediatricians, pediatric medical subspecialists, and pediatric surgical specialists dedicated to the health, safety, and well-being of infants, children, adolescents, and young adults.

American Academy of Pediatrics
PO Box 747
Elk Grove Village, IL 60009-0747
Web site — http://www.aap.org

INFLUENZA VACCINE

WHAT YOU NEED TO KNOW

2001-2002

1 Why get vaccinated?

Influenza is a serious disease.

It is caused by a virus that spreads from infected persons to the nose or throat of others. The "influenza season" in the U.S. is from November through April each year.

Influenza can cause:
- fever
- sore throat
- cough
- headache
- chills
- muscle aches

People of any age can get influenza. Most people are ill with influenza for only a few days, but some get much sicker and may need to be hospitalized. Influenza causes thousands of deaths each year, mostly among the elderly.

Influenza vaccine can prevent influenza.

2 Influenza vaccine

Influenza viruses change often. Therefore, influenza vaccine is updated each year to make sure it is as effective as possible.

Protection develops about 2 weeks after getting the shot and may last up to a year.

3 Who should get influenza vaccine?

People at risk for getting a serious case of influenza or influenza complications, *and* **people in close contact with them (including all household members)** should get the vaccine. An annual flu shot is recommended for these groups:

- Everyone 50 years of age or older.

- Residents of long term care facilities housing persons with chronic medical conditions.

- Anyone who has a serious long-term health problem with:
  - heart disease
  - kidney disease
  - lung disease
  - metabolic disease, such as diabetes
  - asthma
  - anemia, and other blood disorders

- Anyone whose immune system is weakened because of:
  - HIV/AIDS or other diseases that affect the immune system
  - long-term treatment with drugs such as steroids
  - cancer treatment with x-rays or drugs

- Anyone 6 months to 18 years of age on long-term aspirin treatment (who could develop Reye Syndrome if they catch influenza).

- Women who will be past the 3rd month of pregnancy during the influenza season.

- Physicians, nurses, family members, or anyone else coming in close contact with people at risk of serious influenza

Others who should consider getting influenza vaccine:

- People who provide essential community services

- Persons traveling to the Southern hemisphere between April and September, or to the tropics at any time

- Persons living in dormitories or in other crowded conditions, to prevent outbreaks

- Anyone who wants to reduce their chance of catching influenza

4 When should I get influenza vaccine?

Because influenza activity can start as early as December, the best time to get influenza vaccine is during October and November. But getting the vaccine after November can still provide protection. A new shot is needed each year.

- People 9 years of age and older need *one shot*.
- Children less than 9 years old need *two shots*, given one month apart, the first time they get vaccinated against influenza.

Influenza vaccine can be given at the same time as other vaccines, including pneumococcal vaccine.

5 | Can I get influenza even if I get the vaccine this year?

Yes. Influenza viruses change often, and they might not always be covered by the vaccine. But vaccinated people who *do* get influenza often have a milder case than those who did not get the shot.

Also, many people call any illness with fever and cold symptoms "the flu." They may expect influenza vaccine to prevent these illnesses. But influenza vaccine is effective only against illness caused by influenza viruses, and not against other illnesses.

6 | Some people should talk with a doctor before getting influenza vaccine.

Talk with a doctor before getting an influenza vaccination if you:

1) ever had a <u>serious</u> allergic reaction to *eggs* or to a *previous dose of influenza vaccine*
   or
2) have a history of Guillain-Barré Syndrome (GBS).

If you have a fever or are severely ill at the time the shot is scheduled you should usually wait until you recover before getting influenza vaccine. Talk to your doctor or nurse about whether to reschedule the vaccination.

7 | What are the risks from influenza vaccine?

A vaccine, like any medicine, is capable of causing serious problems, such as severe allergic reactions. The risk of a vaccine causing serious harm, or death, is extremely small. Almost all people who get influenza vaccine have no serious problems from it. *The viruses in the vaccine are killed, so you <u>cannot</u> get influenza from the vaccine.*

Mild problems:
- soreness, redness, or swelling where the shot was given
- fever
- aches

If these problems occur, they usually begin soon after the shot and last 1-2 days.

Influenza (4/24/01)   Vaccine Information Statement

Severe problems:
- Life-threatening allergic reactions are very rare. If they do occur, it is within a few minutes to a few hours after the shot.

- In 1976, swine flu vaccine was associated with a severe paralytic illness called Guillain-Barré Syndrome (GBS). Influenza vaccines since then have not been clearly linked to GBS. However, if there *is* a risk of GBS from current influenza vaccines, it is estimated at 1 or 2 cases per million persons vaccinated . . . much less than the risk of severe influenza, which can be prevented by vaccination.

8 | What if there is a moderate or severe reaction?

What should I look for?
- Any unusual condition, such as a high fever or behavior changes. Signs of a serious allergic reaction can include difficulty breathing, hoarseness or wheezing, hives, paleness, weakness, a fast heart beat or dizziness.

What should I do?
- Call a doctor, or get the person to a doctor right away.
- Tell your doctor what happened, the date and time it happened, and when the vaccination was given.
- Ask your doctor, nurse, or health department to file a Vaccine Adverse Event Reporting System (VAERS) form, or call VAERS yourself at **1-800-822-7967.**

9 | How can I learn more?

- Ask your doctor or nurse. They can give you the vaccine package insert or suggest other sources of information.

- Call your local or state health department.

- Contact the Centers for Disease Control and Prevention (CDC):
    - Call **1-800-232-2522** (English)
    - Call **1-800-232-0233** (Español)
    - Visit the National Immunization Program's website at **http://www.cdc.gov/nip**

U.S. DEPARTMENT OF HEALTH & HUMAN SERVICES
Centers for Disease Control and Prevention
National Immunization Program

Reprinted by the American Academy of Pediatrics. Additional copies are available for purchase in pads of 100. To order, contact:
American Academy of Pediatrics
PO Box 747
Elk Grove Village, IL 60009-0747

Web site - http://www.aap.org
Minimum Order 100
3-72/rev0901

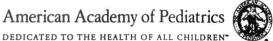

American Academy of Pediatrics

HE0300   DEDICATED TO THE HEALTH OF ALL CHILDREN™

MEASLES MUMPS & RUBELLA VACCINES

WHAT YOU NEED TO KNOW

1 Why get vaccinated?

Measles, mumps, and rubella are serious diseases.

Measles
- Measles virus causes rash, cough, runny nose, eye irritation, and fever.
- It can lead to ear infection, pneumonia, seizures (jerking and staring), brain damage, and death.

Mumps
- Mumps virus causes fever, headache, and swollen glands.
- It can lead to deafness, meningitis (infection of the brain and spinal cord covering), painful swelling of the testicles or ovaries, and, rarely, death.

Rubella (German Measles)
- Rubella virus causes rash, mild fever, and arthritis (mostly in women).
- If a woman gets rubella while she is pregnant, she could have a miscarriage or her baby could be born with serious birth defects.

You or your child could catch these diseases by being around someone who has them. They spread from person to person through the air.

Measles, mumps, and rubella (MMR) vaccine can prevent these diseases.

Most children who get their MMR shots will not get these diseases. Many more children would get them if we stopped vaccinating.

2 Who should get MMR vaccine and when?

Children should get 2 doses of MMR vaccine:

✔ The first at **12-15 months of age**
✔ and the second at **4-6 years of age**.

These are the recommended ages. But children can get the second dose at any age, as long as it is at least 28 days after the first dose.

Some **adults** should also get MMR vaccine: Generally, anyone 18 years of age or older, who was born after 1956, should get at least one dose of MMR vaccine, unless they can show that they have had either the vaccines or the diseases.

Ask your doctor or nurse for more information.

MMR vaccine may be given at the same time as other vaccines.

3 Some people should not get MMR vaccine or should wait

- People should not get MMR vaccine who have ever had a life-threatening allergic reaction to **gelatin**, the antibiotic **neomycin**, or **a previous dose of MMR vaccine**.

- People who are moderately or severely ill at the time the shot is scheduled should usually wait until they recover before getting MMR vaccine.

- Pregnant women should wait to get MMR vaccine until after they have given birth. Women should not get pregnant for 3 months after getting MMR vaccine.

- Some people should check with their doctor about whether they should get MMR vaccine, including anyone who:
  - Has HIV/AIDS, or another disease that affects the immune system
  - Is being treated with drugs that affect the immune system, such as steroids, for 2 weeks or longer.
  - Has any kind of cancer
  - Is taking cancer treatment with x-rays or drugs
  - Has ever had a low platelet count (a blood disorder)

Over . . .

- People who recently had a transfusion or were given other blood products should ask their doctor when they may get MMR vaccine

Ask your doctor or nurse for more information.

4 What are the risks from MMR vaccine?

A vaccine, like any medicine, is capable of causing serious problems, such as severe allergic reactions. The risk of MMR vaccine causing serious harm, or death, is extremely small.

Getting MMR vaccine is much safer than getting any of these three diseases.

Most people who get MMR vaccine do not have any problems with it.

Mild Problems

- Fever (up to 1 person out of 6)
- Mild rash (about 1 person out of 20)
- Swelling of glands in the cheeks or neck (rare)

If these problems occur, it is usually within 7-12 days after the shot. They occur less often after the second dose.

Moderate Problems

- Seizure (jerking or staring) caused by fever (about 1 out of 3,000 doses)
- Temporary pain and stiffness in the joints, mostly in teenage or adult women (up to 1 out of 4)
- Temporary low platelet count, which can cause a bleeding disorder (about 1 out of 30,000 doses)

Severe Problems (Very Rare)

- Serious allergic reaction (less than 1 out of a million doses)
- Several other severe problems have been known to occur after a child gets MMR vaccine. But this happens so rarely, experts cannot be sure whether they are caused by the vaccine or not. These include:
  - Deafness
  - Long-term seizures, coma, or lowered consciousness
  - Permanent brain damage

5 What if there is a moderate or severe reaction?

What should I look for?

Any unusual conditions, such as a serious allergic reaction, high fever or behavior changes. Signs of a serious allergic reaction include difficulty breathing, hoarseness or wheezing, hives, paleness, weakness, a fast heart beat or dizziness within a few minutes to a few hours after the shot. A high fever or seizure, if it occurs, would happen 1 or 2 weeks after the shot.

What should I do?

- Call a doctor, or get the person to a doctor right away.
- Tell your doctor what happened, the date and time it happened, and when the vaccination was given.
- Ask your doctor, nurse, or health department to file a Vaccine Adverse Event Reporting System (VAERS) form, or call VAERS yourself at **1-800-822-7967.**

6 The National Vaccine Injury Compensation Program

In the rare event that you or your child has a serious reaction to a vaccine, a federal program has been created to help you pay for the care of those who have been harmed.

For details about the National Vaccine Injury Compensation Program, call **1-800-338-2382** or visit the program's website at **http://www.hrsa.dhhs.gov/bhpr/vicp**

7 How can I learn more?

- Ask your doctor or nurse. They can give you the vaccine package insert or suggest other sources of information.

- Call your local or state health department's immunization program.

- Contact the Centers for Disease Control and Prevention (CDC):
  - Call **1-800-232-2522** (English)
  - Call **1-800-232-0233** (Español)
  - Visit the National Immunization Program's website at **http:/www.cdc.gov/nip**

American Academy of Pediatrics
DEDICATED TO THE HEALTH OF ALL CHILDREN™

U.S. DEPARTMENT OF HEALTH & HUMAN SERVICES
Centers for Disease Control and Prevention • National Immunization Program

Reprinted by the American Academy of Pediatrics. Additional copies are available for purchase in pads of 100. To order, contact:

American Academy of Pediatrics
Division of Publications
PO Box 747
Elk Grove Village, IL 60009-0747

Web site - http://www.aap.org
Minimum Order 100
(rev1100)

MENINGOCOCCAL VACCINE

WHAT YOU NEED TO KNOW

1 | What is meningococcal disease?

Meningococcal disease is a serious illness, caused by a bacteria. It is the leading cause of bacterial meningitis in children 2-18 years old in the United States. Meningitis is an infection of the brain and spinal cord coverings. Meningococcal disease can also cause blood infections.

About 2,600 people get meningococcal disease each year in the U.S. 10-15% of these people die, in spite of treatment with antibiotics. Of those who live, another 10% lose their arms or legs, become deaf, have problems with their nervous systems, become mentally retarded, or suffer seizures or strokes.

Anyone can get meningococcal disease. But it is most common in infants less than one year of age, and in people with certain medical conditions. College freshmen, particularly those who live in dormitories, have a slightly increased risk of getting meningococcal disease.

Meningococcal vaccine can prevent 2 of the 3 important types of meningococcal disease in older children and adults. Meningococcal vaccine is not effective in preventing all types of the disease. But it does help to protect many people who might become sick if they don't get the vaccine.

Drugs such as penicillin can be used to treat meningococcal infection. Still, about 1 out of every ten people who get the disease dies from it, and many others are affected for life. This is why it is important that people with the highest risk for meningococcal disease get the vaccine.

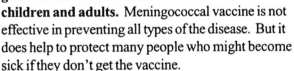

Meningococcal - 3/31/2000

2 | Who should get meningococcal vaccine and when?

Meningococcal vaccine is not routinely recommended for most people. People who *should* get the vaccine include:
- U.S. Military recruits
- People who might be affected during an outbreak of certain types of meningococcal disease.
- Anyone traveling to, or living in, a part of the world where meningococcal disease is common, such as West Africa.
- Anyone who has a damaged spleen, or whose spleen has been removed.
- Anyone who has terminal complement component deficiency (an immune system disorder).

The vaccine should also be *considered* for:
- Some laboratory workers who are routinely exposed to the meningococcal bacteria.

The vaccine may also be given to college students who choose to be vaccinated. College freshmen, especially those who live in dormitories, and their parents should discuss the risks and benefits of vaccination with their health care providers.

Meningococcal vaccine is usually not recommended for children under two years of age. But under special circumstances it may be given to infants as young as 3 months (the vaccine does not work as well in very young children). Ask your health care provider for details.

How many doses?

✓ For people 2 years of age and over: 1 dose (Sometimes an additional dose is recommended for people who continue to be at high risk. Ask your provider.)

✓ For children 3 months to 2 years of age who need the vaccine: 2 doses, 3 months apart

3 | Some people should not get meningococcal vaccine or should wait

People should not get meningococcal vaccine if they have ever had a <u>serious</u> allergic reaction to a previous dose of the vaccine.

People who are mildly ill at the time the shot is scheduled can still get meningococcal vaccine. People with moderate or severe illnesses should usually wait until they recover. Your provider can advise you.

Meningococcal vaccine may be given to pregnant women.

4 | What are the risks from meningococcal vaccine?

A vaccine, like any medicine, is capable of causing serious problems, such as severe allergic reactions. The risk of the meningococcal vaccine causing serious harm, or death, is extremely small.

Getting meningococcal vaccine is much safer than getting the disease.

Mild problems

Some people who get meningococcal vaccine have mild side effects, such as redness or pain where the shot was given. These symptoms usually last for 1-2 days.

A small percentage of people who receive the vaccine develop a fever.

5 | What if there is a serious reaction?

What should I look for?

Look for any unusual condition, such as a severe allergic reaction, high fever, or unusual behavior. If a serious allergic reaction occurred, it would happen within a few minutes to a few hours after the shot. Signs of a serious allergic reaction can include difficulty breathing, weakness, hoarseness or wheezing, a fast heart beat, hives, dizziness, paleness, or swelling of the throat.

What should I do?

- Call a doctor, or get the person to a doctor right away.

- Tell your doctor what happened, the date and time it happened, and when the vaccination was given.

- Ask your health care provider to file a Vaccine Adverse Events Reporting System (VAERS) form, or call VAERS yourself at 1-800-822-7967.

6 | How can I learn more?

- Ask your doctor or nurse. They can give you the vaccine package insert or suggest other sources of information.

- Call your local or state health department's immunization program.

- Contact the Centers for Disease Control and Prevention (CDC):
  - Call **1-800-232-2522** (English)
  - Call **1-800-232-0233** (Español)
  - Visit the National Immunization Program's website at **http://www.cdc.gov/nip**
  - Visit the National Center for Infectious Disease's meningococcal disease website at **http://www.cdc.gov/ncidod/dbmd/diseaseinfo/meningococcal_g.htm**

American Academy of Pediatrics
DEDICATED TO THE HEALTH OF ALL CHILDREN™

 CDC
CENTERS FOR DISEASE CONTROL AND PREVENTION

U.S. DEPARTMENT OF HEALTH & HUMAN SERVICES
Centers for Disease Control and Prevention
National Immunization Program

Vaccine Information Statement
Meningococcal   (3/31/2000)

Pneumococcal Infection and Vaccine

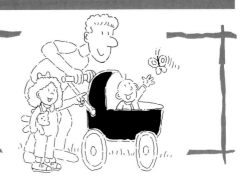

Pneumococcus is a type of bacteria that can attack different parts of the body and cause many serious infections including

- Meningitis (brain)
- Bacteremia (blood stream)
- Pneumonia (lungs)
- Sinusitis (sinus membranes)
- Otitis media (ears)

These infections can be dangerous to very young children, the elderly, and people with certain high-risk health conditions.

Pneumococcal infection

What is pneumococcal infection?

Pneumococcal bacteria live naturally in humans in the back of the nose. Many people carry the bacteria and never get sick. In fact, being a carrier helps boost one's natural immunity to the disease. Others are not immune and can get very sick from the infections caused by the bacteria.

Pneumococcal infections occur most often during the winter months. They spread from person to person the same way a cold or the flu spreads — by droplets passed through the air from coughing or sneezing, and through direct contact such as touching unwashed hands or kissing. The disease may spread quickly, especially in places where there are a lot of children, like child care centers and preschools.

Very young children do not have fully developed immune systems. This makes them more at risk from bacterial infections like pneumococcus. In addition, pneumococcal infections can be life threatening for people with certain health problems such as

- HIV infection or other immune system disorders
- Sickle-cell disease
- White cell cancers like leukemia or lymphoma
- Chronic lung, heart, or kidney disease
- A removed spleen or one that doesn't work properly
- Bone marrow or organ transplants

Common pneumococcal infections and their symptoms

Bacteremia and meningitis

Pneumococcal bacteremia and *pneumococcal meningitis* occur when pneumococcal bacteria get into the bloodstream and/or the central nervous system. Bacteremia is the presence of bacteria in the blood. Meningitis is an infection of the thin lining and blood vessels that cover the brain and spinal cord. Symptoms of meningitis include

- High fever
- Stiff neck
- Headache
- Vomiting
- Extreme tiredness and/or irritability
- Loss of appetite

Pneumonia

Pneumococcal pneumonia is a chest infection in which the lungs become filled with fluid. Symptoms of pneumonia include

- Cough that may bring up thick yellow-green or bloody mucus
- High fever
- Shortness of breath or chest pain
- Extreme tiredness
- Hard and rapid breathing

Sinusitis

Sinusitis occurs when the membranes lining the air-filled pockets in the bone of the face (sinuses) swell. The sinus cavities may fill with fluid. Symptoms of sinusitis include

- Pressure behind the eyes
- Pain in the face
- Trouble breathing through the nose
- Postnasal drip or prolonged runny nose
- Fever
- Toothache

Otitis media

Otitis media is an infection of the middle ear. Young children commonly develop middle ear infections when they have colds, the flu, or other viral respiratory infections. Symptoms of an ear infection include

- Ear pain (very young children may pull at their ears because of the pain)
- Fever
- Restlessness or irritability
- Crying
- Runny nose

Diagnosis and treatment of pneumococcal infections

Your pediatrician will be able to tell if your child has a pneumococcal infection by your child's symptoms, a physical examination, and looking at your child's medical history. X-rays, blood tests, and sometimes a spinal tap also may be done to confirm pneumococcal infection in your child.

Prompt treatment with antibiotics is usually effective. In addition, your child may need bed rest and a lot of fluids. In some cases, your child may need to be hospitalized.

Unfortunately, some strains of the pneumococcal bacteria are developing resistance to the antibiotics usually used to kill them. This means that other antibiotics must be used. Your pediatrician will let you know which antibiotic is best for your child.

Prevention of pneumococcal infections

- Teach your children to wash their hands regularly with soap and water. This helps prevent the spread of infection.
- Avoid dust, tobacco smoke, and other substances that may interfere with breathing and make children more likely to get sick.

Pneumococcal vaccine

A vaccine now offers infants and young children protection against pneumococcal infections. It is most effective against the major pneumococcal diseases — bacteremia, meningitis, and pneumonia. The vaccine is minimally effective in preventing otitis media and sinusitis. Pneumococcal vaccine is safe and can be given as a separate injection at the same time as other immunizations.

Who should receive the vaccine?

The American Academy of Pediatrics recommends that all children younger than 2 years of age receive the Heptavalent Pneumococcal Conjugate Vaccine (PCV7 or Prevnar). A series of doses may be given at 2, 4, 6, and 12 to 15 months of age. A "catch-up" immunization schedule is available for children who get a late start.

Some children between the ages of 2 and 5 years who have certain health problems also need pneumococcal vaccine because they are at higher risk of getting serious infections. Two types of vaccines may be given to children in that group. Your pediatrician can explain which vaccine is best for your child.

Pneumococcal vaccines may be given to some children 5 years of age and older, although the risk associated with pneumococcal infections is much lower in older children.

Are there side effects to pneumococcal vaccines?

Most children have no side effects with pneumococcal vaccines. Those side effects that do occur are mild and temporary. The possible side effects include
- Soreness, swelling, and redness where the shot was given
- A mild-to-moderate fever
- Fussiness

These symptoms may begin within 24 hours after the shot and usually go away within 48 to 72 hours.

Talk to your pediatrician to see if your child should be vaccinated for pneumococcal infection and about the possible reactions to these immunizations.

The information contained in this publication should not be used as a substitute for the medical care and advice of your pediatrician. There may be variations in treatment that your pediatrician may recommend based on individual facts and circumstances.

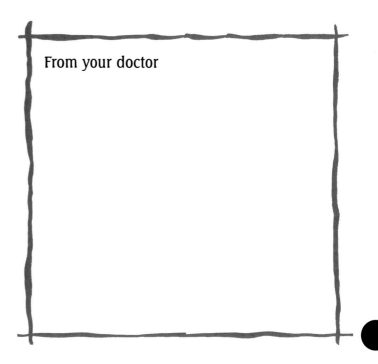

From your doctor

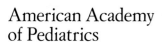

American Academy of Pediatrics

DEDICATED TO THE HEALTH OF ALL CHILDREN™

The American Academy of Pediatrics is an organization of 55,000 primary care pediatricians, pediatric medical subspecialists, and pediatric surgical specialists dedicated to the health, safety, and well-being of infants, children, adolescents, and young adults.

American Academy of Pediatrics
PO Box 747
Elk Grove Village, IL 60009-0747
Web site — http://www.aap.org

Pneumococcal Vaccine Information Sheet

Child's Name _____

Birth Date _____ Date _____

For children up to 2 years of age

- Your child has just been given the (1st, 2nd, 3rd, 4th) dose of the Heptavalent Pneumococcal Conjugate Vaccine (Prevnar or PCV7) for protection against pneumococcal infections.

Immunization Schedule

Prevnar or PCV7   2 months
4 months
6 months
12–15 months

If your child is late getting the first pneumococcal conjugate dose, the total number of doses received may differ from this AAP schedule.

For children between 2 and 5 years of age

- Your child has just been given a single dose of Heptavalent Pneumococcal Conjugate Vaccine (Prevnar or PCV7).
- Your child has just been given a single dose of 23-Valent Pneumococcal Polysaccharide Vaccine (23PS).

Immunization with PCV7 is recommended for children 2 to 5 years of age who are at high risk for pneumococcal infections. 23PS also is recommended for this group. *The type of vaccine and schedule for doses may vary depending on previous immunizations.*

Either pneumococcal vaccine may be given at the same time as other recommended vaccines, but should be injected in a separate site.

Most children have no side effects with pneumococcal vaccines. Those side effects that do occur are usually mild or temporary. Children may experience

- Soreness, swelling, and redness where the shot was given
- A mild-to-moderate fever
- Fussiness

These symptoms may begin within 24 hours after the shot is given and usually go away within 48 to 72 hours.

If you suspect there is a serious problem with your child following this immunization, please call my office. Your child will be examined and treated if necessary.

Dr Name _____

Address _____

_____

Telephone _____

Your child's next immunization for pneumococcal vaccine is scheduled at age _____

The information contained in this publication should not be used as a substitute for the medical care and advice of your pediatrician.
There may be variations in treatment that your pediatrician may recommend based on individual facts and circumstances.

From your doctor

American Academy of Pediatrics

DEDICATED TO THE HEALTH OF ALL CHILDREN™

The American Academy of Pediatrics is an organization of 55,000 primary care pediatricians, pediatric medical subspecialists, and pediatric surgical specialists dedicated to the health, safety, and well-being of infants, children, adolescents, and young adults.

American Academy of Pediatrics
PO Box 747
Elk Grove Village, IL 60009-0747
Web site — http://www.aap.org

POLIO VACCINE

WHAT YOU NEED TO KNOW

1 | What is polio?

Polio is a disease caused by a virus. It enters a child's (or adult's) body through the mouth. Sometimes it does not cause serious illness. But sometimes it causes *paralysis* (can't move arm or leg). It can kill people who get it, usually by paralyzing the muscles that help them breathe.

Polio used to be very common in the United States. It paralyzed and killed thousands of people a year before we had a vaccine for it.

2 | Why get vaccinated?

Inactivated Polio Vaccine (IPV) can prevent polio.

History: A 1916 polio epidemic in the Unites States killed 6,000 people and paralyzed 27,000 more. In the early 1950's there were more than 20,000 cases of polio each year. **Polio vaccination was begun in 1955.** By 1960 the number of cases had dropped to about 3,000, and by 1979 there were only about 10. The success of polio vaccination in the U.S. and other countries sparked a world-wide effort to eliminate polio.

Today: No wild polio has been reported in the United States for over 20 years. But the disease is still common in some parts of the world. It would only take one case of polio from another country to bring the disease back if we were not protected by vaccine. If the effort to eliminate the disease from the world is successful, some day we won't need polio vaccine. Until then, we need to keep getting our children vaccinated.

3 | Who should get polio vaccine and when?

IPV is a shot, given in the leg or arm, depending on age. Polio vaccine may be given at the same time as other vaccines.

Children
Most people should get polio vaccine when they are children. Children get 4 doses of IPV, at these ages:
- ✓ A dose at 2 months
- ✓ A dose at 4 months
- ✓ A dose at 6-18 months
- ✓ A booster dose at 4-6 years

Adults
Most adults do not need polio vaccine because they were already vaccinated as children. But three groups of adults are at higher risk and *should* consider polio vaccination:
(1) people traveling to areas of the world where polio is common,
(2) laboratory workers who might handle polio virus, and
(3) health care workers treating patients who could have polio.

Adults in these three groups who **have never been vaccinated against polio** should get 3 doses of IPV:
- ✓ The first dose at any time,
- ✓ The second dose 1 to 2 months later,
- ✓ The third dose 6 to 12 months after the second.

Adults in these three groups who **have had 1 or 2 doses** of polio vaccine in the past should get the remaining 1 or 2 doses. It doesn't matter how long it has been since the earlier dose(s).

Adults in these three groups who **have had 3 or more doses** of polio vaccine (either IPV or OPV) in the past may get a booster dose of IPV.

Ask your health care provider for more information.

Oral Polio Vaccine: No longer recommended

There are two kinds of polio vaccine: **IPV**, which is the shot recommended in the United States today, and a live, oral polio vaccine (**OPV**), which is drops that are swallowed.

Until recently OPV was recommended for most children in the United States. OPV helped us rid the country of polio, and it is still used in many parts of the world.

Both vaccines give immunity to polio, but OPV is better at keeping the disease from spreading to other people. However, for a few people (about one in 2.4 million), OPV actually causes polio. Since the risk of getting polio in the United States is now extremely low, experts believe that using oral polio vaccine is no longer worth the slight risk, except in limited circumstances which your doctor can describe. The polio shot (IPV) does not cause polio. **If you or your child will be getting OPV, ask for a copy of the OPV supplemental Vaccine Information Statement.**

Polio - 1/1/2000

4 | Some people should not get IPV or should wait.

These people should not get IPV:

- Anyone who has ever had a life-threatening allergic reaction to the antibiotics **neomycin, streptomycin** or **polymyxin B** should not get the polio shot.

- Anyone who has a severe allergic reaction to a polio shot should not get another one.

These people should wait:

- Anyone who is moderately or severely ill at the time the shot is scheduled should usually wait until they recover before getting polio vaccine. People with minor illnesses, such as a cold, *may* be vaccinated.

Ask your health care provider for more information.

5 | What are the risks from IPV?

Some people who get IPV get a sore spot where the shot was given. The vaccine used today has never been known to cause any serious problems, and most people don't have any problems at all with it.

However, a vaccine, like any medicine, could cause serious problems, such as a severe allergic reaction. *The risk of a polio shot causing serious harm, or death, is extremely small.*

6 | What if there is a serious reaction?

What should I look for?
Look for any unusual condition, such as a serious allergic reaction, high fever, or unusual behavior.

If a serious allergic reaction occurred, it would happen within a few minutes to a few hours after the shot. Signs of a serious allergic reaction can include difficulty breathing, weakness, hoarseness or wheezing, a fast heart beat, hives, dizziness, paleness, or swelling of the throat

What should I do?
- Call a doctor, or get the person to a doctor right away.

- Tell your doctor what happened, the date and time it happened, and when the vaccination was given.

- Ask your doctor, nurse, or health department to file a Vaccine Adverse Event Reporting System (VAERS) form, or call the VAERS toll-free number yourself at **1-800-822-7967**.

Reporting reactions helps experts learn about possible problems with vaccines.

7 | The National Vaccine Injury Compensation Program

In the rare event that you or your child has a serious reaction to a vaccine, there is a federal program that can help pay for the care of those who have been harmed.

For details about the National Vaccine Injury Compensation Program, call **1-800-338-2382** or visit the program's website at **http://www.hrsa.gov/bhpr/vicp**

8 | How can I learn more?

- Ask your doctor or nurse. They can give you the vaccine package insert or suggest other sources of information.

- Call your local or state health department's immunization program.

- Contact the Centers for Disease Control and Prevention (CDC):
  - Call **1-800-232-2522** (English)
  - Call **1-800-232-0233** (Español)
  - Visit the National Immunization Program's website at **http://www.cdc.gov/nip**

U.S. DEPARTMENT OF HEALTH & HUMAN SERVICES
Centers for Disease Control and Prevention
National Immunization Program

Vaccine Information Statement
Polio (1/1/2000)   42 U.S.C. § 300aa-26

Reprinted by the American Academy of Pediatrics
Additional copies are available for purchase in pads of 100.
To order, contact: American Academy of Pediatrics
Division of Publications
PO Box 747
Elk Grove Village, IL 60009-0747
Web site - http://www.aap.org
Minimum Order 100   HE0115   Rev 1/00

TETANUS AND DIPHTHERIA VACCINE (Td)

What you need to know before you or your child gets the vaccine

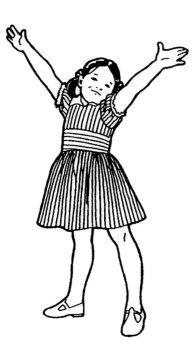

American Academy of Pediatrics

DEDICATED TO THE HEALTH OF ALL CHILDREN™

  CDC
CENTERS FOR DISEASE CONTROL AND PREVENTION

U.S. DEPARTMENT OF HEALTH & HUMAN SERVICES
Public Health Service
Centers for Disease Control and Prevention

ABOUT THE DISEASES

Tetanus (lockjaw) and diphtheria are serious diseases. Tetanus is caused by a germ that enters the body through a cut or wound. Diphtheria spreads when germs pass from an infected person to the nose or throat of others.

Tetanus causes:	**Diphtheria causes:**
serious, painful spasms of all muscles	a thick coating in the nose, throat, or airway
It can lead to:	**It can lead to:**
- "locking" of the jaw so the patient cannot open his or her mouth or swallow	- breathing problems - heart failure - paralysis - death

ABOUT THE VACCINES

Benefits of the vaccines

Vaccination is the best way to protect against tetanus and diphtheria. Because of vaccination, there are many fewer cases of these diseases. Cases are rare in children because most get DTP (Diphtheria, Tetanus, and Pertussis), DTaP (Diphtheria, Tetanus, and acellular Pertussis), or DT (Diphtheria and Tetanus) vaccines. There would be many more cases if we stopped vaccinating people.

When should you get Td vaccine?

Td is made for people 7 years of age and older.

People who have not gotten at least 3 doses of any tetanus and diphtheria vaccine (DTP, DTaP, or DT) during their lifetime should do so using Td, After a person gets the third dose, a Td dose is needed every 10 years all through life.

Other vaccines may be given at the same time as Td.

Tell your doctor or nurse if the person getting the vaccine:

• ever had a serious allergic reaction or other problem with Td, or any other tetanus and diphtheria vaccine (DTP, DTaP or DT)

• now has a moderate or severe illness

• is pregnant

It you are not sure, ask your doctor or nurse.

What are the risks from Td vaccine?

As with any medicine, there are very small risks that serious problems, even death, could occur after getting a vaccine.

The risks from the vaccine are <u>much</u> <u>smaller</u> than the risks from the diseases if people stopped using vaccine.

Almost all people who get Td have no problems from it.

Mild problems

If these problems occur, they usually start within hours to a day or two after vaccination. They may last 1-2 days:

- soreness, redness, or swelling where the shot was given

These problems can be worse in adults who get Td vaccine very often.

Acetaminophen or ibuprofen (non-aspirin) may be used to reduce soreness.

Severe problems

These problems happen **very rarely**:

- serious allergic reaction

- deep, aching pain and muscle wasting in upper arm(s). This starts 2 days to 4 weeks after the shot, and may last many months.

What to do if there is a serious reaction:

✓ Call a doctor or get the person to a doctor right away.

✓ Write down what happened and the date and time it happened.

✓ Ask your doctor, nurse, or health department to file a Vaccine Adverse Event Report form or call:

(800) 822-7967 (toll-free)

The **National Vaccine Injury Compensation Program** gives compensation (payment) for persons thought to be injured by vaccines. For details call:

(800) 338-2382 (toll-free)

If you want to learn more, ask your doctor or nurse. She/he can give you the vaccine package insert or suggest other sources of information.

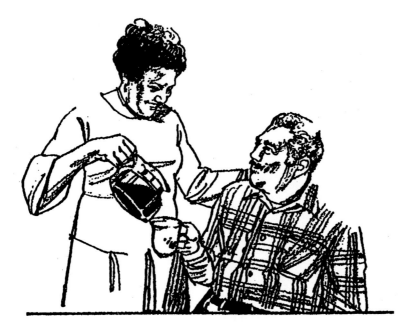

Reprinted by the American Academy of Pediatrics
Additional copies are available for purchase in pads of 100.
To order, contact:
American Academy of Pediatrics
Division of Publications
PO Box 747
Elk Grove Village, IL 60009-0747
Web site - http://www.aap.org
Minimum Order 100
HE0144
(Rev. 6/99)

SECTION TEN

Promoting Pediatric Care

How Special Is Your Child?

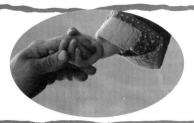

Special enough to be cared for by a doctor who only sees children and youth? Special enough to be cared for by a physician trained and experienced in the physical, mental, emotional, and social development of children and youth?

Special enough to be cared for as a child, not as a small adult?

Special enough to be cared for by a doctor who has had 3 to 6 years of pediatric training after medical school and has passed rigorous tests to be certified as a pediatrician?

Special enough to be treated with respect as an individual and as a person entitled to special care?

If you answered yes to all the above, WELCOME, You've come to the right place.

Your Child Deserves the Best in Pediatric Primary Care and Pediatric Subspecialty Care

Pediatricians spend as much as 3 to 6 years in pediatric training after medical school. That equals up to 24 times more training in the care of children than other physicians who receive an average of 3 additional months of pediatric training after medical school.

More Training in Caring for Children

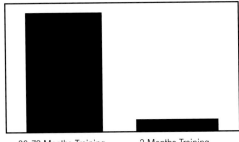

36-72 Months Training - Pediatricians/Pediatric Subspecialists

3 Months Training - Other Physicians

Cutting Edge Knowledge

Pediatricians see only children and youth. Constant changes in medicine can make it difficult to stay up to date. Pediatricians stay current by concentrating their efforts on changes in medicine affecting children.

Quality Primary Care

Pediatricians are trained to provide comprehensive care for children, including preventive care. Pediatricians often work in teams with other professionals, including nurse practitioners, to provide high-quality, cost-effective primary care. High-quality care leads to better outcomes for children and reduced costs for families and society.

Quality Pediatric Subspecialty Care

Pediatric subspecialists have an additional 24 to 36 months of in-depth fellowship training in addition to their 36 to 48 months of pediatric residency, concentrating on clinical and research aspects of specific areas of diseases of children and youth. A child's heart, lungs, kidneys, gastrointestinal system, and nervous system can have different problems than those organs of adults. Children with such problems may require referral by their pediatrician to pediatric medical and surgical subspecialists who have the training and knowledge to take care of these SPECIAL problems in the best manner possible.

Pediatricians Specialize in the Care of Children and Youth

Pediatricians are trained to:

- *Help* you determine healthy lifestyles for your child and useful ways to role model your choices.
- *Offer* advice to prevent illness and injuries.
- *Provide* early and appropriate care of acute illness to prevent its progression.
- *Treat* life-threatening childhood conditions requiring intensive care.
- *Guide* you in anticipating your child's needs from newborn to 21.

Experience

As part of their extensive training, pediatricians are experienced in the physical, emotional, and social development of children. Children may be too young or shy to talk so pediatricians understand the importance of listening carefully to your child, and to you. Pediatricians answer your questions, helping you to understand and promote your child's healthy development. Pediatricians also address issues affecting a child's family and home environment.

Pediatricians understand that children are not simply small adults.

They often present different symptoms from adults. They may need different prescriptions or treatments than adults. Pediatricians are specially trained to recognize the importance of these differences, especially with young children and newborns.

Pediatricians Are Great Advocates!

The American Academy of Pediatrics is highly respected for its child advocacy work. The Academy works to:

- Assure universal health care for all children from birth to 21 years and for all pregnant women.
- See that all immunizations are fully paid for by state and private insurance.
- Reduce the number of intentional and unintentional injuries, including those associated with alcohol and substance abuse.
- Promote healthy lifestyles for children and adolescents.
- Promote health education in schools.
- Increase access to health care for all children, including those with special needs and the homeless.
- Assure health and safety standards in child care settings.

By selecting a Board-Certified Pediatrician, you will have chosen the highest level of medical care for your child.

The information contained in this publication should not be used as a substitute for the medical care and advice of your pediatrician. There may be variations in treatment that your pediatrician may recommend based on individual facts and circumstances.

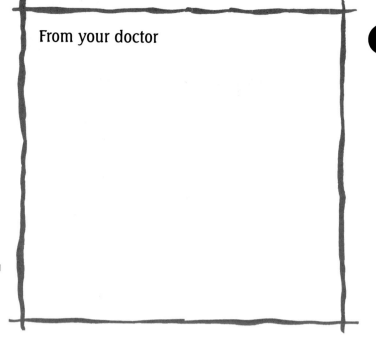

From your doctor

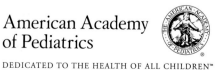

American Academy of Pediatrics

DEDICATED TO THE HEALTH OF ALL CHILDREN™

The American Academy of Pediatrics is an organization of 55,000 primary care pediatricians, pediatric medical subspecialists, and pediatric surgical specialists dedicated to the health, safety, and well-being of infants, children, adolescents, and young adults.

American Academy of Pediatrics
PO Box 747
Elk Grove Village, IL 60009-0747
Web site — http://www.aap.org

Copyright ©1998   American Academy of Pediatrics

What is a Pediatric Allergist/ Immunologist?

If your child suffers from allergies or other problems with his immune system, a *pediatric allergist/immunologist* has special skills to treat your child.

Your child's immune system fights infections. If your child has allergies, her immune system wrongly reacts to things that are usually harmless. Pet dander, pollen, dust, mold spores, insect stings, food, and medications are examples of such things. This reaction may cause her body to respond with health problems such as asthma, hay fever, hives, eczema (a rash), or a very severe and unusual reaction called anaphylaxis.

Sometimes, if your child's immune system is not working right, he may suffer from frequent, severe, and/or uncommon infections. Examples of such infections are sinusitis (inflammation of one or more of the sinuses), pneumonia (infection of the lung), thrush (a fungus infection in the mouth), and abscesses (collections of pus surrounded by inflamed tissue) that keep coming back.

A pediatric allergist/immunologist finds and treats these allergies and immune system problems.

What kind of training do pediatric allergists/ immunologists have?

Pediatric allergists/immunologists are medical doctors who have had
- At least 4 years of medical school
- Three years of primary care pediatric residency training
- At least 2 to 3 more years of study in an allergy and immunology program
- Certification from the American Board of Allergy and Immunology

Pediatric allergists/immunologists treat children from birth through the teenage years. Their choice to specialize in pediatric allergy and immunology equips them to provide the most experience in dealing with the unique medical needs of children who have allergies and immune system problems.

What types of treatments do pediatric allergists/ immunologists provide?

Pediatric allergists/immunologists generally provide treatment for the following:
- Asthma
- Hay fever (allergic rhinitis)
- Sinusitis
- Eczema (atopic dermatitis)
- Hives (urticaria, welts)
- Severe reactions to foods, insect stings, and medications (anaphylaxis)
- Immune disorders that lead to the following:
  - Frequent sinusitis, pneumonia, or diarrhea
  - Thrush and abscesses that keep coming back
  - Severe, unusual infections

Pediatric allergists/immunologists diagnose allergic conditions by using special testing. Newer forms of these tests may be almost painless. Treatment may combine avoiding things that cause symptoms, immunotherapy (allergy shots), or medication. Tests and effective treatments also are available for various causes of a weakened immune system.

Where can I find a pediatric allergist/immunologist?

Pediatric allergists/immunologists practice in a variety of medical settings. These include children's hospitals, university medical centers, large community hospitals, and private offices. Ask your pediatrician or a local children's hospital to help you find an allergist/immunologist who works with children.

Pediatric allergists/immunologists — specialized care for children

Children are not just small adults. They cannot always tell us what is bothering them. They cannot always answer medical questions. They are not always able to be patient and cooperative during a medical examination.

Pediatric allergists/immunologists know how to examine and treat children in a way that helps them relax and cooperate. Their goal is to identify the causes of these disorders in your child, and to offer ways to decrease symptoms so that your child can live a healthier life.

If your pediatrician suggests that your child see a pediatric allergist/ immunologist, you can be assured that she will get expert care. That care will include the most up-to-date treatment and therapy options to improve your child's quality of life.

The information contained in this publication should not be used as a substitute for the medical care and advice of your pediatrician. There may be variations in treatment that your pediatrician may recommend based on individual facts and circumstances.

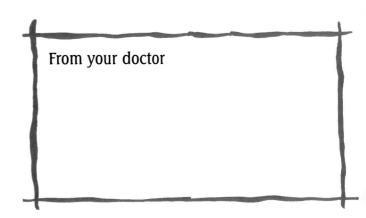

From your doctor

American Academy of Pediatrics

DEDICATED TO THE HEALTH OF ALL CHILDREN™

The American Academy of Pediatrics is an organization of 55,000 primary care pediatricians, pediatric medical subspecialists, and pediatric surgical specialists dedicated to the health, safety, and well-being of infants, children, adolescents, and young adults.

American Academy of Pediatrics
PO Box 747
Elk Grove Village, IL 60009-0747
Web site — http://www.aap.org

What is a Pediatric Anesthesiologist?

If your child has an illness, injury, or disease that requires surgery, a *Pediatric Anesthesiologist* has the experience and qualifications to assist in the treatment and to help ensure a successful surgery for your child.

A pediatric anesthesiologist is a fully trained anesthesiologist who has completed at least 1 year of specialized training in anesthesia care of infants and children. Most pediatric surgeons deliver care to children in the operating room along with a pediatric anesthesiologist. Many children who need surgery have very complex medical problems that affect many parts of the body. The pediatric anesthesiologist is best qualified to evaluate these complex problems and plan a safe anesthetic for each child. Through special training and experience, pediatric anesthesiologists provide the safest care for infants and children undergoing anesthesia.

What kind of training do pediatric anesthesiologists have?

Pediatric anesthesiologists are physicians who have had

- At least 4 years of medical school
- One year of internship and 3 years of residency in anesthesiology
- Additional specialty training in pediatric anesthesiology
- Certification from the American Board of Anesthesiologists

Pediatric anesthesiologists treat children from the newborn period through the teenage years. They choose to make pediatric care the core of their medical practice, and the unique nature of medical and surgical care of children is learned from advanced training and experience in practice.

What types of treatments do pediatric anesthesiologists provide?

Pediatric anesthesiologists are responsible for the general anesthesia, sedation, and pain management needs of infants and children. Pediatric anesthesiologists generally provide the following services:

- Evaluation of complex medical problems in infants and children when surgery is needed
- Planning and care for before and after surgery
- A nonthreatening environment for children in the operating room
- Pain control, if needed after surgery, either with intravenous (IV) medications or other anesthetic techniques
- Anesthesia and sedation for many procedures out of the operating room such as MRI, CT scan, and radiation therapy.

Where can I find a pediatric anesthesiologist?

Pediatric anesthesiologists practice in a variety of medical institutions including children's hospitals, university medical centers, and large community hospitals.

Pediatric anesthesiologists — the best care for children

Children are not just small adults. They cannot always say what is bothering them. They cannot always answer medical questions, and are not always able to be patient and cooperative during a medical examination. Pediatric anesthesiologists know how to examine and treat children in a way that makes them relaxed and cooperative. In addition, pediatric anesthesiologists use equipment and facilities specifically designed for children. Most pediatric anesthesiology offices are arranged and decorated with children in mind. This includes the examination rooms and waiting rooms, which may have toys and reading materials for children. This helps create a comfortable and nonthreatening environment for your child.

If your pediatrician suggests that your child see a pediatric anesthesiologist, you can be assured that he or she has the widest range of treatment options, the most extensive and complete training, and the greatest expertise in dealing with children and their anesthesiology needs.

The information contained in this publication should not be used as a substitute for the medical care and advice of your pediatrician. There may be variations in treatment that your pediatrician may recommend based on individual facts and circumstances.

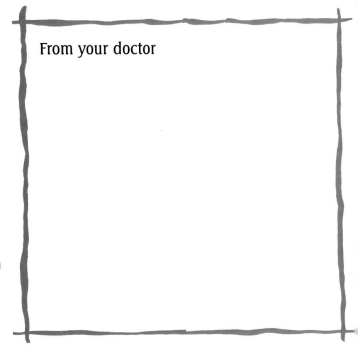

From your doctor

American Academy of Pediatrics

DEDICATED TO THE HEALTH OF ALL CHILDREN™

The American Academy of Pediatrics is an organization of 55,000 primary care pediatricians, pediatric medical subspecialists, and pediatric surgical specialists dedicated to the health, safety, and well-being of infants, children, adolescents, and young adults.

American Academy of Pediatrics
PO Box 747
Elk Grove Village, IL 60009-0747
Web site — http://www.aap.org

What is a Pediatric Neurosurgeon?

If your child has problems involving the head, spine, or nervous system, a *Pediatric Neurosurgeon* has the experience and qualifications to treat your child.

Neurosurgical problems seen by pediatric neurosurgeons are often quite different from those commonly seen by adult or general neurosurgeons. Special training in pediatric diseases as they relate to pediatric neurosurgical diseases is important. Pediatric neurosurgical problems often are present for life. Pediatric neurosurgeons have a special and long-standing relationship with their patients. Children with nervous system problems frequently require ongoing and close follow-up throughout childhood and adolescence.

What kind of training do pediatric neurosurgeons have?

Pediatric neurosurgeons are medical doctors who have had
- At least 4 years of medical school
- One year of surgical internship
- Five or more years of residency training in neurological surgery
- Additional training in pediatric neurosurgery
- Certification from the American Board of Neurological Surgery and the American Board of Pediatric Neurological Surgery

Pediatric neurosurgeons treat children from the newborn period through the teenage years. They choose to make pediatric care the core of their medical practice, and the unique nature of medical and surgical care of children is learned from advanced training and experience in practice.

What types of treatments do pediatric neurosurgeons provide?

Pediatric neurosurgeons diagnose, treat, and manage children's nervous system problems and head and spinal deformities including the following:
- Head deformities
- Spine deformities
- Problems and injuries of the brain, spine, or nerves
- Gait abnormalities (spasticity)
- Birth injuries (weakness of arms and legs)

Where can I find a pediatric neurosurgeon?

Pediatric neurosurgeons practice in a variety of medical institutions including children's hospitals, university medical centers, and large community hospitals. The American Board of Pediatric Neurological Surgery Web site (www.abpns.org) maintains a list of all board certified pediatric neurosurgeons.

Pediatric neurosurgeons — the best care for children

Children are not just small adults. They cannot always say what is bothering them. They cannot always answer medical questions, and are not always able to be patient and cooperative during a medical examination. Pediatric neurosurgeons know how to examine and treat children in a way that makes them relaxed and cooperative. In addition, pediatric neurosurgeons use equipment and facilities specifically designed for children. Most pediatric neurosurgery offices are arranged and decorated with children in mind. This includes the examination rooms and waiting rooms, which may have toys, videos, and reading materials for children. This helps create a comfortable and non-threatening environment for your child.

The pediatric neurosurgeon will provide the diagnostic and surgical interventions in a hospital that has the support services, pediatric physicians, and nurses necessary for the care of your child. Children with special needs require that the pediatric neurosurgeon work closely with the primary care pediatrician and the pediatric specialist to provide coordinated and comprehensive care of the child.

If your pediatrician suggests that your child see a pediatric neurosurgeon, you can be assured that he or she has the widest range of treatment options, the most extensive and complete training, and the greatest expertise in dealing with children and in treating neurosurgical problems.

From your doctor

The American Academy of Pediatrics is an organization of 55,000 primary care pediatricians, pediatric medical subspecialists, and pediatric surgical specialists dedicated to the health, safety, and well-being of infants, children, adolescents, and young adults.

American Academy of Pediatrics
PO Box 747
Elk Grove Village, IL 60009-0747
Web site — http://www.aap.org

American Academy of Pediatrics

DEDICATED TO THE HEALTH OF ALL CHILDREN™

What is a Pediatric Ophthalmologist?

If your child has an eye problem, is having difficulty with a vision screening exam or has difficulty reading or learning, or needs surgery or medical treatment for an illness affecting the eyes, a *Pediatric Ophthalmologist* has the experience and qualifications to treat your child.

What kind of training do pediatric ophthalmologists have?

Pediatric ophthalmologists are medical doctors who have had

- At least 4 years of medical school
- One year of medical or surgical internship
- At least 3 additional years of residency training in ophthalmology
- At least 1 additional year of fellowship training in pediatric ophthalmology

What types of treatments do pediatric ophthalmologists provide?

Pediatric ophthalmologists can diagnose, treat, and manage all children's eye problems. Pediatric ophthalmologists generally provide the following services:

- Eye exams
- Perform surgery, microsurgery, and laser surgery (for problems like weak eye muscles, crossed eyes, wandering eyes, blocked tear ducts, retinal problems, and infections)
- Diagnose problems of the eye caused by diseases of the body such as diabetes or juvenile rheumatoid arthritis (JRA) and other medical and neurological diseases
- Diagnose visual processing disorders
- Care for eye injuries
- Prescribe eyeglasses and contact lenses

Where can I find a pediatric ophthalmologist?

Pediatric ophthalmologists practice in a variety of medical institutions including children's hospitals, university medical centers, and large community hospitals.

Pediatric ophthalmologists — the best care for children

Children are not just small adults. They cannot always say what is bothering them. They cannot always answer medical questions, and are not always able to be patient and cooperative during a medical examination. Pediatric ophthalmolo-

gists know how to examine and treat children in a way that makes them relaxed and cooperative. In addition, pediatric ophthalmologists use equipment specially designed for children. Most pediatric ophthalmologists' offices are arranged and decorated with children in mind. This includes the examination rooms and waiting rooms, which may have toys, videos, and reading materials for children. This helps create a comfortable and nonthreatening environment for your child.

If your pediatrician suggests that your child have his eyes checked, a pediatric ophthalmologist has the widest range of treatment options, the most extensive and comprehensive training, and the greatest expertise in dealing with children and in treating children's eye disorders.

The information contained in this publication should not be used as a substitute for the medical care and advice of your pediatrician. There may be variations in treatment that your pediatrician may recommend based on individual facts and circumstances.

From your doctor

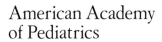

What is a Pediatric Orthopedic Surgeon?

If your child has musculoskeletal (bone) problems, a *Pediatric Orthopedic Surgeon* has the experience and qualifications to treat your child.

What kind of training do pediatric orthopedic surgeons have?

Pediatric orthopedic surgeons are medical doctors who have

- Graduated from an approved medical school
- Graduated from an approved orthopedic surgery residency program
- Completed additional subspecialty training in pediatric orthopedics
  Pediatric orthopedic surgeons treat children from the newborn stage through the teenage years. They choose to make pediatric care the core of their medical practice, and the unique nature of medical and surgical care of children is learned from advanced training and experience in practice.

What types of treatments do pediatric orthopedic surgeons provide?

Pediatric orthopedic surgeons diagnose, treat, and manage children's musculoskeletal problems including the following:

- Limb and spine deformities (such as club foot, scoliosis)
- Gait abnormalities (limping)
- Bone and joint infections
- Broken bones

Where can I find a pediatric orthopedic surgeon?

Pediatric orthopedic surgeons practice in a variety of medical institutions including children's hospitals, university medical centers, and large community hospitals.

Pediatric orthopedic surgeons — the best care for children

Children are not just small adults. They cannot always say what is bothering them. They cannot always answer medical questions, and are not always able to be patient and cooperative during a medical examination. Pediatric orthopedic surgeons know how to examine and treat children in a way that makes them relaxed and cooperative. In addition, pediatric orthopedic surgeons often use

equipment specially designed for children. Most pediatric orthopedic surgeons' offices are arranged and decorated with children in mind. This includes the examination rooms and waiting rooms, which may have toys, videos, and reading materials for children. This helps create a comfortable and nonthreatening environment for your child.

If your pediatrician suggests that your child see a pediatric orthopedic surgeon, you can be assured that he or she has the widest range of treatment options, the most extensive and comprehensive training, and the greatest expertise in dealing with children and in treating children's orthopedic disorders.

The information contained in this publication should not be used as a substitute for the medical care and advice of your pediatrician. There may be variations in treatment that your pediatrician may recommend based on individual facts and circumstances.

From your doctor

American Academy of Pediatrics

DEDICATED TO THE HEALTH OF ALL CHILDREN™

The American Academy of Pediatrics is an organization of 55,000 primary care pediatricians, pediatric medical subspecialists, and pediatric surgical specialists dedicated to the health, safety, and well-being of infants, children, adolescents, and young adults.

American Academy of Pediatrics
PO Box 747
Elk Grove Village, IL 60009-0747
Web site — http://www.aap.org

Copyright © 2000   American Academy of Pediatrics

What is a Pediatric Otolaryngologist?

If your child needs surgical or complex medical treatment for illnesses or problems affecting the ear, nose, or throat, a *Pediatric Otolaryngologist* has the experience and qualifications to treat your child. Many general otolaryngologists provide surgical care for children. However, in many areas of the country, more specialized otolaryngology care is available for children.

What kind of training do pediatric otolaryngologists have?

Pediatric otolaryngologists are medical doctors who have had

- At least 4 years of medical school
- One year of surgical internship
- Often 1 additional year of residency training in general surgery
- At least 3 to 4 additional years of residency training in otolaryngology and head and neck surgery
- Pediatric otolaryngologists often complete additional training in fellowship programs at a large children's medical center

Pediatric otolaryngologists treat children from the newborn period through the teenage years. They choose to make pediatric care the core of their medical practice, and the unique nature of medical and surgical care of children is learned from advanced training and experience in practice.

What types of treatments do pediatric otolaryngologists provide?

Pediatric otolaryngologists are primarily concerned with medical and surgical treatment of ear, nose, and throat diseases in children. Pediatric otolaryngologists generally provide the following services:

- Diagnosis and treatment of ear, nose, and throat disorders, and head and neck diseases
- Surgery of the head and neck, including before- and after-surgery care
- Consultation with other doctors when ear, nose, or throat diseases are detected
- Assistance in the identification of communication disorders in children

Where can I find a pediatric otolaryngologist?

Pediatric otolaryngologists practice in a variety of medical institutions including children's hospitals, university medical centers, and large community hospitals.

Pediatric otolaryngologists — the best care for children

Children are not just small adults. They cannot always say what is bothering them. They cannot always answer medical questions, and are not always able to be patient and cooperative during a medical examination. Pediatric otolaryngologists know how to examine and treat children in a way that makes them relaxed and cooperative. In addition, pediatric otolaryngologists use equipment specially designed for children. Most pediatric otolaryngologists' offices are arranged and decorated with children in mind. This includes the examination rooms and waiting rooms, which may have toys, videos, and reading materials for children. This helps create a comfortable and nonthreatening environment for your child.

If your pediatrician suggests that your child see a specialist for a problem with his ears, nose, or throat, a pediatric otolaryngologist has the widest range of treatment options, the most extensive and comprehensive training, and the greatest expertise in dealing with children and in treating children's ear, nose, and throat disorders.

The information contained in this publication should not be used as a substitute for the medical care and advice of your pediatrician. There may be variations in treatment that your pediatrician may recommend based on individual facts and circumstances.

From your doctor

American Academy of Pediatrics

DEDICATED TO THE HEALTH OF ALL CHILDREN™

The American Academy of Pediatrics is an organization of 55,000 primary care pediatricians, pediatric medical subspecialists, and pediatric surgical specialists dedicated to the health, safety, and well-being of infants, children, adolescents, and young adults.

American Academy of Pediatrics
PO Box 747
Elk Grove Village, IL 60009-0747
Web site — http://www.aap.org

What is a Pediatric Plastic Surgeon?

If your child needs surgery to fix a deformity caused by a birth defect, injury, illness, or tumor, a *Pediatric Plastic Surgeon* has the experience and qualifications to treat your child.

All children become ill or injured at one time or another. Most problems are simple and can be solved by your pediatrician. At times, however, special care from a pediatric plastic surgeon may be needed and may make the difference in achieving the best possible cosmetic result. If you think your child needs this kind of special care, request a visit with a pediatric plastic surgeon.

What kind of training do pediatric plastic surgeons have?

Pediatric plastic surgeons are medical doctors who have had

- At least 4 years of medical school
- Three years of residency training in general surgery, or completion of a residency training program in general surgery, otolaryngology, urology, orthopedic surgery, neurosurgery, or a combined general surgery/oral surgery residency
- Up to 3 years of additional training in plastic surgery
- Additional training in pediatric plastic surgery
- Certification from the American Board of Plastic Surgery

Pediatric plastic surgeons treat children from birth through young adulthood. They choose to make pediatric care the core of their medical practice, and devote 50% or more of their time to the care of children.

What types of treatments do pediatric plastic surgeons provide?

Pediatric plastic surgeons generally provide treatment for the following:

- Birth defects of the face and skull (cleft lip and palate, misshapen skull)
- Birth defects of the ear (protruding or absent ear)
- Birth defects of the chest and limbs (misshapen breasts, webbed fingers)
- Injuries to the head, face, hands, arms, and legs
- Birthmarks and scars
- Burns
- Cosmetic surgery to improve a child's self-image

Where can I find a pediatric plastic surgeon?

Pediatric plastic surgeons practice in children's hospitals, university medical centers, and large community hospitals. Your pediatrician will be able to recommend a plastic surgeon that works with children. Your family, friends, and co-workers may recommend a pediatric plastic surgeon, but it is important that you meet this doctor and review his or her credentials. Check with the plastic surgery department of a nearby university or with the county medical society.

Pediatric plastic surgeons — the best care for children

Children are not just small adults. They cannot always say what is bothering them. They cannot always answer medical questions, and are not always able to be patient and cooperative during a medical examination. Pediatric plastic surgeons know how to examine and treat children in a way that makes them relaxed and cooperative. In addition, pediatric plastic surgeons use equipment specifically designed for children. Most pediatric plastic surgery offices are arranged and decorated with children in mind. This includes the examination rooms and waiting rooms, which may have toys, videos, and books for children. This helps create a comfortable and nonthreatening environment for your child.

If your pediatrician suggests that your child see a pediatric plastic surgeon, you can be assured that he or she has the widest range of treatment options, the most extensive and complete training, and the greatest skill in dealing with children.

The information contained in this publication should not be used as a substitute for the medical care and advice of your pediatrician. There may be variations in treatment that your pediatrician may recommend based on individual facts and circumstances.

From your doctor

American Academy of Pediatrics

DEDICATED TO THE HEALTH OF ALL CHILDREN™

The American Academy of Pediatrics is an organization of 55,000 primary care pediatricians, pediatric medical subspecialists, and pediatric surgical specialists dedicated to the health, safety, and well-being of infants, children, adolescents, and young adults.

American Academy of Pediatrics
PO Box 747
Elk Grove Village, IL 60009-0747
Web site — http://www.aap.org

Copyright © 2000   American Academy of Pediatrics

What is a Pediatric Surgeon?

If your child has an illness, injury, or disease that requires surgery, a *Pediatric Surgeon* has the experience and qualifications to treat your child.

Surgical problems seen by pediatric surgeons are often quite different from those commonly seen by adult or general surgeons. Special training in pediatric surgery is important.

What kind of training do pediatric surgeons have?

Pediatric surgeons are medical doctors who have had

- At least 4 years of medical school
- Five additional years of general surgery
- Two additional years of residency training in pediatric surgery
- Certification by the American Board of Surgery

Pediatric surgeons treat children from the newborn stage through late adolescence. They choose to make pediatric care the core of their medical practice, and the unique nature of medical and surgical care of children is learned from advanced training and experience in practice.

What types of treatments do pediatric surgeons provide?

Pediatric surgeons diagnose, treat, and manage children's surgical needs including:

- Surgical repair of birth defects
- Serious injuries that require surgery (for example, liver lacerations, knife wounds, or gun shot wounds)
- Diagnosis and surgical care of tumors
- Transplantation operations
- Endoscopic procedures (bronchoscopy, esophagogastroduodenoscopy, colonoscopy)
- All other surgical procedures for children

Where can I find a pediatric surgeon?

Pediatric surgeons practice in a variety of medical institutions including children's hospitals, university medical centers, and large community hospitals.

Pediatric surgeons — the best care for children

Children are not just small adults. They cannot always say what is bothering them. They cannot always answer medical questions, and are not always able to be patient and helpful during a medical examination. Pediatric surgeons know how to examine and treat children in a way that makes them relaxed and cooperative. In addition, pediatric surgeons use equipment and facilities specifically designed for children. Most pediatric surgical offices are arranged and decorated with children in mind. This includes the examination rooms and waiting rooms, which may have toys, videos, and reading materials for children. This helps create a comfortable and nonthreatening environment for your child.

If your pediatrician suggests that your child see a pediatric surgeon, you can be assured that he or she has the widest range of treatment options, the most extensive and complete training, and the greatest expertise in dealing with children and in treating surgical disorders.

The information contained in this publication should not be used as a substitute for the medical care and advice of your pediatrician. There may be variations in treatment that your pediatrician may recommend based on individual facts and circumstances.

From your doctor

American Academy of Pediatrics

DEDICATED TO THE HEALTH OF ALL CHILDREN™

The American Academy of Pediatrics is an organization of 55,000 primary care pediatricians, pediatric medical subspecialists, and pediatric surgical specialists dedicated to the health, safety, and well-being of infants, children, adolescents, and young adults.

American Academy of Pediatrics
PO Box 747
Elk Grove Village, IL 60009-0747
Web site — http://www.aap.org

What is a Pediatric Surgical Specialist?

If your child needs an operation, your pediatrician will refer your child to a pediatric surgical specialist. This type of doctor has had special training and is experienced in children's surgical needs from birth to young adulthood.

There are a variety of pediatric surgical specialists including the following:

- Anesthesiologists
- General surgeons (includes neonatal, prenatal, trauma, and cancer surgeons)
- Neurosurgeons (brain and spinal cord surgeons)
- Ophthalmologists (eye surgeons)
- Orthopedic surgeons (bone surgeons)
- Otolaryngologists (ear, nose, and throat surgeons)
- Plastic surgeons
- Urologists (kidney, bladder, and genital surgeons)

Pediatric surgical specialists are the best choice if your child needs any type of surgery because they have the most experience in treating children. This comes from their years of specialized training, which includes

- At least 4 years of medical school
- One year of a surgical or medical internship
- Three to 5 years of residency training in their specialized area of surgery
- One to 2 additional years of fellowship training in their *pediatric* surgical specialty

Brief information on each type of pediatric surgical specialist follows. If you have additional questions, please talk to your pediatrician.

Pediatric Anesthesiologist

If your child has an illness, injury, or disease that requires surgery, a *Pediatric Anesthesiologist* has the experience and qualifications to assist in the treatment and to help ensure a successful surgery for your child.

A pediatric anesthesiologist is a fully trained anesthesiologist who has completed at least 1 year of specialized training in anesthesia care of infants and children. Most pediatric surgeons deliver care to children in the operating room along with a pediatric anesthesiologist. Many children who need surgery have complex medical problems that affect many parts of the body. The pediatric anesthesiologist is best qualified to evaluate these complex problems and plan a safe anesthetic for each child. Through special training and experience, pediatric anesthesiologists provide the safest care for infants and children undergoing anesthesia.

What types of treatments do pediatric anesthesiologists provide?

Pediatric anesthesiologists are primarily concerned with the anesthesia, sedation, and pain management needs of infants and children. Pediatric anesthesiologists generally provide the following services:

- Evaluation of complex medical problems in infants and children when surgery is necessary
- Planning and care for children before and after surgery
- A nonthreatening environment for children in the operating room
- Pain control, if needed after surgery, either with intravenous (IV) medications or other anesthetic techniques

- Anesthesia and sedation for many procedures out of the operating room such as MRI, CT scan, and radiation therapy

Pediatric Surgeon

If your child has an illness, injury, or disease that requires surgery, a *Pediatric Surgeon* has the experience and qualifications to treat your child.

Surgical problems seen by pediatric surgeons are often quite different from those commonly seen by adult or general surgeons. Special training in pediatric surgery is important.

What types of treatments do pediatric surgeons provide?

Pediatric surgeons diagnose, treat, and manage all children's surgical needs including the following:

- Surgical repair of birth defects
- Serious injuries that require surgery (for example, liver lacerations, knife wounds, or gun shot wounds)
- Diagnosis and surgical care of tumors
- Transplantation operations
- Endoscopic procedures (bronchoscopy, esophagogastroduodenoscopy, colonoscopy)
- All other surgical procedures for children.

Pediatric Neurosurgeon

If your child has problems involving the head, spine, or nervous system, a *Pediatric Neurosurgeon* has the experience and qualifications to treat your child.

Neurosurgical problems seen by pediatric neurosurgeons are often quite different from those commonly seen by adult or general neurosurgeons. Special training in pediatric diseases as they relate to pediatric neurosurgical diseases is important. Pediatric neurosurgical problems often are present for life. Pediatric neurosurgeons have a special and long-standing relationship with their patients. Children with nervous system problems frequently require ongoing and close follow-up throughout childhood and adolescence.

What types of treatments do pediatric neurosurgeons provide?

Pediatric neurosurgeons diagnose, treat, and manage all children's nervous system problems and head and spinal deformities including the following:

- Head deformities
- Spine deformities
- Problems and injuries of the brain, spine, or nerves
- Gait abnormalities (spasticity)
- Birth injuries (weakness of arms and legs)

Pediatric Ophthalmologist

If your child has an eye problem, is having difficulty with a vision screening exam, or needs surgery for an illness affecting the eyes, a *Pediatric Ophthalmologist* has the experience and qualifications to treat your child.

What types of treatments do pediatric ophthalmologists provide?

Pediatric ophthalmologists can diagnose, treat, and manage all children's eye problems. Pediatric ophthalmologists generally provide the following services:

- Eye exams
- Prescribe eyeglasses and contact lenses
- Perform surgery, microsurgery, and laser surgery of the eyes (for problems like weak eye muscles, crossed eyes, roving eyes, blocked tear ducts, and infections)
- Diagnose problems of the eye associated with diseases of the body, such as diabetes or juvenile rheumatoid arthritis (JRA)
- Diagnose visual processing disorders
- Care for eye injuries

Pediatric Orthopedic Surgeon

If your child has musculoskeletal (bone) problems, a *Pediatric Orthopedic Surgeon* has the experience and qualifications to treat your child.

What types of treatments do pediatric orthopedic surgeons provide?

Pediatric orthopedic surgeons diagnose, treat, and manage children's musculoskeletal problems including the following:

- Limb and spine deformities (such as club foot, scoliosis)
- Gait abnormalities (limping)
- Bone and joint infections
- Broken bones

Pediatric Otolaryngologist

If your child needs surgical or complex medical treatment for illnesses or problems affecting the ear, nose, or throat, a *Pediatric Otolaryngologist* has the experience and qualifications to treat your child. Many general otolaryngologists provide surgical care for children. However, in many areas of the country, more specialized otolaryngology care is available for children.

What types of treatments do pediatric otolaryngologists provide?

Pediatric otolaryngologists are primarily concerned with medical and surgical treatment of ear, nose, and throat diseases in children. Pediatric otolaryngologists generally provide the following services:

- Diagnosis and treatment of ear, nose, and throat disorders, and head and neck diseases
- Surgery of the head and neck, including before- and after-surgery care
- Consultation with other doctors when ear, nose, or throat diseases are detected
- Assistance in the identification of communication disorders in children

Pediatric Plastic Surgeon

If your child needs surgery to fix a deformity caused by a birth defect, injury, illness, or tumor, a *Pediatric Plastic Surgeon* has the experience and qualifications to treat your child.

What types of treatments do pediatric plastic surgeons provide?

- Pediatric plastic surgeons generally provide treatment for the following:
- Birth defects of the face and skull (cleft lip and palate, misshapen skull)
- Birth defects of the ear (protruding or absent ear)
- Birth defects of the chest and limbs (misshapen breasts, webbed fingers)
- Injuries to the head, face, hands, arms, and legs
- Birthmarks and scars
- Burns
- Cosmetic surgery to improve a child's self-image

Pediatric Urologist

If your child has an illness or disease of the genitals or the urinary tract (kidneys, ureters, and bladder), a *Pediatric Urologist* has the experience and qualifications to treat your child.

A pediatric urologist usually devotes a minimum of 50% of his or her practice to the urologic problems of infants, children, and adolescents.

What types of treatments do pediatric urologists provide?

Pediatric urologists are surgeons who can diagnose, treat, and manage children's urinary and genital problems. Pediatric urologists generally provide the following services:

- Evaluation and management of voiding disorders, vesicoureteral reflux, and urinary tract infections that require surgery
- Surgical reconstruction of the urinary tract (kidneys, ureters, and bladder) including genital abnormalities, hypospadias, and intersex conditions
- Surgery for groin conditions in childhood and adolescence (undescended testes, hydrocele/hernia, varicocele)

Pediatric surgical specialists — the best care for children

Children are not just small adults. They cannot always say what is bothering them. They cannot always answer medical questions, and they are not always able to be patient and cooperative during a medical examination. Pediatric surgical specialists know how to examine and treat children in a way that makes them relaxed and cooperative. In addition, pediatric surgical specialists use equipment specially designed for children. Most pediatric surgical specalists' offices are arranged and decorated with children in mind. This includes the examination rooms and waiting rooms, which may have toys and reading materials for children. This helps create a comfortable and nonthreatening environment for your child.

If your pediatrician suggests that your child see a pediatric surgical specialist, you can be assured that he or she has the widest range of treatment options, the most extensive and comprehensive training, and the greatest expertise in dealing with children and in treating children's surgical needs.

The information contained in this publication should not be used as a substitute for the medical care and advice of your pediatrician. There may be variations in treatment that your pediatrician may recommend based on individual facts and circumstances.

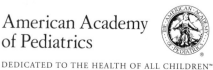

American Academy of Pediatrics

DEDICATED TO THE HEALTH OF ALL CHILDREN™

The American Academy of Pediatrics is an organization of 55,000 primary care pediatricians, pediatric medical subspecialists, and pediatric surgical specialists dedicated to the health, safety, and well-being of infants, children, adolescents, and young adults.

American Academy of Pediatrics
PO Box 747
Elk Grove Village, IL 60009-0747
Web site — http://www.aap.org

What is a Pediatric Urologist?

If your child has an illness or disease of the genitals or urinary tract (kidneys, ureters, bladder), a Pediatric Urologist has the experience and qualifications to treat your child.

What kind of training do pediatric urologists have?

Pediatric urologists are medical doctors who have had
- At least 4 years of medical school
- One year of surgical internship
- At least 3 additional years of residency training in general urology
- At least 1 additional year of fellowship training in pediatric urology

A pediatric urologist must devote a minimum of 50% of his or her practice to the urologic problems of infants, children, and adolescents.

What types of treatments do pediatric urologists provide?

Pediatric urologists are surgeons who can diagnose, treat, and manage children's urinary and genital problems. Pediatric urologists generally provide the following services:
- Evaluation and management of voiding disorders, vesicoureteral reflux, and urinary tract infections that require surgery
- Surgical reconstruction of the urinary tract (kidneys, ureters, and bladder) including genital abnormalities, hypospadias, and intersex conditions
- Surgery for groin conditions in childhood and adolescence (undescended testes, hydrocele/hernia, varicocele).

Where can I find a pediatric urologist?

Today, pediatric urologists can be found in almost every state and in virtually all of the major cities in the United States.

Pediatric urologists — the best care for children

Children are not just small adults. They cannot always say what is bothering them. They cannot always answer medical questions, and are not always able to be patient and cooperative during a medical examination. Pediatric urologists know how to examine and treat children in a way that makes them relaxed and cooperative. In addition, pediatric urologists often use equipment specially designed for children. Most pediatric urologists' offices are arranged and decorated with children in mind. This includes the examination rooms and waiting rooms, which may have toys, videos, and reading materials for children. This helps create a comfortable and nonthreatening environment for your child.

If your pediatrician suggests that your child see a pediatric urologist, you can be assured that he or she has the widest range of treatment options, the most extensive and comprehensive training, and the greatest expertise in dealing with children and in treating children's urinary tract disorders.

The information contained in this publication should not be used as a substitute for the medical care and advice of your pediatrician. There may be variations in treatment that your pediatrician may recommend based on individual facts and circumstances.

From your doctor

American Academy of Pediatrics

DEDICATED TO THE HEALTH OF ALL CHILDREN™

The American Academy of Pediatrics is an organization of 55,000 primary care pediatricians, pediatric medical subspecialists, and pediatric surgical specialists dedicated to the health, safety, and well-being of infants, children, adolescents, and young adults.

American Academy of Pediatrics
PO Box 747
Elk Grove Village, IL 60009-0747
Web site — http://www.aap.org

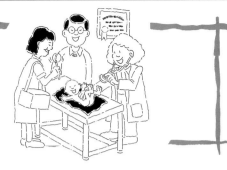

You and Your Pediatrician

The American Academy of Pediatrics (AAP) has developed this information to help you

- Choose a pediatrician.
- Prepare for office visits with your pediatrician.
- Know what to do if you have a question or an emergency health problem.

In choosing a pediatrician, you can know that an expert in children's health is treating your child.

Why your child needs a pediatrician

Children have different health care needs than adults—both medical and emotional. Pediatricians are trained to prevent and manage health problems in infants, children, teens, and young adults. Older patients trust their pediatricians, because they have known one another for many years.

Training

To become trained in pediatrics, a doctor must take special courses for 3 or more years after medical school. This is called *residency*. After residency, a doctor usually takes a long, detailed test given by the American Board of Pediatrics. After passing the test, the doctor is a board-certified pediatrician. He or she gets a certificate that you may see displayed at the office. The doctor can then become a Fellow (or member) of the American Academy of Pediatrics (FAAP). All of this background prepares your pediatrician to manage your child's total health care needs, including the following:

- Growth and development
- Illnesses
- Nutrition
- Immunizations
- Injuries
- Physical fitness

Your pediatrician will also work with you on other issues, such as the following:

- Behavior
- Emotional or family problems
- Learning and other school problems
- Preventing and dealing with drug abuse
- Puberty and other teen concerns
- Television, the Internet, and other media

Pediatricians also work with teachers and other adults in child care centers, schools, and after-school programs. If your child has a very special or complex problem, your pediatrician can refer her to another specialist for further help, if needed.

In addition, your pediatrician can advise you about complementary and alternative medicine treatments and which treatments are safe for children. It is important that your pediatrician be aware of all uses of complementary and alternative medicines. Some can result in serious side effects when used along with conventional medicine.

Finding the right pediatrician for your child

Do not wait until your child is sick or needs a checkup to choose a pediatrician. Even if you recently moved, are changing insurance, or are having a baby, it is best to find a pediatrician as soon as you can. For recommendations about a pediatrician, ask other doctors you know, as well as family, friends, relatives, and coworkers. You may want to contact a nearby hospital, medical school, or your county medical society for a list of local pediatricians. Some health insurance plans may require you to choose a pediatrician from their approved network of doctors.

After you have a list of names, you may visit the pediatricians' offices to help you choose your child's doctor. While you are in the reception area, look around to see if it is clean. (But realize that children have been in it all day long.) Consider whether the office staff seems friendly and helpful.

Ask the office staff some questions, including the following:

- What are the office hours?
- Is emergency coverage available 24 hours a day, 7 days a week?
- Do nurses screen phone calls?
- If I cannot speak with the doctor, who will handle my questions?
- When is the best time to call with routine questions?
- Does the practice have an after-hours answering service?
- Is the after-hours phone service tied in with a university or children's hospital?
- Where are patients referred after hours?
- Is there access to specialists and intensive care if needed?
- Is payment due at the time of visit?
- How does the office handle billing?
- How are insurance claims handled?
- Is this pediatrician accepting new patients with my insurance or managed care plan?

Also prepare a list of questions to ask about the pediatrician including the following:

- What is his or her pediatric background?
- Does he or she have a subspecialty or area of pediatric interest? If so, what is it?
- To what hospital does he or she admit patients?
- Is he or she board certified though the American Board of Pediatrics?
- Is he or she a member of the American Academy of Pediatrics?
- Who are the physicians who will care for my child if my pediatrician is not available?
- Are they on staff at the same hospital? Are these physicians board certified?

These are just sample questions. Ask other questions about things that are important to you.

After your first visit with the pediatrician, ask yourself: Does this pediatrician listen, answer questions, and seem interested? Above all, ask yourself if you like and trust this person. If your instincts say "no," talk with the next pediatrician on your list.

When someone you know suggests a pediatrician, it is also helpful to ask that person some questions about the doctor, such as the following:

- Are all your questions answered by the pediatrician and the office staff?
- Do you think your children like the doctor?
- Does the pediatrician talk with and care about the children, and not just the parents?
- Does the pediatrician seem to know about current issues and advances in pediatric medicine?
- How helpful and friendly is the office staff?
- How well does the office staff manage your telephone calls?
- How does the office handle emergencies?
- Do you have to wait long before seeing the pediatrician?
- Is there anything about the pediatrician or the office that bothers you?

The American Academy of Pediatrics has an online pediatrician referral service for parents. For more information, please go to www.aap.org, click on "You and Your Family," and look for the "Pediatrician Referral Service" link.

Preparing for office visits

Regular visits to the pediatrician are a key part of preventive health care. At each visit, the pediatrician, pediatric nurse practitioner, or pediatric resident will fully examine your child. This checkup will give your child's pediatrician a chance to

- Make sure your child is eating well, growing well, and is healthy.
- Update immunizations.
- Track your child's growth and development.
- Find physical problems before they become serious.
- Help inform you on how to keep your child healthy and safe.
- Answer all of your questions.

Infants and children need frequent checkups during the first 24 months of life. After 2 years of age most children do not need regular visits as often. Your pediatrician will schedule visits based on your child's own needs. Ask your pediatrician how often your child needs a checkup.

Make sure you write down any questions you have before each office visit, so that you do not forget to ask them. Keep up-to-date records on your child's growth and immunizations. Bring this information with you to each visit.

Illnesses and injuries

All children get sick at one time or another. Minor illnesses like colds and coughs are common. This is especially true for children who are in child care or school, where they may be exposed to more infections from other children. It is also common for children to have many minor injuries, as well as other medical problems that will need your pediatrician's attention.

If you are not sure your child needs to see the pediatrician, always call his or her office. The office staff can often tell you over the phone if your child needs to be seen and, if so, can set up an appointment. The pediatrician or nursing staff may give medical advice over the phone if an office visit is not needed.

Calling your child's pediatrician

You should *always* feel free to call your pediatrician's office, either during office hours for routine questions or at any time for an emergency. Call right away if you are worried about your child. Sometimes a parent feels there is a problem

---

Recommended health care visits*

The American Academy of Pediatrics recommends regular health care visits at the following times:

- Before your baby is born (for first-time parents)
- Before your newborn is discharged from the hospital, and again within 48 to 72 hours for babies discharged before 2 full days of life
- During the first year of life—visits at about 2 to 4 weeks of age, and also at 2, 4, 6, 9, and 12 months of age
- During the second year of life—visits at 15, 18, and 24 months of age
- In early childhood—yearly visits from 2 through 5 years of age
- During the early school years—visits at 6, 8, and 10 years of age
- In adolescence and early adulthood—yearly visits from 11 through 21 years of age

*Your own pediatrician may recommend additional visits.

---

before symptoms actually show up. Always call and get proper medical advice. Realize, though, that sometimes your pediatrician may not be able to answer your questions without seeing your child first. When you are not sure whether to call, trust your instincts.

Make the most of the phone. Your pediatrician may prefer that you call with general questions during office hours. Some offices even have special "phone-in" times. Before you call, have a pen and paper ready to write down any instructions and questions. You could easily forget some details, especially when you are worried about your child. Be prepared to provide information about your child's health.

- **Have your child near the phone,** if possible, to help you answer questions when you call your pediatrician. An older child may be able to tell you exactly where it hurts.
- **Take your child's temperature** before you call. If your child has a fever, write down the temperature and time you took it.
- **Remind the doctor about past medical problems.** Do not expect your pediatrician to always remember your child's medical condition. He or she cares for many children each day and may not remember that your child has asthma, seizures, or some other condition.
- **Be sure to mention medications.** If your child is taking any medication, including prescription or nonprescription drugs, inhalers, supplements, vitamins, herbal products, or home remedies, tell your pediatrician.
- **Keep immunization records at hand.** These are especially helpful if your child has an injury that may require a tetanus shot or if pertussis (whooping cough) is in your community.
- **Have your pharmacy phone number ready.**
  Unblock your telephone "call block," and keep phone lines open so that your pediatrician can return your call in a timely manner. Do not leave pager numbers. If you leave your cell phone number, be sure that you have your cell phone on and will be in an area where you can receive calls.

Routine and emergency calls

Routine calls include questions about medicines, minor illnesses, injuries, behavior, or parenting advice. You will usually not need urgent care for a simple cold or cough, mild diarrhea, constipation, temper tantrums, or sleep problems. For these cases you may just need proper medical advice.

However, if your child has any of the following, call to find out if he needs to be seen:

- Vomiting and diarrhea that last for more than a few hours in a child of any age
- Rash, especially if there is also a fever
- Any cough or cold that does not get better in several days, or a cold that gets worse and is accompanied by a fever
- Cuts that might need stitches
- Limping or is not able to move an arm or leg
- Ear pain with fever, is unable to sleep or eat, is vomiting, has diarrhea, or is acting ill
- Drainage from an ear
- Sore throat or problems swallowing
- Sharp or persistent pains in the abdomen or stomach
- A rectal temperature of 100.4°F (38°C) or higher in a baby younger than 2 months of age
- Fever and vomiting at the same time
- Not eating for more than a day

Emergency calls require your pediatrician's prompt attention. But it is best to know what to do before a problem occurs. During a scheduled checkup, ask your pediatrician what to do and where to go should your child ever need emergency medical care. Learn basic first aid, including CPR (cardiopulmonary resuscitation). Keep emergency and poison center phone numbers posted by your telephone.

An infant or child needs emergency medical treatment **immediately** if he has any of the following:

- Bleeding that does not stop after applying pressure for 5 minutes
- Suspected poisoning
- Seizures (Rhythmic jerking and loss of consciousness)
- Increasing trouble with breathing
- Skin or lips that look blue, purple, or gray
- Neck stiffness or rash with fever
- Head injury with loss of consciousness, confusion, vomiting, or poor skin color
- Blood in the urine
- Bloody diarrhea or diarrhea that will not go away
- Sudden lack of energy or is not able to move
- Unconsciousness or lack of response
- Acting strangely or becoming more withdrawn and less alert
- Increasing or severe persistent pain
- A cut or burn that is large, deep, or involves the head, chest, or abdomen
- A burn that is large or involves the hands, groin, or face

Call 911 (or your emergency number) for any severely ill or injured child.

As your child grows

Your pediatrician can continue to be an important resource not only for illness or injury care, but for all sorts of health advice, including the following:

- Exercise
- Nutrition
- Being too thin or too heavy

- Emotional and behavioral problems
- Helping children cope with issues like divorce and death
- School or learning problems
- Family problems
- Media and Internet literacy
- Gun injury prevention

Your pediatrician can respond to your teen's special needs and can offer advice and counseling on

- Body changes during puberty
- Menstruation
- Growth and hygiene
- Coping and being happy with oneself and with others
- Substance abuse
- Dating and sexual issues
- Eating disorders
- Acne
- Birth control
- Violence and related problems
- Gang problems

Immunizations and your child's health

Many childhood diseases can be prevented with regular health care visits and up-to-date immunizations. Children need shots to protect them from diphtheria, tetanus, pertussis (whooping cough), measles, mumps, rubella (German measles), polio, hepatitis A, hepatitis B, *Haemophilus influenzae* type b, chickenpox, influenza, and pneumococcal infections.

Be sure your child is up-to-date with all needed vaccinations. It is the only way to protect your child against many serious diseases.

Your pediatrician can give you the latest information about new vaccines as they become available. At each checkup, ask your pediatrician if your child is fully immunized.

The information contained in this publication should not be used as a substitute for the medical care and advice of your pediatrician. There may be variations in treatment that your pediatrician may recommend based on individual facts and circumstances.

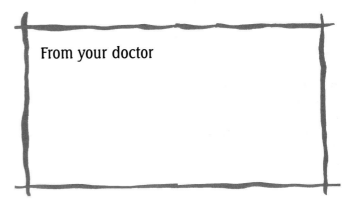

From your doctor

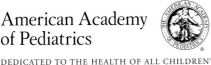

American Academy of Pediatrics

DEDICATED TO THE HEALTH OF ALL CHILDREN™

The American Academy of Pediatrics is an organization of 55,000 primary care pediatricians, pediatric medical subspecialists, and pediatric surgical specialists dedicated to the health, safety, and well-being of infants, children, adolescents, and young adults.

American Academy of Pediatrics
PO Box 747
Elk Grove Village, IL 60009-0747
Web site — http://www.aap.org

Copyright ©2002 American Academy of Pediatrics

Index

Index